Introduction to Clinical Skills

A Patient-Centered Textbook

Introduction to Clinical Skills

A Patient-Centered Textbook

Edited by

Mark B. Mengel, M.D., M.P.H.
Tufts University School of Medicine
Boston, Massachusetts

and

Scott A. Fields, M.D.
Oregon Health Sciences University
Portland, Oregon

Plenum Medical Book Company • New York and London

Library of Congress Cataloging-in-Publication Data

Introduction to clinical skills : a patient-centered textbook / edited
  by Mark B. Mengel and Scott A. Fields.
        p.   cm.
     Includes bibliographical references and index.
     ISBN 0-306-45350-9
     1. Clinical medicine. 2. Physician and patient.   I. Mengel, Mark
  B.   II. Fields, Scott A.
     [DNLM: 1. Diagnosis.   2. Interviews--methods.   3. Physical
  Examination--methods.   4. Medical History Taking--methods.
  5. Physician-Patient Relations.   WB 200 I612 1997]
  RC46.I55   1997
  610--dc21
  DNLM/DLC
  for Library of Congress   96-39432
                                                                  CIP

ISBN 0-306-45350-9

© 1997 Plenum Publishing Corporation
233 Spring Street, New York, N. Y. 10013

Plenum Medical Book Company is an imprint of Plenum Publishing Corporation

10 9 8 7 6 5 4 3 2

Printed in the United States of America

To all those dedicated practitioners who taught us the skills
needed to care for patients well

Contributors

Ric Arseneau, M.D., M.A.Ed., Clinical Assistant Professor and Curriculum Consultant, Departments of Medicine and Educational Studies, St. Paul's Hospital and University of British Columbia, Vancouver, British Columbia V6Z 1Y6, Canada

Ellen Beck, M.D., Assistant Clinical Professor, Department of Family and Preventive Medicine, School of Medicine, University of California at San Diego, La Jolla, California 92093-0622

William M. Chop, Jr., M.D., Associate Professor and Associate Director of Research, University of Texas Southwestern Medical Center, McLennan County Medical Education and Research Foundation, Waco, Texas 76707-2291

Sonia J. S. Crandall, Ph.D., Assistant Professor and Director of Faculty Development, Department of Family and Community Medicine, Bowman Gray School of Medicine, Wake Forest University, Winston-Salem, North Carolina 27157-1084

Larry L. Dickey, M.D., M.P.H., Assistant Adjunct Professor, Department of Family and Community Medicine, University of California at San Francisco, San Francisco, California 94143

Diane L. Elliot, M.D., Professor of Medicine, Division of Health Promotion and Sports Medicine, Oregon Health Sciences University, Portland, Oregon 97201

Kathleen R. Farrell, D.O., Assistant Professor of Medicine and Staff Physician/ Gerontology Section, Oregon Health Sciences University, Portland, Oregon 97201-3098

Linn Goldberg, M.D., Professor of Medicine and Director, Human Performance Laboratory, Section of Health Promotion and Sports Medicine, Department of Medicine, Oregon Health Sciences University, Portland, Oregon 97201

Julie Graves Moy, M.D., M.P.H., Private Family Physician, Austin, Texas 78765

Robert M. Hamm, Ph.D., Assistant Professor, Department of Family Medicine, University of Oklahoma Health Sciences Center, Oklahoma City, Oklahoma 73190

R. Martin Johnson, M.D., Associate Clinical Professor, Department of Family Medicine, Oregon Health Sciences University, Tigard, Oregon 97223

Victoria Kaprielian Johnson, M.D., Assistant Clinical Professor and Chief, Division of Predoctoral Education and Faculty Development, Department of Community and Family Medicine, Duke University Medical Center, Durham, North Carolina 27710

David A. Katerndahl, M.D., M.A., Professor and Director of Research and Education, Department of Family Practice, University of Texas Health Science Center at San Antonio, San Antonio, Texas 78284-7795

John P. Langlois, M.D., Director of Medical Student Programs, Mountain AHEC Family Practice Residency Program, Clinical Assistant Professor of Family Medicine, University of North Carolina, Mountain Area Family Health Center, Asheville, North Carolina 28804

Frank H. Lawler, M.D., M.S.P.H., Associate Professor of Family Medicine, Department of Family and Preventive Medicine, University of Oklahoma Health Sciences Center, Oklahoma City, Oklahoma 73190

Larry B. Mauksch, M.Ed., Clinical Associate Professor and Residency Behavioral Science Coordinator, Department of Family Medicine, University of Washington, Seattle, Washington 98105

Catherine P. McKegney, M.D., M.S., Assistant Professor, Department of Family Practice and Community Health, University of Minnesota Medical School, Hennepin County Family Practice Residency Program, Minneapolis, Minnesota 55408

Mark B. Mengel, M.D., M.P.H., Program Director, The Family Practice Residency Program at Beverly Hospital, and Associate Clinical Professor, Tufts University School of Medicine, The Family Practice Center at The Hunt, Danvers, Massachusetts 01923

Warren P. Newton, M.D., Assistant Professor, Department of Family Medicine, University of North Carolina at Chapel Hill, Chapel Hill, North Carolina 27599-7595

Daniel Pratt, Ph.D., Associate Professor, Adult and Higher Education, Department of Educational Studies, University of British Columbia, Vancouver, British Columbia V6Z 1Y6, Canada

Richard G. Roberts, M.D., J.D., Professor, Department of Family Medicine, University of Wisconsin Medical School, Madison, Wisconsin 53715

John S. Rolland, M.D., Associate Clinical Professor of Psychiatry and Co-Director, Center for Family Health, University of Chicago, Chicago, Illinois 60611

Jeannette E. South-Paul, M.D., Associate Professor of Family Practice and Vice President for Minority Affairs, Department of Family Medicine, Uniformed Services University of the Health Sciences, Bethesda, Maryland 20814-4799

Jeff Susman, M.D., Professor of Family Medicine and Assistant Dean for Primary Care, College of Medicine, and Medical Director of Primary Care Clinics, University of Nebraska Medical Center, Omaha, Nebraska 68198-3075

Kathleen A. Zoppi, Ph.D., M.P.H., Assistant Professor and Associate Residency Program Director, Department of Family Medicine, Indiana University, Indianapolis, Indiana 46202-5102

Preface

Introduction to Clinical Skills: A Patient-Centered Textbook is an introductory textbook focusing on the skills needed by physicians to have the highest likelihood of reaching an optimal outcome in their patients at a reasonable cost and in a humane fashion. Skills described include not only the diagnostic, treatment, and technical skills medical students have previously mastered in Introduction to Clinical Medicine or Physical Diagnosis courses, but also patient-centered skills. These patient-centered or what other authorities describe as generalist skills will help the physician of the future, particularly those going into primary care disciplines, master patient care situations that have previously caused a great deal of discomfort in more biomedically oriented physicians. Mastering these patient-centered skills will also enable physicians to form a lasting partnership with their patients, involving them in their care in a positive fashion and thus improving the likelihood of an optimal outcome and high patient satisfaction. Some of the more advanced skills described in this text will also enable physicians of the future to apply medical research in a more critical fashion to practice, structure their practice so that it supports the use of patient-centered skills, keep up to date in an efficient manner, and advance the discipline of clinical practice through teaching, research, and the development of clinical guidelines.

The description of these clinical skills has been organized into four parts. The first part explores the current dominant model of medical practice, the biomedical approach, contrasting it with an emerging systemic patient-centered care approach, illustrating the skills required for each approach through clinical examples. The second part describes basic clinical skills required of all clinicians, including interviewing, physical examination, appropriate use of laboratory tests, making a diagnosis, instituting treatment, and keeping accurate records. The third part describes skills that will improve clinical expertise in areas of clinical interviewing, decision-making, patient education, negotiating with patients, managing chronic illness, counseling patients for behavioral change, assessing patients' functional status, promoting health and preventing disease, critically appraising the literature, reducing malpractice risks, managing a clinical practice, and developing skills for lifelong medical learning. The final part describes skills clinicians need to advance the discipline of medicine, including medical teaching, research, and a critical new area, the development of clinical guidelines.

Educationally, we hope that these chapters will not simply be read but will be the focus of spirited discussion and practice around skill development. In many first- and second-year generalist clinical experience courses, the cases for discussion at the end of each chapter can serve as a focal point for discussion. These cases can also serve as a vignette for skill practice as well. In other words, when reading the interviewing chapter, don't solely focus on discussion but, through role-playing or actually interviewing live patients, practice interviewing skills with an observer who would be willing to provide you useful feedback. Without such skill practice, these skills are likely to remain but a clinician's dream, rather than a part of each clinician's armamentarian.

As editors, we realize that we could not include all of the skills that successful clinicians will need to care for their patients well. We also realize that developing clinical skills is not an easy process, but one that usually takes years to master depending on the complexity of the skill. For example, many physicians will confess that their skill in examining a fundus was not fully perfected until residency, even though the skill was first described and practice began in the second year of medical school. Thus, we hope that the skills we describe in this text serve as a foundation for future leaning and encourage learners who utilize this textbook to continue practicing skills throughout their career.

Mark B. Mengel, M.D., M.P.H.

Boston, Massachusetts

Scott A. Fields, M.D.

Portland, Oregon

Acknowledgments

Without the aid of many people, this textbook simply would not have been possible. Many of our colleagues have been very supportive of this text even to the point of being chapter authors. Without the warm support and suggestions of these colleagues, this work would not have come to fruition.

Special thanks go to our students, who have stimulated us to continually update and improve our ideas on skill development. Particularly first- and second-year medical students have asked the "embarrassing" questions that have caused us to conceptualize and then reconceptualize our understanding of what skills need to be learned and how best to teach them.

The tireless support of our secretaries, Linda Ready and Becky Settle, is gratefully acknowledged. Chapters have to be edited, authors have to be "nagged," and publishers have to be placated.

We also want to thank the editorial staff at Plenum Publishing headed by Mariclaire Cloutier, who has been very supportive and understanding of our many foibles. They have been particularly helpful in editing our rather long-winded, confusing prose into much briefer, more understandable sentences.

Lastly, we would like to thank our families, without whose support the long hours necessary, usually after work, to put together a book of this size and scope would not have been possible.

Contents

PART I

Introduction

This introductory section will lay the conceptual framework for future skill development. Without such a conceptual framework for skill development, skill development becomes haphazard, unfocused, and, quite frankly, dangerous as physicians are at risk for developing skills that solely benefit themselves rather than their patients. The conceptual framework presented in the chapter that makes up this introductory section is the systemic patient-centered care approach. This approach will enable physicians to focus on that most important recipient of medical care, the patient, and thus remain properly oriented when developing skills. Several basic patient-centered clinical decision-making skills are also described.

CHAPTER 1

The Systemic Patient-Centered Method

Mark B. Mengel

Mastery is central to any scholarly or professional discipline. Mastery of a discipline requires mastery of a method.

Ian McWhinney, M.D., 1989

CASE 1-1

"In Abdera, Anasion, who was lodged near the Thracian Gates, was seized with an acute fever; continued pain of the right side, dry cough, without expectoration during the first days, thirst, insomnolency; urine well colored, copious and thin. On the seventh, in a painful state, for the fever increased, while the pains did not abate, and the cough was troublesome and attended with dyspnea. On the eighth, I opened a vein at the elbow, and much blood, of a proper character, flowed; the pains were abated, but the dry coughs continued. On the twenty-seventh the fever relapsed; he coughed and brought up much concocted sputum; sediment in urine copious and white. Explanation of the characters: it is probable that the evacuation of the sputum brought about the recovery on the thirty-fourth day." (Hippocrates, 1979)

LEARNING OBJECTIVES

At the conclusion of this chapter, the student will be able to:

1. Describe the dynamics in the U.S. healthcare system that are encouraging change

2. Describe the biomedical method of clinical care, including purpose, physician and patient roles, goals of care, strengths, and shortcomings
3. Describe the systemic patient-centered method of clinical care, including purpose, physician and patient roles, goals of care, and shortcomings
4. Describe and demonstrate key systemic patient-centered skills, including responding to patient cues, agreeing on the problem, setting goals, generating options, selection options, and follow-up
5. Discuss other important considerations in utilizing the systemic patient-centered approach, including systemic change, ethics, efficacy, and safety

Since before the time of Hippocrates, people with illnesses, as illustrated in Case 1-1, whom we now call patients, have been coming to their physicians and other healers to cure their distress or at least seek some understanding of it. Hippocrates and his colleagues used largely herbal remedies to restore humoral balance, which did not often alter the natural history of the illness, but neither did they usually cause harm (Hippocrates, 1979). Today, altering the natural history of the patient's bronchitis in Case 1-1 would be easily accomplished with an antibiotic.

Hippocrates and his colleagues greatly respected their patients, seeing them in the patient's home and allowing patients and their families to help concoct medications and make suggestions about needed changes to medication. Given the physician's unique knowledge about the patient's condition, these suggestions were readily agreed to by the physician (else he might not be invited back!). Today, care is largely delivered outside the patient's home. Stripped of this critical context, the patient's family is not so intimately involved in treatment, nor would their suggestions often be welcomed! Looking back at this era through our own scientific, technological, and cultural "filters," as modern providers of healthcare, we wonder why these fathers of our discipline practices were as thriving and busy as ours today, when they apparently had no effective cures, other than lancing abscesses and setting bones.

The scientific and technical advances of the past 150 years have enabled us to develop a staggering number of medications and procedures that can alter the natural history of many diseases, particularly infectious diseases, improving the health of many patients who might previously have died (Reiser, 1978). Yet, surveys of patients indicate decreased satisfaction with personal health as well as dissatisfaction with their interactions with physicians (Barsky, 1988; Shorter, 1985; Simpson *et al.,* 1991). It appears that as medicine becomes more technologically oriented, patients perceive their physicians as less humane. Care is no longer conveniently delivered in the patient's home but in the office or hospital where patients are often viewed from a disease perspective, rather than as an individual with a context, and the patient's and her family's unique values and beliefs are often not taken into account when treatment decisions are made.

Additionally, patient dissatisfactions around issues of access, cost, and quality of healthcare have caused many to cry for reform of the entire U.S. healthcare system (Lundberg, 1992). In some regions of the country, almost a third of citizens lack health insurance (Blendon *et al.,* 1992). Healthcare costs in the United States have climbed to 15% of gross national product in 1994 with no end in sight to cost increases if the current fee-for-service system continues (Lundberg, 1992). Although government efforts to reform the entire U.S. healthcare system failed with the congressional election in 1994, market forces have spawned health maintenance organizations (HMOs) and other managed care plans that try to control costs by reducing unnecessary utilization of medical resources and by restoring the balance between specialists and primary care physicians to a 1:1 ratio. Such plans, however, have not been able to increase access for those who cannot afford the insurance premium. Furthermore, many patients fear that HMOs will deny them needed services in an attempt to control costs (Relman, 1993; Inglehart, 1994; Miller & Luft, 1994).

Unfortunately, the large amount of money Americans spend on healthcare does not seem to provide higher-quality care, as measured by the common indices of the adequacy of healthcare, such as neonatal mortality, age-adjusted mortality rates, and longevity of life (Lundberg, 1992). Other industrialized countries spend much less on healthcare (8–10% of GNP), with much better health outcomes.

Compounding the access problem, U.S. physicians do not distribute themselves adequately. There are too few physicians in urban inner-city areas and rural areas. Of the industrialized countries, the United States has the lowest percentage of its physicians serving as primary care physicians (29.2% in 1992), further reducing access to basic primary care and preventive services (COGME, 1994).

The physician of the future will have to develop the skills necessary to address patient dissatisfactions, particularly regarding the critical areas of access, cost, and quality. Formerly, skill development in medical school and residency programs has focused almost entirely on *diagnostic* skills (accurately performing a complete history and physical exam so that an appropriate list of differential diagnostic possibilities was developed), *treatment* skills (ensuring the proper medication or procedure was selected in a timely manner), and *technical* skills (performing the appropriate test, procedure, or intervention in a correct manner) (Cantor *et al.*, 1993). As will be discussed in the next section, these biomedical skills, although still critical to possess, are not enough to ensure that the physician of the future can produce high patient satisfaction and good outcomes.

To have the highest likelihood of reaching an optimal outcome for their patients at a reasonable cost in a humane fashion, physicians must develop patient-centered skills, in addition to diagnostic, treatment, and technical skills. Patient-centered skills include *interviewing* skills, such as active listening and use of open-ended questions, *negotiation* skills, such as selection of therapeutic options that respect patient values, and *health maintenance and preventive* skills, such as discussion of risks and benefits of screening tests with patients, to name but a few (Rivo *et al.*, 1994; Rubenstein *et al.*, 1994). This chapter, and many subsequent chapters, will focus on the patient-centered skills all physicians need by describing the systemic patient-centered approach to care and contrasting that approach with the current method of patient care, the biomedical model. Skills necessary to both approaches will be described and illustrated through clinical examples.

CASE 1-2

Dr. G. H. is a third-year resident. As a part of residency training, she is assigned to spend 2 months in a rural community working with a group of primary care physicians. It is a rainy Saturday afternoon and G. H. is on call.

Suddenly, G. H.'s beeper summons her to the emergency room. On arrival the nurse informs her that the ambulance has called and is bringing in a 6-year-old boy with marked respiratory distress. Two minutes later the ambulance arrives and the EMTs unload their patient, who has severe inspiratory stridor. His par-

ents have followed the ambulance to the hospital and are pacing anxiously in the waiting room.

As G. H. begins to work on the patient, the boy begins to struggle for breath and becomes cyanotic. He is unable to speak. The nurse tells G. H. that he has a temperature of 103°F. G. H. notices that his pulse is slow and orders cardiac monitoring in addition to oxygen. As the nurse applies the cardiac electrodes, the patient suffers a respiratory arrest. G. H. attempts to ventilate the patient with mouth-to-mouth resuscitation but is unsuccessful. G. H. attempts intubation but find the epiglottis is severely inflamed and swollen, making it impossible to visualize the airway well enough to slide the endotracheal tube into the patient's trachea. As seconds, which seemed like hours, tick by, G. H. realizes that she will have to attempt a cricothyroidotomy.

Using a large-gauge intravenous (IV) catheter, G. H. is successful in performing the cricothyroidotomy. Ventilation of the patient through the IV catheter immediately restores his pulse. As he receives some oxygen, spontaneous respirations begin to return. A general surgeon is consulted so that a tracheostomy can be established.

Treatment of the patient's epiglottis with antibiotics and steroids results in rapid resolution of the illness. Three days later G. H. removes the patient's tracheostomy and allows him to go home. One day later during an office follow-up, the patient is well and has suffered no brain damage as the result of his respiratory arrest. (Contributed by J. Steinbauer, M.D.)

THE BIOMEDICAL MODEL

As McWhinney pointed out at the outset of this chapter, one can learn a great deal about medicine by studying its method, as method is the key to any professional discipline. The most recent method of caring for patients is called the biomedical model. This approach had its origins in the eighteenth century and rested on the foundation of scientific reductionism (Parchman, 1991; White, 1988). The aim of the biomedical model is simple: to interpret the patient's symptoms and signs in terms of physical pathology or physiology. The dominance of the biomedical model is easily understood when its strengths are noted:

1. Its procedures often yield beneficial results for the patient.
2. Procedures are performed in an order that simplifies an otherwise complex and difficult process.
3. Objective data such as laboratory tests, biopsies, and autopsies validate the method.
4. The method enables clinicians to eradicate or cure many previously fatal diseases, as G. H. did in Case 1-2, and successfully control many illnesses for which a cure has not been found (McWhinney, 1989a; Rogers & Blendon, 1977).

Despite its great strength and dominance, the biomedical approach has many shortcomings. Ivan Illich, for example, points out that:

1. Much of what medicine recommends as treatment is based more on tradition than scientific evidence.
2. Many epidemiologic studies have revealed that some medical care provided to patients may actually be inadequate or harmful to health.
3. Extensive resources are devoted to offsetting iatrogenic (physician-induced) damage resulting from overly aggressive biomedical interventions.
4. Medical care encourages patient dependency rather than fostering autonomy (Illich, 1975).

The biomedical model has also been challenged by the consumers of healthcare. Barsky (1988) has noted that although collective health has improved over the past 30 years, surveys of patients continually revealed decreased satisfaction with personal health. Barsky explains this paradoxical finding by the following facts:

1. Despite increased longevity, an increased prevalence of chronic and degenerative disease impairs patients' quality of life.
2. A greater self-scrutiny and overall awareness of symptoms has resulted from patients' consciousness of their health.
3. The widespread commercialization of health has fostered a climate of apprehension, insecurity, and alarm.
4. The medicalization of problems previously thought to be simple matters of daily living has led to unrealistic expectations of cure.

Recent research has also pointed out the inadequacies of the biomedical approach in the primary care setting. Kroenke and Mangelsdorff (1989) reviewed the records of 1000 patients who presented to an internal medicine clinic over 3 years. Five hundred sixty-seven new complaints were noted in these patients' charts. Diagnostic tests were performed on more than two thirds of cases. An organic biomedical disease was discovered in only 16% of these cases. The cost of discovering an organic etiology was high, particularly for patients with headaches ($7778 per patient) and back pain ($7263 per patient). Furthermore, treatment was instituted for only 55% of symptoms and was often ineffective. The authors of this study concluded that "diagnostic strategies emphasizing organic causes may be inadequate."

Yet another shortcoming of the biomedical model is that it does not consider the meaning of the patient's illness (Rabin *et al.*, 1982; Sacks, 1984). As Stetten (1981), a physician afflicted with macular degeneration, a disease of the retina, has written:

> Through all these years and despite many encounters with skilled and experienced professionals, no ophthalmologist has at any time suggested any device that might be of assistance to me. No ophthalmologist has mentioned any of the many ways in which I could stem the deterioration in the quality of life. [T]he purpose of this essay is . . . courteously but firmly, to complain of what appears to be the ophthalmologist's attitude: "We are interested in vision but have little interest in blindness."

Failure to recognize the specific "threats to self" that an illness brings to a particular patient, such as disruption in function, loss of control, or decreased competence, only serves to increase patient vulnerability and alienation, further worsening the experience of the illness (McWhinney, 1989a; Toombs, 1987).

Lastly, the biomedical approach does not allow physicians the opportunity to understand the context in which the patient's illness occurs. Patients' families, communities, work groups, and cultures all have profound effects on patients' health (Mengel & Holleman, 1997). Rather than taking these systemic influences into account, the biomedical model isolates the individual from her context as a diseased organism. Although this focusing clearly allows the physician to concentrate on the biological disease processes, ignoring contextual influences that maintain unhealthy and problem-producing behaviors limits the effectiveness of interventions designed to promote health. Also, a mobilization of resources within the patient's family or community to help the patient function better usually does not occur, as such interventions are not disease "cures" and thus not in the purview of the biomedical model.

Paradoxically, it seems that the success of the biomedical approach has spawned great patient dissatisfaction with medical care. As a result, some clinicians believe that medicine is on the brink of a major transformation in its basic approach to care (Engel, 1977; McWhinney, 1989a; Perkoff, 1985; Stein, 1985c).

CASE 1-3

A 29-year-old white woman who had recently moved to the area presents to Dr. Jones's office complaining of fatigue. Dr. Jones rapidly uncovered her history of hypothyroidism and her story that her previous physician had recommended a reduction in the frequency with which she took her thyroid medication, from every day to every other day, because her laboratory values had indicated that she was taking too much thyroid medication. After about 2 months of taking the reduced dose of medication, she felt more fatigued and wondered if she was now taking too little thyroid medication. Her health goal was to feel more perky, like her old self, as soon as possible.

Even though the patient had noted no weight gain or change in her skin and hair consistent with hypothyroidism, Dr. Jones agreed that her fatigue could be caused by an inadequate intake of thyroid medication. He recommended that her thyroid status be tested and presented her the option of either continuing to take her medication every other day until the test results returned or increasing her medication by taking it once a day for the first 6 days of the week but not on the seventh. Because the patient felt strongly that she was taking too little medication, she elected the latter option.

Dr. Jones, however, was concerned that there might be some other reason for her fatigue, particularly given the fact that she had no findings of hypothyroidism on physical exam. On further questioning, Dr. Jones learned that the patient and her 3-year-old daughter had recently moved in with her sister and was in the process of obtaining a divorce from her husband with whom she had become "incompatible." The patient felt that she was rapidly wearing out her welcome, yet without employment she could not support herself and her daughter. Her ex-husband was not willing to provide child support until the divorce was finalized. Dr. Jones also learned that she was not hopeful that her situation would improve. She was not considering suicide.

Given the patient's history of multiple major life events and her depressed mood, Dr. Jones presented the patient with two further options, either a trial of antidepressant medication or a referral to a counselor to aid her in her adjustment to her new situation. The patient thought that she was on enough medication already and so declined antidepressant medication but did agree that counseling might help.

9

A NEW
FRAMEWORK:
THE SYSTEMIC
PATIENT-
CENTERED
METHOD

The patient's initial laboratory work returned showing that she was minimally hypothyroid. The patient was informed of this by letter and urged to continue her new thyroid regime but to follow up in 6 weeks to ensure that she was not becoming hyperthyroid. Six weeks later, the patient returned for follow-up. Examination at the time by Dr. Jones showed a significant improvement in her mood. Although she still had not found employment, she had been successful in obtaining child support from her ex-husband even though the divorce had not been finalized. The physical examination revealed no findings of hypothyroidism and laboratory tests showed normal thyroid functioning. The patient was very positive about her counseling and wanted to continue. Dr. Jones agreed and then scheduled another follow-up visit in 3 months.

A NEW FRAMEWORK: THE SYSTEMIC PATIENT-CENTERED METHOD

As the shortcomings of the biomedical method have been discovered and understood, many investigators have begun the difficult task of constructing a new method for patient care that preserves the advantages of the biomedical approach yet avoids the shortcomings. While most investigators have focused on one or two shortcomings and developed a limited model to ameliorate some shortcomings, McWhinney and his group from London, Ontario, and Delbanco and his group from Beth Israel Hospital in Boston have developed perhaps the most comprehensive, patient-centered methods of care to date (Gerteis *et al.,* 1993; Stewart *et al.,* 1995). McWhinney's approach is firmly grounded in the traditions of family practice emphasizing primary care and prevention as one of its unique aspects. Delbanco's approach complements McWhinney's by centering on inpatient care. Borrowing from both models, we will present an outline of a systemic patient-centered method of clinical care that centers on the most important aspects of this approach. The term *systemic* is added to emphasize that while partnering with the individual patient is important, taking into account the context of that individual is also highly important and thus a basic tenet of any patient-centered method.

Any new method of care that is proposed should, at a minimum, describe the roles of the participants, the goals of the approach, the process by which those goals are achieved and document the effectiveness of the model, particularly with regard to possible shortcomings. Case 1-3 illustrates some of the new roles, goals, and outcomes of the systemic patient-centered method. First of all, Dr. Jones did not see himself as merely operating under the biomedical method, where physician roles are fairly straightforward, namely,

1. Diagnose illness.
2. Treat disease.
3. Apply preventive strategies based on the age, sex, and risk factors of the patient.

Instead, Dr. Jones expanded his role to include working with the patient to define what health means to that particular patient, obtaining psychosocial and contextual information relevant to the patient's circumstance, facilitating the patient's decision-making process through the formation and prioritization of goals to optimize health, and working with the patient to select the best therapeutic option that will attain the patient's goals while respecting her values.

Patient roles also were expanded in Case 1-3 when compared with the biomedical approach where the patient's role is solely to accept treatment and be as compliant as possible. In Case 1-3, the patient played an active role in decision-making in that she was a seeker of information, was open to a exploration of her own health-related values and preferences, was a risk taker in that she selected some low-cost options, and was willing to share responsibility for her own health by accepting homework assignments from her therapist, which improved her adjustment to her difficult situation.

The goal of the interaction in Case 1-3 was expanded to include not just treating disease and following its pathophysiology but also optimizing patient functioning and satisfaction with care. The process utilized to reach decisions did not just lead straightforwardly from the diagnosis of a disease but relied highly on patient information and preferences to inform the decision-making process. The physician was an educator as well as a recommender, explaining the risks and benefits of certain strategies to the patient in terms that she understood.

CASE 1-4

In April, a 47-year-old wheat farmer came into his physician's office complaining of pain and swelling in his left groin. He told his physician the symptoms had persisted for 3 weeks, were worse when he stood up or coughed, and were less painful when he laid down. The physician was concerned that the farmer might have an inguinal hernia and, indeed, on exam a large reducible inguinal hernia on the left side was discovered. The physician recommended that the farmer come into the hospital the next week to have his hernia repaired, but the farmer flatly refused, saying that harvesttime was approaching and that he couldn't take any time off during that activity. The physician then discussed all of the potential dangers and possible complications of an inguinal hernia, but to no avail. The farmer explained that harvest was the time when the farmer made all of the money required to support himself and the family for the coming year. The physician eventually relented, recommending that the farmer wear a supportive belt and come back for a repair when the harvest was over.

In July, the farmer returned, having sustained no complications from his hernia and asked the physician to repair it. One week later, the physician repaired the farmer's hernia without difficulty.

PHYSICIAN ROLES

There are four new roles that physicians will need to fulfill if utilizing the systemic patient-centered method. Whereas all roles will not need to be fulfilled in depth with each patient, all patients probably will require a certain amount of physician activity within each role, although the depth of that activity will vary with the illness or health problem.

These four new roles are: (1) exploring health-related values, (2) obtaining psychosocial and contextual information, (3) formulating goals to optimize health, and (4) selecting options respecting patient values.

11

A NEW
FRAMEWORK:
THE SYSTEMIC
PATIENT-
CENTERED
METHOD

Exploring Health-Related Values

Under the biomedical model, health is the absence of disease. Under the systemic patient-centered method, health is defined in a much broader, functional way as the totality of the patient's physical, emotional, and social well-being (WHO, 1947). To add to the confusion surrounding the definition of health, sometimes physicians and patients define health differently, even though a congruence of definitions is crucial to shared decision-making.

The dichotomy between the narrower absence-of-disease definition and the broader quality-of-life definition has been recognized over the years by physicians when they talk about curing versus healing. "Curing" implies the elimination of a disease state, whereas "healing" implies the restoration of an individual to his particular role in the family and community. Clearly, some patients can be cured without being healed, such as a woman with breast cancer who undergoes a radical mastectomy that leaves her with feelings of mutilation, grief, and inadequacy concerning sexual functioning. Some patients can be healed but not cured, such as a diabetic patient who effectively maintains her functional status by controlling her disease and actively coping with its ramifications. Obviously, most patients would like to be both cured and healed. The systemic patient-centered method, unlike the biomedical method, recognizes not only the physician's *curative* abilities but also the potential *healing* capacity that physicians can bring to the encounter with the patient.

Just as important as how the patient defines health is the value placed on that health. Is health the number one priority, as most physicians would like, or are other values higher? A related question is: What is the patient willing to invest in order to achieve a certain measure of health? This investment is not just economic but also entails psychological and social costs, such as violations of cultural norms, disruptions of family roles and dynamics, or disruptions of the work environment. Not only do patients value health differently, but there are often limits beyond which they would not go to improve their health, as in Case 1-4, where the farmer was unwilling to suffer the economic loss of missing the harvest in order to have his hernia repaired immediately. Finding and respecting such limits is important under the systemic patient-centered method, as is educating the patient about the health consequences of respecting those limits.

Unfortunately, there are also biological limits in the degree to which health can be improved in some patients. A bicyclist who sustained a cervical fracture resulting in quadriplegia is probably not going to bicycle again. Such limits should be respected, but sometimes they prematurely defeat physicians and patients, who give up hope of ever restoring any measure of patient health, particularly physicians and patients who hold to a narrower absence-of-disease definition of health. In such cases, the patient-centered method allows physicians to help patients, and themselves, by expanding their definition of health and optimizing the patients' health in other ways. The success of many severely injured and disabled patients in achieving happy, productive lives attests to the benefit of this approach.

Obtaining Psychosocial and Contextual Information

Using the processes of interviewing, examining, and laboratory testing, physicians have become very skilled in identifying patients with physiologic and pathological abnormalities that may decrease life expectancy. Physicians operating within the biomedical method, however, often ignore important psychosocial and contextual issues.

Exploration of psychosocial issues allows the patient-centered physician to travel down many potential avenues. McWhinney (1989b) has identified the most important psychosocial areas to explore: (1) the patient's expectations about the illness, (2) her feelings about the illness, and (3) fears that accompany the illness. Open-ended questions should be asked to explore the significance and meaning of the illness: What bothers you about your illness? What can you no longer do that you used to do before you become ill? What sorts of feelings have you noticed since you became ill? What do you fear will happen to you now that you have this illness? Answers to these questions will give the physician a sense of the patient's adjustment to her illness and which issues are important when educating the patient about her disease.

Contextual issues are also important to address. The patient and physician are embedded in a web of social relationships because each is a member of multiple systems, such as family, work, and community (see Figure 1.1). These relationships both affect and are affected by the patient's health because (1) the context often defines healthy and unhealthy behaviors, (2) the context promotes healthy and unhealthy behaviors through behavioral reinforcement and dynamics, (3) context dynamics can have a significant impact on disease outcome through neuroendocrine and immune mechanisms, and (4) contextual issues can have a significant impact on compliance and rehabilitative behavior (Ramsey, 1989b).

By limiting the treatment plan to a disease-oriented framework, physicians risk disruptions of the patients' systems or failure because systemic feedback loops perpetuate unhealthy behaviors or disease exacerbations through psychoneuroendocrine mechanisms. For example, if the family meal preparer is not involved in patient–physician discussions about lowering a heart patient's dietary cholesterol, then dietary instructions to change unhealthy eating habits provided by the physician are less likely to be implemented despite the best intentions of the physician and patient.

Exploring the patient's entire context could be quite time-consuming and could lead to more confusion than clarification. The physician must develop the skill to identify and explore relevant contextual information to gain an understanding of the dynamics within the patient's system that may lead to adverse outcomes. A few simple questions will allow identification of important systemic issues to emerge: What have those around you suggested or tried to do to improve your condition? Which of those suggestions have you tried? Why have you tried those suggestions? What's worked and what hasn't? How has your illness affected those around you? In what way? If those effects are problems for those around you, how did they respond? How did you respond to their response? Further assessment of the patient's systems can then be guided by answers to those questions.

Formulating Goals to Optimize Health

With the biomedical method, goals are defined by the diseases or deficits uncovered. Since there is such a close correspondence between diagnoses and goals under the bio-

13

**A NEW
FRAMEWORK:
THE SYSTEMIC
PATIENT-
CENTERED
METHOD**

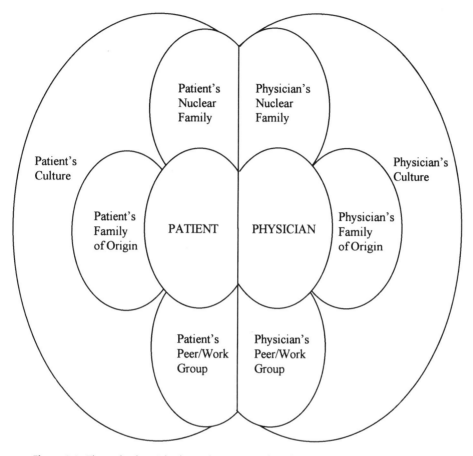

Figure 1.1. The web of social relationships surrounding the physician–patient relationship.

medical method, treatment goals, such as cure or palliation, are not formally mentioned or recorded in the medical record. The systemic patient-centered method, however, acknowledges the functional nature of health and the "trade-offs" that patients often make in order to optimize their health. For example, a diabetic patient may seek better diabetic control by trying the insulin pump, despite the fact that the insulin pump is associated with a decrease in family social activities because of the active management required to utilize the pump (Mengel *et al.,* 1988). In this case, the patient may be willing to trade a decrease in family social activities for better diabetic control. Thus, clearly defined, specific, realistic goals that are mutually agreed on by both the patient and physician (prioritized if multiple or conflicting goals arise) and that acknowledge trade-offs are very important if the systemic patient-centered method is to work.

Goal setting also must take into account what each patient is willing to invest in order to achieve a certain degree of health. If the patient is unwilling to acknowledge and discuss "trade-offs," or if goals set by the patient are incongruent with the physician's beliefs about how best to optimize the patient's health, then a negotiation process, described in Chapter 11, should ensue. Through this process of negotiation the physician and the patient might find that they can work together on only a few desired goals.

Harry Rutherford, a 72-year-old patient of Dr. Jenny Smith, presented with a 3-week history of a decrease in the force of his stream when urinating with occasional hematuria. Harry has been Dr. Smith's patient for the past 20 years and has enjoyed being cared for by Dr. Smith. To evaluate Harry's problem, Dr. Smith ordered a urinalysis, which showed 5–10 red blood cells per high-powered field, and performed a prostate exam, which showed a hard, discrete nodule in the left lobe of that gland. Dr. Smith suspected that Harry might have prostate cancer and so referred Harry to a local urologist, Dr. Binghamton.

Dr. Binghamton performed a prostate biopsy on Harry and confirmed the diagnosis of a nonaggressive form of adenocarcinoma of the prostate that had not spread beyond the capsule. In these situations, Dr. Binghamton preferred aggressive treatment and recommended that Harry undergo a radical prostatectomy. Dr. Binghamton informed Harry that risks associated with the procedure included impotence (20%), incontinence (5%), injury to the rectum or urethra (4%), and deep venous thrombosis (10%) (Hahn & Roberts, 1993; Wasson et al., 1993). Because of these risks, Harry did not feel comfortable electing this procedure without learning more about his other options, and so went back to Dr. Smith.

Dr. Smith counseled him about two alternatives to radical prostatectomy, including radiation therapy and watchful waiting. She counseled Harry that radiation therapy was less effective than radical prostatectomy in preventing death from cancer (23 per 1000 versus 9 per 1000) and had higher rates of impotence (40%), incontinence (8%), and injury to the rectum and urethra (18%), but had much less risk of deep venous thrombosis (Hahn & Roberts, 1993; Wasson et al., 1993). Dr. Smith also told Harry that the annual cancer specific mortality rates for watchful waiting, 9 per 1000, was almost as good as radical prostatectomy, yet had none of the adverse effects on quality of life that were exhibited by either radical prostatectomy or radiation therapy. Lastly, she told Harry that nonaggressive prostate cancer was very common in men his age, often was not the cause of death in these men, and that symptoms could be fairly well controlled with hormonal therapy.

Because he valued his quality of life, Harry chose watchful waiting as his treatment strategy, and tried hormones to reduce his symptoms. He died 3 years later of a heart attack with his nonaggressive prostate cancer still well controlled on hormonal treatment.

Selecting Options that Respect Patient Values

After deciding which goals will optimize health for a particular patient, the patient and physician then need to generate options that have the best likelihood of meeting those goals and respecting the patient's values. Probably the most important skill for the physician during this phase is to be broadminded and not simply recommend to the patient the physician's "favorite" option, as Dr. Binghamton recommended to Harry in Case 1-5. Most physicians usually have one or two favorite approaches to a particular clinical problem that they feel will best meet patients' goals. Sometimes, however, patient preferences and values can make these "favored" options unpalatable to a particular patient, as the twin side effects of incontinence and impotence were unpalatable to Harry in Case 1-5.

Physicians also often don't get into the specifics of a particular option, i.e., when it is to be applied, how it is to be applied, where it is to be applied, how to monitor progress, if and when other healthcare professionals need to be involved for the application of that particular option, and if and when other members of the patient's family need to be involved. The actual specifics of options need to be discussed in depth with the patient, particularly centering on the risks and benefits of each option.

A combination of the scientific information involved in the selection of each option and knowledge of the patient's own values and preferences is needed to make an effective decision about options. For example, a physician may feel that a patient with non-insulin-dependent diabetes mellitus should be placed on a 2200-calorie-a-day diet to control blood glucose values, but if the patient also desires to lose weight, then the physician could reduce the number of calories to ensure adequate weight loss. The major characteristics of medication should be described, including risks, benefits, and cost, so that if the patient does have a difficulty with cost, a less expensive agent may be tried first.

In serving this role the physician can also be a source of encouragement and can suggest strategies that will help the patient carry out the specifics of the plan. A study by Guyatt *et al.* (1984) in 43 patients with chronic obstructive pulmonary disease and congestive heart failure showed that simple encouragement by the physician increased patient performance on a 6-minute walking test similar to the magnitude of performance improvement gained from drug use alone. Thus, the physician's own encouragement and support can have the same effect on outcomes as medication. Likewise, physicians can recommend behavioral strategies or contracts and mobilize family support and community resources that will help the patient perform the necessary behaviors associated with an option, such as taking medicine, exercising appropriately, or staying on a diet. For example, the physician could recommend use of a pillbox in which the patient's pills are placed in an appropriate daily slot, so that the patient can flip open the appropriate slot at the right time to ensure the pills were taken; a visiting nurse, a community resource, could periodically see the patient to ensure that the pillbox system was working well.

Following up is also critical. Despite the best efforts of the patient and physician, a therapeutic plan may not result in achieving the patient's goals. Physicians cannot always predict with accuracy how a patient will respond to a particular treatment. By following up with the patient, the physician can assess the effectiveness of a particular option and change plans if necessary. The frequency of follow-up should be based on the natural history of the disease, problem, or illness in question or the physician's feeling of how frequently she should monitor the patient and support the patient through his change efforts. The patient's own desire for follow-up should also be taken into account.

CASE 1-6

Annette is a bouncy 18-month-old who is brought to the emergency room by her mother, Joan, with a 1-day history of temperature to 103°F. Dr. Martinez examines Annette and cannot find a source for her infection. He orders a urinalysis, the results of which are negative.

Having recently read an article on presenting options to parents of children who have a fever without a source, Dr. Martinez decides to try that approach with Joan, as she appeared very interested in her child's health (Oppenheim et al., 1994). Dr. Martinez stated that two options are available: (1) obtain a blood *culture on Annette followed by an antibiotic injection with frequent follow-up or (2) obtain a finger-stick blood count and then only obtain a blood culture and antibiotic injection if the white blood cell count is greater than 15,000 cells per high-power field. Dr. Martinez explained that the risk of the antibiotic injection is basically pain, allergic reaction, or diarrhea (in about 5% of patients), while the antibiotic injection would be 90% effective in reducing the risk of serious outcomes such as bacteremia (from 4 in 1000 to 1 in 1000) and meningitis (from 1 in 1000 to 4 in 10,000). The first option costs approximately $150 in Dr. Martinez's emergency room while the second varies from $25 to $175, depending on the results of the white blood cell count.*

Joan did not feel that Annette was ill enough to justify the blood culture and antibiotic injection and thus elected the finger-stick white blood cell count, which showed 10,500 white blood cells per high-power field. Joan brought Annette back to her primary care physician the next day and Annette was doing much better.

PATIENT ROLES

The systemic patient-centered method of care will require more from patients. The biomedical model has been dominant for so many years, not only because it spawned a very effective method of care, but also because it is a culturally acceptable model to many patients who view illness very mechanistically. In contrast, the systemic patient-centered method would encourage patients to explore feelings, meanings, and context of illness. Patients would also be encouraged to assume a greater degree of responsibility for their own health and to exercise that responsibility by forming goals and negotiating therapeutic plans with their physicians. Finally, patients would be encouraged to develop an awareness of how their own behavior, feelings, and emotional reactions affect and are affected by their interactions with people around them and work to develop a decision-making process that respects the values of all involved and takes their health and the health of others into account.

Obviously, not all patients will want or be cognitively able to fulfill all of the roles of a patient operating under the systemic patient-centered method. Some patients may not even want to know what disease state they have and may leave decision-making entirely in the hands of the physician. Some patients may want to be educated about their disease or problem and the treatment options available, but may not want to share in the decision-making, relying entirely on the physician's recommendation. Other patients may not want to share risk and will pick options with a minimal risk even if they are not as effective as higher-risk options. Patients with mental retardation cannot accept responsibility for their care and physicians must learn to work with guardians and others who have accepted responsibility for their care. Thus, while all patients will not want to fulfill all of these roles all of the time, most patients will want to fulfill some roles, and it is up to the physician and the patient to negotiate which roles are appropriate under which circumstances.

Seeker of Information

There is little doubt that patients want information about their condition. In a study of cancer patients, over 80% of patients in all age groups wanted information about their condition, whether it was good or bad (Cassileth *et al.*, 1980). The information items that were most desired by the 256 cancer patients in this study included knowledge of all possible treatment side effects, what the treatment would accomplish in realistic terms, whether they actually had cancer, what the likelihood of cure was, whether all or part of their body was involved, exactly what the treatment would do inside their body, and what was the likely day-to-day or week-to-week progress of the treatment.

17

A NEW
FRAMEWORK:
THE SYSTEMIC
PATIENT-
CENTERED
METHOD

Unfortunately, physicians often underestimate the degree to which patients desire information about their condition. In a study of 210 hypertensive outpatients being taken care of by 50 clinicians, 41% of patients preferred more information about their hypertension, whereas clinicians underestimated patient preferences 28% of the time (Strull *et al.*, 1984). Although reasons for physician underestimation of patients' desire for knowledge have not been well studied, several hypotheses have been developed, including physician's lack of skill, i.e., inadequate training to effectively educate patients, lack of time in effectively educating patients, and lack of reimbursement in performing patient education. While patient education itself is clearly effective in improving health outcomes, and while the skills necessary to effectively educate patients are well known and easily learned (see Chapter 10, "Patient Education"), most medical schools still ignore this critical skill area.

It is also important to emphasize that patients do not want to know all there is to know about a specific condition and its treatments. Most patients want to know what a reasonable person would need to know in order to make effective decisions. Thus, physicians can educate patients by "painting" a reasonable picture of the disease and its natural history, highlighting the most important issues, and discussing the most important details of treatment and its potential effects. Such a presentation need not take much time, 3–5 minutes at most, as demonstrated by Dr. Martinez in Case 1-6, and can be supplemented by patient education materials that have been developed by numerous organizations. If more patient education is needed, the physician can send the patient to an appropriate patient education specialist.

Explore Health-Related Values and Preferences

It is almost axiomatic that patients do not think about their health, what their health means to them, and what they would be willing to invest to preserve their health unless they are sick. Once sick, however, health usually surfaces to an important value. For example, it is not uncommon, even in this age of living wills and health proxies, to find a terminally ill patient who is suddenly able to think about the issues involved in deciding "code" status, whereas when they were healthy, such "morbid" issues were far from their minds.

Physicians can be particularly helpful to patients as they begin to explore what is most important to them and what they value in a particular circumstance. For example, if the patient is facing a choice about treatment of his newly discovered prostate cancer, as Harry did in Case 1-5, the physician can help the patient explore effects of treatment on their quality of life and try to balance these effects with the patient's desire to live longer. If the patient has a terminal illness, the physician can explore with the patient the effectiveness of cardiopulmonary resuscitation in those circumstances and can help the patient decide which interventions would be helpful should an emergency situation arise. Family members also should be involved to help the patient. Needless to say, these conversations are often difficult for physicians, as they raise feelings of failure, of not being able to cure a patient's disease.

Involvement in Decision-Making

The extent to which patients would like to be actively involved in the selection and continued judgment about the usefulness of options to improve their health varies widely. While the "patient empowerment" movement has advocated for not only patient involvement but patient preferences reigning supreme, the literature suggests that only one-half of patients prefer to participate in medical decision-making to any great extent and that there is a wide variety of preference with regard to how the patient would like to participate and on which decisions the patient needs input (Cassileth *et al.*, 1980; Strull *et al.*, 1984).

In a study described previously of 210 hypertensive outpatients being cared for by 50 clinicians, 53% of patients preferred to participate in decision-making (Strull *et al.*, 1984). Furthermore, many patients who preferred not to become involved in initial therapeutic decision-making did want to continue to participate in ongoing evaluation of treatment. It is important to note that clinicians *overestimated* patients' desire to make decisions in this study, feeling that patients desired to become involved in 78% of cases rather than 53%. Patients' desire to become involved in decision-making also varied by age, with younger patients being much more interested in participating (87%) versus those over 60 years old only wanting to participate 51% of the time (Cassileth *et al.*, 1980). Patients who wanted to be involved in treatment decisions were significantly more hopeful than those who did not. Thus, physicians must be attuned to and help patients decide whether they want to be involved at all in decision-making, and in what facets of the decision-making process they want to participate. In Case 1-6, Dr. Martinez was able to involve Joan successfully in the decision-making process regarding Annette's case.

Risk Taker

While many authorities would lump this patient role in with involvement in decision-making, I have chosen to extract it from that role and identify it as a specific role for patients. The reason for this delineation is that this is one of the most difficult areas for patients and physicians to explore. In a study of 160 physician–patient encounters in 19 physician practices, researchers found that risk discussion occurred in only 26% of visits and was quantitative in only two cases (Kalet *et al.*, 1994), unlike Case 1-5. Patients initiated only 16% of these discussions. A recent review of the literature on discussions of risk from the patient perspective revealed that both patients and physicians do this poorly, often either over- or underestimating the real quantitative risk involved in a particular treatment option, and often let emotions and other cognitive factors interfere with the rational selection of an option based on weighing risk and potential benefits (Redelmeier *et al.*, 1993). While statistical and other decision-making techniques have been developed to rationalize this process, these techniques have not been well integrated into clinical practice because they are cumbersome and, quite frankly, difficult to understand.

One of the difficulties physicians have in counseling patients about risk is that much of the medical literature has used "relative risk" as a measure of outcome rather than quantifying absolute risk. Patients and their physicians make decisions based on absolute risk, not relative risk; however, medical researchers use relative risk, as findings described in these terms are often more dramatic. For example, case–control studies reveal that the risk of endometrial cancer in women taking unopposed estrogen is five to seven times that of women who take a progesterone medication along with their estrogen (Voight *et al.*,

1991). However, after 5 years the absolute risk of endometrial cancer in women taking unopposed estrogen increases to 20/1000, from 4/1000, still relatively low, with most cancers being of low grade and stage, and thus, with an excellent prognosis (Hulka, 1994). A woman experiencing side effects of progesterone therapy might abandon her estrogen regime entirely if confronted with the five- to sevenfold increase in endometrial cancer, a relative risk; however, she may be more willing to stay on her estrogen replacement therapy and accept the actual small increase in absolute risk of endometrial cancer that would result, if it were presented to her in those terms.

Physicians often take advantage of the uncertainty in risk discussions by presenting their own options as having the less risk under the circumstances and the most likelihood of achieving a certain outcome. Physicians often state risk in very certain terms rather than probabilistic terms, e.g., "You may die of a heart attack if you do not have this cardiac catheterization procedure," leaving the patient feeling scared and uncertain of the true risks involved. Presenting risks in such stark terms, although easier for the physician, may alienate the patient, particularly those patients who understand that risk is probabilistic and not certain.

While all clinicians do not have the skill or desire to become true quantitative clinical decision makers, physicians can adopt several techniques to help their patients in dealing with risks. Physicians should try to be as quantitative as possible, extracting important risk measures from the literature, particularly dealing with treatment options they prescribe or recommend regularly. Risk measures should be based on absolute rather than relative risk. Risk should be linked with outcome and if multiple risks are present, physicians should help patients prioritize their risk, i.e., what side effects or harms does the patient want to avoid the most versus those that are not as important, and select those options that have the highest likelihood of achieving a certain outcome while minimizing unwanted risk. Comparison of risk of side effects with standard activities in which patients often engage, such as driving on a highway, will help them put the risk of a procedure or treatment in perspective. Lastly, there are certain situations, such as emergency surgery in a critically ill person, when risks are high yet the likelihood of death is also high if a specific intervention is not performed immediately. Since patients are largely risk avoiders, physicians can be most helpful in these circumstances by being supportive of patients who must make quite difficult decisions.

Shared Responsibility

While the biomedical approach places the responsibility for patient health squarely on the shoulders of the physician, the systemic patient-centered method takes a more realistic view and recognizes the important contribution to patients' health of their own actions and the systems to which they belong. A recent article on the leading causes of death for U.S. citizens took a "responsibility" point of view rather than a disease-specific point of view and discovered that the top causes of death are all life-style related, i.e., smoking, high-fat diet, sedentary life-style, and heavy alcohol use (McGinnis & Foege, 1993). Thus, it is extremely unrealistic to assume that physicians have total responsibility for their patients' health.

With regard to instituting treatment options, patients and their systems, such as their family, also play a large role in terms of responsibility. Pills must be taken, bandages must be changed, conditions must be monitored, and appointments must be kept. While our societal and governmental institutions have not provided physicians with a clear delineation as to the patient's responsibility in any given clinical situation, it is still unrealistic to place this burden fully on physicians.

Frank discussions of patient responsibility within the context of any therapeutic encounter are the answer to this vexing circumstance. Physicians should be clear with patients as to the areas for which they are responsible and how they should exercise that responsibility. Physicians can give advice, educate patients as to life-style modifications, and ensure high compliance by prescribing treatments in an appropriate manner, but in the end many interventions require the active participation of the patient. Most patients will respond to such a discussion with physicians by acknowledging their responsibility and attempting to carry it out better. However, some will recognize the cost of that responsibility or lack resources or system support to carry out the responsibility and will negotiate with the physician to modify or change in some way the therapeutic plan. The most vexing patients for physicians are those who refuse to accept any responsibility for their health.

CASE 1-7

A 28-year-old white woman is admitted to the labor and delivery unit of a busy tertiary care hospital with premature rupture of membranes (PROM). Her pregnancy is at term, and even though her membranes have ruptured she has no complaints of labor pain. This is her first pregnancy. She has had a benign prenatal course. Examination reveals no signs of infection, a fetus in the vertex position with good fetal heart tones, and a cervix that appears unfavorable for induction. The family physician taking care of this patient obtained a consult from the obstetrician on call, who recommended early induction even though the patient's cervix was not favorable, in order to decrease the risk of intra-amniotic infections in the mother and sepsis in the infant, a known complication of prolonged rupture of amniotic membranes.

The family physician in this case was uncomfortable with the obstetrician's recommendation because he knew that an induction in the face of an unfavorable cervix would greatly increase the chances of C-section and maternal mortality. Despite his discomfort, the physician, fearing medical–legal complications, did go ahead and induce the woman. Eighteen hours later, the woman failed to progress and underwent a C-section. The C-section was productive of a term, viable, male infant who appeared healthy. Mother and baby were discharged 5 days later having suffered none of the complications of an operative delivery.

Despite the good outcome in this case, the family physician continued to wonder if this case should have been managed in a different way so that the woman would not have had to undergo a C-section. Because of his concerns, he consulted a colleague with expertise in clinical decision-making, who agreed that constructing a decision tree, an analysis detailing all possible outcomes with their probabilities given certain clinical actions, might be a useful way to analyze the problem.

21

A NEW
FRAMEWORK:
THE SYSTEMIC
PATIENT-
CENTERED
METHOD

In order to find the probability of the specific events in women with PROM, the physician's colleague did a literature review in which he found three randomized control trials that examined the management of women with PROM in different settings with different interventions. Two early trials done in 1984 and 1986 concluded that expectant management was the correct course, but one recent trail published in 1989 concluded that early induction was better (Duff et al., 1984; Morales & Lazar, 1986; Wagner et al., 1989). Because these trials did not solve the controversy, the colleague felt comfortable in constructing a decision tree using probabilities taken from those randomized control trials in order to see which management strategy reduced risk the most.

A decision tree was constructed comparing four options: induction on presentation at the labor deck, induction 6 hours after PROM, induction 12 hours after PROM, and expectant management (see Figure 1.2). Both maternal and neonatal morbidity and mortality were used as outcome measures. The decision tree produced contradictory results. With regard to maternal morbidity and mortality, the management strategy that best reduced risk and improved outcomes was expectant management, since early induction greatly increased the risk of unnecessary C-sections and maternal mortality.

However, given the hospital's policy of performing a septic workup on all infants born of mothers with PROM for longer than 24 hours, the analysis from the perspective of infant morbidity and mortality revealed that early induction was best, since that significantly reduced the risk of iatrogenic complications from the huge number of septic workups that would be performed on infants delivered of women with PROM for greater than 24 hours. Even when the model was reanalyzed using a more relaxed policy for requiring septic workups on infants, early induction was still found to be the best way to reduce infant risk.

In trying to formulate a coherent approach to this problem, the physician realized that recommending early induction to all PROM patients would no doubt decrease infant morbidity and mortality, but at the cost of increased maternal morbidity and mortality. Likewise, recommending expectant management would reduce maternal risk, but at the cost of infant morbidity and mortality. The physician also realized that to change the outcome of this decision analysis might require a significant relaxation of the septic workup policy, thus going against hospital policy and increasing medical–legal risk.

In thinking further about this problem, the physician realized that a patient's decision could depend on her own unique situation and values. The physician could envision scenarios in which a woman might elect early induction, for example, a woman who was pregnant for the first time after a long course of fertility drugs, versus a woman who might opt for expectant management, for example, a woman with six children who fulfilled the vital family role of the children's caretaker. Despite the fact that it was more time-consuming to explain to each patient the details of the decision analysis, the critical importance of the patient's context and values in helping to make the decision convinced the physician that he should take the time to explain the decision analysis to patients with PROM in order to help them make a decision that best fit their situation and respected their values. (Contributed by D. Marley)

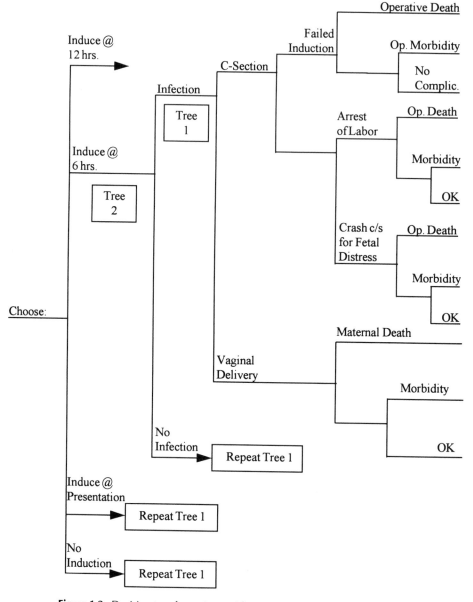

Figure 1.2. Decision tree for patients with premature rupture of membranes.

PATIENT-CENTERED CLINICAL DECISION-MAKING

The systemic patient-centered method approaches clinical decision-making as a partnership between the patient and the physician (see Figure 1.3). Data necessary for this approach include not only traditional biomedical information, but also information helpful

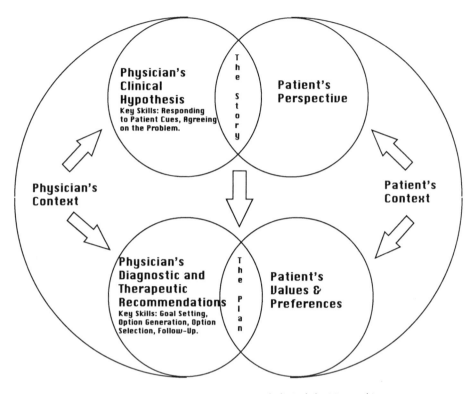

Figure 1.3. Systemic patient-centered clinical decision-making.

in explaining the patient's illness, in setting goals, and in selecting options in planning follow-up. While the data needed and the framework for systemic patient-centered clinical decision-making are not yet as well defined as for the biomedical method, the basic data required and the basic framework are rapidly emerging as research is conducted on this method. The key characteristic of physicians who utilize this method well is that they are not necessarily better "artists" than their biomedical contemporaries, but that they possess more and different skills that enable the systemic patient-centered method to be "workable" with their patients. In other words, successful patient-centered physicians do not need to be born with a certain amount of creative talent, although creativity within the physician–patient relationship certainly will help, but do need to develop the essential skills needed for this approach to be effective.

DATA BASE

A good data base provides all of the information necessary for a medical decision. Obviously no good medical decision can be made in the absence of data; on the other hand, simply gathering data is not the only concern of the patient-centered clinician. How much data to collect is one of the first questions that clinician and patient must answer, since the amount of data that could be collected is vast. The amount of data to be collected can to some extent be determined by the hypotheses that the patient and physician hold with regard to the patient's illness, the amount of psychosocial and contextual information needed to understand the patient's illness and offer the patient an adequate number of treatment options, and the patient's health-related goals.

Also important are data concerning the clinician and the clinician's context. The extent of the physician's medical knowledge and skills is obviously important in making a diagnosis and formulating a therapeutic plan. It is almost axiomatic that unless a physician thinks of a diagnostic possibility, it will not be included in the differential diagnosis. Physician contextual issues are also important. A physician's knowledge of available medical and consultative help, consultant's ability to manage patients, and knowledge of the healthcare system in which the physician operates are all important considerations in the decision-making process, as illustrated in Case 1-7. For example, a physician confronted with a patient who has an acute myocardial infarction may make vastly different decisions in a tertiary care center with rapid access to a cardiac catheterization lab than in a small rural community without access to a cardiologist.

The physician's self-knowledge regarding personal values, attitudes, feelings, expectations, and fears toward specific patients and patients in general is crucial to the physician in understanding her own biases and prejudices. For example, a physician strongly opposed to abortion may not be able to adequately counsel an unmarried adolescent with an unexpected pregnancy who wants to be informed about the abortion option. If the physician understood his values in this case, he might want to refer the patient to a more unbiased counselor.

Health-related values are probably the most important values to explore with the patient. Since an individual's values largely come from family and cultural values and traditions, those contexts may be important to explore as a critical component of the decision-making process.

When values come into conflict in a particular situation, it might be beneficial to explore not only the patient's value context but the physician's value context as well. Physician values, like patient values, largely come from the physician's own family and cultural traditions. In addition, physician values often originate from the healthcare system in which they were trained. By conducting an exploration of their value context, physicians may find that their own values have been shaped by systemic processes that may or may not benefit the current clinical situation. For example, a physician who highly values eradicating disease as a way to benefit patient health and who places health as a top priority might actually exacerbate noncompliance because of the physician's authoritarian manner with patients. An exploration of that physician's values would reveal that they arose from the health-related values of his family and teachers in medical school rather than being formulated individually through his experience as a clinician and his philosophical beliefs. By realizing the origin of his values, the physician might be more willing to explore other options and negotiate rather than demand that patients comply in clinical situations where values are in conflict.

Action constraints are those factors that impose themselves on patients and preclude or demand certain decision-making options. Common action constraints are time and money, but other individual action constraints such as habitual behavior patterns, low motivation, and transference also can block attempts at a solution. Similarly, the individual's context may place action constraints on a particular option or decision, for example, systemic feedback loops that maintain problem behavior, decreased family resources or social support, which preclude complex or difficult decision-making options, and erroneous but powerfully held beliefs that contradict the physician's explanation of the patient's illness.

Action constraints impose themselves on the physician as well. Time and money are action constraints for physicians, as they must see a certain number of patients per day to earn a living. Likewise, lack of medical knowledge or skills in a certain area will preclude certain decision-making options, as will availability of equipment, such as MRI scanners, and personnel. Countertransference can actually be a hindrance not only to the physician–patient relationship but to the decision-making process as well. Physicians may become so frustrated with certain patients because of countertransference arising from family-of-origin issues that they react in ways that preclude rational decision-making and only serve to maintain patient problems (Mengel, 1987). For example, the physician son of an alcoholic father may unconsciously be so angry at his father that he cannot establish enough of a therapeutic relationship to encourage his alcoholic patients to quit drinking.

Finally, the physician's own context might impose action constraints on the decision-making process, such as a recurrent poor communication process among healthcare professionals, consistent disagreements with specific consultants, or systemic feedback loops within the physician's own healthcare system that may preclude certain options. Too many healthcare professionals working on a specific case can actually be an action constraint, as responsibility is so diffused that little active decision-making is performed.

If all health-related information was obtained from all patients, the construction of a patient-centered data base would be a daunting task indeed. Physicians would probably spend 2–3 hours with each patient, significantly reducing access to care for their other patients. Skilled patient-centered clinicians have surmounted this task by utilizing probably the most important clinical skill available to the patient-centered clinician, namely, responding to patient cues. Responding to patient cues allows the patient-centered clinician to construct a data base that is pertinent for that patient at that moment, tailoring it to the specific patient, only utilizing those bits of information that are absolutely essential to the crafting of a therapeutic plan. By using this important skill, researchers have found that no more time is spent with patients by physicians who utilize a patient-centered approach when compared with those who restrict themselves to the biomedical method (Stewart *et al.*, 1995).

RESPONDING TO PATIENT CUES

A patient cue is any bit of information, either contextual or emotional, that if responded to will enable the physician to learn a great deal about the patient's experience of illness. Illness is defined as the patient's experience of having a disease or other healthcare problem that adversely affects her life in some way and provokes feelings and emotions in her, often altering the meaning of her life if it turns out to be a chronic or terminal illness. Patients bring their illnesses, not their disease, to their physicians and then the biomedical clinician attempts to diagnose a dysfunction in an organ system. It's important when using the systemic patient-centered method to focus on the patient's experience of illness rather than solely diagnosing a disease.

Patients often fail to express their ideas or concerns to physicians. Sometimes through long experience with their providers, patients feel that healthcare providers do not want to know their experience of illness. Providers seem busy, harried, often interrupt patients when they are telling their story, and don't spend a great deal of time explaining to patients what they are going to do or try. Patients are often ignorant of the technical terms physicians use and quite frankly fear being embarrassed if they use simple-minded concepts or ideas to explain their own feelings of why they have a particular illness and

Table 1.1
Patient Cues

Direct statement
 • Statement by the patient of explanations, emotions, expectations, and impact of the illness
Expression of feelings about the illness
(Without the patient's naming the specific illness in mind)
 • Direct, projected, or denied expression of feelings or concerns
 • Symptoms described with emotional intensity
 • Repetition of statement or idea about the illness
 • Nonverbal expression of concern
Attempts to explain or understand symptoms
(Without the patient's naming the specific illness considered)
 • Statements revealing active efforts or prior effort to explain, change explanation, or understand
   symptoms
 • Spontaneous description of disease in mind (without naming)
 • A hypothesis that appears incongruous with symptoms, behaviors, or feelings present
Loaded questions, e.g., "Can you get cancer from someone else?"
Spontaneous expression of a personal story
Behaviors indicative of concerns, dissatisfaction, or unmet needs
 • "Routine visit" without specific expressed concern or expectation
 • Presence of other people during the visit who aren't usually there, or absence of people who are usually
   there
 • Reluctance to accept recommendations
 • "By the way, . . ." statements at the close of the visit
 • Seeking a second opinion or an early return visit

what that illness is doing to their daily life. Patients are also quite scared of being ill, fearing that their illness may lead to the diagnosis of something fatal or something that will debilitate them or prevent them from accomplishing a certain life goal.

Healthcare providers have often ignored patient cues because they do not consider them to be within the purview of the biomedical model or fear that focusing on the patient's experience of illness will take more time, require skills in processing that information that they do not possess, or doubt the usefulness of the information they will obtain. Responding to patient cues also requires the physician to stop his own agenda with regard to information collection and allow the patient some time to express her own needs, often a very difficult task in a busy office.

Patient cues usually fall into one of six categories (see Table 1.1). Some of these cues are more difficult to recognize than others, such as expression of feelings about the illness or the "oh, by the way" statement at the close of the visit. Responses need not be sophisticated psychologically but can merely be short statements or questions, such as, "In listening to you chat about your concerns today you seem very sad. Is there something that is upsetting you?" Or, "In hearing you talk, I feel that you may have an explanation for what's causing your symptoms. What do you think is causing your symptoms today?" Taking patient cues and concerns seriously is also important, as patients feel validated and are thus more likely to work with the physician when a therapeutic plan is being negotiated. Once the physician has responded to enough of the patient cues to construct a meaningful patient-centered data base, then the physician and patient can construct a mutually agreeable plan.

Negotiating a mutually agreeable plan requires a certain skill set in order to construct a plan with a high likelihood of success. These skills require the physician to understand and utilize patient preferences, particularly those related to health, costs, and risks. The physician should never expect a patient to engage in a health behavior she thinks will be beneficial for a patient unless the physician can find, with the help of the patient, adequate *reason* to do so. In other words, a change in health behavior needs to be consistent with patient values and have a high likelihood of achieving a goal the patient wants to reach. Fortunately, patients' health perceptions are malleable and the physician can work with the patient to renegotiate strongly held but incorrect health perceptions.

Excessive emotional reactivity during plan construction, either the physician's or the patient's, usually results from how the other party perceives he is being treated and precludes effective communication. Being too "hot" (angry or upset) clouds judgment, while being too "cold" (distant or uncaring) impairs motivation and understanding. Unfortunately, providers are typically perceived by patients as lacking warmth; thus, providers should try to achieve a stance of compassionate neutrality during plan construction.

Effective communication is also important during plan construction. Providers should attempt to use simple terms, not medical jargon, use silences effectively to stimulate patient communication, and judiciously use open-ended questions and use the patient's own words when questioning or explaining something to the patient. Effective communication will facilitate understanding and speed the planning process greatly.

Principles of negotiation and conflict resolution need to be kept in mind. Chapter 11 on negotiation discusses these principles. When conflict arises, some physicians and patients want to avoid conflict, others fight to win. It is important for physicians to remember there is usually more than one reason for conflict, i.e., don't settle for simple solutions, and that most conflicts are fixable as long as key issues are discussed and negotiated.

Lastly, physicians should respect the change process as described in Chapter 13. As physicians, we often ask patients to make changes in their life-style that are difficult. Physicians often underestimate the degree of difficulty involved in such change. By respecting the change process, physicians can take those steps that move the patient through the change process, for example, from contemplation to preparation, rather than always insisting on immediate action.

Constructing a mutually agreeable plan requires four clinical skills: agreeing on the problem, goal setting, generation options, and selecting options (Taylor *et al.,* 1984). Follow-up is also key, particularly the physician's response to plan failure, should that happen.

Agreeing on the Problem

This skill requires the construction of a patient-centered hypothesis that explains the patient's health status. It is important for physicians to realize that most patients have already formed a hypothesis about their illness, and, in fact, have often taken steps based on that hypothesis to improve their health. Failure to discover the patient's hypothesis jeopardizes plan construction. This skill requires the physician to draw on all of the data assembled on the patient to date or to obtain necessary data before formulating a good hypothesis. A good hypothesis requires that both patient and physician follow the usual rules of causality, especially time course. If the patient and physician do agree on the problem, patient outcomes are much improved, as demonstrated in a study of headache patients (Bass *et al.,* 1986).

Goal Setting

Deciding with the patient what realistic obtainable improvement can be made in the patient's health is a critical skill. Achieving a small step, rather than a big gain, is probably more important, as setting unrealistic or very difficult goals often discourages both the patient and the provider. Physicians spend the most time with patients discussing this area and thus goal setting is an easy skill for most physicians to master (Taylor *et al.,* 1984). Because goal setting is a direct reflection of patient values, those values are important to take into account when setting goals. Setting specific realistic goals can also enable both physician and patient to recognize trade-offs and *agreeing* on the goals of therapy often will improve outcomes, as demonstrated in a study of diabetic patients (Greenfield *et al.,* 1988). Setting achievable goals and reaching them motivates both patient and physician to continue their therapeutic alliance.

Generating Options

Once a goal has been constructed, both patient and physician can then generate options that will have the best chance of reaching this goal. Generally, physicians do not spend enough time listening to the patient's opinion about the options generated or explaining to the patient details of the various options described, especially cost and side effects (Taylor *et al.,* 1984). On the other hand, patients want to spend a lot of time on this step and often will exercise a healthy skepticism toward the physician's recommendation unless these details are explained.

Physicians may find this phase difficult, as the medical literature is often not conclusive enough to enable physicians to feel comfortable with the options they generate. Effectiveness data are simply not available, as most studies are flawed and randomized controlled trials are not done over a long enough period of time to yield appropriate clinical information or the outcomes of interest are not included in the studies (Roper *et al.,* 1988). If multiple interventions are available, the most effective or cost-effective is often not determined by research findings. Also, the question of when to begin therapy, for example, at what level of blood pressure or what level of elevated cholesterol, is surprisingly controversial. Thus, physician confusion over options is something that every physician will have to surmount to develop skill in this critical area.

One of the important skills for healthcare professionals to utilize if they have difficulty with option generation is effective involvement of other healthcare professionals. Consultation with clinical specialists, but also other nonphysician providers such as patient educators, therapists, or ethicists, is important. The formation of a multidisciplinary team also seems to be beneficial, particularly when taking care of very vulnerable or frail patients, as such teams are better able to set realistic goals and generate more options than a single physician can.

Selecting Options

Deciding on which options to include in the plan, defining objective measures of success, and appropriate follow-up are also key skills. It is often difficult for physicians to spend much time on option selection, as available data are not up to the task of predicting for the physician which patients will do well with which options and which won't. In other words, it's very difficult for physicians to predict for patients whether they will get a particular side effect or whether a particular trade-off will have to be made; e.g., a drug may decrease the patient's sexual function but will control blood pressure—what is more important to the patient? Therapeutic options often involve other members of the patient's system, so involving those members, for example, through education or mobilization of family support to increase compliance with medication, is important and has been shown to decrease complications in hypertensive patients (Morisky *et al.*, 1983).

In deciding on options, certain characteristics of the patient and physician seem to be important. Is the patient a risk taker, or does he wish to avoid risk at all costs? Is cost a consideration either in terms of money or time, or does the patient want to minimize cost and perhaps select a slightly less effective option? Does either the patient or provider have dominant moral values regarding any of the options being considered?

No matter which options are included in this plan, it is very important that physicians and patients select a measure to judge success that is objective and independent of the will of either party. Most of the time, objective measures of success are readily available, such as glycosylated hemoglobin in patients with diabetes mellitus or the results of a depression questionnaire to determine the effect of antidepressant therapy in a patient with exogenous depression.

Medicine is not a perfect science and thus, even with the best of intentions, the patient and physician may agree on options that simply do not work. When a plan fails, it is important that the patient not be blamed. All too often physicians blame patients by calling them noncompliant, irresponsible, or difficult to manage. However, failure often arises from the failure of the physician to undergo an effective decision-making process and successfully use all of the important patient-centered skills when constructing a mutually agreeable plan. Common reasons for plan failure are listed in Table 1.2.

At this stage, the patient and physician should put their heads together and proceed through the patient-centered clinical decision-making process once again. Often, however, both the patient and the physician will realize that failure, rather than reflecting a short-coming on the part of the physician or the patient, results from the fact that options simply

Table 1.2
Common Reasons for Plan Failure

Failure to agree on the problem
Failure to elicit or respect an important patient preference or emotion
Failure to set realistic, obtainable goals; often more ambitious goals are set than can be reached
Failure to generate an adequate number of options or to educate that patient about available options
Failure to respect patient values or preferences when selecting options
Failure to follow up and support the patient through the change process
Patient or physician emotional reactivity precluding effective communication
Ignoring or not assessing correctly an important system, usually the family, that affects the patient's health

---

are not available for the patient under his current circumstance. Such times are very difficult for physicians, as they often regard themselves as failures or incompetent.

Frequent follow-up cannot be overemphasized. In this age of utilization control, physicians may be reticent to invite the patient back frequently, but without frequent follow-up, failures cannot be detected early and successes cannot be celebrated. Successes need to be celebrated in order to motivate both the patient and the physician to achieve more difficult or costlier goals.

CASE 1-8

A second-year family practice resident became frustrated during his training program when he began to learn how to detect patients who had been beaten or otherwise abused in their home situation. This frustration arose from the fact that he felt his community was not paying attention to this issue and services were not adequate to care for these patients once detected, who were mainly women in abusive relationships.

After several months of thinking about this issue, he realized if he did nothing, his situation would be very similar to several of his patients who remained a victim and returned to their abusive spouses without any real change occurring in their relationships. Not wanting to be a "victim" any longer, this physician organized a meeting with several like-minded health professionals at his hospital and strategized over what they could do. They developed three goals: (1) educating their fellow physicians on how to detect victims of abuse and treat them adequately, (2) raising money to support community organizations that care for abused victims who want to leave their difficult situations, and (3) educating the public on this difficult topic. Their first fund-raiser, a 1950s dance, featuring a group of cardiologists known as the "Arrhythmias," was a huge success and provided the money to begin the development of programs to accomplish the group's goals.

THE SYSTEMIC PATIENT-CENTERED METHOD: OTHER CONCERNS

CHANGING LARGER SYSTEMS

Physicians who use the systemic patient-centered method often try to change dysfunctional systems to improve patient health. Some systems, such as communities or cultural systems, may be so large and powerful that physicians can find themselves frustrated if they attempt to change even a small facet of those systems.

In reality, physicians and other healthcare providers are already attempting to change dysfunctional aspects of systems at many levels. Family therapists have become very successful at changing dysfunctional family systems. Physicians in many communities across this country have taken on the responsibility of educating public school students, community groups, and local parent–teacher associations on various health issues, including AIDS, domestic violence, as in Case 1-8, the unhealthy effects of certain patient life-styles, such as smoking (Doctors Ought to Care), and the medical effects of nuclear war (Physicians for Social Responsibility). Physicians who participate in such activities not only view these activities as part of their professional role as a healthcare provider, improving the health of large groups through systemic involvement, but also view such activity as a duty or repayment to society for the investment society has made in educating them and for the special privileges and respect society has bestowed on them as physicians.

Physicians who attempt to work with small and large systems must continually remind themselves that systems are homeostatic and thus resistant to change. "Burnout" and frustration among physicians occur at a very high rate not only because of the demands of practice but also because of unrealistic expectations in attempting to change patient behavior to improve health. Physicians who lack the skill or motivation to tackle systemic issues should be cognizant of these limitations. Physicians skilled in systemic intervention should work to change systems if they see that such change is a realistic possibility and accept that some systems are simply beyond the power of an individual physician to change. Acknowledging such limitations to patients, which may be difficult for many physicians, will also go far in helping patients to understand the influences of larger systems on their own behavior and perhaps will cause them to entertain systemic change themselves!

ETHICS OF THE SYSTEMIC PATIENT-CENTERED METHOD

There are also ethical implications of systemic involvement. Informed consent, confidentiality, and the physician's duty to other members of the patient's system all need to be explored if the patient and the physician agree that a change in a system is warranted. Many physicians are uncomfortable working with larger systems because they perceive their duty to individual patients as supreme. Since systemic interventions are sometimes paradoxical, particularly in the short term, some physicians may find themselves faced with recommending that patients continue or even increase unhealthy behavior for a short time. For example, a physician caring for an obese woman who is in a complementary conflicted relationship to her mother might actually counsel against a diet initially, anticipating that a straightforward approach would result in noncompliance and failure.

Although difficult, these problems are not insurmountable if approached in an open fashion. If a family system needs to be changed, the physician can obtain consent from the patient to call all family members together, explain the problem, set goals to solve it, and then explain why the involvement of other family members is necessary. The physician can then describe what needs to be done to change the system. All members of the family can then give consent and participate depending on their desires. The envelope of confidentiality would need to be expanded past the individual physician and patient, but that too is not unreasonable as long as the patient agrees.

The physician's duty to an individual patient must still take top priority, but concern, compassion, and professional skills can be directed at other members of the patient's system. Paradoxical systemic interventions can even be used as long as the physician is highly skilled in their use, indications are appropriate, and appropriate follow-up is planned in case the intervention fails. If the physician or patient cannot negotiate these ethical hurdles, then a consultation with an ethicist may be necessary.

EFFICACY OF THE SYSTEMIC PATIENT-CENTERED METHOD

One of the first questions physicians ask about a new test or treatment option is, "Does it work?" In 1989, McWhinney reviewed studies supporting the efficacy of the patient-centered method. Since 1989, more studies have been done, and almost all conclude that the patient-centered method results in improvements in health for a variety of conditions, including acute conditions, undifferentiated symptoms in which a traditional biomedical diagnosis cannot be made, and chronic illnesses (Gerteis *et al.*, 1993; Stewart *et al.*, 1995).

Furthermore, these studies have found few side effects of the patient-centered approach; in other words, the patient-centered approach is not only effective but safe. However, a review of the potential side effects or disadvantages of he patient-centered approach is in order given the early stage of this research.

SAFETY OF THE SYSTEMIC PATIENT-CENTERED METHOD

Viewed from the perspective of the biomedical method, many physicians feel that the systemic patient-centered method may possess some undesirable effects. The breadth of the patient-centered method may dilute physician focus on the biomedical aspects of the cases (Seldin, 1981). Physicians would lose some power within the physician–patient relationship, although their autonomy would continue to be respected. Physicians would have to develop more effective mechanisms for coping with complex conflictional systems. Physicians would need to supplement the sole use of objective validation criteria (such as autopsy results) with more subjective patient-defined outcomes. Additionally, a record system that will document aspects of the patient-centered method has not been fully developed. Finally, physicians and patients wishing to utilize the patient-centered method will be going against cultural and healthcare system precepts that support the biomedical model (Stein, 1990). Thus, patient-centered clinicians may lose respect or even generate anger from colleagues until this new approach is more widely accepted.

Despite these potential disadvantages, the systemic patient-centered method, since it subsumes the biomedical method within its purview and has so much potential for improving patient health, seems to offer many advantages over the biomedical method. In fact, to many clinicians it is even difficult to understand why the patient-centered method has not already gained widespread favor. Perhaps as physicians become more comfortable with nontechnical aspects of clinical care, as governmental agencies and insurance agencies reimburse clinicians more fairly for nonprocedural skills, and as patients realize their own interdependence and how important their psychological state is to their illness, the systemic patient-centered method will gradually transform modern medical practice and be widely adopted by practicing clinicians.

CONCLUSION

Medicine's dominant method of clinical care is still the biomedical method. Despite the great strides medicine has made using this method, it has been severely criticized because some patients being cared for by physicians utilizing this method do not become significantly healthier despite this method's focus on disease states. Many physicians have come to realize that this is not only because health is much more than the absence of disease, but also because the biomedical method does not allow physicians to ask the patient to become involved in the development of a therapeutic plan that is congruent with their feelings, life-style, preferences, values, and systems to which they belong. Because of these shortcomings in the biomedical method, some physicians believe the method they use to care for patients will be undergoing a transformation in response to societal and patients' demands.

Of all of the approaches that have recently been described and analyzed, the one that best fits the new philosophical framework described above is the systemic patient-centered method advocated by McWhinney and others. Under the systemic patient-centered method, the roles of the physician would be significantly expanded to include (1) aiding the patient in deciding what health is and how best to optimize it, (2) obtaining not only biomedical information from the patient but also psychosocial and contextual information, (3) allowing the patient a role in the decision-making process through the formation and prioritization of goals, and (4) guiding the patient through an effective decision-making process to select therapeutic options that have the best chance of achieving the patient's health goals while respecting her values.

This new approach to care would also require much more from patients. Patients would not be able to achieve the complete dominance in the patient–physician relationship that they may want, some patients might have to adapt to a wider view of health than the traditional biomedical model would allow, and patients would be encouraged to allow the physician and perhaps others to help in improving their health. The approach would also demand a greater degree of responsibility on the part of patients as they participate in formulating goals and deciding on therapeutic options. These new responsibilities, rather than harming the patient, would empower patients to be more responsible for their health and thus would be conducive to individual growth and development.

Effective patient-centered clinical decision-making rests on the physician developing new patient-centered skills, including recognizing and responding to patient cues, agreeing on the problem, goal setting, generating options, selecting options, and follow-up. Assessing failure, if it occurs, is also an important skill. While acknowledging failure is difficult for the physician, it must be done without blaming the patient. Often through the assessment of failure, a new patient-centered clinical decision-making process can be begun that will result in success. However, physicians will have certain patients for whom no matter what they do, the patients' health cannot be improved.

Physicians adopting such an approach must be careful to avoid burnout and excessive levels of frustration. Changing patient behavior and changing systems that affect patient behavior can be very difficult. The ethical implications of involving important parts of the patient's context in his healthcare may be difficult to broach at times. Physicians trained solely in using the biomedical method may find it difficult to develop the skills required under a systemic patient-centered method.

However, physicians using this method have generally not found these problems insurmountable. Like-minded physicians have joined together in groups to alter systems that may be reinforcing unhealthy patient behaviors. Support from colleagues, consultation with healthcare providers skilled in systemic issues, and acknowledgment of systemic limitations to patients all help physicians deal with complex matters. Continuing medical education courses are available for physicians who need to upgrade their patient-centered skills. Likewise, ethical issues are not insurmountable as long as they are approached in an open fashion and consensus is reached among all parties concerned.

Studies reveal that the systemic patient-centered method appears to be efficacious with few side effects. Many physicians feel that strategies can be developed to cope with the potential side effects of the systemic patient-centered method and that the advantages of the patient-centered method greatly outweigh its potential disadvantages. However, many aspects of the patient-centered method still need to be adequately studied.

Medical practice is entering an exciting, turbulent time. Not only are patients becoming increasingly dissatisfied with old methods of clinical practice, but physicians too are seeing the disadvantages inherent in the biomedical method. Although a new clinical method has not fully asserted itself yet, many respected scholars and clinicians are undertaking further study and research on the systemic patient-centered method because they believe it will eventually be the desired new method.

CASES FOR DISCUSSION

CASE 1

David, a 16-year-old black teenager, came into his family physician's office with a 1-day history of pain in his lower abdomen, nausea, vomiting, and loss of appetite. Two hours ago, David's pain seemed to be located more in his right lower quadrant. On exam, David was noted to have a temperature of 101°F and to be very tender in his lower abdomen, particularly in the right lower quadrant, where rebound tenderness was present. The physician then ordered two tests: (1) white blood cell count, which returned elevated at 14.8×10^3 cells per hpf, and (2) urinalysis, the results of which were totally normal.

David's family physician made the diagnosis of appendicitis and referred David to a general surgeon, who recommended immediate surgery. On opening the abdomen, the general surgeon found an inflamed appendix, which was removed without complications. David recovered without difficulty and was discharged from the hospital 2 days later. At his 1-month follow-up visit with the general surgeon, David was back to normal.

1. *Which method of clinical care were the family physician and general surgeon using in this case?*
2. *What are some of the strengths of that method?*
3. *What are some of the potential problems associated with this method?*

CASE 2

Mrs. F. Z. is a 68-year-old white woman with mild Alzheimer's dementia who was admitted to an internal medicine teaching service of a busy tertiary care hospital with shortness of breath, right lower lobe pneumonia on chest X ray, and hypoxia on an arterial blood gas. On arrival to the ward, the patient was confused and combative and had to be restrained so that an intravenous line could be started. After the intravenous line was established, appropriate antibiotics were prescribed. Over the next 2 days the patient appeared to be getting better but was still occasionally confused and combative, and so restraints were kept in place.

On the third day, Mrs. F. Z. became acutely short of breath. The resident taking care of Mrs. F. Z. immediately ordered a lung scan, which showed perfusion defects not matched with ventilation defects in the upper left lung field, consistent with a pulmonary embolus. In order to find a source for this embolus, the resident examined the patient's lower extremities and noted that the right calf was swollen and tender. The resident immediately started heparin therapy, which seemed to help the patient, but the patient had to be placed on a larger amount of oxygen in order to decrease her shortness of breath.

One day later the patient refused to eat and complained of abdominal pain. Examination revealed no bowel sounds, bruising around the umbilicus, and hematuria on urinalysis. The resident then obtained an abdominal CT scan, which confirmed his diagnosis of retroperitoneal hematoma. Because of the hematoma formation, heparin therapy had to be stopped.

Two days later the patient still had not improved. On the afternoon of that day the patient became acutely short of breath again and was noted to be more swollen. The diagnosis of pulmonary embolus was again made based on classic findings on a lung scan with swelling secondary to acute renal failure from hypotension. Extremely poor oxygenation was noted on an arterial blood gas, so the patient was transferred to the intensive care unit, where she was intubated and placed on mechanical ventilation. Her blood pressure was supported with pressor agents. Peritoneal dialysis was instituted for the patient's renal failure.

Over the next week the patient continued to do poorly, with many febrile episodes being noted. Despite a change in antibiotics, F. Z.'s lung function continued to deteriorate so that she required larger and larger amounts of oxygen. Ten days after admission to the hospital, she died of a respiratory arrest.

1. What method of clinical care was the resident using in this case?
2. What problem with this method does this case illustrate? Trace out how the resident's actions in this case contributed to the complications that arose.
3. How might this "cascade of unanticipated events" have been prevented?
4. How much do you estimate this hospitalization cost?

CASE 3

Nancy, a 54-year-old successful business executive, presented to her family physician's office with a tired feeling and a chronic cough, which she attributed to her 40 pack per year history of smoking and two recent episodes of hemoptysis. The physician obtained a chest X ray, which showed a large mass in the right hilum that later was diagnosed as an oat cell carcinoma by bronchoscopy. Both the oncologist and the family physician assured Nancy that cure was possible given new radiation therapy and drug treatment protocols that had been recently developed. Nancy gladly consented to these protocols, as she wanted to continue her work as a business executive.

However, after 9 months of painful radiation and chemotherapy, Nancy was becoming more and more depressed. She had to devote increasing amounts of time away from her business for her healthcare, and rather than becoming stronger she was becoming progressively weaker. Nancy began to suspect that her physicians were not telling her the truth and so began reading about oat cell carcinoma in medical textbooks she obtained from her local library. She was devastated to learn that the median survival of patients with oat cell carcinoma was only 1 or 2 years, and even the latest radiation therapy and chemotherapy protocols had not altered that prognosis. Nancy could not understand why her physicians had not been honest with her, but she did not confront them, becoming even more depressed as it became obvious that therapy was not going to cure her.

Despite Nancy's depression, her physicians continued to reassure her that she could maintain an active life as long as she submitted to therapy. Eventually, Nancy became so depressed that she began contemplating suicide. One week later, Nancy was found dead in her garage, all of its doors having been closed and her car left running.

1. What method of clinical care were the physicians in Nancy's case using?
2. What problem arose in this case because of the method the physicians were using?
3. How common is suicide among terminally ill patients? Could this have been prevented?
4. What additional knowledge or information would have been helpful in this case?

CASE 4

Debbie, a 28-year-old factory worker, comes into her physician's office complaining of fatigue of 2 months' duration. In talking with Debbie, her physician learns that she is happily married with two children and considers her family life to be very satisfying. However, 3 months ago she was shifted from assembly line work to piecework at the local shoe factory, resulting in a substantial loss to her income. To make ends meet, both Debbie and her husband have to work, placing the children at a local day-care center during their working hours. Despite this loss of income, Debbie has still not confronted her boss, who would not do anything about it anyway, as Debbie was the only worker who could do piecework well. The physician, having been in this small town for 5 years, knew the boss of the shoe factory where Debbie worked and realized how difficult it was for the boss to find skilled workers.

1. What method of clinical care is the physician operating under in this case?
2. Is it within the purview of the physician to discuss occupational issues with his patients?
3. How would you help Debbie in this case if you were the physician and you knew the boss of the factory? Would you confront the boss directly, or would you encourage Debbie to do so?
4. Would you treat Debbie with antidepressants in this case, psychotherapy, both, or neither?

CASE 5

Barbara, a 33-year-old woman, presented to the labor and delivery service of a busy hospital with a rupture of membranes at 37 weeks estimated gestational age. The obstetrician taking care of Barbara, knowing the results of the decision analysis in Case 1-7, decided to present Barbara with two options, either expective management or induction immediately, even though Barbara's cervix was not favorable for induction. Tom, her husband, was also present in the room when the obstetrician presented the two options and the risks and benefits of both. A heated discussion followed in which Barbara elected one option and Tom elected the other.

1. How might this case have been different if the physician operated under a traditional biomedical method?
2. If Tom and Barbara already had five children and Barbara played a large role in childcare such that if she were injured or dead, Tom would be left taking care of the children, but Barbara felt it was her duty to give her child the best chance of being born healthy and thus wanted an immediate induction, whereas Tom wanted to wait 24 hours to see if Barbara would go into labor on her own, how would you help this couple resolve this issue? Does Tom have any say legally or ethically in any option that Barbara decides on?
3. Would Tom's feelings change, given the ethical theory (duties, rights, or utilitarianism) he is inferred to be using in question 2, if this was their first child after a long infertility workup? Would presenting this scenario to Tom help in the couple's decision-making?

RECOMMENDED READINGS

Gerteis M, Edgman-Levitan S, Daley J, Delbanco TL (eds): *Through the Patient's Eyes: Understanding and Promoting Patient-Centered Care.* San Francisco, Jossey-Bass Inc Publishers, 1993.

This book reviews the literature on patient-centered care from a hospitalized patient's perspective and then presents the results of the author's extensive study of this topic. The book concludes with a practical framework for instituting a patient-centered approach in hospitals.

Stewart M, Brown JB, Weston WW, McWhinney IR, McWilliam CL, Freeman TR: *Patient-Centered Medicine: Transforming the Clinical Method.* London, Sage, 1995.

The most up-to-date discussion of the patient-centered method, particularly appropriate to primary care, is contained in this text authored by a group that has been studying this method for over 20 years. Chapters on learning patient-centered skills and researching the method conclude the text.

RECOMMENDED READINGS

PART II

Foundations of Clinical Expertise

The successful patient-centered physician must develop all of the diagnostic, treatment, and technical skills that are the purview of the biomedical physician. Basic clinical skills are described in chapters in this part from a patient-centered approach, including interviewing, physical examination, ordering laboratory tests, making a diagnosis, instituting treatment, and keeping records.

CHAPTER 2

Interviewing as Clinical Conversation

Kathleen A. Zoppi

Mrs. Dinah Washburn is a 42-year-old woman who has come to the office for the first time. She is experiencing severe abdominal pain, looks pale, and is sweating profusely. Alice, the fourth-year student on a family medicine rotation, is assigned to take her history and to complete a physical examination. She enters the room and begins the interview:

ALICE: *Hi, Mrs. Washburn. I'm Alice Tidwell, a fourth-year medical student, and I'll be taking care of you today.*

MRS. WASHBURN: *Hi. I really feel bad.*

ALICE: *I can see that you're in pain. Is there anything I can do to help you be more comfortable while I talk with you and examine you? I need to find out some basic information before we can give you any medication to help the pain.*

MRS. WASHBURN: *Yeah, if I curl up with a pillow against my stomach it helps a little.*

ALICE: *Then let me get a pillow for you before we begin . . .*

———— EDUCATIONAL OBJECTIVES ————

At the end of this chapter, the student will be able to:

1. Describe the purposes of clinical conversations

2. List the components of communication that can be observed during the interview, including nonverbal cues, topic offerings, follow-ups, and types of responses
3. Describe ways of observing and altering the process of the interview to improve communication with patients
4. Elicit the basic components of the medical history from patients
5. Describe the similarities and differences between a clinical conversation and social conversation
6. Describe a patient-centered approach to interviewing

INTRODUCTION

No skill is more crucial to physician effectiveness than the ability to interview patients. The medical interview has been described as the "cornerstone of the diagnostic process" (Stillman, 1987). In Case 2-1, it is clear that in the first few seconds of interaction, Alice has both gathered important information about the patient's symptoms and created rapport with a patient who is in great pain. These opening interview skills are important, as they facilitate the acquisition of more information later in the interview. Furthermore, Balint (1964) has referred to the physician as a "drug," indicating the therapeutic value of allowing the patients to express fully the problems that are troubling to them and that may or may not be related to the disease. For each patient, the process used to elicit information, arrive at a diagnosis, negotiate treatment, or plan the next visit may be a little different, but knowledge of some common principles about communication with patients will help the physician to effectively interact with each patient.

The quality of the physician–patient interaction also has important consequences for both the clinician and the patient. Physicians who enjoy their interactions with patients are more likely to listen well and to feel more satisfied with their practices (Suchman *et al.,* 1993; Mechanic, 1992). Patients who feel they were able to communicate their problems are more likely to show improvement in symptoms (Headache Study Group of the University of Western Ontario, 1986; Greenfield *et al.,* 1985), are more likely to return to the same physician (Hansson *et al.,* 1988), and are less likely to sue (Lester & Smith, 1993). There may be physiological benefits to satisfying interviews for both patients and physicians as well, including lowered blood pressure and heart rate (Lynch, 1985). In addition, patients who communicate effectively with physicians about the nature of the problem and the treatment are more likely to follow a treatment plan (Ley, 1988), which will presumably improve their health and functioning.

So what makes an interview good? Dr. Gayle Stephens (1994) referred to a good interview as a "clinical conversation," where the goals are to focus on the patient's needs, to improve the patient's health, and to enable the physician to serve as a health consultant to the patient. Physicians and patients probably have different ideas about what makes a "good" interview: Physicians want to get enough information from the patient to accurately understand the patient's illness; patients want to understand why they are ill, whether their illnesses will go away or become worse, and what they can do about their problems. Physicians want to understand the nature of symptoms and the disease that causes them; patients want to understand their illness and suffering, and why it has happened to them. These differences may set up diverging goals for the interview that can cause competition between the patient's and physician's agenda. Part of a good interview is accomplishing a reasonable joint agenda in the amount of time available for the visit.

43

INTRODUCTION

COMPARISON BETWEEN SOCIAL CONVERSATIONS AND CLINICAL CONVERSATIONS

An important step in having good interaction with patients is keeping a clear understanding about the similarities and differences between clinical and social conversations. *Social conversations* are cooperative ventures, characterized by mutual control and reciprocity. Social conversations can range among many topics and can include many emotions. Both participants expect to disclose information about themselves, and each is expected to display interest and regard for the other's disclosures. The purpose of the social conversation is to enhance a relationship, to make a decision, to engage in a ritual, or to end or close a relationship. Participants in conversation usually ask questions of each other in about equal proportions, they each speak and listen about half the time, and they usually match each other in amount of disclosure, rate of speech, and nonverbal behavior (Cappella, 1994).

Similarly, physicians and patients in *clinical conversations* exert mutual control over the interview and respond to each other's bids and cues. They also may match each other's nonverbal behaviors, such as posture, gesture, rate of speech, volume, and intonation—often unconsciously. However, in contrast to social conversations, there is marked inequity in clinical conversations in terms of who talks and who listens, who discloses personal information, who asks questions, and who raises and closes topics. In clinical conversations, while many of the same cooperative principles apply, it is important to note that the focus of the conversation is on the patient's problem, illness, or concern; the goal of the interaction is to arrive at some resolution of the concern, or a plan to treat it; the physician does not disclose as much as the patient and is more likely to talk longer and to ask more questions than the patient. These differences, in addition to the patient's potential physical and psychological dependence on the physician for technical advice and understanding because of illness, fear, or incapacity, are what distinguish clinical conversations from social conversations.

CASE 2-2

Tom, a third-year medical student, is in the ambulatory clinic. It is his first day of seeing patients. He picks up the chart from the door, on which the nurse has written that the patient is there because of a "sore throat." The data sheet indicates that the patient is a 19-year-old male college student. His temperature and blood pressure are normal. Tom knocks on the door and enters the room.

DOCTOR: *(Standing) Hello, Matthew.*
PATIENT: *(Seated on examination table) Hi.*
DOCTOR: *(Still standing) I see you have a sore throat today. How long have you had it?*
PATIENT: *A few days.*
DOCTOR: *Have you had a fever or chills?*
PATIENT: *(Not making eye contact) No.*

DOCTOR: *Any drainage in the back of your throat?*
PATIENT: *No.*
DOCTOR: *You haven't been coughing then?*
PATIENT: *(Squirming on the table) No.*
DOCTOR: *(Reaching for a tongue depressor) Let's take a look then. . . .*
Elapsed time = 17.78 seconds

——— FUNDAMENTAL INTERVIEW SKILLS ———

HOW THE INTERVIEW SHOULD BE STARTED

In our culture, greetings and introductions are ritualized exchanges: People say hello and introduce themselves, usually shaking hands and gauging their physical distance prior to sitting down and beginning to talk about anything more important. Physicians can and should use many of the same social rituals in an encounter with a patient to help set a comfortable pace and tone to the conversation. In most nonemergent situations, clinical conversations are similar to social conversations. The clinician would greet the patient, introduce herself, and invite the patient to sit comfortably while speaking. The provider might also begin a brief social conversation, for example, about the weather, or sport, or some current event, prior to the real "medical business" at hand. When no social exchange occurs, interviews can get off to a difficult start, as in Case 2-2.

Instead, ideally, an interviewer would acknowledge the patient's identified reason for the visit (the sore throat), but would seek to establish a relationship early in the visit and would allow the patient to identify any other concerns early in the conversation. Both the patient and physician would make themselves comfortable, both socially and physically, before beginning the business of the encounter. Notice the differences between the previous interaction and the following:

DOCTOR: Hello, I'm Tom, a third-year medical student working with Dr. Smith today. What do you prefer to be called?
PATIENT: (Seated in chair) My name is Matthew, but I like to be called Matt.
DOCTOR: (Extends hand for a handshake) Nice to meet you, Matt.
PATIENT: (Shakes hand makes eye contact) Nice to meet you, too.
DOCTOR: (Sitting on stool and placing chart on desk) What would you like to tell me about yourself?
PATIENT: Well, I'm here because I've got a big basketball game this Friday night, and my coach is worried I won't be able to play. I've been pretty tired and run-down for a couple of weeks, and now I've got a bad sore throat. I'm a starter, and this is the last game before the playoffs, and I'm really worried I won't be able to play the whole game.
Elapsed time = 31.97 seconds

What differences exist between the initial parts of these two interviews? The initial part of the second interview, which lasted about 10 seconds longer than the first, helped Tom know what the patient prefers to be called, that he's pretty concerned about being ill and potentially missing a game, that he's been sick for a few weeks, and that he only recently developed a sore throat. In comparing the two approaches to the interview with Matt, also notice that there are a number of directions each interviewer could proceed after the initial part. With the additional information acquired in the second interview, the physician might think about anemia, infectious mononucleosis, HIV infection, or cardio-myopathies, rather than centering on the more common cause of sore throat in teenagers, viral pharyngitis and "strep throat."

HOW TO HEAR WHAT THE PATIENT SAYS AND LISTEN TO THE MEANING

In the two versions of the interview in Case 2-2, the difference between hearing and perceptive listening is obvious. The first interviewer physically heard the patient's complaint. He has a sore throat. But did Tom know why Matt was there? What was his actual reason for coming? Do healthy people usually go to a physician after having a sore throat for a few days? Why did he come today, rather than yesterday or tomorrow? Was it just the first time he could get an appointment? Why does Matt's reason for being there matter? Does it affect the treatment plan or recommendations?

In the second version of the interview, it is clear that Matt's concern is not just about having a sore throat, but about how it might affect his ability to play in an important basketball game. He is also quite concerned about his stamina, and his coach is worried, too. It is possible that an interviewer could ask a number of questions that would help uncover these concerns, including "Who else is worried about your illness?" and "Are you having any other problems or symptoms?," but the simple act of listening and not interrupting the patient early in the interview results in more data about the problem, with less additional work on the part of the interviewer.

In fact, an interview style that assumes that patients have concerns beyond the chief complaint, sometimes not related directly to symptoms, has been termed a *patient-centered approach* (see Chapter 1 on the systemic patient-centered approach). This kind of approach relies on several key behaviors: The physician facilitates the early and complete expression of the patient's problem, uses cues and clues from the patient's behavior to identify other concerns or expressions of feeling about the problem, and asks the patient for preferences regarding follow-up or treatment.

Good perceptive listening by the physician is one of the most elusive and sought-after skills, and is possibly the best psychotherapeutic tool in a physician's repertoire. But true listening, without interruption, is a rare occurrence in the first few minutes of the interview. A study of 74 visits to an internal medicine clinic demonstrated that in 69% of visits, physicians interrupted patients after the mention of only one concern, within an average time to interruption of 18 seconds. In instances when patients were allowed to complete their thoughts, the average time they spoke was about 1.5 minutes (Beckman & Frankel, 1984).

It is often difficult to listen if patients seem confused, vague, or unnecessarily descriptive in their use of language. The interviewer may feel confused, bored, impatient, or angry. *It is important to remember that the emotional reactions of the clinician during the interview may be as important a cue about the patient as what is said.* Often, what the physician feels while listening perceptively is similar to the unspoken feelings of the patient. If the physician feels sad, it may be that the patient also feels sad. One of the great advantages of having clinical conversations while a medical student is that a student is often better at listening than is a physician later in training. Patients will often share important information with students they will not tell their physicians, simply because the student is a better listener.

HOW TO DEFINE THE MEDICAL STUDENT'S ROLE

One of the most difficult aspects of interviewing patients during medical school is the ambiguous role the student has in delivering care. While a medical student is part of a healthcare team, her role is also that of a learner. The team may value input about the patient and may include what is told to them by the student in her notes and treatment plan. Unfortunately, medical student input is often not asked for or disregarded if it is offered. A student may, as indicated earlier, hear information from the patient or the family that others do not know and that is important to the patient's treatment. Students may witness treatment of patients that they perceive to be inappropriate or insensitive. And during all of these interactions, the student may be treated by the patient as the person who is responsible for the treatment plan, while the student feels she is still a learner, trying to integrate a great deal of information into organized clinical skills.

Patients may address the student as "Doctor," or conversely, may say the student is too young to know how to help them. Each of these challenges needs to be faced by students participating in patient care. It is important to follow guidelines in your treatment of patients. Students should always identify themselves truthfully as medical students when they begin to talk with patients. If the student is practicing interviewing and is not having a clinical conversation as part of the patient's team, that should be stated explicitly. If a patient asks a student not to tell his physician something, the student should identify herself as obligated to talk with the physician about it, but encourage the patient to tell the physician on his own. The student may also ask the attending physician or resident how he wishes to be informed of what was learned from the patient. It is often the case that the student may learn crucial information, and the patient may benefit from its inclusion in the treatment plan.

CASE 2-3

Nancy, a second-year student, is on rounds with the family practice attending physician and a resident. The team is seeing Nellie Hatter, a 65-year-old woman who is lying across her bed at an angle when you enter he room. She greets the team "Hello, doctors!" and is smiling. Nancy's attending physician begins to ask her how she slept, and whether she is comfortable.

DOCTOR: *Did you have a good night last night?*

PATIENT: *Yes, I slept just fine. I feel much better than last night.*

DOCTOR: *You were in bad shape when you came in. Your blood sugar was over 600 when we saw you in the emergency room. Why do you think that happened?*

PATIENT: *I don't know. My husband gives me my medication every morning before I eat. I'm sure I had it yesterday. Maybe it's due to stress . . .*

In interviewing this patient, how is it decided what to ask next? Questions could be asked about the patient's insulin dosage, and how her husband remembers to give her the shot:

DOCTOR: Could be. Does your husband give you the shot at the same time every morning?

This line of questioning would help determine if the patient is receiving her medication. These questions might also yield some information about their relationship, about the husband's memory, and about her dependence on him for her care. The provider could also pick up her lead about what she thinks caused her blood sugar to be high:

DOCTOR: Stress? Why do you think this could be due to stress?

This question might cause the patient to think her "theory" about stress was subject to scrutiny, and not valid. A similar, yet simpler, approach to following the patient's lead would be:

DOCTOR: Stress? Tell me more about your stress.
PATIENT: Well, yesterday, my son and daughter-in-law and I had some words . . . they live in the downstairs of our house. She's a nurse, a Filipino, and she and my son moved in last year when he lost his job in California. I'm a Jehovah's Witness, and don't like her drinking and smoking.

Simple repetition of the patient's last words can often be an encouraging response to help the patient continue with a particular train of thought. In this case, following the patient's lead resulted in a clearer understanding of what the patient believed affected her blood sugar, as well as some potential resources or impediments to her follow-up care after discharge from the hospital. This information did not directly exclude other causes of her high blood sugar, e.g., infection or a skipped dose of insulin, but did give additional information not available through the first approach of questioning.

HOW A PHYSICIAN SHOULD RESPOND TO PATIENTS' EXPRESSIONS OF FEELINGS

In Case 2-3, the patient gave a clue that she was concerned about the effects of stress on her health. Though she did not appear upset—she was smiling and said she rested well—she did offer what she was thinking on why she had become ill. A wise conversationalist, whether in a social or clinical interaction, will attend to the other person's last remark before changing the subject. For this patient, her worries about her family may have contributed to her physical illness and admission, and may even seem more troubling to her than her hospitalization.

Patients often do not express their feelings directly, even when they are quite distressed. It is important to notice what patients do not say, as well as what they do say. In Case 2-2, when Tom talked with Matt, he might have noticed that Matt looked flushed and avoided eye contact when asked what was wrong. As he reached for a tongue depressor, Tom might have even tried to have some cheery conversation about the local professional team's latest basketball win, and might have noticed that Matt seemed withdrawn or sullen. It is sometimes a useful strategy to observe nonverbal cues or facial expressions and to comment on them directly:

TOM: I notice that you aren't talking too much and that you look uncomfortable when I ask you questions . . .

Sometimes such direct observation or reflection can help the patient identify feelings and trust that the physician is willing to hear more about what is of concern. Occasionally, patients will surprise physicians with strong feelings or expressions about their illnesses, their families, or other physicians. It may take the provider aback to have such an intimate or powerful statement made when questions have barely been asked of the patient at all. And yet, the powerful role of the physician/healer can evoke strong confidences. Sometimes just listening to a patient's expression about her worries, without intervening, and without judging, can be more difficult than "doing," and infinitely more valuable to the patient.

HOW TIMING AND PACING CAN BE GAUGED

Medical lore places a value on quick, efficient, concise interviews that lead to an accurate diagnosis. However, few of *your* conversations with patients feel quick and efficient. One of the important arts of the interview involves the rhythm of the interview, the timing and pacing of the patient's speech, the pauses and silences, the changes of topic, the nonverbal communication, the physical examination, the social conversation, and the farewells. The physician often inadvertently matches the natural rate of speech and movement of the patient, and sometimes wishes the patient would slow down or speed up. It is clear that people in ordinary conversations match their speech and movements to each other more and more as the conversation progresses, but it is often useful to deliberately pay attention to, and try not to match the patient's rate of speech, gestures, or movements. If a patient seems anxious, it may be useful to slow down and see if this also slows the patient's speech. If it does not affect the patient, this failure to change may be useful diagnostic information. If a patient seems very sad, speaking slowly and painfully quietly, it may be inappropriate to overcompensate by smiling, telling jokes, and talking quickly, but it may be useful to change the rate and tone to see if the patient's affect changes when talking about something happy or enjoyable.

It is critical as an interviewer to become familiar with, and aware of, one's own predisposition as a speaker. A provider from a family of fast-talking, interrupting, simultaneous speakers may overwhelm patients whose natural speech patterns require that they wait several seconds after the physician is done speaking before beginning to speak themselves. No one speech pattern is necessarily better or worse than others, but awareness of when style is a catalyst and when it is a barrier to good interaction is integral to the development of a clinical conversationalist.

WHAT TO DO NEXT

One of the hardest developmental tasks of the clinical conversationalist is to structure the interaction, maybe by using a checklist of questions (such as a review of systems checklist) while trying to maintain a normal conversational flow and paying attention to the patient's cues. It is normal to feel torn between these two tasks, and there is no easy solution to the dilemma. The useful principle to remember is equifinality: There are many ways to get there from here! Studies of medical interviewing have shown that highly focused short interviews can be just as effective in gathering information and creating patient well-being as longer, more rambling interviews. The key principles for effective interviews that collect pertinent information and satisfy concerned patients are: they allow patients time to express their worries, fears, or needs; they seem relaxed and unhurried, even if they are not actually very long; they enable patients to express, either verbally or nonverbally, some emotions; they enable physicians to respond to the emotions expressed by patients; they enable patients to leave the interview knowing more about what's wrong and what to do about it than at the start. In addition to gathering sufficient information about the present illness and past medical history, these are the key ingredients to a good clinical conversation. Each patient's clinical presentation will dictate whether asking a few questions and moving to a physical examination, or talking for a while and rescheduling the physical, is the better approach.

HOW THE PHYSICAL EXAMINATION IS NAVIGATED

The physical examination, and the ritual laying on of hands, is one of the primary defining features that distinguishes the clinical conversation from other professional encounters. Touch, outside of a handshake or a shoulder pat on closing, is unlikely to occur with a minister, lawyer, or accountant, whereas touching by the physician of the patient during an examination is an integral part of the visit. Apart from the diagnostic acumen required to distinguish among heart and lung sounds or to palpate and feel physical changes in organs and muscles, the physical examination is a socially challenging experience for both patient and physician. It is useful to make some social gesture to establish contact, such as a handshake, prior to the nonreciprocated touch of the physical examination. It may also be useful for the physician to assist the patient in being seated and getting comfortable for the physical examination, if the patient is elderly or needs such help. The physical examination should be described and prefaced for the patient, not just done to the patient. This might involve the physician saying, "And now I'm going to listen to your heart and lungs . . . ." And physical findings should be described to the patient, who otherwise may misinterpret a squint and silence as cues that something in the breath sounds is horribly wrong. "Your heart and breathing sound perfectly normal." Such feedback is probably better than attempting to distract the patient with social small talk, especially if the patient is anxious. During the physical examination it may be a good time to ask further questions related to the area of the examination, however, since patients may more easily recall symptoms when being touched (e.g., while palpating the abdomen, asking "So you said you have this pain every morning?"). The physical examination should be focused on the systems/regions related to the patient's concerns, unless a full history and physical is being completed (see Chapter 3 on the physical examination).

HOW THE AGENDA CAN BE BETTER MANAGED

Patients often come to the physician with many concerns, which may not be of equal importance. A patient who is concerned about his teenaged daughter, his earache, and the pain in his chest might prioritize what he wants to discuss differently than the physician. He may spend time initially discussing his daughter, whereas the physician may want to focus initially on the chest pain as the most ominous symptom. In this case, a useful skill to practice is the overt identification of priorities. The physician may wish to state clearly that there is a limited amount of time, e.g., 20 minutes, and her desire to know the patient's greatest concern. Planning for a return visit within a short period of time to finish what could not be completed today may be important, as may agreeing with the patient about what can be postponed. This kind of negotiation over the agenda is similar to the negotiation of a plan, discussed in Chapter 11, but may initially seem more difficult because it requires stepping back from the interaction to notice what needs to be discussed.

WHY DISCUSSING THE DIAGNOSIS IS IMPORTANT

Once the physical examination is completed and the history is taken, the physician may recognize the need for more data to confirm her thinking. This may require that some lab test be performed, which may be as simple as a blood test, or may be more extensive and invasive testing. While being uncertain about a diagnosis and gathering more evidence may be routine work for the physician-scientist, such uncertainty may contribute greatly to the patient's anxiety. Tests and procedures are seldom routine for patients, and each one may require a different amount of explanation. It may, for example, be common for patients to have their blood drawn, but to have an MRI or a CT scan can be very frightening. It is important for the physician to help prepare the patient for what she can expect from the experience so the patient will come to the test or procedure less anxious and more cooperative. It is also useful to explain to patients what data the tests may offer, and how the results will contribute to the physician's thinking about what is wrong, and when it may be possible to make a diagnosis about the patient's condition.

CASE 2-4

Kathy is a first-year family practice resident. Her patient, Albert Fuller, is ready to go home from the hospital. He is a 66-year-old male who was admitted for treatment of blood clots in his left leg. Kathy's chief resident planned to send him home on anticoagulants, with a home health nurse scheduled to draw blood weekly to check his clotting. The chief resident just received a page from the social worker, saying Mr. Fuller has refused to take his prescription, and he doesn't want a nurse visiting him at home. The resident asks Kathy to go to the floor to find out what the problem is.

HOW A TREATMENT PLAN SHOULD BE DISCUSSED

Construction of a treatment plan and negotiating that plan with patients will be discussed in detail in Chapters 6 and 11, respectively, but in Case 2-4, it would be useful to know a few pieces of information. It would be helpful to know from Mr. Fuller what he thought was wrong with him, and how he thought it might best be treated. If he thinks that his leg was swollen because he bumped it, and it's better now, he won't be likely to accept a long-term treatment plan. It would also be useful to know when and how the resident discussed the plan for discharge with Mr. Fuller, and with any relevant family or friends. Asking Mr. Fuller what his understanding was of what was to happen after he left the hospital and what he or others thought about the plan may also help. Verifying Mr. Fuller's understanding and correcting any misunderstandings are always useful. If, in fact, he disagrees with the resident's plan, it is possible to start negotiating knowing what Mr.

Fuller has in mind, and by listening carefully to him, Kathy may be able in Case 2-4 to negotiate a plan that meets both Mr. Fuller's health needs and his provider's concerns.

51

**FUNDAMENTAL
INTERVIEW SKILLS**

HOW THE INTERVIEW SHOULD BE CLOSED
PLANNING FOR THE NEXT VISIT

Most interviews will end naturally with the physician and patient finalizing plans for follow-up and treatment. Ask the patient to review, either by repetition or by acknowledgment, the plans for medications, tests, follow-up visits, or treatments. Ask the patient if there are questions or unfinished business before beginning to stand up, closing the chart, or saying good-bye. It is not uncommon for patients to present "doorknob" agendas: When the physician's hand is on the doorknob, ready to exit, patients may have one or more important unresolved concerns that they want to discuss. This pattern can best be averted by asking patients early in the visit about any other concerns, prior to setting the agenda for the day's visit; sometimes even this careful checking will not prevent a last-minute concern. "Doorknob" concerns may be important enough to warrant reopening the discussion, such as with a patient who says she's had trouble breathing the past few days. On the other hand, it may be possible to discuss the problem at an upcoming visit. If the problem can be postponed until the next visit, it is still important for the clinician to acknowledge the patient's concern, while not completely resolving it.

Say good-bye to patients in a way that allows them to return with a sense that the conversation has been important. Assure them of how they can contact you in case of emergency, and touch or shake hands prior to departing. Consider taking a few minutes prior to leaving the room to complete any chart notes or forms.

CASE 2-5

Mrs. Thomas is a new patient to the family practice center. She is a 64-year-old woman who greets the medical student cheerfully as she enters the room. Her chart indicates she is here for a blood pressure check.

MRS. THOMAS:	*Hello, Doctor.*
KARLA JONES:	*Hello, is it Mrs. Thomas?*
MRS. THOMAS:	*Yes, dear, That's fine.*
KARLA JONES:	*How are you feeling?*
MRS. THOMAS:	*Well, fine, although a little tired the last few weeks.*
KARLA JONES:	*Tell me more about feeling tired . . .*
MRS. THOMAS:	*Well, I was here 3 months ago, but since then I've been more tired during the day than before. I think it's my medication.*
KARLA JONES:	*I notice you're on medication for your high blood pressure. Are you on any other medications?*
MRS. THOMAS:	*No. That's all.*
KARLA JONES:	*And tell me about how you're taking your medication each day.*
MRS. THOMAS:	*I was supposed to take a whole pill at night and a half in the morning, but the mornings I often skip or I feel too tired.*

KARLA JONES: *Well, let's check your pressure today and then we'll talk about your medications. Have you been taking your pressure at home?*

MRS. THOMAS: *Yes, and it's been fine.*

KARLA JONES: *Good. Let me take your pressure and listen to your heart today.*

THE MEDICAL HISTORY

The skills used to conduct a clinical conversation with a patient have another purpose: They help the physician to create a clear picture of the patient's illness and the data that support a diagnosis and treatment plan. Notice that the interview, or clinical conversation, is not the same thing as the history. The history is a construction based on the interview, the physical examination, and the observations of the physician. A medical history may be very thorough and comprehensive, or it may be focused on a particular concern of the patient. Medical histories have a structure and sequence, mostly to help keep data well organized and in a familiar pattern (see Chapter 7 on presentation and record keeping). Often, it is of great concern to learners to know what questions to ask and how to ask them in the course of the interview. There are no perfect ways to ask questions of each and every patient, but a few guidelines can apply: The physician should attempt to avoid leading or loaded questions whenever possible (such as: "You don't drink alcohol, do you?" or "How often do you beat your son?"). It may be occasionally useful to ask very focused questions as a way of clarifying information already gathered, but highly structured questions should be reserved until more general questions have been asked. In other words, when gathering information, the physician should attempt to phrase questions in a neutral and nondirective manner.

The medical history begins with the sociodemographic data of the patient and the chief concern (CC) (sometimes called the chief complaint, although not all patients complain). It is often useful to describe the CC using the patient's exact words, which may give clues about what the patient thinks is wrong and what he expects will be done. Next is the history of the present illness (HPI), which elaborates on the presenting symptoms of the patient, including the chronology, duration, alleviation/exacerbation, and temporal course of the symptoms. The patient's own words, which were used in the CC, now are augmented by the physician's assessment of the data, including observations about the patient's appearance, affect, or symptoms. Thus, a patient with a CC of burning in his chest may also be described in the HPI as: ". . . having had this burning sensation for 3 days; after each meal; lasting about 2 hours; unrelieved by antacids, changes in position, or activity. The patient described having this pain during the interview, and appeared to be in acute distress, sweating profusely during this time. While the patient did not report left arm pain in our initial discussion, when asked, he indicated his left arm hurt as we talked."

The past medical and surgical history (PMH) is a thorough identification of major health-related events the patient may have experienced prior to this illness. It should include previous hospitalizations; pregnancies and childbirth; chronic illnesses, including diabetes mellitus; cardiovascular disease (heart attack, heart failure, murmurs, angina); hypertension; pneumonia; tuberculosis; asthma; emphysema; ulcers; liver problems; hepatitis; bladder or kidney problems; arthritis; gout; cancer; thyroid problems; seizures; emotional or psychological problems; suicide attempts; sexually transmitted diseases; and so on. The PMH includes any operations for any of these conditions. It is important to know the dates and places of such surgeries and any additional complications the patient experienced at that time. The PMH is more general than other parts of the history, although it may be focused in relation to the CC. It is also usually useful to have a sense from the patient about the breadth and depth of previous experiences with medical providers.

The next part of the history includes history about the patient's habits. Some authors include this under the rubric of the social history, but the social history properly refers to the patient's interpersonal and familial relationships. The *habits* history should include information about the patient's use of medications (including nonprescription drugs and vitamins) and nonpharmacological remedies (e.g., herbal remedies, acupuncture); use of alcohol, nicotine, and other recreational and injectable drugs; travel; work, especially work conditions and exposures; hobbies; sleep habits; dietary habits; health habits, including examinations and immunizations; use of seat belts, smoke detectors, and bicycle or motorcycle helmets; exercise habits; and sexual practices. Each of these areas is important to assessing risks related to the CC and, more broadly, to helping understand the patient's health practices and behaviors. Not all of these areas will likely be examined in a short, problem-focused visit but all should be part of the physician's model of thinking as a history is developed.

The social history (SH) describes the patient's relationships with significant others, including family, members of the household, friends, work, and community. During a clinical conversation, the social history allows the physician to gain a picture of the patient in the context of her life. It can help the physician to understand how the patient thinks, what she values, and who is likely to be involved in her health-related behaviors, either for better or worse! Since patients with social support fare better than matched controls without the same support in studies, a social history may be more than a way to become acquainted with patients. It may also be a way to help predict and intervene in their care (Spiegel, 1993; Ornish, 1992).

It is useful to preface the habits and social histories with a brief explanation, indicating that these are routine questions asked of all patients to get to know them and their circumstances better. Even more effective is the art of weaving questions in while listening to how the patient describes her life; for example, when a patient says ". . . and my husband thought I wasn't sleeping as well . . ." it may be easy and smooth for the physician to respond: "Tell me more about your husband and his concerns about your sleep. . . ." If questions related to the social history must be introduced later in the interview, it is often useful to begin with a global question ("Tell me about where you live") followed by more specific questions that require a detailed answer ("And who lives with you? How do they get along with each other?"). If using a patient-centered approach, noticing and following up on cues from the patient may help the physician understand what is meaningful and important to the patient as she thinks about her illness: A patient who says she was most upset about being ill and missing her church prayer group has told you several things about herself, including the timing of her symptoms. A patient whose concern is that you rule out a heart attack before the next day because he can't miss a meeting at work has also told you important data. During the social history, it is possible to follow up on cues about work and community activities, asking (for example): "You mentioned a big meeting at work. Can you tell me more about it? Why is it important that you are there?"

The family history (FH) is where the clinician asks specific questions related to disease patterns and illness experiences among other members of the family. Questions about parents' health, illness, or death and the incidence of diseases such as diabetes mellitus, cancer, heart disease, hypertension, mental illness, chemical dependency, or other problems pertinent to the patient's own CC should be asked. Patients may find it difficult to identify all members of the family and their health problems, but a follow-up question asking if conditions run in the family can be useful in clarifying both family patterns and patient concerns about symptoms.

The review of systems (ROS) is the most focused segment of an interview, and usually requires some forethought about the differential diagnosis so that it does not degenerate into an interrogation of the patient by the physician. A complete review of systems asks specific, focused questions about each organ system; these questions should not be too focused on the CC, but rather should be a "net" to catch any unusual or unexpected findings. A complete discussion of the ROS is found in texts by DeGowin and DeGowin (1995) and Billings and Stoeckle (1993).

A good way to preview the ROS for the patient is to explain, "Now I'm going to ask you a series of questions, beginning with the top of your head and going to your toes . . ." or to explain to a patient, "Now I'm going to ask you a series of questions to check some other areas you haven't mentioned. Let's start with your vision." These previews enable the patient to relax a bit, instead of trying to perceive the reason for a seeming barrage of questions unrelated to the reason for the visit. This approach may also help patients to prepare mentally to respond to a list of questions. Care should be given to avoiding the tendency to lapse into fed questions (e.g., "No trouble eating or swallowing?"), which may seem faster to ask but actually presume the patient's response. A list of ROS categories is given in Table 2.1.

All of these questions may be asked in an ROS. In most cases, a positive response will lead to additional, more specific questions about that system. As a physician becomes more experienced, she may restrict the number of questions in the ROS to a more focused group; initially, the student will likely ask an exhaustive list of questions. Be sure the patient is comfortable before beginning the list!

Table 2.1
Review of Systems Categories

Have there been *changes* in:	Type of change
Visual	Disturbances; spots; flashes
Ears	Hearing; ringing of the ears
Chest	Heart troubles; irregular or rapid beating
Bones and joints	Pain; cramping; swelling
Breathing	Pain; shortness of breath; activity; positional; coughing up blood
Digestion	Bowel function; upset stomach; stools; vomiting; bleeding; urination (increased or decreased frequency); incontinence
Head	Trauma; headaches; dizziness; vertigo; syncope; nose; mouth; throat problems (hoarseness, swallowing, pain, swelling)
Motor/memory	Weakness or paralysis; difficulty moving; walking; balancing; difficulty with memory; speaking; mood; enjoyment of life
General health	Sleep patterns; energy; appetite; weight; fevers; chills; skin condition; itching; bruising; bleeding; healing; heat or cold intolerance; excessive thirst
Sexual/urinary/gynecological	Vaginal/penile discharge; pain; masses; menstruation; breast tenderness or discharge; sexual activity; sexual functioning

CONCLUSION

This chapter described the important behaviors of interviewers who are engaging in a clinical conversations with patients. Key behaviors were reviewed, including greeting the patient, attending to the patient's comfort, attending to the patient's chief concern, completing the parts of the medical history and physical examination, and closing the interview. The importance of a patient-centered approach, attending to the patient's words, affect, and nonverbal cues, was stressed.

The medical visit, which includes the patient's presentation of chief concern, the history of the present illness, past medical history, review of symptoms, physical examination, and the negotiation of a treatment plan, was discussed. The importance of key components of the physician–patient relationship such as empathy, responsiveness to feelings, shared control, and timing and pacing was also reviewed. Social and clinical conversations were contrasted.

Students will find it useful to review the concepts in this chapter as they prepare to work with patients, and before each new interview. Research on the development of interviewing skills indicates that, like any physical examination skills, they require rehearsal and practice. Practice may involve role-playing or interviewing with friends or, better still, taping (either audio or video) encounters with actual patients and reviewing those tapes to observe what you do well and what might need improvement.

CASES FOR DISCUSSION

CASE 1

A patient comes to the family practice center. The nurse has written on the chart note that she is there for a sinus infection. You enter the room, seeing a well-dressed woman in a suit. You greet her, introduce yourself, and ask her how she is. She begins to cry.

1. *What could you do or say next?*
2. *If the physician says, "What's wrong?" and the patient responds, "Never mind. I'm here for sore throat," how should the physician proceed?*
3. *Should the physician proceed to ask the patient about her sinus symptoms?*

CASE 2

You are running late in your afternoon on the ward, and you receive a new admission. Your resident tells you to interview the patient; you begin to go to the room. Before you get there, the nurse for the unit grabs your sleeve, rolls his eyes, and says, "This one is a real doozy. You have no idea what a problem he will be. He's already made two of the nursing students angry."

1. *What would be the best strategy for beginning this clinical conversation?*
2. *Why should you be especially aware of any feelings you experience on talking to the patient?*

3. *Assuming this patient talks rapidly and loudly, why would you want to use a matching style? a complementary style?*

CASE 3

You are a medical student on the family medicine service. You enter a room to take a history of a patient who was just admitted. He is lying in bed, with his gown high above his waist, no underwear on, and no covers.

1. *What do you say first?*
2. *How would your **clinical conversation** differ from **social conversation** under some circumstances?*
3. *How could you let the patient know, without shaming or embarrassing him, that you need him to respect you during the interview?*

CASE 4

You are in the clinic and your next patient is a 13-year-old boy who is accompanied by his mother. The reason for the visit is the boy has been having trouble sleeping. When you ask him why, he explains that he often wakes in the middle of the night and screams, sweating and flushed. Usually, his parents come to get him, and he sleeps the rest of the night with them. His mother reports that this has been happening more frequently lately, especially since she was told she needed surgery on her shoulder.

1. *What do you ask next in order to understand what is happening to this boy?*
2. *Given that a 13-year-old boy is not the world's best conversationalist, under what conditions would you want to interrupt him? let him talk?*
3. *How would you prepare the boy (and mother) for physical examination behavior during this encounter?*

CASE 5

You are in the family practice center, and interviewing a new patient. She is a 35-year-old woman who is a mother of three. She seems happy and relaxed as you talk but when you begin to ask her about her marriage, she avoids eye contact and gives shorter answers.

1. *What reasons might a patient begin to change her demeanor?*
2. *How might you reflect to your patient your observation that her affect and eye contact changed?*
3. *The patient responds to your conversation by saying, "I'm fine. My marriage is fine." What hypotheses might you hold in mind for future visits?*

──────────── RECOMMENDED READINGS ────────────

Balint M: *The Doctor, His Patient, and the Illness.* New York, International Universities Press Inc, 1964.

Balint was a British psychoanalyst who worked with general practitioners on their feelings about their patients. In this classic work, he describes the relationship between the patient and the physician as a potential source of healing, comparing the physician's style of interaction to a drug, implying that the interview style is just as therapeutic as the medication prescribed.

Billings JA, Stoeckle JD: *The Clinical Encounter*. Chicago, Year Book Medical Publishers Inc, 1989

This is one of the most comprehensive and thorough references on the medical interview. The chapter on "Eliciting Information for Diagnosis and Management" is a compendium of questions and approaches to the basic history and physical, and offers an excellent range of options for students and residents who desire examples.

Meador C: *A Little Book of Doctor's Rules*. Philadelphia, Hanley & Belfus, 1992.

A delightful compendium of aphorisms distilled from Dr. Meador's own clinical practice. He offers key rules for working with patients that are useful for students and experienced clinicians alike.

CHAPTER 3

Physical Examination

Diane L. Elliot and Linn Goldberg

CASE 3-1

Mrs. R. had delayed finding a new physician for almost a year. Finally, she could not refill her medications without a physician's prescription and made an appointment. She had heard good things about this individual, but a visit with a new physician made her anxious. She wondered what it would be like.

After escorting her into the examination room, the nurse asked her to put on a gown. She had been waiting for 20 minutes when the physician entered. Dr. B. was running late, as a noon business meeting had become bogged down in administrative decisions. There were no last-minute cancellations, and the afternoon schedule was full. It was now 3:30 PM, and Dr. B. was about 30 minutes behind. Pulling the chart off the rack in the office door, Dr. B. read that Mrs. R. was a new patient who had moved to this area about a year ago and now needed refills on her antihypertensive medicines. The nurse had recorded her blood pressure as 145/85 mm Hg.

The interaction between Mrs. R. and Dr. B. lasted about 15 minutes. Dr. B. reexamined her blood pressure, then auscultated her heart and lungs. Mrs. R. had not offered any specific complaints or concerns, and Dr. B. had her sign consents for release of information to obtain prior records, ordered some laboratory tests, refilled her medications, and scheduled her for a return appointment. Dr. B. anticipated that the history would be more focused after an opportunity to review old records and laboratory studies. Dr. B. wished that they could have spent more time establishing rapport and getting to know each other, but nothing seemed urgent.

Mrs. R. was glad that the visit was short. However, Dr. B. seemed so rushed that she felt uncomfortable raising her concerns. She had expected to have a checkup and a more thorough examination. Her former physician had done a "complete examination" every year. She wondered whether Dr. B. was someone she could trust in a crisis.

EDUCATIONAL OBJECTIVES

At the conclusion of this chapter, students will be able to:

1. List, describe, and provide a rationale for maneuvers performed during a "screening" physical examination
2. List unique aspects of examining children and how the physical examination process or findings might differ for a child's physical examination
3. Describe the limitations of physical assessment and methods to decrease examination unreliability
4. Describe how the physical examination affects the physician–patient relationship
5. Describe unique issues related to the breast, pelvic, and genitourinary examinations and relate means to minimize patient distress during these examinations

---
INTRODUCTION

The physical examination is a constant dimension of physician–patient interactions. Although medical knowledge and laboratory assessment are advancing rapidly, the techniques of inspection, percussion, auscultation, and palpation have not changed. Physical examination abilities are critical skills for assessing patients and are of lasting value. When surveyed, practicing physicians indicated that competence in the physical examination, medical interview, and problem definition ranked most important among a long list of clinical abilities (Kern *et al.*, 1985).

In this chapter, we present a rationale for learning a specific physical examination sequence and suggest the content and order for a "screening" examination. Assessment issues unique to pediatric patients are reviewed. In addition to detecting and defining illness, physical assessment also functions to meet patient expectations and enhance physician–patient rapport. We outline "therapeutic" functions of the examination and review components that require high physician sensitivity.

CASE 3-2

M. S. was beginning her third year of medical school. This was her first rotation on the inpatient service. Last year, she had practiced components of the physical examination in her weekly preceptor experience, but she was not sure what the resident had meant when he asked her to "do a complete H and P." She had hoped to watch the intern examine a patient before she had to do one.

Her preceptor, the physician whose office she'd visited weekly last year, rarely did a complete examination. In that ambulatory setting, the examiner focused on aspects relevant to the patient's complaints or maneuvers known to be useful in screening for illness. She had performed all of the examination components, but had not done a "complete" examination. She thought about her music lessons. It seemed like she had learned different passages but had not played the whole composition from beginning to end. She wanted to be able to play without sheet music, which translated into not requiring her physical diagnosis textbook while examining a patient.

Feeling awkward, she resolved that she would practice the complete sequence several times on her roommate before the next admitting day. She needed to memorize an examination sequence. Interpreting findings, deciding when to perform additional maneuvers, paying attention to the patient, and maintaining rapport gave her much to think about during the examination. She could not learn to improvise until she had mastered the basic "composition" of the physical examination.

61

BASIC
GUIDELINES FOR
THE SCREENING
PHYSICAL
EXAMINATION OF
ADULTS

WHY LEARN A PARTICULAR EXAMINATION SEQUENCE?

The physical examination's sequence is designed for efficiency and patient comfort. For example, beginning the examination with attention to a patient's hands and measuring vital signs permits continued eye contact and is less threatening than an initial examination of the eyes and ears. The examination's order progresses from "head to toe," and each anatomic area follows the pattern: inspection, percussion, auscultation, and palpation.

This progression permits using information in subsequent examination procedures. For example, percussing the liver's lower border is used to determine where to palpate for its edge; the eye examination begins with inspection of the external eye structures, followed by assessing visual acuity. Reduced acuity might lead to a more thorough definition of visual fields and additional time observing the optic disk, vessels, and background retina. Patient comfort and examination efficiency are assisted by minimizing position changes and clustering aspects performed with the patient in different positions (sitting, supine, and standing).

BASIC GUIDELINES FOR THE SCREENING PHYSICAL EXAMINATION OF ADULTS

The following is a suggested sequence for the well-patient "screening" physical examination. Maneuvers are outlined in Table 3.1. Although several physical examination texts provide detailed information on examination maneuvers (Bates *et al.,* 1995; Epstein *et al.,* 1992; Greenberger & Hinthorn, 1993; Judge *et al.,* 1989; Novey, 1988; Seidel *et al.,* 1991; Swartz, 1989; Willms *et al.,* 1994), most do not include recommendations for an expedient "screening examination." This probably reflects lack of any order's proven superiority. Suggested sequences, similar to items in Table 3.1, are included in compressed physical examination guides (Macklis *et al.,* 1994; Novey, 1988; Seymour, 1984).

The physical examination commences with the examiner washing her hands, which cleans and warms them. Patient contact begins by touching the patient's outstretched

Table 3.1

Suggested Physical Examination Sequence

Approach the seated patient to perform the following
  General inspection, state of nutrition, and apparent age
  Vital signs (pulse, blood pressure, respiratory rate)
  Inspection hands and fingernails
  Inspection scalp and face
  Inspection scleras and conjunctivas
  Visual acuity
  Pupil reaction to light (consensual and direct)
  Funduscopic examination
  Inspection external ears
  Otoscopic examination tympanic membranes
  Hearing
  Inspection nasal mucosa
  Inspection oropharyngeal mucosa
Move behind or beside the seated patient to perform the following
  Palpation anterior cervical and supraclavicular nodes
  Palpation thyroid gland
  Palpation each carotid artery
  Percussion spine and posterior lung fields
  Auscultation posterior lung fields
Ask the patient to recline supine and cover torso and legs with a drape. Ask the patient to pull up the gown
    so that the chest is exposed and perform the following
  Inspection breasts
  Palpation breasts and axillary nodes, with a woman's hands behind her head
  Inspection neck veins and estimation jugular venous pressure
  Palpation precordium
  Auscultation precordium
  Auscultation carotids
Patient remains supine, gown is lowered, and drape positioned to reveal the patient's abdomen
  Inspection abdomen
  Auscultation of abdomen and over the abdominal aorta, renal, and iliac arteries
  Percussion of abdomen and liver span in the midclavicular line
  Assess for splenomegaly by percussion of left upper quadrant during deep inspiration
  Light abdominal palpation
  Palpation right upper quadrant for liver edge during inspiration
  Deep abdominal palpation all four quadrants
  Palpation inguinal, femoral, and axillary nodes (if last not performed during breast palpation)
Patient's gown is lowered further and drape is positioned to inspect lower extremities, palpate lower
    extremity pulses and assess for edema
Patient resumes the sitting position (if indicated, supine and seated blood pressure can be performed at this
    time)
  Assess remaining cranial nerves (visual fields to confrontation [III]; facial sensation, muscles of
    mastication [V]; facial movement [VII]; palate movement and phonation [IX, X]; shoulder shrug [XI];
    and tongue movement [XII])
  Stretch reflexes: triceps, brachioradialis, patella, Achilles
Patient stands down from the table to demonstrate gate
Genital and rectal examinations are performed as final maneuver (patient dresses after this aspect of the
    examination)
  Males stand for inspection of penis and palpation of the scrotum contents and inguinal ring; patient turns
    to face the examination table for digital prostate and rectal examination
  Females (who emptied their bladder prior to beginning the physical examination) are positioned for the
    pelvic examination

hands and observing the upper extremities. This initial nonthreatening maneuver allows assessment of the patient's reaction to physical contact.

VITAL SIGNS

Vital signs are assessed by palpating the radial pulse for 15 seconds to determine heart rate and rhythm. If irregularities are detected, palpate for a longer interval and establish whether all beats are peripherally transmitted by auscultating the precordium. Assessing respiration involves observing or palpating chest movement as unobtrusively as possible, such as while seeming to palpate the pulse or auscultate the precordium.

Blood pressure can be measured with the patient seated or reclining, and in each position, the artery measured should be at the level of the heart. The examiner should select a blood pressure cuff with a width about 20% greater than the diameter of the arm. Cuffs that are too small can give falsely high readings. The examiner should inflate the cuff while palpating the radial artery to establish the systolic pressure and rapidly deflate it when the pulse is no longer palpable. This initial determination of systolic pressure guides subsequent cuff inflation during auscultation of the pressure. While auscultating the blood pressure, the stethoscope is placed firmly over the brachial artery (medial to the tendon of the biceps muscle), in the antecubital fossae. The examiner reinflates the cuff to about 20 mm Hg above the palpated systolic pressure and then deflates the cuff while auscultating.

HEENT (HEAD, EYES, EARS, NOSE, AND THROAT)

The examiner stands in front of the patient for the majority of the HEENT evaluation. The examiner assesses the sclera and conjunctiva of each eye by asking the patient to look upward, while retracting the lower lid downward. Visual acuity should be checked while the patient wears any corrective lenses. It is evaluated early in the examination using a near vision card or wall chart. Detecting abnormalities of visual acuity can result in additional time spent on other aspects of the eye examination.

Extraocular movements are evaluated as the patient fixes gaze on the examiner's finger. The examiner should ask the patient to look into the distance and then at her finger held 3 inches from the nose, while observing for pupillary constriction and convergence. When observing the direct pupillary response to light, the examiner inspects for pupillary constriction in the same eye. To observe the consensual response to light, the examiner shines the light in one eye and inspects for pupillary constriction in the other eye.

For the ophthalmoscope examination, the patient should be positioned at a height comfortable for the examiner and the room darkened to increase pupillary dilation. The examiner holds the ophthalmoscope with the right hand and uses the right eye when examining the patient's right eye. The examiner should use the left hand and left eye when examining the patient's left eye. From a position of about 15 inches from the patient and about 15 degrees lateral to the patient's line of vision, the examiner shines the light beam on the pupil to elicit the "red reflex." To observe the anterior eye structures, positive diopters (black numbers) are used, and then the examiner moves slowly toward the patient's eye, bringing the optic disk into focus by adjusting the lens disk. The examiner assesses the disk and retinal vessels, and then asks the patient to look directly at the light, so that the macula (located two disk diameters lateral to the optic disk) can be observed.

The examiner should inspect and palpate the auricles and posterior auricular regions. By gently pulling the auricle upward, backward, and slightly away from the skull, the examiner can insert the speculum in a downward and forward position and examine the tympanic membrane and canal. To observe the nasal mucosa, septal location and integrity, the examiner is positioned in front of the patient and gently inserts the short wide nasal speculum through each nostril, while inspecting the nasal passages.

The examiner should inspect the lips, all surfaces of the tongue, gingiva, palate and buccal mucosa. To examine the floor of the mouth, the examiner asks the patient to touch the "roof of your mouth," with the tip of the tongue. To visualize the posterior pharynx and palate movement, the examiner presses a tongue blade firmly down on the patient's nonprotruded tongue and asks the patient to say "ah."

The neck contains several node-bearing areas for palpation: (1) preauricular nodes in front of the ears, (2) occipital nodes at the posterior base of the skull, (3) anterior cervical nodes in front of the sternomastoid muscle, (4) posterior cervical nodes in back of the sternomastoid muscle, and (5) supraclavicular nodes above the clavicle and in the angle formed by the clavicle and the sternomastoid muscle.

The examiner can palpate the thyroid gland while standing in front or in back of the patient. The thyroid gland lies across the trachea below the cricoid cartilage, with the lateral lobes curved around the sides of the trachea. From the front, the thyroid is displaced to one side by applying pressure with the thumb on the thyroid cartilage. With the opposite hand, the thyroid can be palpated between the thumb (held in front of the sternomastoid) and the second and third fingers placed behind the sternomastoid. The procedure should be repeated for the opposite side. From behind the patient, the procedure is similar, except that the thyroid cartilage is displaced with the second and third fingers. The thumb of the opposite hand is behind the sternomastoid muscle, and the second and third fingers palpate the gland. The examiner can palpate and auscultate the carotid arteries with the HEENT examination or defer this portion until examining the heart and blood vessels.

CHEST AND BACK

Moving behind the patient (if not already in that position for the thyroid examination), the examiner palpates the vertebral spinous processes. To examine chest wall movement, the examiner asks the patient to inhale deeply, while observing the extent and symmetry of respiratory movement. The examiner should percuss the posterior lung fields, lateral to both sides of the spinal column. The examiner then auscultates the posterior and lateral lung fields with the diaphragm of the stethoscope. The patient should be asked to breathe deeply through the mouth. Following percussion of the anterior chest, the examiner auscultates those lung fields.

BREAST

For the breast examination, a woman should be disrobed to the waist, and the examiner inspects both breasts with the patient in a sitting position. The patient then reclines, and the breasts are palpated, with the patient's hands behind her head. The examiner should systematically examine all four quadrants and the tail of each breast, using a uniform pattern to ensure a complete examination. A man's breasts should be examined in a similar manner, if a male has breast complaints or when gynecomastia is present on inspection.

The examiner should ask the patient to relax the upper extremity and place the cupped fingers of her hand into the patient's armpit. The right hand palpates the left axilla, and the left hand palpates the right axilla. With the hand moved slowly down over the surface of the ribs, the tissue is compressed against the chest wall. The technique is repeated with the examiner palpating outwardly against the humerus. After palpating the axilla, the examiner should rewash her hands.

CARDIAC

To estimate venous pressure, the patient is positioned so that the highest point of oscillation of the internal jugular veins is visible along the sternomastoid muscle. The vertical distance (perpendicular to the floor) between this point and the sternal angle plus 5 cm is the venous pressure in centimeters of water.

Draping is important to maintain patient comfort. To minimize exposure, the gown is brought up from below and the drape positioned inferior to the area being examined. With the patient supine, the examiner observes the precordium, then palpates the following areas of the chest wall: (1) aortic area (second intercostal space to the right of the sternum), (2) pulmonic area (second and third intercostal spaces to the left of the sternum), (3) tricuspid area (left lower sternal border), and (4) mitral area [apex or fifth intercostal space in the left midclavicular line where mitral murmurs and left ventricular sounds (S4, S3) are heard best]. All four areas are auscultated with the diaphragm and bell. When using the diaphragm (for high-pitched sounds), it should be pressed firmly onto the chest. When using the bell (for low-pitched sounds), it should be applied lightly, with only enough pressure to produce an air seal between its rim and the chest.

ABDOMEN

The examiner should expose the abdomen and inspects its contour. For descriptive purposes, the abdomen is divided into four quadrants (right upper quadrant, left upper quadrant, right lower quadrant, left lower quadrant) by two imaginary perpendicular lines crossing at the umbilicus. In addition, the "epigastrium" (the region between the right and left upper quadrants directly inferior to the sternum) also is used in describing abdominal findings.

The examiner should auscultate the abdomen, while listening for: (1) the frequency and character of the bowel sounds, (2) an aortic bruit (in the midline, above the umbilicus), (3) bruits in the two renal arteries, and (4) bruits in the two iliac arteries. Following auscultation, the examiner percusses lightly in all four quadrants to assess the distribution of tympany and dullness. The examiner begins percussion of the liver in the right midclavicular line at midchest level, percussing downward until reaching the upper border of liver dullness. In the same line, percuss upward from the level of the umbilicus, until reaching the lower border of liver dullness. To assess for splenomegaly, the examiner percusses in the lowest intercostal space in the left anterior axillary line. The examiner then asks the patient to take a deep breath and percusses again. When the size of the spleen is normal, the percussion note remains tympanitic.

Palpation begins with light pressure in all four quadrants, followed by deeper palpation. The examiner watches the patient's face to monitor for expressions of discomfort. Using the palmar surfaces of the fingers, the examiner palpates to identify any masses or areas of tenderness. The epigastrium should be palpated deeply to delineate the margins of the aorta. To palpate the liver, the examiner places her right hand on the right lower quadrant, pressing gently in and upward. The patient then takes a series of deep breaths, while the palpating hand is moved upward toward the right costal margin. The liver edge may be felt as it descends to meet the examiner's fingers as the patient inhales.

To examine the spleen, the examiner's right hand is placed at the lower border of the left rib cage, while gentle pressure is exerted upwards and toward the back. The examiner asks the patient to take a deep breath and then exhale. The examiner may wish to repeat the examination while the patient lies on his right side. In this position, gravity may bring the spleen forward and medially into a more easily palpable position.

LOWER EXTREMITIES

The examiner inspects both limbs from the groin to the toes, noting symmetry, color and texture of the skin, hair distribution, venous pattern, and whether there is edema. To assess for pitting edema, the examiner presses firmly for up to 15 seconds behind the medial malleolus, over the dorsum of the foot or on the anterior tibia.

The examiner should palpate the following pulses: (1) femoral, (2) popliteal (behind the patient's knee; the patient's knee should be slightly flexed, and the examiner should press the fingertips deeply into the popliteal fossa slightly lateral to the midline), (3) posterior tibial (posterior to the medial malleolus), and (4) dorsalis pedis (dorsum of the foot midway between ankle and toes, between the extensor tendon of the first toe and second toe). The examiner should auscultate the femoral pulses for bruits. In addition, the inguinal lymph nodes in the groin, which drain the lower limbs, conveniently are palpated when evaluating the femoral pulses.

REFLEXES

Reflexes routinely assessed are the biceps, brachioradialis, patellar (knee jerk), and tendoachilles (ankle jerk). The biceps (C5–C6) is examined with the patient's arm relaxed in his lap, and the elbow bent at about 90 degrees. The examiner places her thumb against the biceps tendon on the inside of the elbow and taps the thumb with the reflex hammer. The brachioradialis reflex (C5–C6) is performed with the forearm pronated, and the tendon is struck approximately 4 cm proximal to the radial styloid process. The triceps reflex (C6–C8) is accomplished with the elbow flexed, with the upper arm supported by the examiner or with the patient's hands on the hips. The tendon is struck above the elbow. The patellar tendon (L2–L4) is tapped firmly just below the patella, checking for extension of the knee. With the patient sitting, the examiner's fingers support the sole of the patient's dangling foot in mild dorsiflexion, tapping the Achilles tendon just above the heel while observing for plantar flexion at the ankle. Gait is evaluated while the patient walks across the room, turns, and returns. The patient is observed for posture, balance, and symmetry of arm swing and leg movements.

GU EXAMINATION

The pelvic and male GU examination are the concluding examination aspects. Men usually are positioned standing with the examiner seated on a stool, to palpate the penis

Table 3.2
Pediatric Physical Assessment

Vital signs	Chart height, weight, and head circumference; appropriate cuff size for BP assessment; adjust "normal" heart rate and blood pressure for age
Inspection	Skin lesions, bruises, unusual marks (signs of child abuse or neglect); complete skin exam in teens with exposure to sunlight, family history of skin cancer or dysplastic or congenital nevi
HEENT	Visual acuity; evidence ocular misalignment and amblyopia; hearing assessed at 18 months if not previsouly tested and repeated annually if positive family history or condition predisposing to deafness; dentition and oral hygiene; reactive adenopathy common among children, and of concern when localized or nodes > 1.5 cm
Chest	Among small children, respiratory rate can vary widely and be more influenced by illness and emotion, use the small diaphragm or bell for chest auscultation
Cardiac	Until age 7, PMI at or left of midclavicular line, systolic ejection murmurs ("flow" or innocent murmur) and S3 can be normal findings
Abdominal	Liver, spleen, kidneys can be palpated in normal infants, liver often palpable in young children
Genitalia	Males: evidence hypospadias, undescended testes, hydrocele, and hernia; females: pelvic exam if sexually active
Extremities	Newborn hip dislocation; gait; assess back for scoliosis
Neurologic	Observation motor skills; gait; be alert for evidence of behavioral and learning disorders, depressive symptoms and suicide risks (such as divorce, alcohol or other illicit substance use, serious medical disorders and bereavement)

and scrotal contents, and then the patient faces the examination table for the digital examination. For the pelvic examination, women are in the lithotomy position, with their heads elevated at approximately 30 degrees. These examination components require unique attention to patient comfort, and they are discussed further later in this chapter.

ASSESSMENT OF PEDIATRIC PATIENTS

The physical examination of a child emphasizes milestones of growth and development, preventive healthcare, assessment of the social situation, and education of the family (see Tables 3.2 and 3.3). The physical examination is preceded by the examiner and child becoming acquainted, to decrease apprehension associated with the visit. This also allows observation of the interactions between the child and the parent. Clothing should be removed gradually to keep children warm and decrease their stress. During the examination, it is best to begin with areas that will be tolerated easily, rather than adhere to a set sequence. For instance, the ear and throat examination may be saved for last.

The vital signs include charting weight, height, and head circumference, for comparison with standard charts of growth rate. The child's general appearance should be assessed for nutritional status, posture, and gait. Blood pressure measurements require careful attention to cuff size and recognition that normal values differ among age groups. Physical examination components and preventive care aspects unique to pediatric assessment are listed in Tables 3.2 and 3.3.

Table 3.3

Development and Preventive Care of Children

Age	Growth–development	Immunization	Education
Newborn 2 weeks	Lifts head, responds to noise, regards face, follows to midline, turns head side to side and follows to midline	Hepatitis B #1 (Hep B)	Diet: breast, formula, vitamins, fluoride Accident prevention: handling, falling, car seats Behavior: sneezing, hiccups, straining, startle reflex Guidance: spoiling, sib rivalry, pacifer, no bottle in bed, passive smoking
2 months	Vocalizes, lifts head 45°, smiles responsively, follows past midline	Hep B #2 Oral polio vaccine (OPV) #1 Haemophilus influenza B (Hib) #1 Diphtheria/pertussis/tetanus (DPT) #1	Diet: breast, formula, fluoride, iron, vitamins Accident prevention: car seats, toys, rolling over Behavior: crying, thumb sucking Guidance: where sleeping, colds, immunizations, taking temperature, acetaminophen/sponging, babysitters
4 months	Lifts head 90°, squeals and laughs, follows 180°, head steady when sitting, grasps rattle, rolls over one way	OPV #2 Hib #2 DPT #2	Diet: breast, formula, weaning, new foods Accident prevention: falling, aspiration, car seats, sharp objects Behavior: rolls, reaches for objects, drooling, teething Guidance: babysitters, sleeping independently, physician calls
6 months	Pulled to sit without head lag, reaches for object, rolls over both ways, smiles spontaneously, sits briefly alone, gums objects	Hep B #3 OPV #3 Hib #3 DPT #3	Diet: cereal, weaning, no whole milk, new foods Accident prevention: playpen, poisoning, safe high chair, child-proof home Behavior: sitting, crawling, stranger and separation anxiety Guidance: schedule (rising/bedtime), teether, offer cup, no bottle in bed
9 months	Sits without support, feeds self cracker, transfer objects from one hand to another, turns to voice, bangs two cubes, creeps and crawls		Diet: mashed table foods, finger foods, cup Accident prevention: no nuts, candy, or popcorn, electrical outlets, stairs, stove, hot water, pools, car seats Behavior: sitting, crawling, creeping, wants to stand Guidance: appetite, discipline (no spanking)
12 months	Stands momentarily, walks holding (furniture), plays pat-a-cake, mama and dada, thumb–finger grasp, holds cup to drink	Measles-Mumps-Rubella (MMR) #1	Diet: mashed table foods, finger foods, cup Accident prevention: no nuts, candy, or popcorn, electrical outlets, stairs, stove, hot water, pools, car seats Behavior: pulls to stand, nightmares Guidance: discipline (consistency), insurance, wills and guardianship
15 months	Stands and walks alone, builds tower with two cubes, plays pat-a-cake, takes lids off containers, drinks from cup	OPV #4 Hib #4 DPT #4	Diet: table food, milk (1 pint to 1 quart/24 hours), vitamins, candy Accident prevention: childproof home, matches, stove, bathtubs, teach hot and cold Behavior: self-feeding, simple games Guidance: explain temper tantrum, family play, masturbation, don't start toilet training, shoes, bottle

Age	Development	Immunizations	Diet/Guidance
18 months	Mimics household chores (dusting, sweeping), piles three blocks, walks well and climbs, mama, dada, and three words, indicates wants without crying (will point, pull)		Diet: 3 meals/day and snacks Accident prevention: street, refrigerator-freezer, electrical outlets, hot water Behavior: independence/autonomy ("No"), likes action Guidance: toilet training, read to, child temper tantrums, discipline
24 months	Kicks ball, points to body part, simple household tasks, tower of six cubes, scribbles, handles spoon well, plays hide and seek, runs well, walks up and down stairs, two-word sentences		Diet: 3 meals/day and snacks Behavior: runs but falls easily, rough and tumble play, stairs, sharing with others Guidance: toilet training, exercises, peer play, accept negativism, TV programs, dental care
4–6 years	Buttons up (4.2 yr), copies square (4.4 yr), recognizes three colors (4.9 yr), hops on one foot (4.9 yr), throws ball	OPV #5 DtaP (acellular pertussis) #5 MMR #2	Diet: 3 meals/day and snacks Accident prevention: seat belts, street sense Behavior: imitates adults, dresses and undresses, brushes teeth Guidance: TV programs, school, bed wetting, separation, chores, attention span
6–11 years	School progress, grade achievement, sports, peer relationship, hobbies, vocations, stress	Tetanus booster (Td)	Diet, exercise, discipline, home conflicts, sex education, contraception, masturbation, smoking, alcohol, drugs, seat belts, helmets

Table 3.4
Types of Physical Diagnosis Errors

Technique and detection
    Causing patient discomfort or embarrassment
    Improper use of instruments or performance of the examination
    Failure to perform part of the examination
    Missing a finding
Detection and interpretation
    Reporting a finding that is not present
    Incorrect identification or interpretation of findings
    Lack of knowledge or use of confirming signs
Recording
    Forgetting to record a finding
    Illegible handwriting, obscure abbreviations, or improper terminology
    Recording an interpretation rather than the findings

RATIONALE FOR AN EXPLICIT EXAMINATION SEQUENCE

Memorizing and adhering to a specific physical examination sequence and using a standard form on which to record findings increase students' ability to consistently perform an efficient examination (Antonelli, 1993). When studied, learning an explicit pattern decreases both students' anxiety when assessing patients and the time needed for the interaction (Klachko & Reid, 1975).

Physical examination abilities, as with any skill, are improved by practice. Medical educators have identified the types of errors examiners make when assessing patients (see Table 3.4) (Wiener & Nathanson, 1976). Two of the three errors are improved by memorizing a specific examination routine. In addition, abilities are enhanced by watching others perform examinations, practicing maneuvers, and obtaining feedback on technique. Reviewing a patient's findings and their interpretation also will calibrate an individual's assessment abilities.

CASE 3-3

S. Y. had a different preceptor each quarter this year. Although all practiced in an ambulatory setting, each was different. Their "new patient" assessments varied in what examination components were included. Even the same physician did not do similar examinations with each new patient. S. Y. wanted to understand those differences. However, she was reluctant to ask her preceptor about these inconsistencies, because of concern that these questions would challenge Dr. T.'s competence. She wondered what strategy she would use for a complete examination when assigned to the clerkships.

WHY DO PHYSICAL EXAMINATIONS DIFFER?

Although most medical students learn similar physical examination skills, when in practice, the choice of maneuvers differs among physicians. That variability has been documented using standardized patients (SPs). SPs are individuals trained to portray a patient, and interactions with SPs are a method to evaluate assessment abilities. To observe what physicians actually do when examining patients, an SP, simulating a new patient, was seen by multiple primary care practitioners. Despite consistency in the patient's history, the evaluations varied from 5 to 60 minutes in length, and the recommended examination components performed ranged from 16 to 89% (Carney *et al.*, 1993).

Variability among physicians reflects their preferences, visit circumstances, and patient characteristics. For example, the chance detection of an unusual abnormality might bias an examiner to continue that maneuver, despite evidence that it is not a useful part of the examination. Time limitations and anticipation of follow-up examinations also can influence the choice of examination components. In addition, patient characteristics can affect which examination maneuvers are performed. For example, it has been suggested that obese women are less likely to receive a pelvic examination than are nonobese women.

CASE 3-3 (*continued*)

S. Y. had been reluctant to ask Dr. T. about variability in examination components. However, the preceptor had encouraged the student's questions, and finally, S. Y. related her observations about how examinations varied. The observation led to an interesting discussion with Dr. T. They talked about what was known about each examination components' utility, which were advocated by different groups, and how Dr. T. came to include certain parts of the examination. The student brought the issue up with her classmates, and they shared similar experiences. Her physical assessment group even talked about a project to observe their preceptors, gather information about what was done, and define variability in the "screening" examination.

HOW USEFUL AND ACCURATE ARE SPECIFIC EXAMINATION MANEUVERS?

In recent years, investigators have focused on the utility of physical assessment maneuvers in identifying illness (Sox, 1994; Fitzgerald, 1990; Hayward *et al.*, 1991). Studying the physical examination components has been a challenge, as it is difficult to assemble large numbers of appropriate patients, recruit clinicians with similar training, and compare findings against a "gold standard." Table 3.5 lists information about examination maneuvers and whether sufficient evidence exists to recommend them for a well-patient screening examination. "Not recommended" means the component was consid-

Table 3.5

Recommended Physical Examination Practices

	Comments	Canadian Task Force	U.S. Preventive Services Task Force	Oboler & LaForce (1989)	American Colleges of Physicians
Blood pressure	Affected by cuff size and arm position, elevation due to "white coat" hypertension can lead to misinterpretation	At least every 5 years, and after age 65, every 1 to 2 years	At least every 1 to 2 years and annually after age 65	At least every 1 to 2 years	At least every 1 to 2 years and annually if risk factors for coronary artery disease
Height and weight	20% greater than desirable weight for height (using standard tables) defined as obese	If adolescent, women of low socioeconomic status, or unusual dietary habits	Each 1 to 3 years after age 40 and annually after age 65	Every 4 years	Not considered
Visual acuity	Record best corrected vision	Not considered	Annually after age 65	Annually after age 60	Not considered
Hearing	Most accurately assessed using audioscope	If noise exposure, after age 18	Annually after age 65 and begin at age 19, if noise exposure	Annually after age 60 by audioscope	Not considered
Oral cavity	Assess both mucosa and dentition	After age 65 and after age 18, if uses tobacco	After age 18, if uses tobacco or alcohol	Not recommended	Annual dental exam; mouth exam not recommended
Skin inspection	Higher risk if excess sun exposure, dysplastic nevi, > 6 moles more than 5 mm in diameter, or family history of melanoma	Annually after age 18, if excess sun exposure or dysplastic nevi	After age 18, if excess sun exposure, dysplastic nevi, or history of skin cancer	Evaluate for dysplastic nevi at initial visit; annually for high-risk patients	Not considered
Auscultate carotids	Bruits are a marker for ASVD; their absence does not exclude carotid stenosis	Not recommended	Perform if (1) risks for ASVD or symptoms of cerebrovascular disease, (2) each 1 to 3 years after age 40, and (3) annually after age 65	Not recommended	Not considered
Breast	Reinforce self-exam skills and that mammography adds to detection rates	Annually after age 40 and after age 35, if family history of breast cancer	Annually after age 40 and after age 35, if family history of breast cancer	Annually after age 40 and after age 18, if family history of breast cancer	Annually after age 40 and after age 18, if family history of breast cancer
Chest exam		Not considered	Not considered	Not recommended	Not considered

Exam	Comments				
Cardiac	Important component for "sports physical," as hypertrophic cardiomyopathy is most common cause of sudden death among young athletes	Not recommended	Not considered	Auscultate for valvular disease at initial visit and when age 60	Not considered
Abdomen		Not considered	Not considered	Palpate for abdominal aortic aneurysm annually in men over age 60	Not considered
Stool occult blood		Not recommended unless family history of colon cancer, then annually after age 40	Annually after age 40 if family history of colon cancer	Annually after age 50, and begin at age 40 if family history of colon cancer	Annually after age 50 and begin at age 40 if family history of colon cancer
Lymph nodes		Not considered	Not considered	Not recommended	Not considered
Bimanual pelvic exam and cervical cytology		Not considered	Cervical cytology every 1 to 3 years; routine pelvic exams not recommended	Cervical cytology if sexually active; after two negative annual cytological exams, then at least every 3 years; palpation ovaries not recommended	Pelvic exam not considered; cervical cytology every 1 to 3 years
Digital prostate palpation	American Cancer Society and National Cancer Institute recommend annually after age 50, and if increased risk prostate cancer, annually after age 40	Not recommended	Not recommended	Not recommended	Not considered
Musculoskeletal exam		Not recommended	Not considered	Back exam not recommended	Not considered
Mental status	Several studies document that dementia often missed	Not recommended	Not recommended	Not recommended	After age 65

ered, but evidence supporting its performance was weak. "Not considered" indicates evidence for the maneuver was not evaluated by the authors or expert panel.

Few patient encounters are exclusively "well-patient" or "screening" examinations. Most interactions are shaped by both the patient's complaints and the prevalence of disorders in the patient's demographic group. For example, an individual complaining of dyspnea would receive close attention on the cardiac and pulmonary examinations, because those systems are likely to reveal the complaint's etiology. A teenager being seen for a "sports physical" would be assessed for abnormalities of joint range of motion, an examination aspect that might not otherwise be performed. Using the history to select examination components is analogous to relying on a patient's history and physical examination findings to choose which laboratory tests to perform.

CASE 3-4

Presenting a patient's history and physical examination at the bedside made the student, N. S., feel uneasy. N. S. was concerned that he might say something that the patient would misinterpret or find embarrassing. However, the attending physician demanded bedside rounds, and the student had practiced the presentation with the team's senior resident. The student was surprised when the attending asked the patient a question identical to his and received a different answer. And, he was embarrassed when he could not remember the liver span in centimeters, as he only had written "normal." His uneasiness was heightened when the murmur he had heard the night before was not heard on rounds. He wondered what had gone wrong and what he could do to avoid these events happening again.

WHY DON'T EXAMINERS AGREE ON THEIR ___ PHYSICAL EXAMINATION FINDINGS?

Clinicians frequently disagree about physical examination findings. Agreement between observers (interobserver reliability) relates to patient factors, examiner influences, and the clinical setting (see Table 3.6) (Department of Clinical Epidemiology and Biostatistics, McMaster University, Part I, 1980; Koran, 1975). The reliability relates to how much confidence or diagnostic certainty can be placed on a finding. Percent agreement is not an accurate index of interobserver agreement. Disagreement is measured better by concordance, which takes into account both the "true" agreement of observers and the amount of agreement that would occur by chance. Table 3.7 presents an example illustrating the difference between percent agreement and concordance (measured by the kappa statistic). After examining the same 100 men (85 of whom have true prostate enlargement), two different examiners' findings are shown. The percent agreement is misleadingly high because of the high prevalence of the abnormality.

When evaluating studies of physical examination reliability, look for measures of concordance. The kappa statistic is often used (Maclure & Willett, 1987), and a kappa of $+1$ is perfect agreement, 0 is chance agreement, and -1 is total disagreement. When used to assess interobserver agreement, a kappa greater than 0.6 is substantial agreement, 0.2 to 0.6 is fair to moderate agreement, and less than 0.2 is slight or poor agreement.

75

WHY DON'T
EXAMINERS
AGREE ON THEIR
PHYSICAL
EXAMINATION
FINDINGS?

Table 3.6
Causes for Clinical Disagreement

Examiner
  Biologic variation in the senses
  Tendency to record inferences or classifications rather than evidence
  Bias from prior experiences
  Incorrect use of diagnostic tools
Patient
  Biologic variation in organ systems
  Changes related to illnesses' natural history and management
Setting and equipment
  Disruptive examination environments
  Malfunction or absence of examination equipment

EXAMINER FACTORS

A physician's performance is not constant, and that variability is a source of examination unreliability (Table 3.6). This inconsistency has been shown by having interns read ECGs when tired and well rested. Their skill in interpreting ECG rhythms was shown to differ with the amount of physician rest (Asken & Raham, 1983). Among busy clinicians, fatigue, transient physical limitations, such as a serous otitis affecting hearing, and other distractions can impact on physical assessment abilities.

In addition, practitioners often record "interpretations," rather than specific examination findings. These inferences lose objective clinical information and can be misinterpreted. For example, "no hepatomegaly" conveys less information than recording the liver's percussion span. A normal-sized 8-cm liver could enlarge 2 cm and still its size would be "normal." Similarly, writing "normal mental status" omits results of specific mental status components and assumes examiners share common tests and standards.

Prior experiences and biases also influence clinicians' interpretation of findings. The effect of bias was shown when investigators trained two female patients to present the same information concerning their chest pain. When the first woman was dressed in a business suit and calmly articulated her symptoms, half of the physicians felt that she needed further diagnostic studies. However, when the second woman was dressed less

Table 3.7
Calculating Agreement and Concordance of Two Physicians'
Examination Findings

	Observer B's exam finding		
Observer A's exam findings	+	−	
+	75	10	85
−	9	6	15
	84	16	

Percent agreement = $\dfrac{75 + 6}{100}$ = 0.81 (81%)   Calculated kappa = 0.13

"professionally" and appeared more flamboyant in her manner, only 13% advised further testing, despite identical verbal information. Although risk factors and description of symptoms were similar, the patient's style and physicians' interpretation of the patient's style affected management (Birdwell *et al.*, 1993).

PATIENT COMPONENTS

An individual's biologic variability affects physical assessment findings (Table 3.6). In addition, the effects of an illness and the resultant examination observations are not constant. For example, pleural and pericardial rubs vary with patient position, and distribution of rhonchi can change after a deep cough. The effects of medication, for example, using a narcotic analgesic, and other treatments further compound physical findings' inconsistency.

EXAMINATION SETTING

The clinical environment impacts on the examination reliability. Background noise level and examination equipment affect one's ability to perform portions of the examination and recognize abnormalities. For example, "white coat hypertension" can be resolved in a more relaxed setting. Detecting jaundice or pallor in a dimly lit room and auscultating cardiac findings in a noisy clinic are difficult. A high examination table can result in assessing paretic individuals in their wheelchairs, rather than the examination table, because of time constraints or lack of ancillary help.

CASE 3-4 (*continued*)

N. S. could have decreased the chance that physical assessment findings would vary by minimizing effects of the patient, examiner, and setting. As he reflected back on the patient encounter, N. S. remembered that his examination had been interrupted twice to deal with other issues. He may not have focused his full attention on the interaction. He decided that, in the future, he would record precise findings. Because the student had limited clinical experience, he was not subject to its bias. However, he recognized that examinations recorded in the old chart biased his assessment. Next time, he would reexamine the patient prior to attending rounds and compare his results with other examiners. In addition, he was convinced that it was time to buy a better stethoscope.

___ WHAT CAN EXAMINERS DO TO REDUCE ___ EXAMINATION VARIABILITY?

There are several ways to reduce clinical disagreement and increase an examination's reliability (see Table 3.8) (Department of Clinical Epidemiology and Biostatistics, McMaster University, Part II, 1980). It often is useful to ask a colleague to repeat portions of the history or physical examination to confirm findings. The second examiner assesses the patient with limited historical information, to remove the effects of bias. Relating

77

HOW DOES THE
PHYSICAL
EXAMINATION
AFFECT THE
PHYSICIAN–
PATIENT
RELATIONSHIP?

Table 3.8
Strategies Minimizing Clinical Disagreement

Examiner limitations minimized by
  Practice skills and calibrate the examination with a broad range of findings
  Seek corroboration of key findings (repeating oneself and examination by others)
  Ask "blinded" (nonbiased) examiners to assess the patient
  Confirm key clinical findings with appropriate tests
  Report evidence rather than inferences
Patient limitations minimized by
  Repeat assessments to evaluate tempo of an illness and expected changes
Setting limitations minimized by
  Match the environment to the diagnostic task
  Establish appropriate rapport prior to the examination
  Use appropriate examination tools

---

findings to a "gold standard" also will refine an examiner's abilities. For example, comparing the examination for ascites with abdominal ultrasound, chest findings with the radiograph, and cardiac auscultation with echocardiography increases an examiner's abilities. In addition, repeatedly assessing patients over time acquaints practitioners with the potential variability of findings.

CASE 3-5

During hospital rounds, things moved quickly. His role as third-year clerk was to preround and obtain vital signs, review the chart for any new developments, and be prepared to briefly report his findings. Although he did not say much else, the student tried to observe all he could about patients and others on the team. The staff physician, Dr. T., always checked a patient's pulse as the first thing. He usually would check the pulse with his left hand, while clasping the patient's hand in his. Dr. T. had related that it was something that he began doing as a resident and continued to do. He felt that it was a way to make physical contact and connect with the patient, rather than directly go to examining the wound. The student was trying different styles and ways to interact, and this was one that he wanted to try.

HOW DOES THE PHYSICAL EXAMINATION AFFECT THE PHYSICIAN–PATIENT RELATIONSHIP?

The physical examination provides information and enhances physician–patient rapport. Study of physician–patient interactions indicates that time spent on the physical examination is positively correlated with patient satisfaction (Robbins *et al.,* 1993). Extrapolating from studies of the interview, maintaining patient comfort, avoiding patient embarrassment, and demonstrating facility with the examination enhance patient satisfaction. A clear rationale for performing specific physical examination components allows acknowledging variability among practitioners and helps explain to a patient why examination items were omitted or performed.

Physical contact during the examination may have therapeutic benefits. The use of "manual therapy" or "therapeutic" touch has generated extensive literature and national and international organizations to share experiences (Carruthers, 1992; Fishman *et al.*, 1995; Krieger, 1979). Data substantiating the use of touch primarily are anecdotal, and these techniques' utility has not been assessed rigorously. Touch also is a nonverbal behavior that can have negative effects. When objectively assessed, more touching during an office visit correlated with lower patient satisfaction (Larsen & Smith, 1981). However, these investigators did not differentiate new from follow-up visits nor determine whether the touch was a response to patient distress. Nevertheless, the findings show that nonverbal actions influence the physician–patient relationship.

CASE 3-6

Ms. F. did not like these annual examinations, but she knew that they were important. Now that she was in her 40s, she had some questions about "menopause." The nurse had asked her to remove her clothing, and she waited in the room dressed only in a gown, with a paper drape across her lap. She was surprised when Dr. K. entered the room with a student, although she had seen the sign concerning medical students being in the office. Perhaps the surprise on her face resulted in Dr. K.'s attempt at humor as he prepared for the pelvic examination and asked, "Did you remember to bring your cervix?"

WHICH PHYSICAL EXAMINATION ——— COMPONENTS REQUIRE SPECIAL ——— ATTENTION TO PATIENT COMFORT?

The breast, pelvic, and genitourinary examinations can result in patient embarrassment and feelings of vulnerability. These examinations require special attention to patient comfort. Physicians also report anxiety when performing these examinations. Examiner distress has been shown to decrease when these feelings are acknowledged as common and discussed with colleagues (Lang, 1990). Talking about these feelings is preferable to more maladaptive behaviors, such as avoiding the examination or attempts at inappropriate sexual humor.

PELVIC AND GENITOURINARY EXAMINATIONS

In the last 15 years gynecologic teaching associates or standardized patients have come to medical schools to teach the complex motor and verbal skills of the pelvic and breast examination (Beckmann *et al.*, 1992; Wallis *et al.*, 1983). Teaching associates are similar to SPs, in that their examination findings are known, and they can provide feedback on an examiner's skills. Teaching associates educate students and provide explicit instruction on students' examination abilities. Importantly, teaching associates can teach and discuss appropriate verbal and nonverbal behaviors during performance of the history and physical examination.

79

WHICH PHYSICAL
EXAMINATION
COMPONENTS
REQUIRE SPECIAL
ATTENTION TO
PATIENT
COMFORT?

Features of a pelvic examination that reduce women's anxiety include obtaining a history while the patient is dressed, rather than when she is disrobed on the examination table (Weiss & Meadow, 1979). Distress is decreased further by performing the examination in an unhurried manner and informing patients about findings (Weiss & Meadow, 1979). Monitoring a woman's comfort is facilitated by elevating the head of the examination table. Allowing a woman to dress before discussing findings reduces her feelings of vulnerability.

Physicians' practices vary concerning the presence of a chaperon during the pelvic examination. This variability is paralleled by surveys of patients' preferences (Patton *et al.*, 1990; Penn & Bourguet, 1992). Although women did not want a chaperon with a female examiner, approximately half preferred one with male examiners. When being evaluated by a male examiner, women (especially teenagers) should be given the option of a chaperon.

BREAST EXAMINATION

An examiner's actions during the breast examination are important for detection of abnormalities. In addition, the examination can influence a woman's behavior regarding self-examination and obtaining mammography. It is an opportunity to review breast self-examination recommendations and technique. This review should not be limited to women who admit a lack of skill, as research documents that women's self-rating has a low correlation with measured abilities (Stratton *et al.*, 1994).

Paradoxically, studies indicate that an increase in self-examination skills may decrease the rate of mammography. To avoid this result, it is important to address both self-examination and mammography. The factor most affecting mammography rate is the physician's personal recommendation and enthusiasm about mammography's importance (S. A. Fox *et al.*, 1994; Friedman *et al.*, 1994; Johnson & Meischke, 1994). To avoid decreasing self-examination, the examiner should emphasize that it adds to mammography, and a normal self-examination does not negate mammography's utility and vice versa.

MALE GENITOURINARY EXAMINATION

The U.S. Preventive Services Task Force recommends a genitourinary examination for men with a history of cryptorchidism, orchiopexy, or testicular atrophy. However, most individuals with a testicular malignancy have none of these risks, and others recommend that this procedure and education about testicular self-examination be included during all routine examinations (Vogt & McHale, 1992).

Unlike the pelvic examination, male patients' reactions to a genitourinary examination have not been well studied. Current recommendations are an extension of findings from women's pelvic examinations. Men differ from women in their preference for chaperons during the examination. When studied, 46% of female adolescents wanted a chaperon during the pelvic examination; however, male teens preferred that no chaperon be present during the genitourinary examination (Penn & Bourguet, 1992).

—————————— CONCLUSION ——————————

Physical examination abilities are important for confirming diagnostic impressions, detecting abnormalities, documenting progression of illness, and enhancing the physician–patient relationship. As with any diagnostic test, or maneuver, physical assessment has its limitations. Being aware of those limits can allow minimizing factors that decrease examination reliability. A beginning student benefits from learning a basic examination sequence. The basic sequence will remain constant, and it forms a framework on which practitioners will refine their patient assessment abilities throughout their careers.

—————————— CASES FOR DISCUSSION ——————————

CASE 1

Mr. T. is a 58-year-old man complaining of leg pains. His history is remarkable for 12 years of diabetes and 8 years of hypertension. A. S. is a second-year student working with his preceptor, and he has first contact with Mr. T. today. The student was thinking that seeing this patient was "great," as he had learned about diabetic neuropathies just last week. The student began with a neurologic examination, including assessment of light touch and vibratory sense. He finished the neurologic assessment with gait testing and a Romberg test. While Mr. T. got back on the examination table, A. S. rewashed his hands, then obtained vital signs and began the head and neck examination. After the abdominal examination, the student asked the patient to stand for the rectal. While Mr. T. returned to the table, the student washed his hands again and completed his examination of the extremities and peripheral pulses.

1. A. S. thought that the "money" (that is, the examination that was most likely to have findings related to the patient's complaint) was in the neurologic examination. What is wrong with that approach?
2. Why is it useful to learn a specific physical examination sequence?
3. How do you think the examination was perceived by Mr. T.?

CASE 2

Y. R. is a man who just turned 40 years old, and at the insistence of his wife, he comes in for a "checkup." He also is motivated to make the appointment because a neighbor his age had died recently of a myocardial infarction. Mr. R. has not seen a physician for many years. He has no history of medical problems, and he is feeling well. You are about to begin the physical examination.

1. What aspects of the physical examination are of "proven" value for Mr. R.?
2. What aspects of the physical examination would you perform? Why?
3. How could you define what aspects of the examination Mr. R. thinks would or should be performed? How can you avoid accomplishing that task without appearing as though you don't know what to do? What would you say or do if after completing what you think is indicated, Mr. R. asks, "Is that all you're going to do? I had wanted a complete exam."

CASE 3

The student reentered the examination room with her preceptor. She had explained that Ms. P. was at the clinic for follow-up of her treatment for hypertension. Today, the student had measured the blood pressure as 160/90 mm Hg. The physician began by rechecking the pressure and called out a value of 132/80 mm Hg. He also auscultated the patient's precordium, and holding the diaphragm of the stethoscope to Ms. P.'s chest, he handed the student the earpieces, saying, "Do you hear this systolic murmur?"

1. *Did the student take the blood pressure incorrectly?*
2. *What factors contribute to unreliability of the examination and how might they relate to this situation?*
3. *The student listened, but couldn't hear a murmur, but she did hear the preceptor advising her to "listen hard." What are the student's options in the situation? If she says that she can't hear a murmur, will the patient think that the preceptor is an ineffective teacher?*

CASE 4

The student was aware of universal precautions to prevent transmission of HIV disease. Ms. J. (an asymptomatic patient who is HIV positive) had no open skin lesions, but the student had fingertip eczema, with plaques and cracking of fingertips of his right hand. The student wondered whether he should put on gloves before beginning the physical examination.

1. *Should the student put on gloves? How might their use affect Ms. J.?*
2. *How does physical contact affect the physician–patient relationship? How could it enhance the relationship? How might it adversely influence physician–patient rapport?*

CASE 5

R. D. is a 2-year-old boy who is brought in by his mother for follow-up of otitis media. It is his third episode this winter. You do not know it, but the mother particularly is worried, as she just saw a TV show that investigated a young boy's death during myringotomy tube placement. R. D. is rambunctious during the history, and his mother lets him make a mess of the examination room. He squirms during the examination and won't cooperate with the otoscopic assessment. He keeps shaking his head and turning away from you.

1. *Give examples of how a toddler's behavior and parent interactions would provide "diagnostic information" for the physical assessment.*
2. *What could have been done to make the examination easier? Should you comment on the child's behavior? How would you do that?*

CASE 6

H. D. is a 14-year-old boy whom you are seeing at your preceptor's office. He is here for a "sports physical" examination, which often includes a GU examination to identify two descended, normal testes (at least that's what F. D., a first-year student, thinks she remembers). Things start out well, and the student thinks her prolonged small talk with H. D. will make the examination easier. However, when she reaches the point for the GU examination, H. D. says, "No way."

1. *What aspects of the interaction influenced H. D.'s reaction (both positively and negatively)?*
2. *What could have been done to make the patient's reaction less likely? The only other male on the clinic staff was a high school work study student. Should the student have gotten him as a chaperon?*

RECOMMENDED READINGS

Bates B, Bickley LS, Hoekelman RA: *Physical Examination and History Taking,* ed 6. Philadelphia, JB Lippincott Co, 1995.

> Initial edition was published in 1974; it provides explicit guidelines on physical examination maneuvers. The text is large and bulky, and it is similar in size to several other books (such as Greenberger & Hinthorn, 1993; Seidel *et al.,* 1991; Swartz, 1989; and Willms *et al.,* 1994); a videotape series and a pocket-sized edition ("baby Bates") also are available.

DeGowin RL: *Diagnostic Examination.* New York, McGraw–Hill Book Co, 1994.

> Original edition was by Richard DeGowin's father, and the book is in its sixth edition; this 4 by 6-inch soft-backed book is organized by systems and findings; its structure makes it an efficient, useful source for looking things up but not as helpful when trying to learning the examination.

Elliot DL, Goldberg L: *The Clinical Examination Casebook.* Boston, Little, Brown & Co 1996.

> This book does the best job of bridging the gap between the basic physical examination guides and medical textbooks (we might be biased); brief patient vignettes, accompanied by a narrative text and tables, show how patient assessment is used to define abnormalities.

Judge RD, Zuidema GD, Fitzgerald FT: *Clinical Diagnosis: A Physiologic Approach.* Boston, Little, Brown & Co, 1989.

> This is a basic text; it is a medium-sized (8 by 9 inches) soft-backed book; its organization follows the physical examination sequence; although its guidelines for examination maneuvers are less explicit than Bates, it is accompanied by a narrative text discussing selected abnormalities.

Macklis RM, Mendelson ME, Mudge GH Jr: *Introduction to Clinical Medicine: A Student-to-Student Manual.* Boston, Little, Brown & Co, 1994.

> Several different paperback books attempt to meet the needs of beginning clerks; along with physical examination information, they contain advice about ward routine, presenting cases and medical "work-ups."

CHAPTER 4

Appropriate Use of Laboratory Tests

Victoria Kaprielian Johnson

CASE 4-1

A 20-year-old white female presents to her physician's office complaining of increasing nonproductive cough for 1 week. She reports a low-grade fever (100° F) and malaise, but no other respiratory symptoms. In addition, in the past 2 days she's developed some chest pain with coughing. She is otherwise healthy, does not smoke, and is on no medications except an over-the-counter cough syrup, which has given little relief. She has no personal or family history of asthma or other lung problems. On physical examination, she appears slightly uncomfortable but in no distress. Her temperature is 99.5° F, and HEENT assessment is unremarkable except for slight erythema in the oropharynx. Lung examination reveals scattered rhonchi, but no rales or wheezes, including on forced exhalation.

The physician suspects the patient has atypical pneumonia or bronchitis. He orders a chest X ray, the results of which are unremarkable, and a blood count, which shows a slightly elevated number of white blood cells. After a positive cold agglutinin study confirms the likely diagnosis, he prescribes a course of erythromycin.

——————— **EDUCATIONAL OBJECTIVES** ———————

After completion of this chapter and the accompanying exercises, the student will be able to:

1. Describe three reasons for performing diagnostic tests

2. Discuss two guiding principles for selection of laboratory tests to be used in patient care
3. Describe appropriate uses of common basic laboratory tests, including complete blood counts, urinalyses, electrolytes, and simple X-ray studies
4. Demonstrate awareness of the costs and risks inherent in diagnostic testing
5. Discuss the influences of disease prevalence and test sensitivity and specificity on interpretation of test results
6. Demonstrate understanding of the concepts of positive and negative predictive value, and their application in the use of diagnostic tests
7. Given a case scenario, suggest diagnostic studies necessary and appropriate for the care of the patient described

INTRODUCTION

Most physicians currently practicing in the United States trained in an environment of seemingly endless resources. Any diagnostic test or approved treatment could be used for any patient, with little regard for cost to the patient or the system. Students and residents were rarely faulted for ordering unnecessary studies, but frequently criticized for not ordering tests of even marginal potential utility. Studies were commonly ordered "just to know," even if they would have little or no impact on treatment or prognosis. In Case 4-1, for example, $150 worth of studies only confirmed the physician's initial impression, and did not change the treatment or outcome.

The realization that our resources are not limitless has prompted dramatic change in the U.S. medical environment. Managed care has come forward as the predominant system for providing care while limiting costs. In this system, physicians are discouraged from performing or ordering any but the most helpful and necessary studies. In order to prepare to practice in such an environment, today's physicians in training must develop a very cost-conscious approach.

There are two major steps in the appropriate use of laboratory tests and other studies. The first, selection of studies, requires careful consideration of alternatives and thinking ahead to the potential usefulness of results. The second step, interpretation of results, requires understanding of several basic principles of epidemiology.

CASE 4-2

A 21-year-old male presents to his physician with a history of physical examination results essentially identical to those of the patient in Case 4-1. The physician orders no tests, and prescribes a course of erythromycin.

SELECTION OF STUDIES

Tests may be used for three basic reasons:

1. To screen for subclinical disease in asymptomatic individuals

2. To identify or clarify diagnoses in symptomatic individuals
3. To monitor status of known disease

In order to select studies and use them appropriately, clinicians should be certain of the reason for ordering tests in the specific patient under consideration. This chapter will focus primarily on the use of tests to pursue a diagnosis; see Chapter 15, "Health Promotion and Disease Prevention," for a discussion of the use of studies for screening of asymptomatic individuals.

The differences between Cases 4-1 and 4-2 raise several questions. Are laboratory tests or X rays necessary for the care of these patients? What studies are available for the physician to order? How might they influence the treatment plan? The patient is clearly symptomatic and the precise diagnosis is uncertain, so the first physician orders an X ray and blood tests. The second physician considers whether further testing is warranted before treatment. The history and physical examination are consistent with an atypical pneumonia. A complete blood count (CBC) is commonly done in this situation, as it was in Case 4-1. However, it is unlikely to change the diagnosis or treatment plan. Ordering a chest X ray is also an option, but findings in atypical pneumonias are inconsistent, and in the absence of other risk factors, an unexpected finding is highly unlikely. Therefore, a course of erythromycin may be prescribed empirically, based on clinical findings only. This inexpensive and effective treatment will adequately treat the several most likely causes of the patient's illness (mycoplasma pneumonia, pneumococcal pneumonia, and acute bronchitis), so absolute identification of the causative organism is unnecessary. In telephone follow-up, the patient reports rapid improvement on the medication. On re-examination 2 weeks later, his symptoms are totally resolved and his lungs are clear.

This chapter proposes two questions to be used as the guiding principles of the approach to choice of laboratory tests. Before performing or ordering any study, the student or physician should consider the following:

1. *Will the results of this study affect the plan of care for this patient?* In Case 4-2, both the CBC and chest X ray were decided against because the physician felt the treatment would, in all likelihood, have remained the same regardless of the results.
2. *Is this the least invasive and least costly means of getting the necessary information?* If a study meets the criterion of influencing the plan, then the physician must decide whether an alternative study may be preferable because of lesser risk or cost. For example, bronchoscopy can be very useful in the assessment of some lung infections, and in Case 4-2 could provide specimens to more accurately determine the causative organism. However, the risks, patient discomfort, and costs involved in this procedure preclude its use except in cases in which less invasive methods fail to provide the necessary information.

These questions will be discussed in more detail and applied in the following sections.

CASE 4-3

A 34-year-old married female presents to her physician with a 1-day history of urinary frequency, urgency, and dysuria. These symptoms closely resemble those she had with two prior episodes of uncomplicated cystitis, most recently 18 months ago. She has no fever, back pain, nausea, or other symptoms. Her LMP was 2 weeks ago and normal. On examination, she has mild suprapubic tenderness and no CVA tenderness.

WILL THE RESULTS INFLUENCE THE PLAN?

The first decision a physician must make in appropriate use of laboratory tests is whether to use them at all. Before ordering or performing any study, it is the physician's responsibility to decide what will be done with the results, by answering the following questions:

- "What relevant results could this test provide?"
- "If the results are positive (or abnormal), what will I do?"
- "If the results are negative (or normal), what will I do?"

If the answers to the last two questions are different, the test may be worthwhile. If they are the same, it probably is not.

Case 4-3 demonstrates this well. In this case, the history and examination are classic for uncomplicated cystitis in an otherwise healthy, sexually active woman. This diagnosis is common (and indeed, the patient has had prior episodes) and not likely to indicate more serious disease, especially in the absence of frequent recurrences. The physician appropriately considers ordering a urinalysis and/or culture, and decides against both. A 3-day course of trimethoprim–sulfamethoxazole is prescribed, and the patient's symptoms resolve without difficulty.

Consider these tests individually.

Urinalysis

A urinalysis (UA) is actually a set of tests performed on a single urine specimen. Its typical cost is approximately $15. The UA can provide a variety of useful information:

1. *Specific gravity*–a measure of urine concentration, which indirectly provides information as to the patient's hydration status.
2. *pH*–indicates the degree of acidity or alkalinity of the urine.
3. *Color and clarity*–these are subjective judgments made by the technicians and are not always useful.
4. *Dipstick results*–a set of colorimetric reactions on sticks manufactured specifically for this purpose, testing for the presence of glucose, protein, blood, ketones, and other items in the urine. This is often used as a screen to determine whether microscopic examination is worthwhile.
5. *Microscopic examination of sediment*–the urine is spun in a centrifuge, and the clear supernatant is poured off, leaving a sediment of cells and solids. This is examined and the results quantified in terms of elements seen per high-power field. Important elements include:
   a. *White blood cells* (WBCs)–greater than 5 generally suggests infection.
   b. *Red blood cells* (RBCs)–normally not present; in the absence of menses, considerable numbers of RBCs may indicate infection, inflammation, or presence of tumor or stones.

c. *Casts*–presence of multiple casts suggests renal disease, either pyelonephritis or glomerulonephritis of some type.

In Case 4-3, a urinalysis could document pyuria (presence of WBCs), but the patient's symptoms are classic enough that the diagnosis is clearly likely and empiric
treatment could be recommended even in the absence of many white cells. Similarly, it
could show casts, but without fever or costovertebral angle (CVA) tenderness, the likelihood of ascending infection is vanishingly small. A high specific gravity may indicate that
the patient needs to increase her fluid intake, but this can be safely recommended without
the test results. Therefore, it is appropriate and acceptable to treat without the test. If
symptoms had not resolved as anticipated, or if any indications of more extensive infection developed, the patient would return and tests could be performed at that time.

This should not, however, be taken to infer that testing is never necessary for
assessment of urinary tract infections. If the patient in Case 4-3 had diabetes mellitus or a
history of structural abnormality in the urinary tract, she would be at increased risk for
complications, and testing would be important. Similarly, if symptoms included fever
and/or flank pain, the possibility of ascending infection would be more significant, and a
UA would be warranted to look for indications of this (i.e., the presence of casts). Every
patient and each incident must be considered individually.

Urine Culture

There are two common forms of urine cultures: the office screening culture and the
formal culture with sensitivities.

The office screening culture, also commonly called a dipslide, is a relatively inexpensive ($20), semiquantitative method of determining bacterial content in the urine. A small
plate coated with growth medium is dipped into the urine specimen and incubated for 24
hours. The density of colonies on the plate is then used to estimate the bacterial concentration, by visual comparison with illustrative photos. This provides evidence of the presence
of bacteria, but does not identify the organism(s) present, nor can it indicate the response
of these bacteria to specific drugs. The office culture is most useful when an equivocal UA
requires clarification, or as a test of cure after treatment.

In a formal urine culture with sensitivities, a measured amount of urine is plated on a
growth medium and incubated. Colonies are counted to provide quantitation of the bacterial concentration. These colonies are further tested and replated on various media to
identify the specific organism(s) present. Plating of the organism with various antibiotic-
containing disks allows measurement of the sensitivity of the organism to specific antibiotics. This more costly study ($35) is a necessary step in the care of high-risk patients
and those with recent antibiotic or hospital exposure, to rule out the presence of resistant
organisms that might not respond to the usual antibiotics used to treat urinary tract
infections (UTIs).

In Case 4-3, the patient is a healthy woman with no known risk factors for complications. In this situation, the vast majority (80%) of UTIs are caused by *Escherichia coli*
(Isselbacher *et al.,* 1994), a common intestinal organism, and therefore a urine culture is
unnecessary. This organism is typically responsive to a number of common antibiotics,
including trimethoprim–sulfamethoxazole, as was used in this case.

As noted earlier, however, differences in the patient's history and risk factors could
make more intensive evaluation necessary. If she had been diabetic or had a history of
complicated UTIs, UA and some form of culture would be appropriate. If she had been

recently hospitalized or catheterized for any reason, identification of the infecting organism and documentation of its sensitivity to the chosen antibiotic would be necessary.

CASE 4-4

A 12-year-old boy is brought in by his father, who reports that the child twisted his right ankle while playing basketball with friends yesterday. The child noted immediate pain and left the game; they used ice and Tylenol last night, but he's still unable to bear weight on the leg because of pain in the ankle. He is otherwise healthy, and has no history of significant injuries to this limb in the past. On examination, the right ankle shows substantial swelling and ecchymosis laterally, around and below the malleolus. The child reacts strongly to any palpation of the lateral malleolus or the areas adjacent to it. With coaxing, he demonstrates a limited range of motion in all directions, and will stand lightly on the foot, but cannot bear enough weight to walk on it. The physician orders an X-ray series of the right ankle (AP and lateral views), with contralateral views for comparison. These are negative for fracture; the initial diagnosis of second-degree ankle sprain is made. Treatment includes brief immobilization (3 days), ice, anti-inflammatory medication, and an exercise rehabilitation program.

Bone X Rays

Of course, appropriate use of laboratory tests does not always mean nonuse. Case 4-4 illustrates a situation in which X-ray studies of two joints are necessary for proper assessment of injury to only one joint.

In this case, the physician is faced with the determination of whether this child has sustained a soft-tissue injury or a fracture. The differentiation is important, since early mobilization is desirable for the former, but prolonged immobilization may be necessary for the latter. Simple X rays of the bones (i.e., "plane films") can clearly show the bony anatomy and clarify the presence or absence of fracture.

A complicating factor in this case is the age of the patient. Twelve-year-old boys have not yet reached full skeletal height, and thus have cartilaginous growth plates at the epiphyses of many bones. Since cartilage is radiolucent (i.e., allows X rays to pass through it), X rays cannot directly show injuries to growth plates. Views of the opposite (uninjured) limb are used for comparison, and growth plate injuries can be indirectly identified by asymmetries in the width of the lucent band and/or position of the bones on either side.

As always, a careful history and physical examination are necessary before the decision to order studies can be made. Several findings, if present, can indicate the increased likelihood of bony injury and should encourage consideration of radiographic study:

- Visible deformity of a limb or joint
- Tenderness that is greater over bone than over soft tissue
- Inability to bear weight (lower limbs)
- Pain out of proportion to apparent injury

These general principles have been more precisely delineated for ankle injuries in the Ottawa rules (Stiell *et al.*, 1994). In Case 4-4, both the bony tenderness and the child's inability to bear weight on the injured leg support the need for study.

Since growth plate injuries are difficult to identify by physical examination alone and can have significant impact on later growth, X rays are often important in evaluation of injuries in children. Once the growth plates have closed (age 16–18 in girls, 18–20 in boys), examination-based criteria are more important in determining whether radiographic studies are indicated.

X rays increase in importance again when evaluating injuries in patients at the other end of the age spectrum. In the elderly, osteoporosis or malignancy can lead to fractures with minimal or no causative trauma. In addition, the inflammatory response to bony injury is often less in the elderly than might be expected, so fractures may not be remarkable on physical examination except for tenderness. Therefore, physicians should have a lower threshold for ordering radiographic studies of injuries in the very old and the very young.

CASE 4-5

A 40-year-old male smoker is in for his third visit about upper abdominal pain. About 7 weeks ago he presented with a classic history of burning epigastric pain before meals and late at night, relieved with eating or antacids. Given his smoking, frequent use of ibuprofen, and moderate alcohol intake, the physician felt the pain was most likely acid-peptic in origin, and prescribed 6 weeks of H2 blocker therapy. The patient took his Zantac as prescribed, but did not decrease his use of cigarettes, ibuprofen, or alcohol. His pain disappeared as long as he took the medication, but returned promptly when he ran out of it last week.

At this point, the physician feels a study is warranted to determine if ulcers are indeed present, and to help guide choice of further therapy. He considers upper gastrointestinal (GI) endoscopy versus GI X-ray series, and discusses the options with the patient.

IS THERE A BETTER WAY TO GET THE INFORMATION?

The decision of which test is optimal is often a difficult one, without absolute right or wrong answers. As in this case, the alternatives are usually not equivalent, and the physician and patient must balance issues of cost and risk against the degree of accuracy and precision needed. In Case 4-5, the X-ray study and the endoscopy each have advantages and disadvantages, and the physician felt that neither was absolutely preferable over the other. Allowing the patient to make the choice is often the best course in this situation.

Consider each of these studies in more detail.

Radiographic Contrast Studies

The upper GI series is one of a class of radiographic studies that use a contrast medium to visualize the structures in question. Since soft tissues and organs are generally radiolucent, plane films without added contrast are of limited use in examining soft tissues. To expand on the information obtainable, radiopaque contrast media of various types can be injected or ingested before the films are taken. The X rays are blocked by the contrast, and thus the structures containing the contrast are clearly visible on the resulting films.

For an upper GI series, the patient drinks a contrast medium (usually containing barium), which allows the esophagus, stomach, and duodenum to be visualized. By using fluoroscopy, taking films with the patient in various positions, and compressing various structures by external pressure, the radiologist can examine the lining of these structures in fair detail, demonstrating the presence or absence of masses, ulcerations, or strictures.

While patients may complain about the chalky texture and taste of the contrast, this study is generally much less uncomfortable for the patient than an upper endoscopy. Its typical cost of $300 is also less than that of the fiber-optic study. However, this test also involves considerable X-ray exposure, which may be a long-term health risk, and its ability to detect ulcer disease (sensitivity; later in this chapter) is less than that of endoscopy.

Endoscopy

Upper endoscopy is the visual examination of the esophagus, stomach, and first segment of the duodenum by the use of a fiber-optic scope. The endoscope, a long flexible tubelike instrument about 2 cm in diameter, is introduced through the mouth and guided into the desired structures with direct visualization. This does not generally involve radiation, but often requires sedation to minimize patient discomfort from triggering of the gag reflex. The cost (approximately $800) is substantially greater than that of an upper GI series. The endoscope can be used to obtain biopsies and specimens to culture for *H. pylori,* which has been implicated in cases of recurrent ulcers.

Endoscopy can be used to examine many other organs. With scopes specifically designed for each, properly trained physicians may examine the sigmoid colon (sigmoidoscopy), the entire colon (colonoscopy), the lungs (bronchoscopy), the nasopharynx and larynx (nasopharyngoscopy), and the uterus (hysteroscopy). In addition to biopsies, some of these scopes allow removal of lesions in their entirety (e.g., colon polyps), eliminating the need for surgery. Developments in this field are ongoing, and the development of smaller scopes is rapidly expanding the possibilities for diagnosis and intervention.

None of these studies is without risk, however. Whenever a scope is introduced, there is risk of damage to the internal organs. Perforation of a hollow viscus is possible, especially if the wall is weakened by ulceration or tumor. This is a serious complication that often requires major surgery for repair.

In Case 4-5, the patient had multiple risk factors for duodenal ulceration, including his use of tobacco, alcohol, and ibuprofen. Thus, the physician did not feel strongly that biopsies or cultures were necessary. Either study would be likely to provide the desired information as to whether or not an ulcer was present. In skilled hands, the risks of the procedures are acceptable, though more acutely evident for the endoscopy. Since the physician cannot always predict patients' priorities in such a situation, it is appropriate to involve them in the decision. This patient, having heard a friend last year describe endoscopy as "the worst thing I've ever been through," was most concerned about potential discomfort, and opted for the radiographic study. The upper GI series showed a duodenal ulcer and no other abnormalities. With continued ranitidine, avoidance of ibuprofen, and efforts by the patient to discontinue alcohol and tobacco use, the symptoms resolved completely.

A thin 63-year-old woman comes in for a routine check of her hypertension. She takes 12.5 mg of hydrochlorothiazide daily, as she has for years, without any problems. Her blood pressure today is 130/84; she brings with her several outside readings with systolic levels of 124 to 138 mm Hg, and diastolics of 80 to 86. She also was tested for potassium level last week at the physician's request; the lab reports the result as 5.6 meq/liter (normal 3.5–5.0).

Since the elevated potassium level is completely unexpected, the physician decides to repeat the test. Knowing that changes in renal function can affect potassium levels, she decides to get a chemistry panel to check that also. The results come back in 2 days:

> *Sodium 144 meq/liter (normal 135–145)*
> *Potassium 4.0 meq/liter (normal 3.5–5.0)*
> *Chloride 100 meq/liter (normal 98–107)*
> *Creatinine 1.0 mg/dl (normal 0.6–1.2)*
> *BUN 18 mg/dl (normal 8–20)*
> *Glucose 103 mg/dl (normal 60–115)*

INTERPRETATION OF TEST RESULTS

When a physician decides to order a study, she must then analyze the results. This case illustrates important points to consider when interpreting test results:

1. Unexpected results may be mistakes
2. No test is perfect
3. Always consider results in the context of the specific patient

UNEXPECTED RESULTS MAY BE MISTAKES

The initially elevated potassium level of the patient in Case 4-6 is completely unexpected. Patients on diuretics such as hydrochlorothiazide lose potassium at a higher rate than normal. Without potassium supplements, elevated levels are highly unusual. Thus, the step of repeating the test is critical before any action is taken. The normal result on the second study is reassuring and within the range of expectation.

What is a "normal" test result? For most tests with numerical results, the normal range is defined statistically as a 95% confidence interval. That is, if a population of healthy people were tested, for tests with a normal statistical (bell-shaped) distribution of results, 95% of the results would fall within the designated "normal" range (plus/minus two standard deviations from the mean; see Figure 4.1). By definition, this means that 5% of the normal population will have results outside the range defined as normal. Therefore, not all values outside the normal range indicate pathology. This is most often true for results that are just outside the range in asymptomatic individuals. The physician must think carefully about any abnormal values and their relevance to the patient in question before deciding that they indicate a problem.

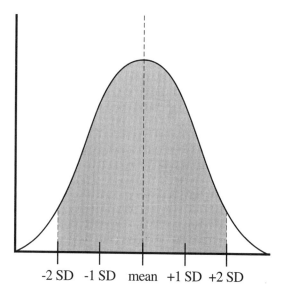

Figure 4.1. Bell-shaped distribution of normal results, illustrating 95% of values falling within two standard deviations (SD) of the mean.

What was the cause of the first result in Case 4-6? We may never know exactly, but there are several possibilities. Since the repeat test fell within the reference range, it is unlikely that this patient is one of those 5% at the extremes of the normal distribution. There may have been chemical error or artifact in the analysis. Specimens or results may have been mixed up with those of another patient. If the phlebotomy was difficult, there may have been hemolysis in the sample tube; since intracellular potassium levels are much higher than extracellular levels, hemolysis can cause significantly elevated results. Finally, the patient might have had a true but temporary rise in her potassium level, especially if she uses KCl-containing salt substitutes and missed a few doses of her medication. If careful history regarding diet and medication use makes the last of these unlikely, one can generally attribute the value to error or artifact.

In general, with the exception of emergency situations where time is of the essence, it is prudent to recheck unexpected results before making major decisions based on them. Most labs have protocols that require recheck or verification by dilution for substantially abnormal values; however, since that would not eliminate the chance of a contaminated or mislabeled specimen, it is often important to repeat the study on a new specimen as well.

Electrolytes

Electrolyte levels are very commonly ordered blood chemistry studies. These include the concentrations of sodium, potassium, chloride, and bicarbonate ions in the blood, usually the serum poured off a clotted specimen. These results can be used individually and in combination for a variety of purposes and calculations, which are beyond the scope of this chapter. Abnormal electrolyte levels can reflect dehydration, acid–base imbalances, and endocrine abnormalities.

Potassium levels are frequently affected by antihypertensive medications. Because of this, and the ion's critical role in cardiac physiology, monitoring of potassium levels is important for patients with cardiovascular disease on medications.

The set of electrolytes described here is an example of what is commonly referred to as a "panel." Specified lists of chemistry tests can be ordered in sets including as few as 2 or as many as 24 or more separate assays. The ordering convenience of these panels is tempting and has led to routine use of multichem panels for a variety of weak indications. In addition to the monetary cost of the panels themselves, these may lead to unexpected "abnormal" values requiring further assessment. Statistically, if 20 or more tests are performed on a normal individual, at least one result will fall outside the reference range and require further testing to determine its significance (or lack thereof). Thus, one should order only those tests necessary, and use caution in the selection of panels of tests.

BUN and Creatinine

The blood urea nitrogen (BUN) and creatinine levels are indirect measurements of renal function. Since both of these substances are waste products normally cleared by the kidneys, their blood levels rise when kidney function deteriorates. Normal kidneys have substantial excess capacity, however (a person can survive quite well with the functional capacity of less than half of one normal kidney); these tests do not become abnormal until renal function is greatly impaired. Other tests must be used to detect early stages of kidney impairment.

Loss of kidney function can affect a multitude of other blood chemistries, including potassium, calcium, phosphorus, and magnesium. As noted earlier, when serum potassium rises unexpectedly, it is reasonable to check BUN and creatinine levels to rule out renal failure as the cause.

CASE 4-7

A physician reviewing lab reports notices identical results for two of her patients.

Mr. Smith, a 50-year-old healthy white man, had requested a "blood test for prostate cancer" after reading a magazine article about it. Despite reassurances that his negative family history and other factors put him at low risk, he insisted, and the physician had agreed to order a prostate-specific antigen (PSA) level.

Mr. Jones, a 68-year-old healthy black man, had expressed concern about prostate cancer because his brother had recently died at age 71 of that disease. Since his race and family history placed him at high risk for prostate cancer, the physician had recommended PSA screening, and the patient agreed.

Both patients have PSA levels of 6 ng/ml (normal <4). Does this result have the same significance for both of these men?

NO TEST IS PERFECT

Every laboratory test has its own characteristics and limitations. No test is 100% accurate. As described in Case 4-6, even when perfectly performed, a test may indicate disease in a patient who is, in fact, normal (called a false-positive result). Similarly, a test may appear normal in a patient with disease (called a false-negative result). The frequency

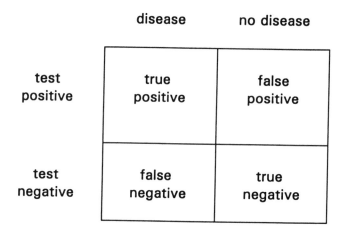

Figure 4.2. Structure of a 2 × 2 table of test results.

of these results is used to define certain epidemiologic terms that are essential in proper interpretation of test results.

Given two possible categories of test results (positive/abnormal and negative/normal) and the presence or absence of disease, all possible results from a single test can be placed in one of four cells in a 2 × 2 table, as illustrated in Figure 4.2. We will use this 2 × 2 table to define a few terms, and then apply them to Case 4-7.

Sensitivity and Specificity

Sensitivity describes the ability of a test to detect the disease in question. It is defined as the percentage of patients with the disease who correctly test positive. Using the 2 × 2 table in Figure 4.2,

$$\text{sensitivity} = \text{true positives}/(\text{true positives} + \text{false negatives})$$

A test with high sensitivity will miss few cases of disease (few false negatives).

Specificity is the percentage of patients without the disease who will correctly test negative. From the 2 × 2 table in Figure 4.2, it is calculated as

$$\text{specificity} = \text{true negatives}/(\text{true negatives} + \text{false positives})$$

A test with high specificity will rarely give an abnormal result in the absence of disease (few false positives).

Sensitivity and specificity are characteristics of the test assay itself. Obviously, it is desirable to have tests with both high sensitivity and high specificity. Because of practical limitations, that is not always possible. Improving sensitivity often results in a decrease in specificity, and vice versa. For example, the distribution of PSA results may be illustrated as in Figure 4.3.

The selection of the cutoff point for the upper limit of normal determines the sensitivity and specificity of the test. If point A is used, very few patients with disease are missed (those to the left of the cutoff), so the sensitivity is high. This is achieved, however, at the cost of including a large number of patients without disease (to the right of

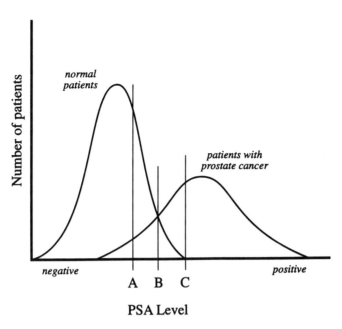

Figure 4.3. Hypothetical distribution of PSA results in patients with and without disease.

the cutoff), which lowers the specificity. Specificity can be raised to 100% by using point C at the cutoff, but then many patients with disease will be missed, lowering the sensitivity. Usually a point in between (such as point B) is used, allowing a limited number of both false positives and false negatives.

For current PSA tests, using a cutoff of 4 ng/ml, sensitivity is estimated at 73%, while specificity is about 91% (Gann *et al.*, 1995).

Predictive Value

In clinical situations, even more important than sensitivity and specificity is the concept of predictive value. Faced with an abnormal test result, the physician needs to know the likelihood that the patient truly has disease. Similarly, when results are normal, the provider needs to know the likelihood that the patient is truly disease-free. These likelihoods depend on the prevalence of the disease (the number of persons with the disease) in the population being tested.

Positive predictive value (PPV) is the probability that a person has the disease, given a positive test result. From the 2 × 2 table in Figure 4.2, this is calculated as

PPV = true positives/(true positives + false positives)

Negative predictive value (NPV), then, is the probability that, given a negative result, the patient is free from disease. This is calculated as

NPV = true negatives/(true negatives + false negatives)

Let us return to Case 4-7 to see how these are affected by disease prevalence.

	prostate cancer	no cancer	Total
PSA positive (>4)	14,600	7,200	21,800
PSA negative (<4)	5,400	72,800	78,200
Total	20,000	80,000	100,000

Figure 4.4. Hypothetical 2 × 2 table for PSA screening of prostate cancer in a low-risk population.

Mr. Smith is in a low-risk group for prostate cancer. Available prevalence data are limited, because determination of absolute values would require biopsy or autopsy results on a large asymptomatic population. It has been estimated that latent, microscopic prostate cancer is present in at least 30% of all men over age 50 (Gann *et al.*, 1995); however, prevalence data for specific population groups are not available. For the purpose of illustration, let us assume that the prevalence in a group of men comparable to Mr. Smith (white 50-year-olds without family histories of prostate cancer) is approximately 20%. Using the sensitivity and specificity estimates given above, the hypothetical 2 × 2 table shown in Figure 4.4 can be constructed for this population.

The positive predictive value of Mr. Smith's PSA result is 67.0%. On the other hand, the negative predictive value of a normal result in this population is 93.1%. In low-risk populations, the test is much more able to correctly predict the absence of prostate cancer than its presence.

Mr. Jones is in a high-risk group, given his race and family history. If we assume a prevalence of 50%, the hypothetical 2 × 2 table for this population is as shown in Figure 4.5.

	prostate cancer	no cancer	Total
PSA positive (>4)	36,500	4,500	41,000
PSA negative (<4)	13,500	45,500	59,000
Total	50,000	50,000	100,000

Figure 4.5. Hypothetical 2 × 2 table for PSA screening in a high-risk population.

value of a normal result would be 77.1%. In a high-risk population, a test is better able to rule in disease than exclude it.

The use of PPV and NPV illustrates the importance of careful consideration of disease likelihood before deciding to order a study. If the prevalence of the disease is very low, even a good test will more often give false-positive than true-positive results.

CASE 4-8

A 27-year-old type I diabetic patient has been hospitalized for cellulitis of the left forearm resulting from a cat bite. At his initial presentation, he had a temperature of 39°C; his WBC count was 19.8 thousand/mm³ (normal 5–10) with 32% bands on manual differential. After 2 days of IV antibiotics, he is afebrile, and the swelling and erythema are much decreased. Repeat blood count shows WBCs 15.4 thousand/mm³ with a differential of 87% polys, 2% bands, 10% lymphs, and 1% monos. His fasting glucose is 135 mg/dl (normal 60–115), in comparison with 312 mg/dl at admission.

CONSIDER RESULTS IN THE CONTEXT OF THE PATIENT

All test results must be interpreted in the context of the clinical situation of the particular patient being tested. In Case 4-6, the patient's medication history made the initially elevated potassium level unbelievable, and the repeat level confirmed the clinician's suspicions. In Case 4-8, the second set of WBC and glucose results, while clearly outside the normal range, signify a substantial *improvement* for this patient. These cases illustrate the importance of considering the clinical situation and the patient's past lab values in interpreting results.

Case 4-8 illustrates the importance of looking at trends rather than isolated values. A WBC count of 15.4 is well above normal, and could be worrisome, especially for a diabetic patient. A clinician seeing this result for a patient on IV antibiotics could become concerned about the effectiveness of the drug treatment. However, in comparison with the result of 19.8 two days earlier, this actually shows substantial improvement and confirms that the treatment is working well. Similarly, while the fasting glucose of 135 is higher than desirable, it is much better than the previous level of over 300.

Complete Blood Count

The complete blood count (CBC) is a set of counts and measurements of blood cells of various types. This analysis is generally performed by an instrument called a Coulter counter. While the specific values provided may differ slightly between institutions, all CBCs generally include:

1. *White blood cell count* (WBC)—the number of white blood cells, in thousands per cubic millimeter (normal 5–10). Elevated values generally indicate infection or some other stressed state. Abnormally low values may occur with immunosuppressed states.
2. *Red blood cell count* (RBC)—the number of red blood cells in millions per cubic millimeter. Because women lose blood monthly with menses, the reference

range for this and several other blood measurements is determined by gender (normal 4.5–6 for men, 4–5.5 for women). The RBC count can be helpful in assessment of anemia, but is used less often than the following two values.

3. *Hemoglobin* (Hgb)—the concentration of hemoglobin in grams per deciliter of whole blood (normal 14–18 for men, 12–16 for women). This is below normal in anemia and hemoglobinopathies.

4. *Hematocrit* (Hct)—the percentage of blood volume filled by red blood cells (normal 40–54 for men, 37–47 for women). This can be determined without a Coulter counter by centrifuging a small tube of blood and comparing the height of the RBC column to the total height of the fluid in the tube. This is an important value in assessment of anemia and blood loss.

5. *Mean cell volume* (MCV)—the average volume of RBCs in the sample (normal 80–100 fl). Cells are abnormally small in iron deficiency, lead poisoning, and hemoglobinopathies (e.g., sickle cell, thalassemia, hereditary spherocytosis). Heavy smoking, alcoholism, and vitamin deficiencies can increase cell size.

6. *Mean cell hemoglobin* (MCH)—the average amount of hemoglobin in each RBC, in picograms. This is influenced by both the size of the cell and the concentration of hemoglobin inside it.

7. *Mean cellular hemoglobin concentration* (MCHC)—the average concentration of hemoglobin in the RBCs, in grams per liter. This and the MCH are decreased in iron deficiency, hemoglobinopathies, and other states impairing hemoglobin synthesis.

8. *Platelets*—the number of these tiny cells, in thousands per cubic millimeter. Since these are the shortest-lived of all blood cells, platelet counts are often a reflection of bone marrow activity; they can fall during acute illness, and rebound thereafter. If they get extremely low, the risk of bleeding is increased.

An adjunct to the CBC that is often requested with it is a "differential"—a delineation of the proportions of the different types of WBCs present. While automated estimates are available, most physicians prefer a manually performed count, since current technology does not allow the same precision in automated counts. Proportions of specific cell types may help in interpretation of abnormal WBC counts, or show infection even in the presence of a normal total number of WBCs. Reference ranges vary by age; normal values shown below are for adults.

1. *Segmented neutrophils* (polys or segs)—normally 37–80% of the total; increases in the percentage of these cells suggest bacterial infection.

2. *Band neutrophils* (bands)—an immature form, normally not seen in peripheral blood except in the presence of infection or stress.

3. *Lymphocytes* (lymphs)—normally 10–50%; increases suggest viral infection.

4. *Monocytes* (monos)—normally 0–12%.

5. *Eosinophils* (eos)—normally 0–7%; may be increased in allergic states.

6. *Basophils* (basos)—normal cells usually seen in small numbers (0–1%).

7. *Other immature forms,* such as myelocytes, metamyelocytes, and blasts, may be seen in leukemias or perhaps in times of extreme physiologic stress.

In Case 4-8, the presence of a large number of bands in the first blood count indicates the presence of severe infection. While some bands are still present in the follow-up count, the decrease in their proportion reassures us that the treatment is effective, and the patient is improving.

99

CASES FOR DISCUSSION

Glucose

The blood glucose (BG) is perhaps the most frequently used chemistry test. Elevated glucose is the hallmark of diabetes mellitus, and this test is used in both the diagnosis of this disease and the monitoring of known diabetic patients. It may be performed on venous blood using a laboratory chemistry analyzer. Patients may also monitor their own levels at home using an electronic glucometer; these utilize colorimetric reactions from a drop of blood, obtained by fingerstick, on a test strip to provide reasonably precise measurements of whole blood glucose levels. While the fingerstick measurements are less reliable than venous blood testing, the convenience and capability of monitoring at multiple times each day make this test an essential part of modern diabetes management.

Glucose values in a single individual vary greatly over the course of the day, based on timing in relation to oral intake; therefore, it is best measured in the morning after an overnight fast. In Case 4-8, the patient's first fasting glucose was dramatically elevated, as a result of the acute infection. As the infection improved, so did his fasting BG, though it was still higher than desired at the second testing.

CONCLUSIONS

Appropriate use of laboratory tests requires consideration of the characteristics of each individual patient and of the tests in question. In selection of laboratory tests and other studies, always make certain that whatever you choose will make a difference in the patient's care, and be sure that the test is the optimal (including most cost-effective) choice for your purpose. In interpretation of results, be aware of test and population characteristics that influence the reliability, accuracy, and meaning of the results. Finally, before acting on results, always be sure they correlate with the clinical situation.

CASES FOR DISCUSSION

CASE 1

A 12-year-old girl is brought in by her mother, who reports that her daughter is complaining of a sore throat. The child has had a runny nose and sore throat for 3 days, and she seems to be feeling a bit worse today. She's been drinking fluids well, but solid food is uncomfortable to swallow. The child is otherwise healthy, and has no significant chronic or past illnesses. On examination she has a temperature of 99.7°F; her throat is red but the remainder of the results of her examination are normal. The mother expresses concern that this might be strep throat.

1. *What possible diagnoses are you considering?*
2. *What tests might be used? What are the pros and cons of each?*
3. *If your suspicion of strep is low, which test is best suited to reassuring the mother?*

CASE 2

An 88-year-old woman is brought in by her husband because she's "not feeling well." The woman says that for the past 2 days she's felt tired and not very hungry, but she can't define any more specific symptoms. Her husband says she's also not thinking quite as clearly as usual, being a little more forgetful. She's generally a remarkably healthy woman. She's on no medications except a multivitamin. Her chart indicates she's been treated in the past 5 years for one episode of pneumonia, and one UTI. Physical examination is unrevealing, except that she doesn't look quite as well as she usually does.

1. *What possible diagnoses are you considering?*
2. *What tests might be helpful?*
3. *Urinary tract infections are a very common cause of general decline in elderly women, and don't always present with symptoms relative to the urinary tract. How might this change your approach?*
4. *Is a urine culture indicated in this case? If so, are full identification of the infecting organism and sensitivities needed?*

CASE 3

A 23-year-old male comes in reporting that he twisted his knee playing soccer yesterday. While running, he attempted to make a sharp turn, and had immediate pain and a single pop in his right knee. He had to stop playing, and went home and put ice on it. This morning it's swollen and hurts to bend, and he can only walk with a limp. He's never had trouble with the knee before.

1. *What possible diagnoses are you considering? Which are most likely?*
2. *Will plane films help to differentiate between the likely diagnoses?*
3. *What physical examination findings might make you want X rays of the knee?*
4. *Might other radiographic studies be helpful?*

CASE 4

Two patients come in independently requesting HIV tests. The first is a 34-year-old married woman, who has told you previously that she's used some IV drugs in the past and had multiple sexual partners before getting married. The second is the same age and also married; she and her husband each had one prior partner before their marriage, and neither has a drug history. Neither woman has any symptoms, nor have they been tested for HIV before.

1. *How would you classify the risk levels of these two patients? What other information might you need?*
2. *What tests are currently used to test for HIV? What is known about their sensitivity and specificity?*
3. *Before ordering the tests, what would you discuss with the patients about interpretation of the results?*
4. *Both results are negative. How might your discussion of this differ between the two patients?*

CASE 5

A 69-year-old man presents reporting he had several episodes of visible blood in his stool about a week ago. This was painless and not associated with any other symptoms. It has now resolved and his bowel movements are normal. He's had hemorrhoids before, but notes that this bleeding was different. Neither he nor his family have any history of colon cancer or polyps, but he is overweight and doesn't eat a very healthy diet.

1. *What diagnoses are you considering?*
2. *What studies could help in determining the cause of the bleeding? What are their risks and costs?*
3. *Assuming his physical examination is negative, how might you proceed?*

———— RECOMMENDED READINGS ————

Detmer WM, Nicoll D: Diagnostic testing and medical decision-making, in Tierney LM, McPhee SJ, Papadakis MA (ed): *Current Medical Diagnosis and Treatment.* Norwalk, CT, Appleton & Lange, 1994.

Clear, brief review of uses and interpretation of diagnostic tests, with additional information on therapeutic drug monitoring.

Grossman ZD, Katz DS, Santelli ED, *et al: Cost-Effective Diagnostic Imaging: The Clinician's Guide,* ed 3. St. Louis, MO, CV Mosby Co, 1995.

A concise and usable discussion of appropriate selection of radiographic studies, with cost information. While the authors occasionally recommend studies in situations with low likelihood of findings, they otherwise promote a very rational approach.

Mulley AG: The selection and interpretation of diagnostic tests, in *Primary Care Medicine: Office Evaluation and Management of the Adult Patient,* ed 3. Philadelphia, JB Lippincott Co, 1995.

A concise review of the necessary epidemiologic principles and their application in determining and revising diagnostic probabilities.

Sox HC Jr (ed): *Common Diagnostic Tests: Use and Interpretation,* ed 2. Philadelphia, American College of Physicians, 1990.

More detailed discussion of specific tests, with ACP guidelines for their use in both inpatient and outpatient settings. Chapters by Shapiro and Greenfield (on CBCs), Komaroff (on UAs and cultures), and Beck and Kassirer (on electrolytes, BUN, creatinine) are particularly relevant.

CHAPTER 5

Making a Diagnosis

John P. Langlois

CASE 5-1 (Part I)

Dr. Nolan, a family physician in private practice, began using her diagnostic skills almost as soon as she awoke. At 6:00 AM the hospital called telling her that Mr. Ingle, a 64-year-old patient on the telemetry unit who had been diagnosed with a myocardial infarction yesterday afternoon, was having an unusual cardiac rhythm that the nurses were having trouble interpreting. After a few quick questions to assess that the patient had a stable blood pressure and no signs of shock and to be sure that supportive measures of oxygen and intravenous fluids were in place, she ordered an electrocardiogram (ECG) and headed for the hospital. During the 10-minute ride she reviewed in her mind the diagnostic possibilities. On arrival she found a stable patient with a rapid heart rhythm (tachycardia) with a wide complex on the ECG. Through an organized and stepwise approach she was able to correctly diagnose and treat Mr. Ingle's ventricular tachycardia, while arranging for his transfer to the intensive care unit. After a quick breakfast she completed her hospital rounds, including a complete history and physical on a new patient admitted with abdominal pain.

After a hectic start to the day Dr. Nolan has a full schedule at the office. She was 30 minutes late getting to the office, but has made up a little time on her first 3 patients: an OB recheck at 38 weeks, a truck driver with hypertension, and a child with a fever and otitis media. She has an additional 9 patients on her morning schedule and 14 for the afternoon. She takes a deep breath and prepares to see her next patient.

─────────── **EDUCATIONAL OBJECTIVES** ───────────

After completion of this chapter and the accompanying exercises the student will be able to:

1. Identify and describe the basic characteristics of four diagnostic methods—exhaustive, algorithmic, pattern recognition, and hypothetico-deductive
2. List the major steps in the hypothetico-deductive approach to clinical reasoning
3. Identify several pitfalls and optimizing strategies for each step
4. Define the concept of differential diagnosis and discuss its usefulness

─────────── **INTRODUCTION** ───────────

Clinical practice presents a challenge of a widely varying spectrum of patients and problems with which to deal. Behind each door is an unknown, a question in search of an answer, and before the door is opened, the possibilities of what that answer will be are nearly endless. The patient may present for a simple health maintenance visit or with symptoms suggesting an acute myocardial infarction, a simple cold, or a complication of AIDS. In addition, the first-contact physician often sees diseases present for the first time and in their earliest and most confusing stages. It is in the "front line" trenches of patient care that well-developed skills for making an efficient and accurate diagnosis are essential, as in Case 5-1. A practicing physician is continually challenged to use every technique available to make the correct diagnosis for her patient.

There are a number of techniques that physicians use to arrive at the correct diagnosis (Curtis, 1993). One technique that is often taught early in medical school is the *exhaustive* method, where every possible question is asked and every available piece of data is collected and organized to help arrive at the diagnosis. In Case 5-1, Dr. Nolan's admission history and physical included the components of a complete workup—chief complaint, history of present illness, past medical history, current medications, allergies, family history, social history, review of systems, vital signs, complete physical, laboratory values, X-ray results, assessment, and plan. Although this degree of completeness is important for the hospitalized patient, she does not have the luxury of time or the energy to be able to employ that method for every patient on today's schedule.

A second method is the *algorithmic* method. In this approach, the decision options are already laid out based on a proven strategy. The physician then follows the steps making decisions at preselected branch points, based on the clinical data available. Dr. Nolan used this method this morning in assessing and caring for Mr. Ingle by following an Advanced Cardiac Life Support (ACLS) algorithm for tachycardia (Figure 5.1) that she had learned in her residency. Unfortunately, algorithms have not yet been developed for all medical problems, and many presentations are too complex to lend themselves well to this approach.

A third diagnostic method is *pattern recognition.* In this technique a pattern of clues or clinical characteristics trigger a memory response in the physician of something that he had seen or learned previously. Dr. Nolan used this technique when she recognized a brown rash on the cheeks and forehead of her pregnant patient as melasma, a skin change

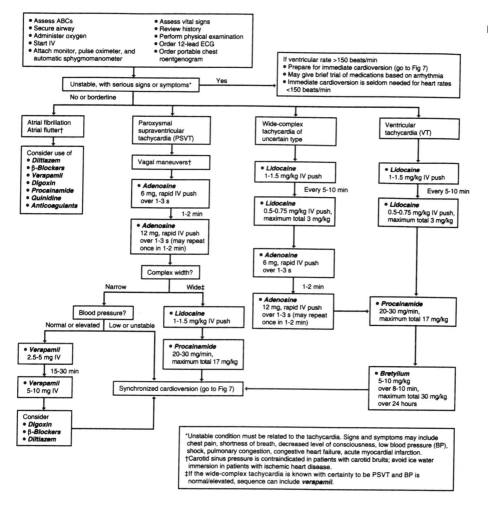

Figure 5.1. Tachycardia algorithm, from Emergency Cardiac Care Committee and Subcommittees, American Heart Association. Guidelines for cardiopulmonary resuscitation and emergency cardiac care, III. Adult advanced cardiac life support. *JAMA* 268:2223, 1992.

related to the increased estrogen level in pregnancy. Pattern recognition takes considerable clinical experience, and often the clues are partial and may be too incomplete to trigger awareness of the pattern.

The technique that is used most often by physicians is the *hypothetico-deductive* method. In this method, clues and hunches are used in a systematic way to guide a focused inquiry and the development of a rank-ordered list of hypotheses. This list is known as a differential diagnosis or "diff." The method consists of a series of steps, some of which occur essentially simultaneously (see Figure 5.2). Each of these steps has distinct characteristics, potential pitfalls, and possible shortcuts. By optimizing each step, avoiding the pitfalls, and taking advantage of any shortcuts, the physician can arrive efficiently and accurately at the correct diagnosis.

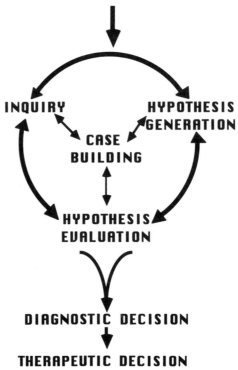

INITIAL CLUES/ INITIAL HUNCHES

INQUIRY

HYPOTHESIS GENERATION

CASE BUILDING

HYPOTHESIS EVALUATION

DIAGNOSTIC DECISION

THERAPEUTIC DECISION

Figure 5.2. Schematic of the steps in the hypothetico-deductive process.

The systematic but problem-focused nature of the hypothetico-deductive method particularly lends itself to the primary care setting, where the population and their potential medical issues represent a broad spectrum of problems. Diagnosis of these "undifferentiated patients," who are not preselected into an organ-specific clinic population, requires a high level of diagnostic skill. The purpose of this chapter is to review in detail the characteristics, pitfalls, and shortcuts in each step of this approach to making the diagnosis, in order to help you to be a more efficient, accurate, and skillful diagnostician.

CASE 5-1 (Part II)

The next patient is a 58-year-old woman named Betty with a complaint of "cough" as recorded by the nurse. Vital signs are recorded as: temperature 100.2°F orally, blood pressure 138/92 mm Hg, pulse rate 60 beats per minute, and 20 respirations per minute. While reviewing the chart outside the door, Dr. Nolan hears a persistent cough. As she enters the room she sees a tired-looking woman who has just finished a spasm of coughing. She has already begun the diagnostic process and has developed some initial hunches to help direct and focus her approach to making the correct diagnosis.

Even before Dr. Nolan has asked Betty a single question she has used available clues and observations to form initial hypotheses that focus and organize her approach. Before obtaining these early data, the diagnostic possibilities were nearly endless. Now the clinician has an initial list of possibilities. Although not all clinicians will admit to forming hunches quite this early in the encounter (before the patient is seen), forming hunches occurs very early and guides further steps in the reasoning process. Table 5.1 outlines the characteristics, pitfalls, and shortcuts of this first step in the hypothetico-deductive method.

Isn't the clinician "jumping to conclusions" by forming a list of diagnoses before laying eyes on the patient? Jumping to conclusions is a potential pitfall in this step of the diagnostic process. If the clinician places too much value on a single diagnosis and he is unwilling to consider other options, this will subvert the diagnostic process. An example of premature closure is when a physician, during a flu epidemic, assumes that a patient with a fever and achiness automatically has the flu and is unwilling to consider or to look for evidence of other possibilities, such as pneumonia or pyelonephritis. These initial hunches must be flexible and expendable as the situation requires. Note that the plural *hunches* is always used. By developing more than one initial hunch, you automatically make it difficult to become overly focused on one idea.

Initial clues can be misleading. Early in the diagnostic process the clinician must be alert and be prepared to change his approach. For example, a male patient may be embarrassed to tell the female nurse that the true reason for his visit is sexual dysfunction, and may instead give "headache" as a chief complaint. Beginning the visit with an open question such as, "What brings you to the office today?" may elicit the patient's true agenda.

It is imperative that the clinician clarify the reason for coming into the office, but, at times, the patient's stated reason for coming may not seem to make sense. If the patient has had mild, occasional headaches for 6 months, why has he come to the office today? In these situations it may be useful to ask yourself, "Why now?" The patient may recently have learned of a coworker who has been diagnosed with a brain tumor. The terminology used by the patient can be misleading. A patient's idea of "diarrhea" may be very different from the medical definition, and your diagnostic approach must vary accordingly.

Table 5.1
Initial Clues/Initial Hunches

Characteristics
  Early information leads to very early hypotheses
  Involves initial rapid focusing
  Gives initial direction to encounter
Pitfalls
  Premature closure
  Failure to recognize patients' true reason for seeking medical care
  Failure to clarify initial confusion (e.g., "What do you mean by 'diarrhea'"?)
Shortcuts
  Always generate more than one initial hunch
  Clarify chief complaint
  Ask yourself, "Why now?"

Numerous potential pitfalls in this stage of the diagnostic process can be avoided by working at being clear and accurate about the reason why the patient is presenting. At this point, the clinician should have more than one early diagnostic "hunch" that will direct the next steps in the diagnostic process.

CASE 5-1 (Part III)

Dr. Nolan's initial hunches about Betty's illness are bronchitis versus reactive airway disease. After confirming the patient's chief complaint of "cough," she questions the patient about her recent history. The patient reports that she began getting sick about 10 days ago. At first she thought it was a chest cold that would pass, but it has not gotten better. The cough is nonproductive (no phlegm), "hacking," and seems to be worse at night when she lies down. She has tried a humidifier and cough medicine but they don't seem to help. Initially there was some nasal congestion but this resolved after 2 days. The patient states she has noticed some wheezing and that her chest feels tight. She does not have a history of asthma or allergies. No one at home has been sick but several people at the office have been sick with similar symptoms. Their illness did not last this long. When asked if there are any other symptoms associated with this illness, the patient reports that her feet have been swelling a little more than usual. The patient speaks in short but complete sentences. Dr. Nolan notices a smell of tobacco smoke and a quick glance at the chart reveals a history of hypertension for which the patient is taking captopril, 50 mg twice a day, an angiotensin converting enzyme (ACE) inhibitor.

THE DIAGNOSTIC CYCLE

It is at this point that the clinical reasoning process appears to become very complex and to appear almost random and haphazard. The concept of a stepwise, definable process seems to break down. The reason for this apparent chaos is that several steps are occurring almost simultaneously. Once a question is asked (inquiry), the answer is used to evaluate the existing hunches (hypothesis testing). In addition, the answers to the questions can generate additional possibilities (hypothesis generation). These hypotheses bring new questions to mind and the cycle continues. At the same time, the clinician is modifying her differential diagnostic list as well as generating an abbreviated summary of the clinically relevant history (case building). The result is a series of interdependent events occurring rapidly (see Figure 5.1) and, in some experienced physicians, nearly subconsciously. Although it may seem confusing when taken as a whole, by analyzing each component individually, a method for understanding and optimizing each step will become clear.

INQUIRY

With the first question a cascade of events is started, initially guided by the starting hunches (see Table 5.2). There are specific strategies and types of questions that are employed. A *search* strategy employs questions that are aimed toward obtaining specific information. During initial questioning, Dr. Nolan was obtaining specific information on

Table 5.2

Inquiry

Characteristics
  Guided by hypotheses
  Two techniques of inquiry that give initial direction to encounter:
    1. Search—seeking additional data to support or refute existing hypotheses
    2. Scan—randomly or routinely ordered questions to explore further
Pitfalls
  Limited focus on one hypothesis
  Too much random or routine choice of items
  Rigidity of style or approach
Shortcuts
  Gather data in blocks, a series of questions that clarify a complaint
  Choose and develop high-yield questions
  Be flexible in approach, e.g., do early physical for complaint of rash

---

the present illness by means of an organized approach. A look back at the case will show that she obtained information on the following areas of importance related to the symptom of cough: duration, quality, exacerbating or relieving factors, therapeutic attempts, and associated symptoms. This was not accidental, but a deliberate attempt to obtain as complete an understanding of the primary symptom by intentionally asking questions on the short list of symptom characteristics she felt was relevant. The list of relevant issues may vary depending on the type of symptom. For example, a list for a complaint of pain might include: duration, quality, location, radiation, exacerbating/relieving factors, therapeutic attempts. Note that this list could be used for any type of pain—chest pain, head pain, foot pain—and that not every clinician's approach need be exactly the same. The systematic gathering of a block of needed information can make processing of the data easier and makes it less likely that an important facet of the history will be missed.

A *scan* strategy is also used. The purpose of this inquiry is to explore other clues or hypotheses that have not been brought to light by more focused questions. Scan strategies include random exploration of other systems, or a more ordered but routine "review of systems" approach to questioning. Open-ended questions can be useful in scanning for additional information. Dr. Nolan asks the vague question, "Have you noticed any other symptoms that we haven't discussed yet?" and learns about the foot swelling, a new clue that may be important.

HYPOTHESIS TESTING

The majority of Dr. Nolan's questions in Case 5-1, Part III, were of the "search" type. This is characteristic of a mature and efficient reasoning style. The questions asked are carefully thought-out and designed to clarify important points of the history and to "test" the existing hypotheses. When we think of tests in medicine, we are quick to think of laboratory tests or imaging studies. It is important to remember that questions are tests and have similar characteristics of sensitivity, specificity, and predictive value. The questions that you ask of patients are the principal means you have to evaluating and ordering your hypotheses to make the correct diagnosis of your patient.

With what questions did Dr. Nolan begin to evaluate her initial hypotheses? Even her initial series of questions, which clarified the details of the chief complaint, provided

Table 5.3
Hypothesis Testing

Characteristics
  Each question is a test of existing hypotheses
  There are several strategies for hypothesis testing:
    1. Confirmation—presence of finding supports disease
    2. Elimination—absence of usually present finding goes against presence of disease
    3. Discrimination—discriminates between two or more hypotheses
    4. Exploration—a search for evidence of the disease in other systems
Pitfalls
  Inaccurate data
  Overreliance on the weight of evidence
Shortcuts
  Use carefully selected high-yield questions
  Consider and optimize the accuracy of the data

clinical information that will help in ordering hypotheses. For example, the 10-day duration of the illness makes a pure viral process less likely. This protracted time course and the nonproductive nature of the cough diminish the likelihood of a typical bacterial process, such as a pneumococcal infection. After getting these initial data, she focuses on the hypotheses she has developed by asking questions related directly to reactive airway disease or asthma and infectious causes or exposures. Table 5.3 outlines the characteristics of the hypothesis testing process.

Questions can be used in several ways to evaluate hypotheses, each involving a different strategy (Kassirer & Gorry, 1978). In the strategy of *confirmation,* a question is used to elicit *a finding that supports the disease.* An example is to ask about exertional chest pain to evaluate the possibility of stable angina, the presence of which supports the diagnosis of stable angina.

A second strategy is *elimination,* where *the absence of a finding goes against the presence of a disease.* The same example of chest pain can be used: If exertional chest discomfort is not reported, then stable angina is less likely. Note that the phrase "less likely" is used. Just as there are false-negative lab test results, there are few answers to medical questions that are 100% sure. It is best to base your decisions on several corroborating factors.

A third strategy for hypothesis testing is *discrimination.* In this approach, the answer to *a question can discriminate between two or more hypotheses.* A very useful "discriminating" strategy in the patient complaining of "dizziness" is to differentiate "light-headedness" from true vertigo. One approach is to ask, "Does the room seem to spin around during these episodes, such that you have to hang onto something to keep from falling?" (If the patient can tell you which direction the room is "spinning," that is even more convincing!). Determining that the patient's dizziness is true vertigo results in a very different list of possible hypotheses from a symptom of light-headedness or near syncope.

A fourth questioning strategy is *exploration,* where the goal is to *search for evidence present in other organ systems that may support the hypothesis.* In a patient who presents with a complaint of fatigue, the hypothesis of hypothyroidism may be considered. Proper evaluation of this hypothesis will involve exploration of many organ systems, asking about skin changes, changes in voice, excessive menstrual flow, constipation, and so forth.

A number of disease processes may have a primary symptom involving one organ system, but additional supporting findings may be revealed when other systems are explored.

Hypothesis testing does have its pitfalls. The most common is inaccurate data. Both patient and laboratory may unintentionally mislead the clinician. As a result, it is wise to use a variety of strategies in evaluating your hypotheses. Sometimes the weight of evidence can seem greater than it is in reality when two or more tests demonstrate the same finding. An example from radiology may illustrate this point best. A patient with abdominal pain is shown to have gallstones on an ultrasound study. The diagnosis of cholecystitis (gallbladder inflammation) as the cause of the pain is not made more likely if the gallstones are also seen on an abdominal CT scan, as both studies only reveal the same data by a different technique. Evidence of a blocked duct and inability to visualize the gallbladder on a nuclear medicine study does give new information and lends additional support to the diagnosis. A large number of positive tests, or a number of positive answers to similar questions, may not lend additional support to the hypothesis if they reveal the same information in a different way.

All questions are not created equal. As seen in the examples here, some questions have a very high yield of useful information. A single, well-asked, carefully selected "high-yield" question can dramatically change your differential diagnosis list. Learning high-yield approaches that have worked for others and developing your own list of quality questions to use in commonly encountered clinical situations will improve your diagnostic efficiency. In addition, well-developed interviewing and interpersonal skills will improve the sensitivity and specificity of your questions.

HYPOTHESIS GENERATION

At the same time that questions are being asked, and hypotheses are being tested, new data result in the generation of new hypotheses (see Table 5.4). Any question has the potential to both evaluate and generate hypotheses simultaneously. Dr. Nolan asked about other symptoms associated with Betty's illness in Case 5-1, Part III, and got a history of foot swelling, raising the new hypothesis of congestive heart failure (CHF), which can present with coughing and wheezing. This would be an important diagnosis not to miss

Table 5.4
Hypothesis Generation

Characteristics
    Additional data lead to new hypotheses
    Data are only clues when their significance is recognized
    Data may come from many sources
Pitfalls
    Missing key clues
    Not developing a broad enough differential
    Familiarity can cloud vision
Shortcuts
    Use all sources of available data
    Learn and watch for key clues
    Be alert for familiarity bias and other biases
    Use differential diagnosis broadening tools, when needed

since CHF would not be expected to go away on its own or to respond to treatment for reactive airway disease or bronchitis.

Hypotheses may be generated by clues other than responses to questions. During a medical encounter, the physician is being literally bombarded with information such as sights, sounds, smells, emotional affect, body language, and so on. Dr. Nolan made a note of the patient's speech pattern as a manifestation of difficulty breathing at rest. Also, the smell of tobacco smoke raises the hypothesis that an exacerbation of an underlying chronic obstructive pulmonary disease (COPD) may be the cause of the patient's symptoms. One side effect of an ACE inhibitor is a cough, so another hypothesis is generated from a new source.

Valuable sources of clues, and hence hypotheses, may be overlooked at times. In fact, medical students are often concentrating so hard on the next question that much of these valuable data are missed. Experienced clinicians may be so adept at using these data that they occur nearly automatically and are incorporated into their thinking without their conscious awareness. Cultivating and practicing an awareness of these other clues is a valuable clinical tool.

As with the other steps in this clinical reasoning process, there are potential pitfalls in the hypothesis generation step. Never generating the hypothesis that is the correct diagnosis is the end result of these pitfalls. Missing key clues is one pitfall. The significance of an essential bit of information may not be apparent to the inexperienced clinician who has not yet learned that "flashing lights" may be a warning symptom of an impending migraine or of a tear in the retina. Key clues for common and important diseases can be learned and their use in generating hypotheses practiced by producing broad differential diagnosis lists.

Failure to produce a broad enough differential is another pitfall. But how can you tell when it is broad enough, or how can you work to make it broader when you have run out of questions and ideas? There are a number of strategies that can help when you need to broaden your differential (see Table 5.5). An anatomical approach to the cause of a problem may be useful (Byyny & Adams, 1981), using your knowledge of the anatomy of the symptomatic area and the diseases of those structures to help broaden your differential. For example, if the complaint is right upper quadrant abdominal pain, you can start with skin problems that might cause pain (such as early shingles, even before the rash), move to musculoskeletal chest pain, then consider diseases of the lower lung, liver, gallbladder, duodenum, pancreas, back, and so on. This systematic approach can help you discover possibilities that you might not have considered.

Another approach to broadening the differential is to use a pathophysiologic approach to the symptom (Byyny & Adams, 1981). Consider each of the classes of disease. For example, could an infectious process be responsible for the symptom of right upper quadrant pain? Could it be a traumatic process? An inflammatory process? A congenital process? Continue until you have considered all of the major types of disease process. Since this list can be rather long and you want to consider all potential causes, some people have developed mnemonics to help (see Table 5.5). Note that the first letter of each word in the pathophysiology list combines to make a single word (Collins, 1987). Whatever strategy you use, use one that you will remember and be able to use consistently. Some of the unusual infectious causes of disease such as rickettsias or parasites may not jump readily to mind. Organizing a list of infectious agents in order of size (see Table 5.5) and reviewing it may help bring to mind some of the more unusual causes of a symptom complex (Collins, 1987).

Table 5.5
Differential Diagnosis Broadening Tools

Have you considered . . .
  • Common diseases?
  • Uncommon presentations of common diseases?
  • Life-threatening/serious/treatable diseases?
  • Rare diseases?
Anatomical approach
  What structures are in the region that could produce the symptoms?
Pathophysiologic approach
  V—vascular
  I—inflammatory
  N—neoplastic
  D—degenerative
  I—intoxication
  C—congenital
  A—autoimmune
  T—trauma
  E—endocrine
Infectious agents (Smallest to largest)
  Viruses
  Rickettsias
  Bacteria
  Spirochetes
  Fungi
  Parasites
Don't forget the great imitators . . .
  Syphilis, tuberculosis, HIV/AIDS, pulmonary embolus

Some diseases are confusing, with multiple and varied manifestations that can mimic many other diseases. These have been referred to as the "great imitators," and the classic representatives are syphilis and tuberculosis. A modern addition to this list is the HIV virus and AIDS. Characteristic of all of these diseases are their subtlety, especially in the early stages of disease, and their wide range of manifestations. If you do not consider them often, you will likely miss an opportunity to diagnose them early. You may want to customize your list of "imitators" and not just rely on the classics. Pulmonary embolus can have varied and subtle presentations, and early recognition is very important. Mono-nucleosis (Epstein–Barr virus infection) is another candidate for the list. This list can be used in reviewing your diagnoses to see if any of these masqueraders might warrant consideration. Another approach is to learn several key clues for each of these diagnoses and look often for those clues, when the clinical situation is appropriate.

Bias on the part of the clinician is another potential pitfall in generating hypotheses. A bias may be negative—for example, a reluctance to take seriously a patient who may have exaggerated symptoms in the past. It may also be positive—for example, not want-ing to consider cancer as a possibility in someone of whom you are very fond. This bias is called a "familiarity bias" and is one important reason why physicians should be very cautious when evaluating friends, colleagues, employees, or family members. There are many who would advocate avoiding these situations completely, but it is not always possible. Biases can be very subtle in their effects on the clinical reasoning process. Awareness of their presence or the possibility of their presence is a first step, and a willingness to get impartial help is essential.

If the diagnostic cycle of three processes occurring together seems too complicated, there is a fourth component that is simultaneous with inquiry, hypothesis testing, and hypothesis generation. This component of the process is called case building. The human brain, although the most efficient data-processing instrument known, has its limitations. For example, evidence suggests that clinicians can only maintain up to seven active hypotheses on their differential diagnosis list (Kassirer, 1989). Likewise, there are limitations to the amount and detail of data that can remain under active consideration, although this is harder to quantify. Case building is a technique that streamlines and condenses the clinical material. The clinician almost naturally assembles the key facts and clues about the case, in such a way that a brief concise summary is usually possible.

A look at an example of case building will help to shed some light on the process. Table 5.6 demonstrates how this "thumbnail sketch" is continually evolving during a clinical encounter. During her last weekend on call, Dr. Nolan was called to see a patient who presented to the emergency room with severe shortness of breath. If you could read her mind every 10 to 30 seconds during the encounter, the results might look something like Table 5.6. After the chief complaint Dr. Nolan's next key clues are visual: that the patient cannot lie down without worsening of his shortness of breath (orthopnea) and that his neck veins are distended [jugular venous distention (JVD)]. To keep her sketch manageable, she takes these three clues and collapses them into the category "symptoms of congestive heart failure." The timing of the symptoms is a key clue. Sudden onset of CHF is usually caused by an acute insult to the heart. Focused questions lead to the history of recent chest pain. In this acute and unstable situation, rapid progress to a focused physical examination followed by an ECG is appropriate. These additional clues are added and are then collapsed into a hypothesis of a ruptured papillary muscle. This hypothesis will be further tested as a stat echocardiogram is ordered and a call to a cardiologist is made while emergency stabilization of the patient occurs.

Case building is assembling the key facts and clues in a case and simplifying and modifying them as new information develops in order to keep the complexity of this case description manageable. The resulting sketch is longer and more complex than when the case started, but because of condensation of several facts into an interim hypothesis, it is not merely a sequential list of all data obtained. This process does have potential problem areas (Table 5.7). As we mentioned previously, not obtaining or recognizing key facts or clues will affect the quality and utility of the case description. Inquiry, hypothesis evaluation, and hypothesis generation all feed into and affect the quality of the case building

Table 5.6
Case Building: An Example

Middle-aged man with shortness of breath

Middle-aged man with shortness of breath, orthopnea, and JVD

Middle-aged man with symptoms of CHF

Middle-aged man with new-onset symptoms of CHF today

Middle-aged man with new-onset symptoms of CHF today, with history of chest pain 2 days ago

Middle-aged man with new-onset symptoms of CHF today, with history of chest pain 2 days ago, and new murmur

Middle-aged man with new-onset CHF, history of chest pain, new murmur, and ECG C/W recent anterior myocardial infarction

Middle-aged man with new-onset CHF, recent anterior MI, and possible ruptured papillary muscle

---

Table 5.7

115

THE DIAGNOSTIC
CYCLE

Case Building

Characteristics
    "Case building" is a system to manage data
    Streamlining and condensation of facts
    The reasoner retains relevant high-priority data
    Generation of a thumbnail sketch that is added to and modified
Pitfalls
    Missing key points
    Condensation bias
    Narrowing of focus too early
Shortcuts
    Keep your thumbnail sketch true to the facts
    Avoid condensing to a hypothesis too early
    Be careful not to throw out potential valuable data

process. The more effective and efficient the clinician is in these steps, the more relevant and useful the summary will be.

The step in case building where several steps or clues are combined or condensed is another potential source of problems. If the reasoner combines clues incorrectly, an error occurs. For example, if a physician sees a person who is suddenly unable to move her arm and leg on one side, condensing this presentation to a "hemiparesis" may be appropriate, but to automatically label this a "stroke" may be incorrect. The differential for a hemiparesis may include stroke, but there are other possibilities that should be considered, such as a spinal cord lesion or injury. This type of error is called a "condensation bias." In order to avoid it, it is important to maintain an adequate differential diagnosis and to be careful not to overinterpret available data.

CASE 5-1 (Part IV)

Further questions by Dr. Nolan reveal that Betty denies paroxysmal nocturnal dyspnea—suddenly awakening with the feeling of shortness of breath, a symptom associated with CHF. She reports some shortness of breath with exertion. The patient attributes her foot swelling to sitting up in a chair at night because she coughs more when she lies down. She denies shortness of breath with lying down (orthopnea). There is no history of chest pressure or chest pain. Her only risk factor for heart disease is high blood pressure, which has been well controlled. The patient has been taking captopril 50 mg twice daily for her blood pressure for 2 years. She does not smoke and has not smoked in the past, but her husband smokes in the home and it aggravates the cough.

A focused physical examination confirms the absence of nasal congestion and postnasal drip. Wheezes are present with forced expiration on lung examination and physical signs of pneumonia or CHF are absent. A peak flow determination of 275 liters per minute demonstrates that the patient is able to move air somewhat less rapidly than expected, indicating a mild to moderate airway obstruction. An albuterol nebulizer treatment, to administer a bronchodilating medication directly to the airways, is given by the nurse as a therapeutic trial while Dr.

Nolan sees her next patient. Twenty minutes after the treatment, the peak flow has increased to 325 liters per minute. Dr. Nolan has made a diagnostic decision and returns to the patient to inform her and to begin planning and implementation of treatment.

—————— A DIAGNOSTIC DECISION ——————

In most clinical encounters a moment arrives where the clinician makes a diagnostic decision. The preceding steps with their pitfalls and shortcuts are all directed at getting you to this point effectively and efficiently, but how do you know when you have arrived? Unfortunately, there is no bell or alarm that goes off when you have gathered enough information to alert you that all of the important pieces of information have been obtained. The diagnostic decision occurs when uncertainty about the diagnosis has been reduced to an acceptable level for the clinician (see Table 5.8).

How does the clinician reach a decision? There are some tools that are commonly used. The first is the *representativeness heuristic,* a process where the clinician matches his patient's symptoms with a classic or textbook descriptions of disease (Reigelman, 1991). The basis for this process occurs during the hypothesis testing phase, where the physician is obtaining specific data to compare and contrast hypotheses and to compare these hypotheses to the characteristics of disease processes that he has learned. There are a number of pitfalls with this process. Not every disease has "read the textbook." Patients often present with incomplete or modified disease manifestations. This problem can be especially significant in primary care, where patients often present early, before the "classic" manifestations described in the textbooks are detectable. An uncommon presentation of a common problem occurs more often than a rare disease.

Table 5.8
A Diagnostic Decision

Characteristics
  A diagnosis requires that the cause, the disease, and the clinical manifestations fit together and have an adequate and coherent explanation
  Reasoner decides that there are enough data to adequately reduce uncertainty
  Diagnostic decision usually made by 10 minutes into the visit
  Representativeness heuristic—a matching process where reasoner matches patient's symptoms with those of classic or textbook descriptions
  Principle of parsimony—put together as many of the clues as possible into one disease process
Pitfalls
  Patient may present with incomplete or modified disease manifestations
  Patient may engage in denial or fail to convey the key points
  A disease process uncovered may not be the one involved in production of the symptoms, e.g., gallstones and RUQ pain, hemorrhoids and rectal bleeding
Shortcuts
  Acknowledge any uncertainty that remains in the diagnosis
  Maximize and evaluate the reliability of the data
  Find out what the patient's concerns are
  Provide a "safety net" for the patient

Physicians must be alert to the marked variation that may occur in the presentation of the same disease process in different patients. One patient with a myocardial infarction may have severe, crushing substernal pain radiating to the jaw and left arm, associated with nausea, sweating, and palpitations. Another patient with the same amount of damage to the same area of the heart may present with a vague complaint of "chest discomfort, like heartburn." The "disease" is the same but the "illness" is a function of the patient's personal, biologic, and emotional response to the process. Patients may intentionally or unwillingly engage in denial and fail to openly convey critical information necessary to make the diagnosis. Awareness of this possibility and, if available, prior knowledge of the patient and his response to disease can help to overcome this pitfall.

Another useful approach in making the diagnosis is the *principle of parsimony,* the process of trying to put together as *one* disease process the clinical manifestations of the patient (Reigelman, 1991). In some cases it may appear that the patient has more than one disease process occurring, as in a patient with burning on urination and a sore ankle, where both problems may be caused by Reiter's syndrome. Another patient with pelvic and right upper quadrant pain may seem to have two separate processes but actually has pelvic inflammatory disease with perihepatitis (the Fitz–Hugh–Curtis syndrome). Searching for a potential explanation for all of the symptoms with one diagnosis forces you to broaden your differential and consider disease processes that affect multiple sites and systems. An obvious pitfall for the principle of parsimony is the fact that a patient *may* have more than one disease occurring simultaneously. Two common diseases occurring simultaneously may be more likely to occur than one very rare disease.

Dr. Nolan employed both approaches to making a diagnostic decision in Case 5-1. Her initial hunches of "bronchitis versus reactive airway disease" continued to remain near the top of her differential diagnosis list, although by the end neither fit a "classic" or typical case description. The acute onset, associated fever, and exposure to others with similar symptoms support a diagnosis of bronchitis, but the long duration of the illness and the documented presence of bronchial obstruction do not fit with the typical case. On the other hand, although evidence of wheezing and reversible bronchospasm support the diagnosis of reversible airway disease, new-onset asthma in an older adult without a significant allergic history is unusual, and the acute onset and presence of an elevated temperature are not supported. Fortunately, Dr. Nolan is able to use the principle of parsimony in this case. Occasionally, an infectious bronchitis can trigger bronchospasm and a symptom complex similar to asthma in a patient without an allergic history or other prior evidence of lung disease, asthmatic bronchitis. For Dr. Nolan, this is the most adequate and coherent explanation that best combines the cause, the clinical manifestations, and the disease, an essential definition of the diagnosis.

Can physicians be 100% sure of their diagnosis? In many clinical situations this is not possible. Reasonable doubt often persists despite the most effective diagnostic process. Awareness of this residual uncertainty is essential. Often a "final diagnosis" might best be considered a "working diagnosis." It is incumbent on the physician to create a "safety net" for the patient in order to reduce the risk to the patient of residual uncertainty. The "safety net" might consist of a scheduled follow-up visit to assess efficacy of the therapy, instructions to the patient on what to expect from the therapy, and when to call if symptoms are not improving or getting worse. Physicians and patients must learn to live with some uncertainty, but the negative impact can be minimized by careful and thoughtful planning and communication.

MAKING A
DIAGNOSIS

Dr. Nolan reenters Betty's examination room to find her appearing more comfortable and coughing less. A brief lung examination reveals improved air movement and less wheezing. Dr. Nolan informs Betty of the diagnosis of asthmatic bronchitis, and relates this to her symptoms and the improvement seen with the nebulizer treatment. She writes a prescription for an albuterol metered dose inhaler, two puffs 15 minutes apart, every 4 to 6 hours and instructs her in the correct use of the inhaler. Another prescription is written for enteric-coated erythromycin, 333 mg to be taken with food three times a day for 7 days. Betty is informed of the possible side effects of stomach irritation from the erythromycin and jitteriness from the albuterol. She is encouraged to avoid exposure to her husband's cigarette smoke, and states that she has already planned to have him smoke outside. She is asked to call if her symptoms worsen or are not significantly better in the next day or two and to come back for a follow-up visit in 5 days. Betty demonstrates understanding of the instructions and leaves the office more comfortable, both physically and emotionally.

CONCLUSION

We have examined the steps in the hypothetico-deductive reasoning process. Beginning with some initial hunches, we have analyzed our way through a whirlwind of inquiry, hypothesis testing, and hypothesis generation—each part feeding off and contributing to the others in a complex circular waltz. As if this was not enough, at the same time it was necessary to build and modify a brief but accurate and complete outline of all of the pertinent facts and maintain and modify a list of possible diagnoses. Eventually this process reduced diagnostic uncertainty to an acceptable level and a diagnosis was selected, a complex process in itself. It is no wonder that for many years the clinical reasoning process was seen to be too complex to describe and teach.

The reasoning process needed to make the correct diagnosis can seem to be an overwhelming quagmire of simultaneous processes, gaping pitfalls, and shortcuts that appear to have as many limitations as they have benefits. When taken step by step, each component can be learned, practiced, and optimized to improve the success and efficiency of the whole process. The lists of characteristics, pitfalls, and shortcuts outlined here are not intended to be comprehensive or complete. They are intended to serve as examples, as bricks for a foundation that you will build on, both consciously and unconsciously, throughout your medical career.

There is more to making the right diagnosis than following a collection of steps. Clinical reasoning brings all of your medical knowledge and experience, all of your skill at interviewing and physical examination, all of your interpersonal skills and insights, in essence your entire being, and uses this to bear on the problems of your patient. As you gain increased knowledge, skills, and experience in all facets of medicine, it will contribute to your ability to make the correct diagnosis.

There is an old joke: "Why do they call it the 'practice' of medicine? Don't doctors ever get it right?" Like many jokes, there is more than a grain of truth. There is always room for continued growth and improvement as a physician, a continual search to learn from your experiences and to do better the next time. Physicians' diagnostic skills may not peak until their mid-50s. I believe that a majority of these physicians would tell you that they are still trying to improve their skills, to learn more and to do better the next time. As you progress in your medical career, I encourage you to follow their example and keep "practicing," in the fullest sense of the word.

————————— **CASES FOR DISCUSSION** —————————

CASE 1

Outside of the examination room, you pick up the chart of Mr. Black, a 42-year-old man whose chief complaint is "headache." According to the chart, he has a history of hypertension. And his blood pressure today is 180/110 mm Hg. The lights are off in the room and you find Mr. Black lying on the examination table.

1. *What clues have you identified in the scenario above?*
2. *List several initial hunches that could guide your initial questioning and reasoning.*
3. *What are some potential pitfalls at this early stage of this encounter?*

CASE 2

Mr. Antonelli is a 50-year-old truck driver who was last seen in your office 5 years ago for a broken ankle. The nurse obtained the chief complaint of a "sore shoulder," and the patient states that it has been sore off and on for 6 months. It usually bothers him after he has played catch with his son and is not particularly painful. The examination reveals normal strength and range of motion with minimal tenderness over the bicipital tendon on the right.

1. *What are your hypotheses at this point?*
2. *Are there clues that may suggest that "shoulder pain" may not be his primary reason for coming to the office?*
3. *What questions might help you uncover an alternative reason for this visit?*

CASE 3

Mrs. Clay is a 21-year-old woman who complains of abdominal pain. Pain has been present for 2 days but has worsened this morning and is located in the right lower quadrant. She vomited once last night and feels nauseated and has not eaten. Her last menstrual period was 5 weeks ago.

1. *What hypotheses have you formed from the above information?*
2. *Using the differential diagnosis broadening tools (anatomic approach, pathophysiologic approach, "great imitators"), see if you can expand your differential.*
3. *What additional questions would you ask now to test your hypotheses?*
4. *Write a thumbnail sketch of this case in one or two lines that would quickly and accurately communicate the essentials of this case to a colleague.*

CASE 4

Abbie is a pretty, 2-year-old child whom you had delivered and cared for. You are called to the emergency room to see her because she had a 1-minute, generalized seizure this evening. She was confused and lethargic for several minutes after the event, and was found to have a temperature of 104.2°F rectally. She was given acetaminophen and taken to the ER. On examination she is quiet but alert, has a right otitis media (middle ear infection), and does not have a stiff neck.

1. *What are your current hypotheses?*
2. *What additional history would you obtain now? physical examination? laboratory studies?*
3. *Would you obtain a lumbar puncture (spinal tap) on this patient? What are the risks and benefits of doing it? of not doing it?*
4. *Are there any potential sources of bias that you need to be aware of in making your clinical decisions?*

CASE 5

Mr. Diorio is seen in the office as a work-in patient for acute chest pain. The pain occurred in his left anterior chest while he was at work. He smokes a pack of cigarettes a day, is 40 pounds overweight, and is very concerned that he is having a heart attack because his mother and father both have a history of "heart trouble."

1. *What is your differential diagnosis at this point?*
2. *What additional information is needed to give you a complete clinical description of his pain? Of his risk factors for cardiovascular disease?*
3. *On completion of his history, physical, and review of an ECG, you are 95% certain that this patient has musculoskeletal chest pain from lifting at work. Recognizing that there is a 5% chance that you are wrong, how would you deal with that uncertainty in caring for this patient?*

—————— RECOMMENDED READINGS ——————

Kassirer JP, Kopelman RW: *Learning Clinical Reasoning.* Baltimore, Williams & Wilkins Co, 1993.

> This text includes a very detailed description of the clinical reasoning process, backed up by a series of excellent clinical cases, each illustrating a specific point. Appropriate for early clinicians as well as more advanced clinical reasoners.

Rakel RE (ed): *Essentials of Family Practice.* Philadelphia, WB Saunders Co, 1993.

> This general, primary care-oriented text presents much of its clinical content in problem-oriented chapters, focusing on clinical cases. This helps readers improve their knowledge base, while testing their current knowledge and problem-solving skills.

Reigelman RK: *Minimizing Medical Mistakes: The Art of Medical Decision Making.* Boston, Little, Brown & Co, 1991.

> This is a very readable book, filled with practical hints and tips that are illustrated by realistic clinical examples. Recommended as a next step in reading about practical clinical reasoning techniques.

CHAPTER 6

Instituting Treatment

Jeff Susman

CASE 6-1

D. G., a 68-year-old gentleman, presents with nocturia and increasing urinary urgency. He is on no medications and has been in good health. He must get up at night at least every 2 hours and finds it difficult to sit through an entire meeting without making a hasty exit for the restroom. He must strain to initiate urination and has found the urinary stream to be less forceful. D. G. presents to his physician asking if anything can be done to alleviate his distressing symptoms.

——— EDUCATIONAL OBJECTIVES ———

By the end of this chapter, the reader will be able to:

1. Understand the issues relevant to instituting patient-centered medical therapy
2. Describe the negotiation of treatment with the patient, including the balancing of benefits, harms, and costs of therapy in today's healthcare environment
3. Discuss the role of the family and community in treatment decisions
4. Describe the importance of the balance between patient and physician needs with regard to therapy decisions
5. Define the role of watchful waiting, trials of therapy, and "n of 1" trials
6. Discuss the factors influencing the initiation of treatment
7. Describe how uncertainty affects treatment decisions and the trade-offs this entails
8. Outline methods for enhancing adherence with medical therapy

INTRODUCTION

The decision to institute treatment should be made thoughtfully and in concert with the patient. This decision is ideally based on a combination of physician, patient, and family preferences and an educated estimate of likely outcomes. An accurate history including the functional and psychosocial impact of the problem, a targeted physical examination, and judicious ancillary testing will help inform decision-making. In Case 6-1, D. G. is found to have a history of significant life-style compromise and a physical examination consistent with BPH. There is no suggestion of prostate cancer. Further workup would be prudent.

CASE 6-1 (*continued*)

D. G.'s physician administers the American Urological Association Symptom Index (McConnell et al., 1994). D. G. scores in the severe range. A physical examination including a focused neurological examination is remarkable only for an enlarged, smooth prostate. Results of urinalysis and serum creatinine are normal. D. G. is eager to begin therapy immediately, "Anything which will allow me to make it through my conference calls."

In some instances, the physician may choose to observe the natural history of a problem, so-called "watchful waiting." For example, a physician may choose to closely follow a patient with fatigue, arthralgias, or mild mood disturbance rather than immediately performing an elaborate workup or instituting aggressive treatment. In Case 6-1, however, D. G. clearly desires immediate treatment.

CASE 6-1 (*continued*)

D. G.'s physician discusses treatment options including surgery or the initiation of an alpha blocking agent or finasteride. While the success rate for surgery is greater, D. G. opts for a trial of medication given the potential complications of surgery (McConnell et al., 1994). Terazosin is chosen.

When therapy is begun, the physician should initiate measures to enhance adherence and guarantee follow-up. In Case 6-1, the physician has asked D. G. to keep track of serial symptom scores. An office nurse checks with D. G. after 1 week to confirm that he is tolerating the terazosin without undue side effects. An office follow-up visit is scheduled in 1 month. At that point therapy will be reassessed and modifications made. The clear plan for follow-up and measurable outcomes of therapy should allow an accurate assessment of therapy.

Attention should also be paid to the unique needs of special populations, including elders, patients with chronic illnesses, and individuals whose cultural or social background may impact their treatment. A 27-year-old homeless drug addict with AIDS may have significant difficulties adhering to a multidrug treatment regimen. Significant social, psychological, and medical supports would be required to achieve optimal therapy.

Thus, each individual poses a unique challenge when instituting treatment. The physician must balance the patient's needs and preferences, the likelihood of benefits and harms, and the costs and functional impact of therapy.

123

TREATMENT
INITIATION

CASE 6-2

J. B., a 44-year-old black male, presents with lightheadedness, fatigue, and blurred vision. His history is positive for polydipsia and polyuria. His father suffered a heart attack at age 57, and his mother has a history of diabetes mellitus and hypertension. The patient smokes two packs of cigarettes per day. On physical examination his blood pressure is 140/92 mm Hg, weight 84 kg, and height 5 feet 7 inches. The rest of the examination results are normal. Initial laboratory testing discloses a blood glucose of 302 mg/dl, a total cholesterol of 257 mg/dl, a low-density-lipoprotein (LDL) cholesterol of 154 mg/dl, and a high-density-lipoprotein (HDL) of 35 mg/dl. Other laboratory results are normal.

—————————— TREATMENT INITIATION ——————————

DECIDING TO BEGIN TREATMENT

The decision if and when to begin treatment bears careful consideration. When a patient presents to the physician, active intervention is not always necessary. Indeed, many patients simply want reassurance that the condition will spontaneously remit. For example, the patient with a cold or a minor injury often warrants such an approach.

In other conditions, only certain patients need active treatment. For a patient presenting with a sore throat, the decision to treat is based on the probability of the individual having a streptococcal infection, since the results of a throat culture usually take 1 to 2 days. Certain features are associated with an increased or decreased probability of streptococcal infection. For example, the presence of tender cervical adenopathy, fever, tonsillar exudate, and lack of cough increase, the likelihood of streptococcal infection to 42.5% based on an overall prevalence of group A streptococcal pharyngitis of 10% (Centor *et al.,* 1986). Centor and colleagues recommend empiric treatment when the clinical signs predict a probability of streptococcal infection greater than 47% without testing, in order to optimize outcomes, including the prevention of rheumatic fever, the quicker resolution of symptoms, and the avoidance of unnecessary antibiotics. If the patient has none of the above features, the likelihood of a strep infection is less than 3% (Centor, *et al.,* 1986). Most physicians and patients would defer therapy in such patients given the low probability of infection.

The decision to initiate therapy will be influenced by the seriousness of the problem and its prevalence. For example, a physician is apt to initiate anticoagulant therapy for a 68-year-old who presents with pleuritic chest pain, a tender calf, atrial fibrillation, and mitral valvular disease. In this instance, the possibility of a serious disease, pulmonary embolism, is high, as the patient has multiple findings making this diagnosis more likely. On the other hand, a well 27-year-old who presents with upper respiratory symptoms and pleuritic chest pain would be far less likely to have a pulmonary embolism. Few physicians would begin anticoagulant therapy for this individual without further evidence.

In practice, many factors influence therapy. A physician's previous experience, particularly critical incidents where a treatment had a spectacularly good or bad result, may overshadow reason. For example, if the afore-mentioned 27-year-old who presented with pleuritic chest pain ultimately had an occult neoplasm and a pulmonary embolism, the physician might be much more aggressive in evaluation and treatment. Many physicians will poorly estimate the prevalence of disease states and the potential benefits and harms of treatment. Indeed, such outcomes are often unknown in the typical office setting. Finally, patients clearly influence physician choices of therapy.

Even in instances where the physician believes treatment is of low probable benefit, some patients may request therapy. It is not unusual for a patient (or the patient's parent) to "demand" treatment despite a low probability of benefit. In the end, there are trade-offs of costs, the possibility of adverse outcomes, and the use of unnecessary medication or procedures (DeNeef, 1987). Such decisions become dependent on a subjective weighing of patient preference. Most practitioners would acquiesce to treatment when the harms are relatively infrequent or of limited magnitude. Where each practitioner draws this line is an individual decision.

The decision to initiate any treatment is even more complex in individuals, such as J. B. in Case 6-2, with a chronic disease such as diabetes mellitus. In the patient with diabetes mellitus, the threshold for treating hypertension may be lower because of the synergistic effect of hypertension and diabetes mellitus in accelerating renal and vascular disease. In a frail elder, the decision to treat mild hyperglycemia may be forestalled because of the risks of hypoglycemia and questionable benefits. In Case 6-2, treatment appears warranted; the question is which options to use and how to begin.

CASE 6-2 (continued)

In discussion with the patient, J. B. is willing to meet with the dietitian. J. B.'s physician suggests that his wife join this meeting since she does most of the cooking, and J. B. agrees. An appropriate diet is prescribed. The patient is also willing to use his lunch hour to play basketball at the gym where he works. He does not want to quit smoking at the present time. After discussing the options of beginning insulin versus an oral hypoglycemic agent, J. B. responds that "I would rather be dead than on the needle."

TAILORING TREATMENT DECISIONS

Once a decision to initiate treatment is made, the focus and form of therapy should be tailored to the patient. In Case 6-2, J. B. has expressed important preferences concerning treatment. Understanding the patient's perspective can enhance adherence to a treatment plan (Cohen-Cole, 1991). Moreover, the physician treating the patient with multiple problems would be advised to ascertain the issues of most interest to the patient. Thus, in an initial visit, recommendations to quit smoking, lose weight, reduce salt intake, limit fat intake, exercise, begin insulin, and begin an antihypertensive medication would be overwhelming and all would likely be ignored. A more effective strategy would be to have a discussion concerning the options for treatment and their potential harms and benefits. It should be remembered that negotiating a plan for care in patients with chronic problems often takes time and usually occurs over a series of visits.

After 3 months of dietary therapy, J. B.'s physician places J. B. on glipizide 5 mg daily and schedules a return visit in 1 month. At that time his BP is 136/86 mm Hg, glucose 215 mg/dl, and his weight is down 2 kg. He has been very compliant with diet, a fact corroborated by his spouse.

USING CONTINUITY TO ADVANTAGE

In some cases, a long-term physician–patient relationship built on trust allows the physician and patient to mutually agree on a treatment plan that was initially untenable. For example, in the treatment of depression, many individuals are loath to initiate anti-depressant medications. In one poll, 70% of individuals would take a medication for a headache while only 12% would take an antidepressant (Roper Reports, 1986). Recent investigations suggest that physicians actively negotiate with patients with regard to the "right" time to begin antidepressant therapy (Susman *et al.*, 1995). Moreover, many practitioners will use "watchful waiting" or a "tincture of time" approach. In managing minor depressive symptoms, many physicians indicated that they followed patients to see if their mood disturbance resolved or worsened, and initiated further treatment on this basis. Thus, continuity of the physician–patient relationship is important.

The initial response to treatment in Case 6-2 has been successful. By respecting the patient's wishes to concentrate on diet modification rather than smoking and respecting his concern about injections and prescribing an oral hypoglycemic agent, patient trust and initial treatment progress have been accomplished. While alternative or additional therapy may be appropriate in the long run, rapport building is important when treating any patient, especially an individual with a chronic disease.

CASE 6-2 (*continued*)

J. B. returns after 2 months. He is continuing on a program of diet and exercise modification. He is happy with his slimmer self, having lost 3 more kg. His BP is 138/87 mm Hg, glucose 225 mg/dl, and an initial HbA$_1$C 11.4%. J. B.'s physician continues to discuss the importance of diet and exercise, gently reminds him about smoking cessation, and schedules a follow-up in 1 month. He will have his blood pressure checked weekly at a worksite clinic and report on his home-monitored blood glucose to your office nurse.

NONPHARMACOLOGIC TREATMENT MODALITIES

While sometimes relegated to second-class status, nonpharmacologic therapy can be effective for many conditions. Nonpharmacologic approaches have important places in the management of such common disorders as hypertension, hyperlipidemia, and diabetes mellitus (weight control, diet, exercise, smoking cessation), mood disorders (counseling), and even conditions such as obstructive sleep apnea [weight control and nasal continuous positive airway pressure (CPAP)]. While life-style modification may prove challenging, it is important to set reasonable goals for therapy and allow time for these interventions to be effective. A potential pitfall for physicians is urging patients to make multiple life-style changes simultaneously in a very short time. When patients are "unsuccessful," the physician will then place them on an alternative pharmacologic treatment because of the "failure of conservative therapy." Again, a longer-term perspective, months to years as in J. B.'s case, should be taken.

CASE 6-2 (continued)

J. B. follows up in a month accompanied by his wife. He appears to be doing excellently based on his physical examination and laboratory results: BP today is 128/80 mm Hg and at work all readings have been under 134/86 mm Hg. His blood glucose level is gradually decreasing with the most recent readings between 104 and 210 mg/dl. Nonetheless, J. B.'s physician senses some unresolved problems. After some initial pleasantries, it turns out that Mrs. B. is quite concerned because of problems in their marital relationship. J. B. has had gradually increasing problems with impotence, getting and maintaining an erection, over the past year. He is quite embarrassed and says that he still loves his wife very much, but "things just don't seem to work like they used to." While a comprehensive review of systems had been performed as part of the initial evaluation, his physician is not surprised to have "missed" this issue.

ARRANGING FOLLOW-UP

An important part of initiating therapy is scheduling follow-up. Follow-up can be done by phone, in the office by another staff member, at the home, or at another community venue. For example, in Case 6-2, J. B. is asked to attend a worksite program so that further data can be gathered on his blood pressure control, and so as to maintain regular contact with the office nurse. Other common follow-up providers might include visiting nurses, home health aides, and physical therapists. Particularly for individuals who are older or require protracted skilled care, such as prolonged antibiotic therapy, home visits may be important. Many worksites have programs emphasizing wellness, occupational issues such as back care, and employee assistance programs for individuals with substance abuse or mental health problems. A large number of volunteer and community agencies offer programs, support groups, and educational materials. Moreover, as in J. B.'s case, adequate follow-up allows the physician to support the patient through difficult life-style changes and enhances adherence to recommendations.

INITIATING TREATMENT IS AN ONGOING ISSUE

It is not uncommon for a richer understanding of a patient's medical and psychosocial problems to unfold over time (Cohen-Cole, 1991). Even direct questioning about a particular issue, such as sexual problems, may fail to elicit the full story until a patient and his family gain trust in the physician, as in Case 6-2. Thus, initiating treatment is an ongoing process that requires careful vigilance to changes in the patient's status and demeanor and thoughtful mobilization of the involvement of the family and significant others.

Office systems can also play an important role in supporting the physician in decisions to monitor and initiate changes in therapy (Pommerenke & Weed, 1991). For example, flow sheets can be quite helpful in monitoring the course of a chronic illness.

Peak expiratory flow rates can be monitored in patients with asthma, HbA_1C measurements followed in patients with diabetes mellitus, and blood pressure determinations tracked in those with hypertension. Nursing staff can complete inventories geared to specific problems. In Case 6-2, an office nurse could inquire about foot and skin care, monitor hypoglycemic episodes, and monitor regular ophthalmologic evaluation. A midlevel practitioner or nurse may play a key role in education and monitoring of chronic illness. Staff can also use questionnaires or instruments to screen for certain conditions and guide the physician to consider the initiation of treatment. For example, a Beck or Zung depression inventory may be helpful to initially find those with depressive symptoms who might benefit from a more complete history and physical (Depression Guideline Panel, 1993). More and more evidence suggests that developing an office environment that promotes health is an important part of medical care.

CASE 6-2 (*continued*)

After taking further history and in consultation with J. B., his physician offers a urology evaluation for his impotence. He is scheduled for follow-up in 3 months. During the next months, J. B. learns more about diabetes mellitus by attending meetings of the local chapter of the American Diabetes Association. He learns about a program through the local hospital for patients with diabetes and enrolls. The local nurse, dietitian, endocrinologist, and retinal specialist discuss the importance of preventive care and a stable long-term relationship with a primary care physician.

USING THE HEALTHCARE TEAM

Many times, a team or collaborative approach to care is useful. Judicious consultation and referral can help provide comprehensive state-of-the-art care. By acknowledging the strengths of the healthcare team, both within the primary care office and in the greater community, a patient can receive support from a group of experts, coordinated by the primary care physician. Good communication, mutual respect, and an open mind make for added value in collaborative care.

CASE 6-3

A. S., a 74-year-old male, has a history of benign prostatic hypertrophy, mild congestive heart failure, and diabetes mellitus. He is widowed and lives at home. His medication regimen consists of glyburide 10 mg daily and enalapril 5 mg daily. Following the death of his wife last year, A. S. has gradually withdrawn from his social activities. He no longer plays cards at the senior center, has given up tending his vegetable garden, and complains he is just too tired to engage in outside activities. He goes to bed at 9 PM, awakens at 4 or 5 AM, and tends to nap during the days. He just doesn't feel like cooking. He denies being depressed, but allows he just isn't interested in life anymore. While he has thought it would be a relief to "have it all over with," he denies active suicidal intent. His physician makes a presumptive diagnosis of depression. After discussion, A. S. is willing to initiate antidepressant therapy, "Anything to alleviate this fatigue, but I'm not going to some shrink."

— MAKING INFORMED TREATMENT DECISIONS —

INITIATING TREATMENT WITH CONCOMITANT MEDICAL CONDITIONS

In Case 6-3, A. S. is willing to initiate pharmacologic treatment for his depression. Now, the physician must initiate treatment with a holistic care plan in mind. Such planning should consider the patient's overall medical status, risk for medication-induced side effects, and the costs of therapy. A recent summary of the literature suggests that counseling and medication are equally efficacious in the treatment of mild depression (Depression Guideline Panel, 1993). In this instance, the patient has clearly decided against formal counseling and is willing to initiate antidepressant therapy. His current conditions may significantly influence the choice of antidepressant. Common tricyclic antidepressant side effects include sedation, anticholinergic problems, postural hypotension, and cardiac problems. With A. S.'s history of heart failure, diabetes mellitus, which might predispose to orthostatic hypotension, and benign prostatic hypertrophy, it would appear he is at risk for tricyclic-induced side effects. Probably the best tricyclic choice for A. S. is nortriptyline (Pamelor), which has relatively low anticholinergic and cardiac side effects. Newer antidepressants also avoid most of these potential problems. For example, the selective serotonin reuptake inhibitors, e.g., fluoxetine (Prozac), paroxetine (Paxil), and sertraline (Zoloft), have little or not anticholinergic and postural problems and low potential for cardiac problems (Shaughnessy, 1995).

CASE 6-3 (continued)

Based on these considerations, A. S.'s physician decides to prescribe fluoxetine. The physician performs an initial Beck inventory and hopes to see a drop in score of at least 10%. The physician explains that unlike other medications, fluoxetine takes approximately 4 to 8 weeks to become effective. Potential side effects such as wakefulness are described and the physician suggests A. S. begin at 10 mg, each morning. A. S. is told that up to 70% of individuals improve on their initial antidepressant and the physician schedules a phone call in 3 days to discuss any progress. If the patient notices any significant problems or increasing depression, he is advised to call immediately.

A. S. calls within an hour. "I tried to get that medicine and my insurance plan won't cover it. I decided I would just go ahead and buy it, but what is it made of—gold? I can't afford to take it!" Sheepishly, A. S.'s physician apologizes and ascertains that paroxetine is covered under the patient's managed care plan.

RECOMMENDATIONS ON INITIATING THERAPY

On initiation of any therapy, certain guidelines should be followed. A clear explanation of the medication's intended action and possible side effects is important. Many medications have significant drug–drug, drug–disease, or drug–nutrient interactions. Clear prescribing instructions should be given, including when the dose is to be taken and under what conditions. The initial course of treatment should be outlined and plans for follow-up should be arranged. Guidelines for earlier follow-up should be given. In many patients, an "n of 1" trial is initiated: An intervention is tried and a principal outcome measure is monitored before and during therapy (Kazdin, 1982). In Case 6-3, the effect of an antidepressant on A. S.'s Beck score will be monitored. Occasionally, the physician may choose to withdraw therapy and see if the intervention truly accounts for the noted improvement in outcome.

CONSIDERING COSTS

In today's medical environment, cost is an important aspect of medical care. Unfortunately, calculating costs can be challenging. It is important to consider not only the actual medication cost, but also the cost of monitoring and ongoing medication management and from whose perspective costs are being viewed. Clearly, from A. S.'s perspective, a medication that is not covered under his insurer's formulary will be personally quite expensive and, without clear evidence of differing efficacy, of unwarranted expense. The "Red Book" is a list of average wholesale prices (AWP) and can be useful in considering drug acquisition costs. However, other costs are important to consider. For example, will drug levels or laboratory tests need to be monitored, and will follow-up visits or procedures be needed? Moreover, total costs are significantly related to real-world effectiveness as opposed to theoretical efficacy (Wilson, 1992). For example, reserpine is quite inexpensive and is effective as an antihypertensive. However, its side effect profile may lead to discontinuation or medication-induced problems. Similarly, one recent study looked at the effectiveness of imipramine and desipramine, older tricyclic antidepressants, versus fluoxetine, a newer SSRI. This study found that patients randomized to fluoxetine were more likely to receive adequate treatment when compared with the tricyclics (Simon *et al.,* 1994). Finally, in today's world of managed care, it becomes an ethical issue of whose perspective costs are accrued. Many plans place the physician at risk for expenses. Under such a plan, a practitioner could choose a less costly medication at the expense of patient convenience or side effects. Thus, consideration of costs is an important part of practicing medicine today.

CASE 6-3 (*continued*)

A. S. returns after 8 weeks. He says his fatigue is improving and he has noticed a significant improvement in his sleep routine. He is thinking about returning to the senior center to play cards. He is grateful to his physician for her ongoing help.

ENHANCING ADHERENCE

Methods to enhance adherence are an important part of initiating and maintaining therapy. Adherence is compliance with the clinician's instructions and may be influenced by the patient's motivation, the problem being treated, the medication's benefits, harms, and costs, and the quality of the physician–patient relationship. Nonadherence is very common; for example, up to 50% of individuals with hypertension are not taking their medication at the end of 1 year of treatment. Adherence may be improved by simplifying instructions, simplifying medication regimens, discussing common side effects, enhancing the patient's feeling of self-control and choice, understanding the illness from the patient's perspective, providing the tools to implement self-monitoring, and developing ways to enforce therapy or deal with barriers to ongoing treatment (Ruffalo *et al.,* 1985). In Case 6-3, prescribing a medication once a day, providing written instructions, involving caregivers and significant others, discussing side effects before and during therapy, and continuing to explore the patient's feelings were all done to enhance adherence.

CASE 6-4

G. M., a 32-year-old factory worker, presents with low back pain. He said he injured his back on the job while working on the assembly line. He is responsible for tightening two bolts and installing a filter in a truck assembly plant. He has had shooting pains down his right leg and complains of some mild tingling. He denies bowel or bladder complaints and says that other than the pain, his strength is unchanged. He denies any other medical problems, constitutional symptoms, drug abuse, risk factors for HIV infection or immunocompromise, or trauma.

On physical examination, G. M. is in some obvious discomfort. The straight leg raise is equivocally positive on the left and positive at 35 degrees on the right. He has a minimally diminished ankle reflex on the right, and diminished light touch and sensation on the lateral aspect of the right foot. Results of the rest of the examination are unremarkable.

Dr. C. M. makes the presumptive diagnosis of an S1 radiculopathy and begins to discuss treatment options when the patient inquires, "You mean to tell me you aren't going to do an X ray, aren't recommending bed rest, and won't authorize traction and a TENS unit like the last time I was out?"

DEALING WITH UNCERTAINTY AND BALANCING SCIENCE WITH HUMANITY

DEALING WITH UNCERTAINTY AND THE USE OF CLINICAL POLICIES

Medical practice changes. What was once accepted as dogma falls aside with the acquisition of new knowledge. While traditionally, patients were placed on strict bed rest, put in traction, and offered a wide variety of exotic therapies, recent literature has demonstrated the lack of effectiveness of such interventions for patients with back pain, as G. M. has in Case 6-4 (Bigos *et al.*, 1994).

One of the great challenges for the family physician is keeping up with the medical literature. Especially when medical practice has changed significantly, or different physicians' practices vary widely, the clinician may look for help in making informed decisions. Many organizations, such as the Agency for Health Care Policy and Research (AHCPR), are developing clinical policies, practice parameters, or practice guidelines. These policies provide explicit summaries of the literature, including the latest in diagnosis and management strategies. Moreover, the policies currently available through the AHCPR, covering conditions ranging from low back problems to pressure sores, are accompanied by well-written patient guides. As discussed, a key task in initiating therapy is to negotiate with patients and address their understanding of their illness. A clinical policy, therefore, not only can help guide physician decision-making, but also can support patient adherence and improve education (see Chapter 22, "Development of Clinical Guidelines").

The physician shares the AHCPR low back problems patient brochure with the patient. She explains that bed rest is recommended for no longer than 4 days, that there is no evidence that traction is helpful, and that a TENS unit is of unproven benefit in the treatment of acute low back pain. Although G. M. is skeptical, he is willing to discuss options recommended as effective. The physician decides together with G. M. to try a nonsteroidal anti-inflammatory drug (NSAID) and to touch base over the next couple of days.

After 48 hours, however, the pain has increased and the patient notices increasing numbness. He goes to his local chiropractor and experiences significant relief of his discomfort after a week of manipulative therapy. He returns to his physician's office in 2 weeks saying he continues to have pain, but found it impossible to take the NSAID because of stomach upset. The manipulative therapy has helped somewhat, but there is still considerable numbness. The physician discusses further options and decides to switch the medication to acetaminophen and instructs the patient to apply cold packs at home. After 7 weeks, the patient continues to experience pain and activity limitation. He continues to have numbness and the results of his physical examination, while stable, are consistent with an S1 radiculopathy. A CT scan of the spine discloses an S1 nerve root entrapment. The physician offers referral to a spinal surgeon, who after discussing options with the patient, recommends chymopapain treatment.

SHARING UNCERTAINTY WITH OTHERS

It is important for the primary care physician to maintain continuity of care both in the initial treatment phases and during any ongoing consultations or referral. Decisions to order further diagnostic tests or treatments should be based on the patient's response to therapy, his ongoing preferences, and the opportunity to influence the course of illness. The vast majority of patients with low back problems, even with radiculopathy, recover uneventfully (Bigos *et al.*, 1994). Initiating treatment requires a knowledge of the natural history of the disease in question, an understanding of the effect of various treatment strategies, and the trade-offs of each. While surgery for herniated discs is effective, the long-term outcome for most patients following more conservative therapy is the same. The question becomes how much does the patient value shorter-term improvement at the risk of a surgical complication.

In this instance, the surgeon has recommended a treatment option that has significant risks and is not as effective as other surgical options such as discectomy (Bigos *et al.*, 1994). Again, the physician should be able to act as an advocate and interpreter for the patient and family members with consultants. In Case 6-4, the physician might suggest other treatment options that are more appropriate and act as an intermediary between the patient and the surgeon.

CASE 6-4 (*continued*)

After a standard discectomy, the patient continues to have pain and applies for workmen's compensation. G. M. says that he is fed up with his job and things are not going well at home, either. In fact, G. M. is drinking up to 12 bottles of beer each day and he and his wife are nearing a divorce. Assessment of the physical examination is remarkable for multiple pain behaviors but there are no new findings. A follow-up MRI is unremarkable, and the orthopedist consultant says there is nothing further to be done: "He will just have to live with it." The patient wonders if he should be placed on Percodan or a stronger medication.

UNPROVEN OR RISKY TREATMENTS

Unproven or even risky treatments are sought by some individuals, especially those with chronic or incurable diseases. It is important for the physician to react to such patients with equanimity, offer support and hope, and suggest more appropriate alternative measures. Individuals such as G. M. in Case 6-4 with chronic pain or concomitant psychiatric problems offer special challenges to the physician. When initiating ongoing therapy, such circumstances test the mettle of even the most experienced clinician. Clearly negotiating boundaries of care, working with a multidisciplinary team, and developing an empathetic but firm approach are needed. Involving the family, coworkers, and significant others in an intervention can be more effective than trying to treat such patients alone.

CASE 6-4 (*continued*)

G. M. returns after undergoing counseling and working with a multidisciplinary pain management team. After much self-reflection, he has retrained for another job, moderated his alcohol use, and patched up his marriage. He is extremely grateful for his physician's help, and grateful that his father, B. W., has come for evaluation of his own back problems. B. W. is 78 years old and has had increasing back problems over the past 3 months. Other than a history of prostate cancer, B. W. has been remarkably well. He has noted a 10-pound, unintentional weight loss over the past month. Physical examination is remarkable for some tenderness at the L2 vertebra.

The physician is concerned about B. W.'s history of prostate cancer, unintentional weight loss, and back tenderness. The physician's worse fears are confirmed when a bone scan and subsequent MRI discloses metastatic cancer, presumably from the prostate.

TREATING SPECIAL POPULATIONS

When initiating therapy the physician must remember to assess the whole patient, her personal history and unique background. This assessment should consider the epidemiology, culture, and beliefs of the patient and her community. For example, the astute clinician in Case 6-4 recognized the different epidemiology of back pain in B. W. While his son's presentation was similar, B. W. has a much higher risk of having a serious underlying cause of his back discomfort.

In elders, the physician must consider changes in the distribution, absorption, metabolism, protein binding, pharmacokinetic, and pharmacodynamic action of medications. For example, the half-life of benzodiazepines may be significantly longer in elders. Elders may also have significant comorbidities that make them susceptible to medication side effects. Moreover, they may lack the social supports, sensory or motor facilities, or capability to adhere to optimal therapy.

Functional outcomes become increasingly important, rather than curative goals, in the elderly (see Chapter 14, "Functional Assessment"). While a diuretic may improve blood pressure, the precipitation of orthostatic hypotension and falls, a common side effect, could be devastating. Modifying cardiac risk factors, such as cholesterol, may have less influence on a patient's longevity and significantly impact a patient's quality of life.

Other special populations have important needs. For example, in today's diverse society, understanding the patient's cultural, ethnic, and racial background can also be crucial. An individual with G6PD deficiency will be intolerant of certain medications. A Jehovah's Witness may refuse blood products on religious grounds. An elderly Czech farmer may have certain dietary preferences. And an individual who is homeless will face significant barriers to adhering to many treatment regimens. Understanding the patient's needs and sociocultural perspective is important to tailoring therapy appropriately (Helman, 1994).

CONCLUSION

The decision to institute therapy should be considered judiciously. Many patients will warrant watchful waiting. Others will benefit from nonpharmacologic treatment. The initiation of therapy will depend on the seriousness of the problem, the probability of treatment success and complications, and patient preference. In many cases, a series of treatment options will be outlined and an initial therapy chosen.

When beginning treatment, measures to enhance adherence and plans for follow-up should be enacted. The physician should set outcome goals and discuss ways to monitor for possible complications. Involving the patient in treatment will enhance adherence. The partnership between the clinician and patient is important to ongoing treatment success.

Special care should be paid to the patient's unique needs. Many patients will have preexisting conditions, extenuating social or economic circumstances, or particular ethnic or cultural preferences. Acknowledging and respecting these differences will also enhance adherence to treatment. By carefully considering the whole patient, the astute physician can help guarantee favorable outcomes.

CASES FOR DISCUSSION

CASE 1

P. M., a 25-year-old IV drug abuser, presents because of fatigue, night sweats, and an oral rash. During the course of the history, the physician learns he has had multiple same-sex partners and has been engaging in "risky" sexual activities, i.e., is at high risk for sexually transmitted diseases. P. M. has had a positive HIV test. On physical examination the physician finds an oral rash suggestive of candida infection and generalized adenopathy. A CD4+ lymphocyte count is 150 cells/μl.

1. Does this patient have AIDS?

2. When should treatment with antiretroviral therapy be started? Does such therapy forestall the development of AIDS, prolong an asymptomatic phase, or increase life span?
3. Are there particular illnesses to which this patient is susceptible? What interventions are appropriate to prevent these illnesses?
4. What nonpharmacologic treatments should be instituted?
5. What role do family, community support groups, and other counseling resources play in this patient's treatment?

CASE 2

J. M., a 36-year-old woman, presents with a 3-month history of a distinct mass in her right breast. She has a history of fibrocystic changes and underwent aspiration of a benign breast mass 3 years ago. Her mother and a sister have a history of breast cancer. Examination discloses a discrete 2-cm mass in the right upper quadrant of the right breast. An attempt at aspiration is unsuccessful.

1. What further diagnostic evaluation, if any, would you recommend before instituting treatment in this patient?
2. How would your recommendations differ if the patient were 26 or 76? if the patient had no family history of breast cancer? if the mass first appeared 2 weeks ago?
3. If the mass turned out to be an adenocarcinoma, and there was no evidence of distant metastasis, what options would you recommend? Construct a list of the pros and cons of various treatment options.

CASE 3

D. C., a frail 89-year-old, presents with urgency, hesitancy, and difficulty maintaining a good urinary stream. The patient has a history of moderate Alzheimer's disease, diagnosed 3 years ago, coronary artery disease and congestive heart failure, osteoarthritis, and diabetes mellitus. Evaluation by your urologic consultant discloses prostate cancer with an equivocal area of bony metastasis to the spine on bone scan. The patient's daughter has flown in from California and wants to know what you recommend as treatment.

1. What factors influence treatment decisions in this patient?
2. What is the natural history of prostate cancer in this patient?
3. How would you make treatment decisions for a cognitively impaired individual?
4. What if the patient had never clearly expressed wishes regarding treatment and you and the daughter's judgment concerning the best course of action differed?

CASE 4

L. S., a 64-year-old with mild Parkinson's disease and diabetes mellitus, presents to your office having "passed out." The patient is a vice president at a major corporation and a vigorous and mentally sharp individual. He was rising to go to the bathroom yesterday evening when he "fainted," just missing hitting his head on the nightstand. He said he didn't really lose consciousness, but felt light-headed. He returned to bed, rested, and after sitting up for a short period of time, was able to make it to the bathroom without incident. His wife was away on a business trip, but on her return, "made him" come to your office for assessment. She is quite concerned, and wonders if his heart is acting up. The patient takes levodopa/carbidopa 100/25 TID and glipizide 5 mg po qd. Examination reveals an alert, cooperative gentleman in no distress.

- *BP 130/70 mm Hg, pulse 67/minute, respirations 12/minute*
- *HEENT: normal*
- *Neck: supple, no bruits*
- *Lungs: clear to A and P*
- *Cor: S1, S2, no murmurs, clicks, or rubs*
- *Periphery: remarkable for minimal distal sensory peripheral neuropathy in toes*
- *Results of neurologic examination are normal except for a slight tremor and minimal rigidity in the upper extremities*
- *HbA$_1$C is 8.1%, results of the chemistry profile and EKG are normal*

1. *What is the differential diagnosis in this patient?*
2. *How useful is the clinical history and examination in narrowing down the possibilities?*
3. *Are there are any other historical or physical findings you would seek?*
4. *How much further evaluation (if any) is prudent?*
5. *What would you tell this patient about driving or operating his Rototiller this spring?*
6. *How likely is the patient to experience another "spell"?*

CASE 5

A 17-year-old high school gymnast presents to the office with a painful right ankle. She fell off the parallel bars earlier today and now complains of discomfort and swelling along the lateral aspect of the ankle. She believes she bent her ankle inward, but is not sure. She is extremely upset because the state tournament is tomorrow.

On examination there is obvious swelling and early bruising. There is pain on palpation in a diffuse area along the lateral aspect of the ankle. There is no point tenderness along the posterior edge or tip of either malleolus. There is no tenderness at the base of the metatarsals or at the navicular. The patient limps, but can cautiously bear weight with assistance.

1. *Did this patient break her ankle? Did she sprain her ankle? Do you remember the anatomy of the ankle ligaments?*
2. *Is an X ray needed? Will treatment be influenced by the findings on X ray?*
3. *Are there some guidelines that might help in ordering an X ray?*
4. *How would you manage this patient?*

CASE 6

A 7-year-old presents with earache. An examination discloses a red ear with a poorly movable tympanic membrane. You believe the patient has otitis media.

1. *What factors would you consider in initiating therapy?*
2. *What are the costs of various alternative treatments?*
3. *How would you deal with a parent requesting an effective, but costly, pharmacologic treatment when less costly alternatives were available?*

————————— RECOMMENDED READINGS —————————

Brody DS: The patient's role in clinical decision-making. *Ann Intern Med* 93:718–722, 1980.

  Clearly articulates the primary role of the patient in clinical decision-making.

136

Helman CG: *Culture, Health and Illness*. London, Butterworths–Heinemann, 1994.

A classic work of medical anthropology describing the interaction of culture, well-being, illness, and disease.

Hilfiker D: *Healing the Wounds: A Physician Looks at His Work*. New York, Viking Penguin, 1987.

An insightful, often heartwrenching look at an individual's practice, including the challenges of diagnosis and treatment and facing the limits of knowledge and ability.

Howell JD, Lurie N, Woolliscroft JO: Worlds apart: Some thoughts to be delivered to house officers on the first day of clinic. *JAMA* 258:502–503, 1987.

This article shares useful philosophy about the role of the clinician in the outpatient arena, including the importance of communication, the savvy use of time, and the consideration of a broad range of outcomes.

Pauker SG, Kopelman RI: Some familiar tradeoffs. *N Engl J Med* 331:1511–1514, 1994.

This article describes the decision-making process used to initiate anticoagulant therapy, including the trade-offs balanced in management. The clinical problem-solving series in *NEJM* is an excellent resource for thinking about the initiation of therapy.

Reilly B: *Practical Strategies in Outpatient Medicine*. Philadelphia, WB Saunders Co, 1992.

Centered around common ambulatory problems, this book combines helpful hints on the physical examination, useful tables, and practical advice.

CHAPTER 7

Record Keeping and Presentation

William M. Chop, Jr.

CASE 7-1

Trembling, Mr. Madigan opens the door of his home to Dr. Harrison. Mr. Madi-gan's wife Mary is deathly ill with fever and shortness of breath. Dr. Harrison examines her, diagnoses pneumonia, and drives her to a small-town hospital in the next county.

After a bumpy ride, Dr. Harrison presents Mrs. Madigan's case to Dr. Bell, a physician practicing at the county hospital. A few words about Mary's past poor health and her difficult life on a run-down old farm help complete the picture for Dr. Bell and the night nurse, who both commit the story to memory. No paper records are exchanged. The physician examines Mrs. Madigan and gives verbal orders to the nurse, who helps the new patient into a bed on the ward. Dr. Bell writes the patient record by simply recording Mrs. Madigan's name and diagnosis in the ward's large ledger book. She miraculously survives the pneumonia, and after 3 weeks of prayer, care, and fresh air her husband takes her home. Dr. Bell records the final outcome of the case on the same line of the same ledger, and the case is closed. Her hospital record consists of one line of text. The year is 1911.

—————— EDUCATIONAL OBJECTIVES ——————

After reading this chapter, students of medicine should be able to perform the following:

1. Discuss users and uses of patient records
2. Explain the advantages and disadvantages of source-based and problem-oriented records

3. Given a patient encounter, author a data base, a problem list, and an assessment and plan
4. Given a patient encounter, write an untitled "SOAP" note and a true problem-oriented record, and explain the advantages and disadvantages of each
5. Explain the advantages and disadvantages of traditional, problem-based, and newspaper-style case presentations
6. Given a patient encounter or record, a particular audience, and a purpose, give a verbal presentation that efficiently and effectively conveys the patient's story and achieves the purpose for that audience
7. Produce records and presentations that are accurate and honest, but favorably portray each patient as a person worthy of empathy and care

INTRODUCTION

Skills in record keeping and presentation add leverage to other clinical skills. It is through patient records and presentation that other clinical skills are most acutely displayed to mentors, to other clinicians, and to posterity. The process of preparing records and presentations yields insight into a patient's case, protects against clinical oversights, and provides feedback that will advance clinical expertise. Record keeping and presentation are primary means by which general and case-specific medical knowledge and wisdom are transmitted over time and space to other physicians. The ability to capture and transmit the story of each patient is fundamental in maintaining the professional literature and preserving the art of medicine.

Writing about patient cases is an ancient medical tradition, but in the past it was done only infrequently, mostly to support investigation and education rather than to support direct patient care. The one-line record of Case 7-1 was typical in small rural hospitals. Today, patient records are authored mainly because they are so helpful in the care of individual patients. They have become multicomponent documents that serve numerous users and uses, with a complexity such that computerized patient record systems are becoming necessary to medical practice. Expertise in the creation and use of patient records is one of the hallmarks of a good physician. This chapter will increase appreciation for the variety of types and purposes of patient records and help develop strong skills in using and keeping patient records.

The importance of excellent oral presentation skills has also grown during the twentieth century. Presentations of a patient's case remain an important part of the grand tradition of medicine, especially in medical education settings. In the past, physicians had a slower pace and a relatively small menu of available diagnostic modalities and treatments. Simple communications sufficed. Dr. Harrison's presentation to Dr. Bell in Case 7-1 was simple and direct compared with the communication that often occurs between two physicians today. As the complexity of medicine increased, so did the need for frequent, rapid, and concise communication of accurate and precise patient information. Division of labor occurred, and medicine became "industrialized." Nurses, pharmacists, technicians, researchers, and physicians of every kind now practice in a wide variety of both general and highly specialized facilities. Consultation and teaching also depend heavily on quality verbal presentations of patient cases. This chapter will focus on the importance of strong skills in listening to and presenting patient cases.

In approaching this subject, remember that charting and presentation skills depend on medical knowledge and experience. An excellent patient record or presentation will only result from excellent data collection and analysis. Do not become discouraged if it is initially difficult to produce smooth, useful records and presentations. Also, be aware that presenting patient cases is a higher-order skill than writing patient records. A patient record depends on a patient data base and on medical knowledge and experience. It represents an understanding of the complex intersection of medical observations and previous interventions with current wellness, illness, and the patient as a person with a life. A case presentation depends on a patient record. It takes into account everything in the complete patient record, but must also be audience specific and concise as it conveys the significant knowledge and wisdom represented by a particular patient case. The ability to skillfully present a case depends as much on ability to skillfully author a patient record as it does on the other presentation skills.

CASE 7-2

Mrs. Smith thoughtfully completed the health forms the nurse gave her. She listed her diabetes mellitus, her hypertension, and the births of her children. She explained her possible allergy to sulfa drugs. On the review of systems form she checked the appropriate boxes and explained all of the symptoms she was experiencing. The nurse took her vital signs and complaints, and led her to an examining room.

Dr. Susan Jones picked up the chart of this new patient from the rack on the examination room door, and began to read it. New patient . . . 47-year-old woman . . . diabetes mellitus . . . hypertension . . . makes a living as an artist. She entered the examination room, and started the visit. After the visit, Dr. Jones wrote a two-part prescription form, gave the original to Mrs. Smith, and filed the copy in the chart. She had Mrs. Smith sign releases to get records from her previous physicians. She completed the problem list in the chart, filled in the top of the flow sheet with a preventive health plan, and wrote the new medication and dose at the bottom. She then dictated a progress note. The next afternoon, after the transcribed progress note returned, Dr. Jones reviewed and signed it, and a nurse placed it in Mrs. Smith's chart. When copies arrived from Mrs. Smith's previous physicians, Dr. Jones reviewed them, updated the chart with a brief note, and filed them in the "old record" section. Two weeks later, Mrs. Smith's insurance company requested a copy of her chart, and it was sent. A month later Mrs. Smith's chart was randomly selected by the clinic's quality assurance committee for review. It passed. Three months later the chart was reviewed as part of a retrospective research study of antihypertensive medications. When Mrs. Smith returned for a sprained ankle 4 months later, Dr. Jones's detailed note allowed her partner to more quickly appreciate Mrs. Smith as a person, and to take better care of her and her family.

PATIENT RECORDS

Sigurdsson describes the purpose of patient records simply, stating that they are "aids to the treatment of the patient," "instruments of teaching, learning, and research," and "a source of statistics." Sigurdsson also warns clinicians that "the ultimate test of a system for collecting and handling data in primary health care should be whether such a system helps us to understand better the special relationship between healer and patient; not just the interaction between the two, but the relationship itself in its full sociocultural context" (Sigurdsson, 1984). Prompted by the exploding popularity of computerized patient record systems, the Council on Scientific Affairs of the American Medical Association (1993) cited seven categories of users and 13 broad uses of patient records. This chapter focuses on uses of patient records in the provision of patient care, and on the role patient records play in the patient–physician relationship. A brief discussion of the full spectrum of important users and uses for patient records will help to set the stage.

At its essence, the patient record is a tool to facilitate the complex process of caring for patients in sickness and health. The process of care involves many people, including patients, families, students, residents, physicians, consultants, nurses, educators, researchers, psychologists, lab technicians, radiology technicians, insurance companies and other third-party payers, financial staff, managers, reviewers, licensing and accrediting agencies, and professional associations. All of these people interact with the patient, the patient record, and each other, in different ways, and for many purposes, as illustrated in Case 7-2.

The most obvious purpose of the patient record is to serve as a memory device to foster continuity of care. Even when a patient sees only a single physician, that physician cannot afford to rely on simple memory for all of the important details about that particular patient. At a second visit the physician uses the record to gain a clinical and personal foothold based on the information recorded at the first visit. Even in less desirable clinical settings where the patient sees a new physician at each visit, good records help each different physician to gain a more rapid and complete understanding of the patient as a person and of the patient's medical needs. Through each physician's contribution, a historical record for the future is maintained that is much more accurate and comprehensive than memory.

The record also helps clinicians to visualize the patient's clinical situation to support intelligent diagnosis and treatment. Even if no illness is identified, a record helps the physician to assess and manage health risks in providing preventive care to both individual patients and communities.

Patient records document the patient's case management for billing and legal purposes. Because of legal and economic pressures, an unfortunate line of thinking has been allowed to arise in medical management circles that "if it's not documented, then it didn't happen." Of course this statement is not true, but for medicolegal purposes it's a wise statement to keep in mind. If a physician bills an insurance company for a service rendered to a patient, but does not produce a record that documents and justifies the service, it could be claimed that the physician did not actually render the service, or the service was unnecessary, and that the bill was at best a mistake and at worst fraud. Also, if a patient feels that a physician was negligent and sues the physician, the patient record is considered objective evidence of what actually happened. Physicians are especially sensitive to the tension between the need for records to be concise and clinically relevant and the need for records to serve these somewhat arbitrary legal purposes. Misunderstandings arise from this area of tension when people who have a single-minded view of the patient record do not appreciate the multiple priorities of the physician.

Patient records also are a window into a physician's past experiences. Records are ideal for use in teaching and in gathering research information. Records support case-based reasoning in which specific past cases help solve new cases and collections of past cases are used to formulate future practice guidelines. Utilization review, quality assurance, and licensing entities use patient records to assess physician performance, and medical students and residents are constantly evaluated through their patient record keeping.

Finally, in considering the ubiquitous nature of patient records in healthcare today, it is critical to remember that *patient information must be kept confidential.* Those directly caring for the patient usually should have access to the entire patient record, but other people and organizations should only have limited access on a need to know basis after explicit permission has been granted by the patient. All parties with access to information must carefully protect patient confidentiality.

CASE 7-3

First the intern, then the chief resident, and finally the pediatric floor nurses interviewed the mother and poked and prodded the little girl late into the night. Five hours later the sun was rising. The on-call team assembled at morning report to present their admission of the 6-year-old girl with pneumonia and a pain crisis resulting from sickle-cell disease. Soon afterward, James Johnson, MSII, the medical student assigned to the service, was dispatched to introduce himself, examine the patient, and write a problem-based progress note. The student read the admission H&P, examined the patient, and wrote this "untitled SOAP note":

3/27/95   0815   Student Note

(S)ubjective: *Pain is decreased in legs and feet. Still complaining of pain in her right chest when she coughs. Not hungry this morning, but thirsty and drinking juice.*

(O)bjective: *Vital signs: T 101.6°F, HR 115, BP 100/54, RR 34. Medications: Oxygen 28% mask, IV: D5½NS at 100 ml/hr, oral morphine, cefazolin 300 mg IV q8h. Input 800 ml, output 300 ml urine, no bowel movements. General: Alert, fussy but cooperative. Lungs: Patient splinting the right side of chest. Decreased breath sounds, dullness and rales are noted in the right posterior lung field. Heart: Tachycardic; regular rate and rhythm; no murmurs, gallops, or rubs. Abdomen: BS normal, no tenderness, masses, or hepatosplenomegaly. Extremities: Tender diffusely in the legs. Lab: Pending.*

(A)ssessments: *(1) right lower lobe pneumonia; (2) Sickle-Cell Disease with Pain Crisis.*

(P)lans: *Continue hydration, antibiotics, morphine, oxygen, and check lab.*

TYPES OF INFORMATION AND RECORDS

Medical information about a patient may be discovered through direct observation or from another source, such as the patient, a parent, a nurse, another physician, or a previous medical record. The information may pertain to health or disease, to one or more systems, and to one or more pathologic conditions. Medical information of any type from any source is subject to various biases.

In the past patient records were almost exclusively "source oriented," arranged according to the source authoring or providing the information. This orientation did not facilitate analysis of patient problems very well, so another method of structuring the same data base, called the problem-oriented medical record (POMR), was developed by Weed (1968) and is still in extensive use. The essential element of the POMR system is the *titled progress note*. A data base is collected and recorded, and then a separate note is written for each problem identified. Each problem-oriented note is comprised of relevant history, physical, and lab data abstracted from the patient information data base, followed by an assessment of its significance, and by a three-part plan detailing the diagnostic, therapeutic, and educational options needed to address that problem. A list of active and inactive problems is kept at the front of the chart to serve as a table of contents to the dated, titled notes in the chart. Since each problem is separately addressed and recorded along with supporting data, analysis, and plan, the logic and thinking behind the plan is quite evident for each problem. Other record keeping systems that do not abstract history, observations, assessment, and plan for each problem into a single context do not clearly and overtly reveal the thinking and logic behind the plan.

Untitled SOAP Notes

In Weed's problem-oriented system, the note describing each problem is arranged by history ("Subjective"), physical and laboratory findings ("Objective"), Assessment, and Plan. These problem-based notes have thus become known as "SOAP Notes." If a patient has five problems addressed at a single visit, then five separately titled SOAP notes should be written—one for each problem. The essence of the POMR is not the arrangement of information in a SOAP fashion, but titled progress notes—a clinical data base abstracted into data pertinent to problems and indexed to a problem list. But ironically the SOAP arrangement has become more popular than titled progress notes. Many physicians who write notes arranged in a SOAP fashion think that they are using problem-oriented records, when in fact they are not. Case 7-3 exemplifies such an *untitled SOAP note*.

It is so easy for physicians to gravitate toward the use of untitled SOAP notes that they deserve to be discussed explicitly. Although physicians are continually "foraging for data" in caring for patients, constant time pressure limits the opportunity to optimally synthesize additions to the patient record (Tang *et al.*, 1994). At each patient encounter, information tends to be gathered in a parallel fashion, not by problem. A physician may also obtain data from other sources, such as the current chart, an old chart, a nurse's clipboard, a family member, the patient, the laboratory computer, a verbal report from a radiologist, and so forth. All of this information must be collated and considered in addressing the patient's problems. It seems natural to record this information as it is collected in a source-oriented data base, but after doing so, many physicians find it burdensome to duplicate portions of the data in the separately titled problems of a true problem-oriented system. Instead the data base is followed by a simple list of assessments and a simple list of plans that are not tied to the data base. Anyone reading the record is forced to glean from the data base any information that would seem to support the assessments and plans. In untitled SOAP notes the thought process behind the assessment is not well preserved.

In summary, untitled SOAP notes are not ideal, but they are often used, are often adequate, and are often the best record that a physician can be expected to produce given the intense time pressures of medical practice. A well-constructed and defended POMR is ideal because it preserves both the data and the rationale of the clinician's diagnoses and plans, but it involves redundancy and increased effort.

Later that morning the student made rounds with the chief resident, who showed him how to rewrite the note in problem-oriented fashion so that the thinking and decision-making process would be displayed more clearly. The chief advocated using "History" and "Observations" instead of "Subjective" and "Objective" because they were more accurate terms.

3/27/95   0815   Medical Student Note

PROBLEM #1: *PNEUMONIA, RIGHT LOWER LOBE*

History: *Still complaining of pain in her right chest when she coughs.*

Observations: *Vital signs: T 101.6°F, HR 115, BP 100/54, RR 34. On oxygen 28% mask and cefazolin 300 mg IV q8h. Lungs: Patient splinting the right side of chest. Breath sounds are decreased and dullness and rales present in the right posterior lung field, and clear elsewhere.*

Assessment & Plan: *Pneumonia clinically is slightly better, and does not seem to have spread. Patient has not developed respiratory distress. Almost certainly bacterial. Sputum studies pending. Initial films without effusion, but risk of emphysema present. Diagnostically, get sputum studies, CXR tomorrow to document response and exclude effusion. Therapeutically, continue cefazolin and oxygen, add respiratory therapy. Educationally, try to keep patient and parents informed about progress.*

PROBLEM #2: *SICKLE-CELL DISEASE WITH PAIN CRISIS*

H: *Pain is decreased in legs and feet. Not hungry this morning, but thirsty and drinking juice.*

O: *Medications: Oxygen 28% mask, oral morphine, hydration per problem #3. Heart: Tachycardic with regular rate and rhythm with no murmurs, gallops, or rubs. Abdomen: BS normal, no tenderness, masses, or hepatosplenomegaly. Extremities: Tender diffusely in the legs.*

A/P: *Pain improved. No evidence of other complications thus far. No current diagnostic plans. Therapeutically, continue hydration, oxygen, and morphine as necessary. Treatment of pneumonia should also help. No educational plans at present.*

PROBLEM #3: *FLUID/ELECTROLYTES/NUTRITION*

H/O: *Drinking fluids well, not hungry. IV: D5½NS at 100 ml/hr. Input 800 ml. Output 300 ml urine, no bowel movements. Good skin turgor. Electrolyte panel pending.*

A/P: *Not dehydrated, but has higher fluid requirement due to fever, increased respiratory rate, and need for hydration due to sickle crisis. Diagnostically, obtain pending electrolyte panel now and daily while on IV to guide additional IV fluids. Watch input and output. Therapeutically, continue IV but encourage oral intake. Decrease IV rate as oral intake increases.*

The Titled HOAP Note

The medical student in Case 7-4 could see that more work was involved in authoring the titled progress notes of the problem-oriented medical record, but after writing precisely about each problem, he had a better understanding of his patient's situation, an easier time following the patient's course, and an easier time presenting the case to his attending physician. The revised note also revealed his thinking much more clearly to his supervisors.

Case 7-4 also illustrates how physicians sometimes write progress note assessments and plans in proper POMR fashion, but do not write a separate source-oriented data base. Instead, data are included only in the problem-oriented abstracts of the data base supporting each related assessment and plan. This method preserves both data and logic, and is concise, but may make the data harder to find. Usually this method is used only for progress notes where less data are recorded, or when a data base has been previously recorded in the chart, perhaps by another physician. Compared with untitled SOAP notes, titled notes are superior sources for verbal presentations. But although this system encapsulates each problem unto itself, the lack of a source-oriented data base as in Case 7-4 forces another clinician foraging for data to read each individual problem until the information of interest is located. If the results of a chest examination and X ray are only recorded under the problem "TB exposure" and not in a data base, then a cardiologist evaluating the patient for chest pain must read the TB problem in order to find a description of the chest examination. Moreover, the use of a titled note implies that there is no need to search the data base for additional support. Therefore, if a titled note incompletely abstracts the supporting information from the data base, it can make a case look artificially weak. An untitled SOAP note might actually be preferable to a poorly written titled note.

Since physicians are not always able to produce an ideal POMR, how should charting be approached? In general, physicians should strive toward an ideal POMR by using clinical judgment to create the most important "views" of each case. Ideally there should be an overall data base, a view by problem, perhaps a view by medication, a chronological view, and so forth. Much of this involves writing the same information over and over in different parts of the chart, although a computer-based record system may obviate this chore. Sometimes a mere reference to another part of the chart, e.g., "see Social History," is sufficient. Redundancy is expensive in terms of physician and transcriptionist time, so in reality only the most useful redundancies can be incorporated into charts. It is up to physicians to do this in a clinically meaningful manner. As long as physicians honestly attempt to address the needs of potential future audiences, useful charts generally are produced.

CHARTING

The term *charting* is used by physicians to refer to the maintenance of a patient record in a chart. A chart is an integrated record that includes a number of preprinted forms, dividers, and other devices to improve the utility of the information we record. Although there are many different types of charts, physicians typically use two types.

Hospital charts are episodic, typically covering only one discrete episode of care over one block of time. Such charts tend to be divided into many sections, sometimes 15 to 20. Typical sections are admission history and physical, orders, progress notes, vital signs, nurses' notes, consultations, lab, radiology, ECG, and so forth. This format is convenient for people who deal with only one aspect of patient care, because they can focus on only that section of the chart. Chart subdivisions may also make it easier to follow trends; for example, a physician can flip through the radiology section to see how an infiltrate is progressing on serial chest X-ray reports. However, storage of these records all over the chart in a source-oriented manner makes it difficult for physicians to view a case chrono-logically by problem. For this reason, results stored in other sections are often transcribed by the physician into the daily physician progress notes, permitting the progress notes to stand more coherently by themselves. All too often, however, physicians fail to record all meaningful results tied to specific problems. Reviewing such a chart is difficult and time-consuming. It is clinically unreasonable to expect physicians to transcribe and comment in the progress notes on every single test and study reported elsewhere in the chart, but at least the significant results should be referred to and discussed.

Unlike hospital charts, *outpatient charts are not episodic,* but cover the patient over time through periods of health and disease. Charts in an outpatient primary care setting typically have five to ten source-oriented sections. The sections might be progress notes, intake forms and flow sheets, lab and X-ray results, consultations, and so forth. A number of special forms are used to facilitate long-term continuous care of the patient. Usually, some forms called "intake forms" are completed by the patient, such as a survey of past medical history and a written review of systems. While it may be suboptimal to rely on these forms instead of a personally taken history, these forms prime the patient's memory and serve as an excellent starting point for discussion.

Progress notes are the key component of the outpatient primary care chart. They are supported by lab tests, radiographs, outside reports and records, and other third-party paperwork filed chronologically. Problem lists and flow sheets are especially important components of the outpatient chart. These are preprinted forms, usually with grids, on which to record problems, medications, and important serial observations like blood pressure and target lab values. Preventive interventions can also be tracked easily with a flow sheet. Problem list forms allow physicians to list the patient's major problems for quick reference and review during follow-up visits. It is important that these forms actually be used. If they are not kept consistently up to date, they will not be trusted, they will not be referred to, and they will become even less likely to be maintained.

The form and function of charts has important implications for medical care (Donnelly, 1988). For example, there are some parts of the data base that tend to be collected or updated infrequently, and other parts that are updated almost every time the patient comes to the office. A patient's living conditions may be recorded only once, if at all, on a sheet kept in the back of the chart, whereas a patient's blood pressure may be recorded at the top of each visit. Bias may result from this, since the physician may concentrate on the medical information close at hand rather than looking back into the chart to find something of greater importance to the patient's care. To ensure that such a problem receives due attention, many physicians record any significant aspect of a pa-tient's data base in the problem list. If "very poor housing" is recorded as a problem on the problem list, it will be far more likely to receive due consideration from the physician as plans are made at future visits.

Bias also occurs because of the artificial subjective/objective dichotomy introduced by Weed's problem-oriented medical record. In reality the distinction between subjective and objective information is fuzzy. Usually the story of the patient, the history, is the most important and useful part of the data base. Yet by definition the patient's story is consid-ered "subjective." Ironically, some physician observations contain considerable subjec-tivity, but are classified as "objective." Use of the latter term obscures the physician's fallibility and humanity. So instead of "SOAP," Donnelly and Brauner (1992) advocate thinking and writing in terms of "HOAP," meaning, "History, Observations, Assessments, Plans," an example of which is given in Case 7-4. *History* is a more honorable term than *subjective*. It makes it clear that the patient's observations, the previous observations of the current physician, and the observations of other physicians and institutions all belong together in the history section. The *observation* section is reserved only for the current observations of the authoring physician, including current lab results and tests.

The subjective–objective dichotomy so entrenched in the SOAP mnemonic has also been reinforced by a change in the meanings of the terms *symptoms* and *signs*. Modern use of the term *symptom* refers to an abnormal phenomenon experienced by an individual. A *sign* is an abnormality discovered by the physician during an examination. However, prior to 1900 the term *symptom* generally referred to "any manifestation of a disease whether perceived by a patient or a physician" and *sign* to "a perception that led to a meaningful inference about the patient and his or her disease." Signs were considered to be symptoms with meaning. It was not the source of information that distinguished between these two (Donnelly & Brauner, 1992). Nonetheless, in modern usage symptoms are recorded in the history or subjective section of the data base and progress notes; signs noted by others are also recorded in the history or subjective section; and only the observations of the authoring physician are recorded in the observation or objective section.

CASE 7-5

It was a hectic afternoon in the student clinic. Maria Brown, MSII, was feeling rather stressed. She walked to examination room No. 2, slipped the thick chart quietly out of the rack on the door, and opened the chart of Margaret Green, another patient she'd never met. She scanned down the problem list: obesity, diabetes mellitus, hypertension, ethanolism, tobaccoism, depression, and many more. The flow sheet showed a series of elevated blood pressure readings, and a series of equally elevated glucose readings. At least ten medications were on the flow sheet, most no longer active. And then, on the top progress note, she read the final note written by the outgoing MSIV assigned to Ms. Green. It began, "This is a difficult, noncompliant 47-year-old alcoholic who comes to clinic frequently with multiple somatic complaints." The other notes indicated many attempts to diagnose and treat her complaints, most of which failed. The new patient intake forms that Ms. Green had completed 3 years ago were sparsely completed and were not helpful.

Maria dreaded seeing a "difficult, noncompliant alcoholic," but she took a deep breath, letting it out slowly. She cleared her mind of distractions, pictured Ms. Green as a suffering, perhaps confused person, and set a learning goal for herself for this visit: find out who Ms. Green the person really is. With a calm demeanor she entered the room, allowed her patient to speak without interruption, and addressed her concerns. She gleaned from the chart that several preventive interventions were overdue. A plan was negotiated. Soon the visit was complete, with a recheck scheduled in 2 weeks. As Ms. Green left, she told Maria that it was the first visit where anyone really listened to her.

Sitting at the physician's workstation, Maria completed the chart, adding new problems to the problem list: illiteracy, loneliness, grief, poverty. She would scarcely be able to address these problems as a student physician, but now they wouldn't be forgotten. And she added a neatly printed picture of Ms. Green's life to the chart as insurance against a future student dreading her patient on a future

hectic afternoon: "Margaret Green is a pleasant 47-year-old woman. She was
orphaned as a baby and was raised in a series of foster homes. She was physically
and mentally abused in many of the homes, until finally at the age of 13 a woman
took her in who loved her, cared for her, and adopted her. Since she was hard of
hearing she did poorly in school, finally dropping out at age 16 because she could
not keep up and because so many children made fun of her. For the next 20 years
she was employed cleaning buildings but after she turned 40 her adopted mother
suddenly died. Her health deteriorated, and she quit working. . . ." Maria paused,
sad at seeing such a story in black and white, but pleased that Ms. Green's chart
was no longer "poisoned."

REVIEWING PATIENT RECORDS

It is important to be skilled in reviewing patient records. Unfortunately, physicians
and especially new students of medicine frequently do not review patient charts adequately. Osheroff *et al.* (1991) found that 52% of patient care-related questions arising in
an internal medicine teaching program "requested a fact that could have been provided
using the patient record or hospital information system." Students should review the
patient record more effectively prior to seeing patients and prior to presenting those
patients to other physicians. Reviewing charts is also an effective way to learn about
writing charts. In a thick patient chart there are frequently three or four notes that prove to
be especially helpful. Look carefully at these key notes, decide what it is about them that
makes them especially helpful, and when appropriate, try to emulate them.

There is almost always some type of record to review before seeing a patient. Even
when the patient is new, it is likely that some sort of intake history form has been
completed. Remember that the physician is responsible for the information the patient
discloses on intake forms. If a patient writes that she is taking birth control pills, but the
physician fails to read it and prescribes an antibiotic that reduces the effectiveness of those
pills, then the patient may become pregnant. The same thinking applies to information in
previous progress notes in the clinic chart. The physician *must* consider those notes during
the current episode of care. Review the chart and be up to date on the patient before
entering the examination room.

Reviewing the chart does not mean reading the entire chart. If previous authors have
been keeping up with problem lists and problem-oriented notes, medication lists, and flow
sheets, then it is easy to review the patient's chart. Often a previous note summarizes
important past information in such a way that both data and thinking are reliably preserved. Sometimes, though, the previous notes are sparse and disorganized, requiring the
physician to "read between the lines," and "forage for data" in the patient intake forms,
past notes, and old records.

The method used to review a chart also depends to some extent on the review's
purpose. If the patient already has a physician and presents to a Saturday morning walk-in
clinic with an acute sore throat, then a review of past abdominal surgeries is unnecessary.
However, an infectious disease specialist must carefully search the entire patient record
for clues when consulted about a patient with fevers that remain unexplained despite a
well-directed workup.

In learning to review charts, notice helpful and unhelpful features and take a lesson
from them. Legible handwriting and typed notes speed chart review. Redundant records
and serial records of irrelevant information inhibit chart review. A complete data base is

important, but excessive amounts of redundant normal observations obscure important past observations. When problem lists, medication lists, and flow sheets are not maintained, they cannot be trusted and physicians are forced to review the entire chart.

It is helpful to adopt a consistent agenda to try to extract *functional* information about the patient from the chart. Review the activities of the patient—occupation, hobbies, exercise, typical days. A note documenting that a patient is a volunteer who delivers meals to homebound people 3 days a week tells something about the patient and establishes a baseline that can be used as a basis for comparison later. Reviewing patient activities will also raise awareness of how often physicians neglect to record functional information. Too often it is impossible to tell from a chart how a patient is really doing. Two patients may have virtually identical charts from a disease standpoint, yet one is doing very poorly in life, while the other scarcely notices poor health. The lack of a good record of function makes it very difficult to effectively address a patient's needs.

Finally, take special notice of how the patient record is able to either humanize or dehumanize the patient. Prior to reading a chart and entering an examination room, each physician should "suspend judgment" so that she is prepared to interact with the patient as a person in need and not as an abstract "case." If the chart berates the patient or inappropriately leads a reviewer to conclude that the patient is "difficult," as in Case 7-5, there is a risk the physician will be "poisoned" by that information and establish a less satisfactory relationship than would have occurred if the chart had portrayed the patient more humanely. Patient records should ideally establish that the patient is a person with a life and family who should be treated with respect and compassion. However, many progress notes are simply sterile; often little social history has been recorded other than something like, "smokes two packs per day." Before meeting any patient, shake off any "poison" noted in the chart by scanning for narratives that establish the patient as a person. Take time to read the social and family histories, and scan the progress notes for "stories" about the patient. Enter the examining room prepared to be compassionate and empathetic. And if the chart does not contain an adequate narrative of the patient as a person, add one!

AUTHORING PATIENT RECORDS

General Considerations in Authoring Records

An important clinical skill is authoring excellent patient records in an efficient manner. The author of a patient record creates a legacy that may follow the patient the rest of her life and represents the author's skills and logic in a form that may be reviewed and used by many future physicians. The record is a literary work and a tool specifically designed to benefit that patient in the future. Consequently, physicians have a profound responsibility to be complete, accurate, precise, and concise—and an equal responsibility to present the patient as a person worthy of respect. It's a difficult and time-consuming task. Physicians in primary care specialities can easily spent 5 to 10% of their working time authoring patient records.

Patient records must be legible, so they should be typed whenever possible. Many physicians find that dictating notes for later transcription is both faster and less expensive. Unfortunately, students commonly are not taught how or permitted to dictate. Dictating is faster, captures more detail, and is compatible with computerized record systems. The time saved can then be devoted to other activities. Dictated notes are more comprehensive. It is much easier and faster to dictate the flourishes and details that establish the patient as a person, and to leave a clear starting point for the next patient encounter. Future physicians can review typed notes much more easily and quickly. Physicians typically review transcribed dictation and sign it before placing it permanently in the patient's chart. Although this requires the physician to handle the chart a second time, it also provides a second chance to think about the patient and notice any potential problems with the previous care.

It is always important to know and document the sources of information and opinion about the patient. A major write-up such as an admission history and physical examination should reference the source of information and its estimated reliability. When the source is a person, such as the patient or the patient's parent, that person is called an "informant." Histories are not taken, but created. The author of the history—the "historian"—is the physician, established by a signature at the end of the write-up.

When the source of information is a "third party" such as lab or X-ray reports, or records from another facility, be sure to verify the information with names, ID numbers, dates, and times. Be sure to date, time, and sign all notes. Physicians with illegible signatures should type or print their name underneath. If the note occupies more than one physical sheet of paper, then sign at the end of each sheet and note that the write-up is continued to another page. Record the date and time on each continuation page.

Any changes made to the medical record must leave an "audit trail" by writing any new information, crossing out incorrect information with simple lines that leave the old information legible, and dating, timing, and signing the change. In many cases an explanatory addendum can be added to a chart, but sometimes it's safest to directly edit an old note. For example, if a patient develops a drug allergy it might be good to note it, with the current date, on previous notes that stated "no allergies." In cases known to concern litigation, however, it is best not to make any changes, even if they are signed and dated, without first discussing it with a lawyer.

In using patient records, remember that they must remain accessible. For that reason, most facilities do not permit records to be taken off premises for any reason. It is preferable to make a photocopy if the record is truly needed elsewhere. For the same reason, all charts not in proper storage should be left out in the open where they can be seen. They should never be hidden in a drawer, a cabinet, or a locked room. Forms and papers important to the record must be handled carefully, preferably by fixing any loose forms in the chart. Each sheet of paper should have the patient's unique chart identifier written on it so that if it is separated from the chart, it can be refiled later. The addition of photographs of the patient to the chart can serve as a useful patient identifier with the advantage that they simultaneously add a human dimension to the patient's record.

CASE 7-6

3/15/95   1640   **Resident Admission Note (RAN)**

ID: *Jane Smith is a 51-year-old female from Smallville, Texas. She is a commercial artist, mainly a painter, married with four children, three still living at home. She has hypertension and adult-onset diabetes mellitus. This is her first hospital admission since her youngest child was born. The history is obtained from the patient, who is a reliable informant, and by phone from Dr. Susan Jones, her attending family physician.*

CC: *"I'm coughing up blood and my chest hurts." She is admitted by Dr. Jones for treatment of a right lower lobe pneumonia.*

HPI: *Mrs. Smith felt well until about 8 days ago when she developed fever, chills, headache, body aches, sore throat, and nonproductive cough. She began taking over-the-counter cold medications and acetaminophen. After 2 days she went to see her family physician, Dr. Susan Jones, who diagnosed influenza A and prescribed amantadine 200 mg STAT followed by 100 mg twice a day. Her glucose was normal. By the next day she began to feel better and her fever resolved. She continued to have a dry cough until 2 days ago when she began to feel achy again and began coughing up small amounts of yellow sputum. Yesterday chills and fever reappeared and a pain in the lateral right chest developed that was worse with coughing and deep breathing. Her discomforts continued today and she also began to feel somewhat short of breath. At about 10 AM, she started coughing up dark blood. The appearance of the blood frightened her so she came to the emergency room (ER). After evaluation in the ER, Dr. Jones was called, and admitted the patient.*

Mrs. Smith smoked one pack per day for 15 years, but quit 10 years ago as a health measure. She has no history of pneumonia, lung disease, TB, cancer, or asbestos or other exposures; there is no history of coagulopathy. She has never had either influenza or pneumococcal vaccines.

The hemoptysis was especially frightening to Mrs. Smith because her brother has lung cancer. She feels embarrassed that she did not seek attention earlier. She is tired of having to worry about her health and take medications, so she just kept hoping that this problem would go away.

PMH:

1. Diseases:

   Diabetes mellitus: *15 years ago she developed polyuria and fatigue, was found to have a fasting blood glucose of 286 mg/dl, and was diagnosed with adult-onset non-insulin-dependent diabetes mellitus. She weighed 223 pounds at the time. She took the news positively and went on a diet (2500 calories per day), began taking an oral hypoglycemic, and learned to check her own glucose values. She began a water aerobics class, which she continued up until last year. Her very best friends are all members of this class. Her weight dropped to 145 pounds and she was able to stop taking the oral hypoglycemic. In the last year she has been nursing her ill brother frequently, and had to stop her aerobics classes. Her weight rose to 169 pounds, glucose into the low 200 range, she developed polyuria, and last month Dr. Jones recommended that she resume glyburide 5 mg every morning. Her glucose readings then decreased to the 120 mg/dl range, but when she became ill they increased again to the low 200 range. She is unaware of any complications of her diabetes mellitus, and sees an ophthalmologist annually.*

   Hypertension: *Diagnosed 15 years ago at the same time her diabetes mellitus was discovered. She has always taken a diuretic, no apparent side effects, with good blood pressure control.*

2. Trauma and Operations: *None significant. G4P4 with four normal vaginal deliveries.*

3. Transfusions: *None.*
4. Immunizations: *Had usual childhood immunizations. No hepatitis B series. No influenza or pneumovax.*
5. Medications:
   Glyburide 5 mg qd for the last month for diabetes mellitus, no side effects.
   HCTZ 25 mg qd for 15 years for hypertension, no side effects.
   Amantadine 100 mg bid for influenza A, currently on day #6, no side effects.
   Acetaminophen recently for pain and fever, and an over-the-counter cold medication.
6. Allergies: *Long ago a sulfa medication caused a "rash."*

Family History:

Grandparents: Paternal grandfather died, 87, old age; paternal grandmother alive, 86, has diabetes mellitus, hypertension, hypothyroidism, lives out of state; maternal grandfather died, 74, stroke; maternal grandmother died, 73, colon cancer.

Parents: father died, 60, heart attack, emphysema; mother died, 70, kidney infection, diabetes mellitus.

Siblings: Brother age 53, alive with terminal lung cancer, hypertension.

Children: Bill, 20, attending college 100 miles away; Adam, 17; Amy, 16; Lisa, 15. All are in good health. There is no history of other cancers, congenital diseases, TB, mental disease, or any other serious diseases.

Social History:

Mrs. Smith was born and raised in a suburb of Dallas, attended the University of Texas graduating with a degree in art. Her parents and brother later moved to Smallville, so she settled there also. She lived at home and was employed in commercial art until she married 21 years ago. When her children all were in school she went back into commercial art, lately working out of her home. Her husband is in a stressful construction job presently. She has remained monogamous. She considers her marriage good but not very supportive. Her children are very active in school activities.

Hobbies are reading and sculpture—she makes metal welded statues and has a lot of noise exposure from a grinder—has not done much in the last year.

Habits: Drinks at least 12 cups of drip coffee per day. Drinks alcohol only occasionally. Smoked one pack per day cigarettes for 15 years, but quit 10 years ago as a health measure. No illicit drug use.

Has been very preoccupied with caring for her terminally ill brother who has lung cancer. He lives in Mrs. Smith's guest room. She does not want to be here in the hospital because she is afraid he will need her help. She handles all his medication, feeds him all his meals, bathes him, and does some respiratory therapy. Caring for him is very time-consuming.

She has always tried to minimize her own health needs. She grieved quite a bit when diagnosed with diabetes mellitus, but soon accepted the need to take better care of herself, so quit smoking and started water aerobics classes and a weight loss program. When she began caring for her brother she was forced to quit her classes. She gained weight, her diabetes mellitus became symptomatic again, and she became discouraged. Her husband is very stressed himself, and provides little help. She refuses to ask her children to help her. Most of her friends were in her aerobics class and she has no one to talk to now. She used to attend church, and does pray about her situation, but stopped going about 6 months ago.

ROS (review of systems):

General/Systemic: gained about 25 pounds over last year; generally tired lately; no hot or cold intolerance; no abnormal bleeding.

HEENT: No visual problems, sees ophthalmologist; thinks her hearing is a little worse, has had much noise exposure to metal grinder, did not use hearing protection; occasional hay fever symptoms; sees dentist, no current dental problems.

Neck/Nodes: No lumps or pain.

Chest/Breasts: No chest pain except as in HPI; checks breasts a few times a year, but has never had a mammogram, no lumps or discharge noted.

Respiratory: No breathing problems except as in HPI.

Cardiovascular: BP typically runs around 135/85 on her diuretic; no chest pain except as in HPI; no palpitations, dyspnea (except as in HPI), orthopnea, or paroxysmal nocturnal dyspnea. No claudication or edema.

GI: no nausea, vomiting, heartburn, dysphagia, diarrhea, constipation, hematemesis, hematochezia, melena.

GU: sometimes she loses urine when she coughs; last menstrual period 6 weeks ago; has had some hot flashes over the last year and menses have been irregular, not on hormones; Pap smear 3 years ago was normal, has never had an abnormal one; no hematuria, dysuria, frequency, but has had some polyuria lately.

Musculoskeletal: no muscle or joint pain or swelling except (1) for years has had tight, tense neck and headaches when she works a lot at her art; currently not flared; and (2) has tingling, paresthesias, and some pain in her right wrist and forearm worse when she is working a lot.

Neurologic: as per musculoskeletal section above, otherwise no loss of consciousness, tremors, seizures, or neurosensory changes.

Skin: a bit dry recently; no rashes or lesions.

Psychiatric: has had difficulty falling asleep and early morning awakening for at least a year; appetite has been increased and she eats to relax; frequent crying spells for no particular reason; does not enjoy any activities anymore; no past diagnosis or treatment for depression; denies suicidal ideation.

PE (physical examination):

Vital signs: T 102.5°F, BP 150/92, HR 110, RR 32; wt 169 pounds, ht 64 inches.

General: alert, oriented, ill woman who tries to be helpful; initially dyspneic but improved with oxygen.

HEENT: no head trauma; no facial tenderness; pupils equal, round, and reactive to light and accommodation; extraocular muscles intact without nystagmus; fundi with some arteriolar narrowing; nose congested; TMs and canals clear, hearing grossly intact but perhaps a bit hard of hearing; mouth with good dentition, pink mucosa with normal lips, tongue, and throat.

Neck: supple; full range of motion; no jugular venous distention; carotid upstrokes normal without bruits; no thyromegaly.

Nodes: no abnormal nodes appreciated in neck, supraclavicular, axillary, epitrochlear, or inguinal areas.

Breasts: no masses, skin changes, retraction, or discharge.

Chest: mildly increased AP diameter, no tenderness; tachypneic, no retractions but splinting right chest; breath sounds slightly decreased diffusely; no wheezing, rales, rhonchi, or dullness except for the right lower posterior lung field which is dull to percussion and has tubular breath sounds and rales.

Heart: mild tachycardia with S1, single S2, and no murmurs, gallops, or rubs appreciated.

Abdomen: BS normal; soft, nontender; liver 8 cm by percussion; no masses or splenomegaly.

Genital: externally normal, vagina normal, cervix multiparous, bimanual with normal uterus size and position, no adnexal enlargement or tenderness appreciated. Pap smear taken, result pending.

Rectal: normal tone, no masses; stool brown, occult blood negative.

Neurological: normal mental status; cranial nerves 2–12 intact; deep tendon reflexes at biceps, triceps, patellar, and Achilles are 2+ bilaterally; motor examination intact in mass, tone, and strength; sensory examination intact to light and sharp touch, but mild vibratory loss in feet bilaterally; gait and coordination intact; Romberg and Babinski signs absent.

Skin: fair skinned with actinic changes on face and shoulders, but no lesions noted; skin somewhat dry.

Lab: Chest X ray shows a dense right lower lobe infiltrate without effusion, otherwise normal. Remainder of lab tests are pending.

Problem List:
1. Pneumonia, right lower lobe, postinfluenza
2. Diabetes mellitus, adult-onset
3. Hypertension, chronic essential
4. Obesity
5. Perimenopausal
6. Stress urinary incontinence, palpable bladder
7. Hearing loss, mild, history of noise exposure
8. Depressive syndrome, etiology undetermined
9. Psychosocial stress
10. Excessive caffeine use, 12 cups coffee per day
11. Actinic skin
12. Breast cancer prevention
13. Allergic to sulfa medications

Assessments/Plans:

Problem #1: *PNEUMONIA, RIGHT LOWER LOBE, POSTINFLUENZA*

H/O: By history patient had an influenza syndrome that improved with treatment, but later flared with a productive cough, hemoptysis, pleuritic chest pain, fever, and dyspnea. On examination she is febrile, tachypneic, splinting her right chest, and has signs of right lower lobe consolidation. Chest X ray confirms a right lower lobe infiltrate.

A/P: This is likely a secondary bacterial pneumonia, possibly caused by Strep-
tococcus pneumonie, Haemophilus influenzae, *or* Staphylococcus au-
reus. *The hemoptysis in this context is consistent with pneumonia, but
must be watched carefully. At risk for development of empyema. Plan to
check pending lab, including sputum Gram stain. Start broad-spectrum IV
antibiotics, pulmonary toilet, pain meds to help her cough and breathe
more deeply. Monitor carefully. See orders. Since patient is a former
smoker and has a family history of lung cancer will need to be sure
infiltrate improves and resolves completely and is not related to a tumor.
Also needs pneumococcal vaccine and annual influenza immunizations.*

Problem #2:   *DIABETES MELLITUS, ADULT-ONSET*

*H/O: Began as an adult 15 years ago (per PMH) and initially required oral
hypoglycemic, later was controlled by diet (2500 calories per day) and
exercise (water aerobics), but patient stopped exercising, gained weight,
became symptomatic, and 1 month ago reinstitution of oral hypoglycemic.
Has not had obvious complications. On examination (undilated) has no
diabetic retinopathy, but does have palpable postvoiding bladder and loss
of some vibratory sensation in feet. Blood glucose pending.*

*A/P: Overall patient has had a fairly benign course because of her previous
efforts. Control has been worse in the last year, mostly for psychosocial
reasons, and probably glucose is even worse now because of the stress of
the pneumonia. Plan to monitor and control glucose acutely, and to address the psychosocial problems to try to permit patient to resume diet and
exercise program.*

Problem #3:   *HYPERTENSION, CHRONIC ESSENTIAL*

*H/O: Mild hypertension for 15 years on diuretic without side effects or compli-
cations. Current blood pressure 150/92. Fundal examination shows arteriolar narrowing. Lab pending.*

*A/P: Hypertension has been mild and controlled by history, and there is
scarcely any evidence of end-organ damage. Nonetheless, because she also
has a positive family history and diabetes mellitus she is at even higher risk
for strokes and heart disease, so it is important to control her BP. Plan to
continue the diuretic and consider starting an aspirin per day to reduce
risk of strokes and heart attacks.*

Problem #4:   *OBESITY*

*H/O: Has gained weight over the last year as discussed in #2 above. Thyroid
gland normal.*

*A/P: Probably the weight gain was related to the effects of life-style changes
and possibly depression, but because patient has also had dry skin and
fatigue, hypothyroidism should be ruled out. Plan to address the psychosocial issues, encourage proper diet and exercise, and check thyroid function
tests.*

Problem #5:   *PERIMENOPAUSAL*

*H/O: Lately has had irregular menses and hot flashes, age is compatible with
menopause.*

*A/P: May be menopausal. At risk for osteoporosis. Continued estrogen would
be beneficial from a cardiovascular standpoint, also. However, obesity or
thyroid could also be affecting menses. Plan to check thyroid function*

tests, and Pap smear for estrogen index. Will consider estrogen replacement with patient after hospitalization.

Problem #6: *STRESS URINARY INCONTINENCE, PALPABLE BLADDER*

H/O: Long-standing problem, off and on. Four vaginal deliveries.

A/P: May be related to childbirth, but may be retaining urine because of diabetic neuropathy and may be at risk of infection. Could also be related to menopause. Anticholinergic effects of whatever cold preparation she is currently taking could have contributed too. Plan to check pending lab including urinalysis, and treat as indicated. Also will quantitate postvoid residual with bladder ultrasound.

Problem #7: *HEARING LOSS, MILD, HISTORY OF NOISE EXPOSURE*

H/O: Becoming hard of hearing and has excessive noise exposure without protection.

A/P: Hearing loss may well be related to noise exposure. Will quantitate as outpatient, and recommend hearing protection. Will make sure patient able to hear discussions during this hospitalization.

Problem #8: *DEPRESSIVE SYNDROME, ETIOLOGY UNDETERMINED*

H/O: Anhedonia, sleep disturbance, appetite changes, crying spells, much stress and grief related to her terminally ill brother. Appears depressed, denies suicidal ideation.

A/P: Depressive syndrome. May be situational and there are several other problems that could be related such as possible hypothyroidism or menopause. She is also acutely ill. Depression could be important if it caused loss of control of diet and exercise and exacerbated her diabetes mellitus. Plan to observe carefully, discuss with patient, and consider treatment after acute problems have stabilized.

Problem #9: *PSYCHOSOCIAL STRESS*

H/O: See social history.

A/P: Stress is definitely contributing to the deterioration of this patient's health. Initially, if agreeable to family and brother will ask hospice program to consult for additional support of brother.

Problem #10: *EXCESSIVE CAFFEINE USE, 12 CUPS COFFEE PER DAY*

H/O: 12 cups of drip coffee per day chronically.

A/P: At risk for caffeine withdrawal headaches and dysphoria while here. May be contributing to sleep disturbance, also. Allow reduced amount of coffee, and encourage patient to reduce amount more.

Problem #11: *ACTINIC SKIN*

H/O: Fair skinned with significantly actinic skin, face and shoulders.

A/P: At risk for skin cancers. Encourage sunscreen use, limit solar exposure. Needs regular skin examinations.

Problem #12: *BREAST CANCER PREVENTION*

No risk factors and examination normal, but due for baseline mammogram. Will obtain while here.

Problem #13: *ALLERGIC TO SULFA MEDICATIONS*

Will not use sulfa drugs, and will be careful with related compounds.

Signature

Table 7.1
Traditional Format for the History and Physical Examination

Component	Information included
Heading	Date, Time, Type of Note
ID	Patient identification, Informant/Source of history, Estimate of reliability
CC	Chief Complaint
HPI	History of Present Illness
PMH	Past Medical History
	Diseases (active and past), trauma, and operations (chronologically)—describe all relevant details
	Other relevant risk factors and problems
	Transfusions
	Immunizations
	Medications (significant past, currently prescribed, currently OTC)
	Allergies/adverse reactions
FH	Family History (includes ethnic, genetic, and familial risk factors)
SH	Social History (personal profile, support systems, travel history, exposure and occupational history (including hobbies), health promotion habits, substance use/abuse, sexual history, etc.)
ROS	Review of Systems
PE	Physical Examination
Lab	Laboratory tests, X rays, etc.
Problems	Problem list (including "health maintenance")
A/P	Assessments and Plans for each problem
Signature	

The History and Physical Examination

Traditionally one of the first clinical tasks medical students face is to author a complete history and physical examination on a patient being admitted to the hospital. Case 7-6 represents such a write-up. Students now participate in outpatient clinical experiences much earlier in medical school. In outpatient settings a "complete H & P" is rarely done at a single visit. However, it remains the standard for an ideal *initial* data base, even for outpatients.

The complete patient data base should include identifying information, a chief complaint, a history of the present illness, a past medical history (including meaningful descriptions of current and past medical conditions, operations, medications, allergies, risk factors, and other important historical information), a family history, a social history, a review of systems, a physical examination, and the results of lab and other special studies. The history and observation data base is followed by a problem list, and then by a note for each problem excerpting, in SOAP or HOAP fashion, the supporting history and observation data from the data base, with narrative assessments and plans for diagnosis, therapy, and patient education, as outlined in Table 7.1. Any risk factor identified should be included in the problem list and be addressed in the assessments and plans.

CASE 7-7

The resident who admitted Mrs. Jane Smith, Case 7-6, gave the following comprehensive presentation at a busy morning report session. Note the strategic omissions and summarizations.

"For our next admission I would like to present Mrs. Jane Smith, who is a 51-year-old woman admitted to Dr. Jones's service for pneumonia. She is a married 51-year-old from Smallville, Texas, employed as a commercial artist. She has hypertension and adult-onset diabetes mellitus. This is her first hospital admission since her youngest child was born. History is obtained from the patient, who is reliable, and by phone from Dr. Susan Jones, her attending family physician.

"She presented to the emergency room stating that her chest hurt when she breathed and that she was coughing up blood. She felt well until 8 days ago when she developed a fever, chills, headache, body aches, sore throat, and dry cough. She began taking over-the-counter cold meds. After 2 days she went to see her family physician, Dr. Jones, who diagnosed influenza A and prescribed amantadine. Her glucose was in good control. By the next day she began to feel better and her fever resolved. Two days ago she developed myalgias and the cough became productive. Yesterday she developed chills, fever, and right lateral pleuritic chest pain. Today she felt dyspneic and at 10 AM started coughing up some dark blood. The appearance of the blood frightened her so she came to the emergency room.

"She has a 15 pack-year smoking history, quitting 10 years ago as a health measure. She has no history of pneumonia, lung disease, TB, cancer, or asbestos or other exposures; there is no history of coagulopathy. She has never had either influenza or pneumococcal vaccines.

"The hemoptysis was especially frightening to Mrs. Smith because her brother has lung cancer. She feels embarrassed that she did not seek attention earlier. She is tired of having to worry about her health so she just kept hoping that the problem would go away.

"Her past medical history is remarkable for 15 years of diabetes mellitus. At first it was treated with oral meds, then she lost a lot of weight and was able to control it well with diet and exercise. A year ago she had to quit her aerobics class to care for her brother. She started gaining weight and a month ago Dr. Jones had to start her back on glyburide. She also has a history of hypertension well controlled for 15 years on hydrochlorthiazide.

"Family history includes diabetes mellitus, hypertension, stroke, MI, and colon and lung cancer. Her husband and children are well. Socially she is a commercial artist whose husband is in a stressful construction job. One child is in college, and three are at home, ages 17, 16, and 15. She drinks 12 cups of coffee per day. It's significant that she is preoccupied with caring for her terminally ill brother who has lung cancer and now lives in the patient's guest room. Caring for him is very time-consuming and stressful. Her support systems are poor at present.

"Her review of systems is most significant for a 25-pound weight gain over the last year. She's not exercising, has increased appetite, and finds herself eating to relax. She also has difficulty falling asleep, early awakening, frequent crying spells for no particular reason, and inability to enjoy the activities she used to like.

"On examination this is an alert but ill woman who is cooperative. She was initially dyspneic, but improved with oxygen. She was febrile at 102.5°F, with BP 150/92, HR 110, and RR 32. She is 5 feet 4 inches tall and mildly obese at 169 pounds. Her head and neck were normal. No abnormal nodes were appreciated. Her chest was nontender with a mildly increased AP diameter. She was tachy-

pneic, with no retractions but splinting her right chest. Breath sounds were slightly decreased diffusely and no wheezing, rales, rhonchi, or dullness were present except for dullness, tubular breath sounds, and rales in the right lower posterior lung field. The only other remarkable examination findings were a palpable bladder, mild vibratory sensation loss in the feet, and actinic skin. Her chest X ray confirmed a right lower lobe infiltrate without effusion. Other lab is pending.

"Mrs. Smith has the following problem list:"

The resident then gave the full problem list from Case 7-6, and then presented the history, observations, assessment, and plan for the most important problems of pneumonia, diabetes, depressive syndrome, and psychosocial stress. The final summation was as follows:

"I will be pleased to elaborate on any of the less relevant problems that I was only able to mention. In summary, Mrs. Smith is a functional, hardworking woman admitted with a severe, acute postviral right lower lobe bacterial pneumonia and adult-onset diabetes mellitus that is no longer in dietary control because of the effects of psychosocial stress and possible depression. I will be happy to entertain questions."

CASE PRESENTATIONS

TYPES OF CASE PRESENTATIONS

While patient records are relatively audience independent, presentations are always audience dependent. Although there are audiences and situations where a complete data base is presented, verbal presentations are usually brief, and present a developed point of view, not just a recitation of information. The style of presentation also depends on the clinical situation. An admission presentation made by a new medical student will tend to be much more comprehensive than a presentation made at rounds on a patient who has been in the hospital for several days.

Early in clinical training, medical students are often expected to give "complete presentations." These often are the equivalent of reading the written history and physical examination since the goal is to verify that the student has collected and analyzed a complete data base on the patient. After gaining experience, presentations will be shortened by omitting findings that are not positively or negatively relevant to the patient's problems. While rotating with a subspecialty, students are often asked to focus only on findings pertinent to that subspecialty.

The purpose of a presentation also determines the style and depth. "Morning report" presentations are often conducted as much for academic as for communication purposes. Therefore, the cases are often presented as unknowns, mainly concentrating on data, with the attending physician asking questions to cause the audience to think about the diagnostic possibilities. Another type of morning report is simply to present information most pertinent to the case to launch a discussion of the diagnoses or problems. Often this type of presentation is like reading the assessment and plan without the data base. A brief overview of the patient is given, followed by a presentation of each problem, the data supporting that problem, and the plans for that problem.

Other presentations involve "checking out" a case to another physician who is going to assume care of the patient for the night or the weekend. These presentations are problem oriented, brief, and focus on pitfalls and plans. Presenting to consultants is another important skill. A presentation to a busy consultant should give the most important information first and then add the details. Do not present the patient as an "unknown" where the consultant must keep listening and waiting for the punch line. Tell the consultant who is calling, and then what, why, and how, followed by who, where, and when. It is very helpful to listen to experienced physicians present cases in order to learn how to present salient points of a patient's story without boring the audience with a recitation of irrelevant details.

GIVING CASE PRESENTATIONS

Case presentations are fun for those who are prepared, but stressful for the unprepared. Develop skill in both planned and spontaneous case presentations. Know the importance of each particular presentation for patient care, for education, and for grades! Know the purpose of the presentation and the intended audience. Consider rehearsing the presentation either actually or mentally. Be prepared to deliver the presentation the audience needs and expects.

Presentations should be short, no longer than 5 minutes, even for complicated cases. According to Cutler (1985), "A case presentation should consist of sifted, selected, and processed data and must be delivered in a lucid, brief, precise manner. It ought to include only the most important positive findings and a few pertinent negatives." There may be instances when for the purpose of educational gamesmanship students are expected to present a case as an "unknown," without selling the audience on any particular diagnosis. However, in most situations simply present a cogent argument supporting the best positions and refuting any less plausible alternative positions.

The best way to decide what information needs to be presented, given the requirement for brevity, is to "think backwards." Each diagnostic or therapeutic plan should have a supporting problem or diagnosis. For each significant problem or diagnosis identified and excluded, be able to identify the historical, clinical, and lab observations that provide a rationale for including or excluding that diagnosis or problem. These data, along with a general description of the patient and the vital signs, are the *core case data*. Present *only* the core case data, the problems and plans they support, and nothing else. If these data are reduced to compact, technical language, it is quite likely that the entire case can be presented in 5 minutes or less, as was done by the resident in Case 7-7.

Decide whether to do a traditional presentation, a problem-oriented presentation, or a "newspaper-style" presentation for a busy consultant. If a full problem-oriented assessment and plan has already been written using excerpts from the data base, then the case can be directly presented by problem from that write-up. If the traditional format is to be used in which the core case data are presented followed by the problem list and plan, then the core case data from each problem must be combined back into one abbreviated data base that can be presented as a unit. Case 7-7 was presented in this manner. It is a good idea for presenters to have something written as a guide, especially if tired or distracted. It can be helpful to "highlight" the core case data on a photocopy of the write-up, so that only core data are presented, in order, as a unit. Notecards or other working notes are also helpful. Neither the traditional nor the problem-oriented approach is difficult if the case has already been written up and the core case data are selected by working backwards.

The newspaper-style presentation to a consultant is different and will be discussed separately.

Begin the presentation with a brief description of the patient that sets the stage for the audience to regard the patient as a person and not just a case. Mention the informant and the reliability of the information. State the chief complaint in the patient's exact words if they facilitate understanding of the case, but if clinical judgment indicates no distortion would result, it is acceptable to restate the chief complaint more succinctly. For hospitalizations the reason for admission is stated up front, as the resident did in Case 7-7, although some attending physicians prefer not to hear the reason for admission until the plan is discussed.

After the opening of a traditional presentation, go through all of the core case data in the same order that they would appear in the patient record. Stick strictly to the core case data that were selected by working backward through the case. Follow the HOAP arrangement, presenting the history, personally made observations, and tests. After presenting the data, give the problem list, followed by a separate assessment and plan for each significant problem.

Do not let the audience erroneously think that the presentation is jumping around, as may happen if the patient's history includes historical observations or tests. Make it obvious that they are historical. For example, after presenting most of the history, say, "After Mrs. Bennett's arrival at the ER, she was evaluated by Dr. Casey, who observed that Mrs. Bennett was tachypneic and splinting her right chest. He ordered a chest X ray that showed a right lower lobe effusion, so prior to calling us, he performed a thoracentesis removing 250 ml of pus." If instead it was simply stated that a chest X ray and thoracentesis were done, without mentioning Dr. Casey, it might appear that the presentation skipped straight from history to observations. Someone would probably interrupt wanting the rest of the history, the vital signs, and the examination.

After the opening of a problem-oriented presentation, launch right into the problem list, starting with the problem related to the chief complaint. State the entire list, then for each problem germane to the presentation, describe its specific core history, observations, assessment, and plan. Include the general description of the patient and the vital signs with the first problem, even if they are not particularly important to that problem, because it helps in portraying the patient as a person and because the vital signs are always relevant to the overall case.

Conclude either type of presentation by summarizing the case. Restate the most important problems and plans to help consolidate major points of the case, and help the audience focus on the meat of the case instead of on whatever minor details were presented last. The goal should be to present all of the core case data and analyze them so well that the audience is left speechless, without questions!

Skill in less formal types of presentations will develop naturally, but the "newspaper-style" presentation is especially worth discussing. It is an "all business" type of presentation designed to present specific facts and requests as efficiently as possible. It is used most often with consultants. Like it or not, there are always some consultants who will seem intimidating. Others are very busy and preoccupied. By knowing the patient's core case data and following a few simple rules, even medical students can be confident and do quite well at presenting to consultants.

If a consultant likes cases presented in a certain manner, then present them that way. Otherwise, use the newspaper-style presentation format. Imagine a general surgeon who is paged while beginning a cholecystectomy. A nurse dials the number on a speaker phone.

An intern answers, and launches into a story, "We've got a patient, Mrs. Green in room 315, who is a 65-year-old female with diabetes mellitus and hypertension who was admitted with a right cerebral infarction. We've had a lot of trouble controlling her hypertension." By this time the surgeon is annoyed. It is not even clear why the intern is calling so it's especially unclear what data are important to try to catch from the intern's presentation. The surgeon is also occupied with the operation and wants the intern's presentation to get to the point. It would have been much better if the intern had said, "This is Dr. McCoy with the resident service. We would like to consult you on a patient who may have a perforated duodenal ulcer. May I tell you about the case?" With permission granted, the intern continues, "At exactly 6 AM this morning the patient suddenly developed intense epigastric pain that is now generalized. The abdomen is silent, rigid, and has a rebound. Abdominal X rays are pending. The patient is tachycardic and has a low-grade fever. She's 65 and has already been in the hospital for a week because of a right cerebral infarction and hypertension. We feel she needs a surgical opinion as soon as possible."

This type of presentation gives the most important and dramatic facts first, up front. It's very efficient to listen to this type of presentation, even when busy and preoccupied. Moreover, after only three sentences the preoccupied surgeon has enough information to tell the intern that it would be best to call someone else.

CASE 7-8

Even before the phone rings, the caller-ID system pops Mrs. Vaughn's record onto the receptionist's computer screen. "Hello, Mrs. Vaughn," she says. The reason for visit, "back pain," is soon entered into the scheduling system. When Mrs. Vaughn arrives, her name appears on the nurse's workstation. The physician reads her chart on a workstation, shows her a digital video of low-back exercises on a computer in the examination room, and orders blood tests and prescriptions that are electronically sent to the lab and the pharmacy. When the patient arrives at the checkout counter her bill has already been processed, and the physician is dictating the progress note directly into the computer system. Problem lists, medication lists, and flow sheets are automatically and transparently maintained as the note is created. The next day the lab results are electronically routed to the physician, working from home, who consults an on-line textbook, adds a new problem to the patient's list, automatically calls the patient to discuss the result, and clicks in an addendum to the chart documenting it all. Later in the year, reminders for preventive care are automatically generated and sent to the patient by electronic mail.

CONCLUSIONS

Computer systems like that described in Case 7-8 are reality. Even more sophisticated systems are on the way. The future of patient records and case presentations is exciting. Computer systems are making it possible to easily record, classify, and store large amounts of detailed patient information, to view that information in creative, helpful ways, and to share and communicate information with others involved in the care of the patient. A whole new series of skills will be needed by the physicians who participate in the medical informatics revolution and in computer-based patient record systems. It will be up to those physicians to create record templates, initiate clinically desirable practice guidelines, present patients and charts over video links, and otherwise initiate the features of record systems in a humane, professional manner that preserves the art and humanity of medicine.

Authoring patient records and presenting cases are skills critical to a physician's career. Over a career, much time and energy is spent authoring and reviewing patient records. There are important technical considerations involved in optimally using and creating patient records and presenting cases. It is equally important, however, that records remain confidential and portray a true and accurate story of each patient as a person.

CASES FOR DISCUSSION

CASE 1

A previously healthy 40-year-old man is paralyzed from the shoulders down because of a motor vehicle accident. During his acute hospitalization his problems included spinal shock, urinary retention, two operations on his neck, pulmonary edema, pneumonia, kidney infection, fecal impaction, bedsores, and depression. He has health insurance through an HMO, disability insurance through his employer, and is suing the person who caused the accident. After he is more stable he is transferred to a rehabilitation unit where he receives physical and occupational therapy. When he returns home he requires home visits.

1. *Who are some of the most important users of this gentleman's patient records?*
2. *What are some of the important uses for his patient records?*
3. *How could inadequate or distorted records adversely affect this patient?*

CASE 2

A physician wrote the following untitled HOAP note:
   H: 6-year-old here because of right ear pain and fever for 3 days. Also, chronically has runny nose and rubs eyes a lot. Has chronic itchy rash on arms. Developed a new rash on chest last week. Severely sunburned on face recently. Has wheezing problems during soccer; has been out of previously prescribed medications for 6 weeks including albuterol and cromolyn sodium inhalers because mother thought they were no longer needed. Overdue for immunizations. No known medication allergies.
   O: Fussy, Well-hydrated. T 101.9°F. Bags under eyes. Left TM clear, right TM bulging and red. Nose with boggy, weepy nasal mucosa. Neck supple. Lungs with diffuse end-expiratory wheezing, otherwise clear. Skin with scaly, secondarily excoriated patches in the flexor areas, and ringlike scaly reddish lesions on torso. The torso lesions have hyphae on KOH preparation.
   A: #1—Acute otitis media (OM), right
      #2—Allergic rhinitis
      #3—Atopic dermatitis
      #4—Tinea corporis (ringworm)
      #5—Sunburn

#6—*Asthma, mildly flared off meds*
#7—*Needs immunizations*
P: #1—*Amoxicillin 250 mg tid × 10 days for OM*
 #2—*Clemestine fumarate 1.34 mg bid for allergic rhinitis and atopic dermatitis*
 #3—*Clotrimazole cream applied bid for tinea corporis*
 #4—*Albuterol and cromolyn inhalers qid for asthma*
 #5—*Recheck in 14 days and as needed*

1. How could the above note be rearranged into a true problem-oriented note?
2. What are the advantages and disadvantages of this note compared with a problem-oriented version?
3. What are the three components of an excellent plan section? Which are missing in the above note?

CASE 3

An elderly male patient arrives at the emergency room unconscious. According to family members, over the last week he gradually became more lethargic. They were unable to arouse him that morning. Many interrelated diagnoses are noted on old charts, including ethanolism, alcoholic liver cirrhosis, ascites (fluids in the peritoneum), coronary artery disease, hypertension, prostatic hypertrophy with history of urinary retention, and several others. He is on a long list of medications. A family member reports the patient had rectal bleeding yesterday. A nasogastric tube is inserted, and gross blood is found in the stomach. The case is so complex and the patient so critical that it seems best for the intern to appraise the chief resident about the case before fully evaluating the patient.

1. What approach should the intern take in presenting the situation to the chief? Why?
2. How should the intern present the case in consulting a busy gastroenterologist about the GI bleeding?

After additional study, it is confirmed that the patient has hepatic encephalopathy precipitated by bleeding esophageal varices. At morning report the next day the intern wants the audience to mentally work through the differential diagnosis of the initial presentation.

3. What approach should the intern use for the presentation at morning report? Why?

All problems are addressed, and the patient is ready for discharge. To better convey the patient's current status, the intern decides to call the out-of-town family physician who will assume care for the patient.

4. How might the intern best present this complex case to the physician assuming care?

CASE 4

A medical student picks up a chart in clinic to review prior to a visit, notes the two problems ethanolism and hypertension, and reads the previous note written by a resident who previously saw the patient:

 Subjective: *Anxious, demanding 49-year-old alcoholic hypertensive who returns wanting more medication refills. Noncompliant with propranolol. Denies being on any other medications. Claims she's not drinking. Complains of insomnia and fatigue. Unemployed. Sits around all day apathetic and doing nothing.*

 Objective: *Dirty 49-year-old woman with rotten teeth but no alcohol on breath.*

1. *What could the effects of such a note be on the patient's care?*
2. *How could the above note be revised to portray the patient truthfully but more positively?*
3. *What steps could the student take to keep from being "poisoned" by this note even before meeting the patient?*

CASE 5

A group of primary care physicians using paper records has become busier and busier and must expand its capabilities. The group's main priority is to continue to provide excellent, comprehensive, personal care to its large number of patients and families. At the same time, the group wants to be able to practically review its own medical records in order to conduct quality assurance and community research activities and to become more effective in providing preventive care services. To accomplish its goals, the group has decided to convert to a computer-based patient record system. In deciding what system to use, some physicians are extremely concerned that the new system not disturb the patient–physician relationship. Some are concerned that the system capture the true stories of their patients rather than forcing the use of simplistic boilerplate stories pre-programmed into the system. Others want all of the convenience features of such a system, such as chart sharing, electronic communications between all members of the healthcare team, interfaces to lab equipment and the hospital, and so forth.

1. *How should this group best balance the needs and desires of the patients and physicians in deciding how to implement a computer-based patient record system?*
2. *Where should terminals for the system be placed? In examination rooms? In workstations outside the examination rooms? Both? How might terminal placement affect charting and the patient–physician relationship?*
3. *What are some of the risks and benefits of implementing a computer-based patient record system?*

—————— RECOMMENDED READINGS ——————

Council on Scientific Affairs, American Medical Association. Users and uses of patient records: Report of the Council on Scientific Affairs. *Arch Fam Med* 2:678–681, 1993.

> This article will not be very helpful in developing skills, but it will provide a very solid sense of the wide world of medical records, and how the physician's component of records is now only one part of a much larger system.

Cutler P: *Problem Solving in Clinical Medicine: From Data to Diagnosis,* ed 2. Baltimore, Williams & Wilkins Co, 1985.

> This entire book is a medical gem. I recommend reading it cover to cover toward the end of the second year of medical school to prepare for intense clinical activity. Although Cutler advocates a more detailed and lengthy data base than is generally practical, his material on records and presentation is as wise and helpful as the rest of the book.

Donnelly WJ: Righting the medical record: Transforming chronicle into story. *JAMA* 260:823–825, 1988.

> This is a readable and important article that makes a strong case for including "the voice of the patient" in the medical narrative. As information technology advances, clear thinking like Donnelly's is needed to provide a defense against those who would have us produce illness narratives using only sparse, limited language that can be processed even by unsophisticated computer systems.

Weed LL: Medical records that guide and teach. *N Engl J Med* 278:593–657, 1968.

> This is the classic article introducing problem-oriented medical records that is still useful for those wanting to understand and learn more about them.

PART III

Improving Clinical Expertise

While the acquiring of basic clinical skills described in the previous part is important, the patient-centered physician should not stop there. As the definition of what health is to patients has broadened, as patients have been more active in terms of demanding information about their health and being involved within clinical decision-making, and as physicians have had to face new challenges such as medical malpractice, the skills required to meet these challenges have been developed by clinicians. The development of these more advanced clinical skills will enable the physician to function more effectively in the clinical arena.

CHAPTER 8

The Difficult Clinical Conversation

Kathleen A. Zoppi and Catherine P. McKegney

CASE 8-1

Dr. Smith's first patient of the day is a 63-year-old woman, Mrs. Meyer, who has persistent diarrhea and a weight loss of 10 pounds (from 92 pounds to 82 pounds) over 2 months. She is widowed and has three daughters who live in town. When Dr. Smith asked about her past medical history, she indicated that she smokes about two packs per day, consumes about two drinks per day, and has been hospitalized once for an appendectomy and for the births of her three children.

—————— EDUCATIONAL OBJECTIVES ——————

At the end of this chapter, the student will:

1. Describe situations or topics that may contribute to difficult clinical conversations
2. Describe possible helpful responses to difficult conversations with patients
3. Describe and demonstrate insight regarding patients or situations that are difficult because they evoke particular responses from the student, which may be related to difficulties or family issues of the learner
4. Describe resources for managing the feelings patients evoke in the student
5. Describe common patterns in difficult encounters
6. Define content and relational aspects of communication processes

——————————— **INTRODUCTION** ———————————

When Dr. Smith saw Mrs. Meyer in Case 8-1 for the first time, many different diagnostic possibilities came to her mind, including infection, inflammation, nutritional deficiencies, gastrointestinal disease, or malignancies. But Dr. Smith had a funny sense of missing something important, and that this patient's picture was more complicated than it appears. She considered running some tests to rule in, or rule out, certain possibilities.

DR. SMITH: I'm curious about what you think might be causing you to lose weight. Do you have any ideas?

MRS. MEYER: No. I'm eating the same as I have been. I think maybe it's because I've been nervous lately.

DR. SMITH: Nervous. Tell me more about being nervous.

MRS. MEYER: I don't know, I just feel jumpy all the time. Like something is about to happen. But everything is just fine. So I don't know what's wrong.

DR. SMITH: Has anything changed in your life recently?

MRS. MEYER: No. Like what?

DR. SMITH: Changes at home?

MRS. MEYER: No.

DR. SMITH: Changes at work?

MRS. MEYER: No.

DR. SMITH: Any new stresses that you can think of?

MRS. MEYER: No, none. I think I'm fine, it's just my stomach and this diarrhea that are slowing me down.

DR. SMITH: Well, I think that we need to find out a little more about why you're having this weight loss. I'd like to order some blood tests for starters, and to see you back next week. Is that okay with you?

MRS. MEYER: That's fine.

CASE 8-1 (*continued*)

Mrs. Meyer's lab tests came back, and showed she had elevated liver function tests, including AST and ALT. Her GGT was 2.5 times normal. Her hepatitis studies were negative. She was slightly anemic. She kept a diet diary, and at her next office visit Dr. Smith reviewed it with her. Nothing in the diary could explain why she might have lost 10 pounds in 2 months. Dr. Smith has a funny feeling of something missing. She asked Mrs. Meyer to begin some nutritional supplements, and return in 2 weeks. A week later, she was admitted in the evening with pneumonia. Her daughters were with her in the hospital.

In Case 8-1, what one might not know about the patient may be as useful to the diagnosis and treatment as what one does know about her. In this chapter, we will try to outline frequently encountered difficult interviewing situations, and offer some ways of working within them to better meet the goals of caring for the patient while maintaining balance and poise. We will describe these difficult situations using a relational model of communication in clinical conversations.

An interaction between patient and physician can become difficult when both parties feel unable to understand the other, when there is incongruity between the patient's and physician's goals, or when the patient and the physician battle for control. Sometimes difficulties arise because patients and physicians treat each other as though they were significant people, such as parents or teachers, from their past, rather than as the people they are now. Such difficulties related to countertransference (the physician's feelings toward the patient) or transference (the patient's feelings toward the physician) can distort the relationship and create difficult communication (Stein, 1985b). This phenomenon may mean that caring for an elderly female patient is more difficult for a physician who had difficulties with his grandmother, and easier for a physician whose grandmother died at a younger age. Each physician will find different types of patients who push his or her buttons: One of the key skills to managing difficult encounters is to use self-awareness of what kinds of patients or problems are likely to "push one's buttons," and then to employ strategies to use that knowledge for the patient's improved care and one's own professional development (Ellis, 1983). This self-knowledge and the skill to use this self-knowledge does not happen automatically: Real improvement in interactions with patients takes concerted effort. The experienced clinician will become increasingly sensitive to feeling her buttons being pushed, will hear a "warning bell" earlier in the interaction, and will seek help from colleagues or teachers.

RELATIONAL COMMUNICATION IN DIFFICULT CLINICAL CONVERSATIONS

In any interaction between two people, there are two levels of message exchange: One is at the content level, where the message is encoded in words or nonverbal cues such as gestures. Sometimes communication difficulties occur when people misunderstand each other at the content level: They do not clearly understand each other's words or cues. However, more often difficulties arise when there are differences between what is said and what is meant or interpreted. This difference between message and meaning occurs at the relational level, in which nonverbal cues, context, or relationship history may be congruent with, or may contradict, the content level of the message. Suppose that two longtime friends are talking, and one comments to the other: "Hey, nice haircut!" If this message is delivered with a straight face, a sincere expression, and unwavering eye contact, it may be heard by the recipient as a compliment. However, imagine a relationship where both parties frequently tease each other. If the speaker uttered the same words (content) but instead rolled his eyes and smirked, the meaning (relational) level would be different. The first instance would have been a compliment, where the content and relational levels were congruent, but the second an insult, where the content and relational levels contradicted each other. In any interaction, meaning is created and negotiated at the relational level, and often this level is more important than the content or what is actually said.

In the course of clinical conversations, noticing what is occurring at the relational level is critical for understanding and resolving difficult interactions. In the process of attending to the patient's relational message, the physician may be able to choose a different way of responding than usual. In noticing that the patient is saying he is angry, but that his voice in whiny, it is possible to acknowledge his need for reassurance rather than responding with anger or defensiveness. In addition, noticing what relational messages the physician is giving, through body language, facial expression, distance, or movement, is important, particularly when the physician is using her own self as a diagnostic and therapeutic instrument to improve the health of the patient.

One of the inherent contradictions in medical education is the admonition to use yourself as a diagnostic tool, attending to your own feelings as a barometer of the interaction (Balint, 1964), while much of the experience in medical school trains one to ignore internal feelings and reactions (Smith & Kleinman, 1989). Throughout this chapter, we will identify situations in which both the patient's and the physician's feelings contribute to the quality of the interaction: Neither person is free from affecting the interaction. Paying close attention to when patients evoke certain feelings can be one of the best (and most challenging) ways of learning about what issues or problems in your own life are important or unresolved. It is also useful to include more sources of information, including family members, nursing staff, or others who can help provide missing pieces of the puzzle.

CASE 8-1 (continued)

Dr. Smith was stumped by Mrs. Meyer's problems: She'd been in practice 7 years, and was still not able to figure out the linkages among Mrs. Meyer's weight loss, her "feeling jumpy," her pneumonia, her anemia, and her liver function tests. She met with Mrs. Meyer and her daughters in the hospital late one afternoon after she was admitted.

DR. SMITH: *Well, I'm glad you are all here today. I'm quite concerned that you, Mrs. Meyer, are still not feeling well, and that we can't seem to find what's wrong. I wonder if there is anything that I've missed, or that we haven't talked about.*

DAUGHTER: *Well, we were wondering that too. Mom's been sick for 2 months, and she looks weak and tired. She keeps telling us that she's been eating, and we take turns stopping in to see her and feed her lunch, but it doesn't seem to help. I think sometimes she smokes and drinks herself to sleep, and can't remember to eat.*

MRS. MEYER: *That's not true. I told you I haven't been drinking that much since I haven't been well. You just hush up.*

DR. SMITH: *Mrs. Meyer, when we talked about your drinking, you told me you had one or two drinks in the evening. (Daughter snorts.) How has that changed since we talked?*

MRS. MEYER: *I guess I sometimes have a little one in the afternoon.*

DAUGHTER: *She's usually passed out by four in the afternoon. Little one my foot!*

MRS. MEYER: *I just have a small glass . . .*

DR. SMITH: *Mrs. Meyer, it's really important that I understand every detail of what you are drinking. Tell me about a typical day. What do you drink and when?*

MRS. MEYER: *Well, I usually pour myself a paper cup of vodka while I'm watching my soaps at 11, and doing housework. And then I just have another about 1 PM.*

DAUGHTER: *Mom, you usually have about a full bottle of vodka a day. Usually by about 7 PM. And you've been doing that since dad died. . . .*

TALKING ABOUT ALCOHOL OR OTHER CHEMICAL DEPENDENCIES

In Case 8-1, Mrs. Meyer presents the physician with a difficulty: Should Dr. Smith confront her about her drinking directly? She now suspects Mrs. Meyer knows she's drinking too much, but never brought it up directly as a possible problem. Rather than accusing Mrs. Meyer of lying, Dr. Smith uses a simple set of screening questions, the CAGE questions, to gauge Mrs. Meyer's perception of the problem (see Table 8.1).

The CAGE questions have been identified as a more sensitive and specific screening test for alcohol abuse than either liver enzymes or blood tests (Kitchens, 1994). While the patient may deny drinking often or in great quantity, he is less likely to be able to deny the consequences of drinking, on which the CAGE questions focus.

THE PHYSICIAN'S OWN REACTION AS A CUE

The physician's response to the patient while carrying on a clinical conversation can be a useful source of data. While it is difficult for a physician to simultaneously listen to the patient, pay attention to the interaction, and monitor herself, it may be most worthwhile for the physician to use her own reactions as a source of data. In Case 8-1, the physician was not clear about what feelings were evoked by Mrs. Meyer, but was clear (and communicated this to the patient) that she was confused and needed to ask some questions again. The systematic repetition of parts of the history may help confirm the feelings evoked the first time, or may help resolve what was unclear during the preceding interview.

Skilled clinicians will notice their own feelings at the same time as observing the patient's behaviors. If one feels overcome with sadness, and this sadness is only present when the clinician is with the patient, it may be that the patient is sad, or that something about the patient's situation has triggered some sadness in the clinician and may be a useful clue about what's going on with the patient. An angry patient in the office may be a very angry, rageful person in many situations. The physician may be only one of many recipients of her anger. Knowing this, through talking with her about other parts of her

---

Table 8.1
The CAGE Questions[a,b]

---

1. Have you ever felt the need to Cut down on drinking?
2. Have you ever felt Annoyed by criticism of drinking?
3. Have you ever had Guilty feelings about drinking?
4. Have you ever taken a morning Eye-opener?

---

[a]From Mayfield D, McLead G, Hall P: The CAGE questionnaire. *Am J Psychiatry* 131:1121–1123, 1974.
[b]Note: One positive answer should lead to further inquiry; two is strong evidence of alcoholism.

life, may actually help the physician understand her anger and work with her more easily, with more empathy for her as a person.

It may also be helpful to tune in to what the patient is *not* saying, such as when a patient says she is doing just fine, and isn't upset about the death of her sister, but the longer the physician is in the room, the sadder and more lonely the physician feels. Sometimes the physician who is attuned to the patient's cues may detect feelings the patient isn't even aware of yet; for example, perhaps the patient is smiling tensely as she talks about her husband working long hours, but her fists are tightly clenched, betraying anger she may be feeling. It may be therapeutic for the physician to merely reflect the incongruity observed; for example, by stating, "I noticed that you said your marriage was fine, but when you talked about your husband, your fists were clenched."

Finally, a physician's emotional response may provide useful clues about who in the physician's life the patient represents: perhaps the gray-haired sweet lady reminds the physician of his grandmother, or the angry patient brings up memories of an aunt who was disliked. The recognition of the countertransference, or the feelings evoked by the patient, is important to separating fact from fiction. The care of the patient depends in part on the physician's ability to *accurately* recognize the patient's needs and behaviors, rather than assuming the patient is like another person from the past. This accurate perception cannot be accomplished if a physician reacts unconsciously, unaware that his reaction is really a reaction to a patient or other person from the past.

Often, the awareness of a particular countertransference toward a patient can be a clue about undiscovered features of the patient which may be useful in working more constructively with that person. For example, in Case 8-1, the physician may reflect that Mrs. Meyer reminds her of her aunt, whom she likes a great deal. However, this resemblance begins to dissolve as Dr. Smith gets to know Mrs. Meyer better and realizes she is different in significant ways from her aunt. She is cantankerous and difficult with her daughters, and not really a cheerful person.

CASE 8-2

Ms. Hall is a 36-year-old woman who was admitted to the impatient service with a concussion and a broken arm. She said she fell down the stairs off a stepladder after trying to change a light bulb at the top of the stairs. An X ray of her fractured arm is consistent with an injury caused by a blow to the forearm with a large object. She is cooperative until the interviewing resident tries to ask questions about her fall. She becomes sullen and silent and tells him it is none of his business.

MS. HALL: *I already told you what happened.*

RESIDENT: *Yes, but I think it is important to be sure about what really happened so we don't treat you the wrong way. I think this injury looks more like you were hit than like you fell down the stairs.*

MS. HALL: *Well, you're wrong. I told you the truth. Why can't you just take care of me?*

RESIDENT: *How can you expect me to take care of you when you are lying to me?*

WHEN THE PATIENT AND PHYSICIAN DIFFER
IN THEIR AGENDAS

173

WHAT MAKES AN
ENCOUNTER
DIFFICULT?

When confronted with a patient who is not interested in divulging more of her history, the physician may be tempted to stop questioning, out of respect for the patient's privacy and perhaps out of fear of evoking the patient's anger. In effect, Ms. Hall in Case 8-2 is saying, "Just take care of me, don't ask me why . . ." (Ness & Ende, 1994). And yet, without additional questioning, it may be unclear what really happened to the patient to cause her injuries. However, confronting Mrs. Hall directly, implying that she was lying, would likely be counterproductive. On the other hand, accepting her story without questioning might allow her to go home to a potentially violent situation, where the harm done to her next time might be even worse.

In fact, each year 2–8 million women in the United States experience physical violence in their homes, which often escalates after the woman seeks medical attention (Sassetti, 1993). Thus, it is important to proceed deliberately but carefully in gathering information and in documenting information gathered, because such data may also be used later in police or legal proceedings. Since the patient and physician may begin the encounter with different goals for the relationship, attending and identifying the relational levels of the interaction may be important when negotiating with the patient.

One important beginning point is for the physician to negotiate the relationship and responsibilities with the patient prior to obtaining a detailed history. Ms. Hall will be very concerned about the confidentiality of what she tells the physician. Thus, it is important to clarify with her the privacy afforded her in the patient–physician relationship. It is also important for her to know what is written within the medical record, and who might have access to the record, including insurers and third-party reviewers.

Beginning with some general screening questions as part of a routine psychosocial history can be useful when assessing whether a person is likely the object of abuse. It is crucial that the interviewer maintain a calm, nonreactive nonverbal stance: It may be helpful to put down pen and paper and take a relaxed listening posture.

RESIDENT: Tell me about the people who live in your house.
MS. HALL: Well, there's my husband, the two kids, and our dog, Max.
RESIDENT: How do they all get along?
MS. HALL: Okay most of the time.
RESIDENT: What about the rest of the time?
MS. HALL: Well, the kids fight like they all do, and my husband gets mad and takes it out on me.
RESIDENT: How does he do that?
MS. HALL: Well, he yells and throws things around a lot.
RESIDENT: Do you ever feel that you and your sons are not safe?
MS. HALL: Well, sometimes.
RESIDENT: That must be hard for you.
MS. HALL: I'm used to it.

It might be tempting to move more quickly here, to ask the patient whether she has ever considered leaving her husband, or whether today's injuries represent an outburst by her husband. It is important to attend to signs of discomfort, since the patient has just indicated that the abuse she described is not a big problem for her. The wise physician will move along at the patient's pace, or gently leave the door open to return to the topic later.

RESIDENT: Do you feel you would be safe if you went home today?
MS. HALL: I guess so.
RESIDENT: What could you do to feel safe?
MS. HALL: I guess I could take the phone number of the hotline and keep the car keys outside so I could leave if I need to . . . .

The therapeutic benefits of seeing the physician as a resource, not another (albeit psychological, not physical) dominator, is critical to the patient's improvement. Since domestic violence is a disease that often escalates when the patient makes a move to become independent of the abuser, it is critical for the physician to acknowledge and support the patient in her attempts to move slowly enough to be on solid ground with each new step.

Confrontation of the patient who seems to be giving contradictory information can also be a useful therapeutic strategy. This must be handled gently and respectfully, but it helps the physician to better understand what help the patient is seeking.

PHYSICIAN: The last time I saw you, you told me your husband was drinking a lot and hitting you. Today, you are saying he's fine and you are doing well. I'm curious about how this has changed since we last spoke.
MS. HALL: Well, it's better than it was. I just want it all to be okay right now, all right?
PHYSICIAN: I want it to be okay, too. But in case it isn't okay again, I also want you to know I am here to help you if you want me to.
MS. HALL: I know that. Thank you. I just hope he can behave well enough that I don't have to move out. I'll let you know how we're doing.

CASE 8-3

Mr. Fisher is a 68-year-old man with end-stage renal disease. He has had several visits to the nephrologist, who has said that there was nothing more that could be done for him. He has had dialysis three times each week for the past 4 years. His children, who are married and live close by, take turns driving him to the appointments. Mr. Fisher is increasingly disoriented and unable to care for himself. He was admitted to the hospital and needs a complete history and physical. The nephrologist did not discuss the prognosis with the patient or his children but felt the primary care physician should begin to help them prepare for his death. The patient's family physician is out of town. Dr. Monon, a first-year resident, is assigned the care of Mr. Fisher. He is startled by the resemblance of the patient to his own grandfather.

DR. MONON: *How are you feeling today, Mr. Fisher?*
MR. FISHER: *Fine. Where am I?*
DR. MONON: *You are in the hospital. Do you know what day it is?*
MR. FISHER: *It's Sunday. Can I go home now?*
DR. MONON: *Not yet. We are still concerned about why you were sick yesterday. Do you remember coming to the hospital?*

MR. FISHER: *No. My son comes to see me every Sunday. I need to be home when he comes . . .*

175

WHAT MAKES AN
ENCOUNTER
DIFFICULT?

TALKING ABOUT TERMINAL ILLNESS

There are some major difficulties facing the physician, Dr. Monon, who treats Mr. Fisher in Case 8-3. When caring for an unfamiliar patient, it is often hard to assess what behavior is normal and routine and what is unusual and the result of stress or illness. In Case 8-3, an additional source of difficulty is that the patient and family are not aware of the seriousness of his illness or its likely terminal outcome. This unawareness not only affects them in their decision-making about the aggressiveness of treatment but likely also affects the physician and how open she feels she can be with the family. Some of what may need to be discussed with this patient and family involves code status and about anticipating the death of the patient. Mr. Fisher's confusion makes communication more problematic: It would be easiest and best to talk directly with him, and yet he seems to be able to be oriented at some times and not others. The physician would be prudent to document the waxing and waning of mental status through a series of mini-mental status examinations at each visit to demonstrate improvement or decline (see Table 8.2). In addition to the difficulties of talking with the patient about his diagnosis and prognosis, it is difficult to manage and help support the family members in their feelings about their father's impending death. And yet, in order to help the family cope and plan appropriately, it will be necessary to help them decide, with Mr. Fisher, how he wishes to be treated and what kind of care he'll receive.

All of these issues are complicated by the countertransference of the physician, who is reminded of his own grandfather when he talks with Mr. Fisher. The physician finds himself feeling more emotional and sad, and even more angry when one of the patient's sons wishes aloud that his father would just die quickly and quietly. After talking with a behavioral preceptor, Dr. Monon realizes that his own feelings of wanting to save Mr. Fisher at all costs are related to his feelings for his grandfather and are interfering with his ability to listen to the family members in this situation. He finds greater equilibrium as he listens with greater care to what this family wants for Mr. Fisher.

CASE 8-4

Ms. Graves is a 35-year-old multiparous homemaker who was referred by her OB-GYN for a routine set of screening tests, including a CBC for anemia, a VDRL, and an HIV screening test. Her OB-GYN felt that routine screening was important for all of his pregnant patients. She is returning to the office today for her test results. Her results indicate she is HIV positive. When the test was discussed with her on her last visit, she expressed no concern at all that she had any risks for exposure to HIV. She and her husband have been married for 10 years; however, 5 years ago, they separated for 3 months. Each had different sexual partners at that time. They since reconciled, had three other children, and have been monogamous. She has had no occupational exposures, has never used IV drugs, and cannot recall any exposures to blood or blood products. Today's visit will require discussion of the risks to her and of the 30% likelihood of her child being HIV positive. (U. S. Public Health Service, 1995)

Table 8.2
The Folstein Mini-Mental Status Examination[a]

Give one point for each correct response.		Score	Points
Orientation			
1. What is the	Year	———	1
	Season	———	1
	Date	———	1
	Day	———	1
	Month	———	1
2. Where are we?	State	———	1
	County	———	1
	Town or city	———	1
	Hospital/nursing home/other building	———	1
	Floor	———	1
Registration			
3. Name three objects, taking one second to say each. Then ask the patient to repeat all three. (Give one point for each correct answer. Repeat the answers until patient learns all three.)		———	3
Attention and calculation			
4. Serial sevens: Ask the patient to count backwards from 100 by sevens, as 93, 86, 79, etc. (Stop after five answers; give one point for each correct answer.) Alternative: Spell WORLD backwards.		———	5
Recall			
5. Ask for names of the three objects learned in question 3. (Give one point for each correct answer.)		———	3
Language			
6. Point to a pencil and a watch. Ask the patient to name each as you point.		———	2
7. Ask the patient to repeat "No ifs, ands, or buts."		———	1
8. Ask the patient to follow a three-stage command: "Take a paper in your right hand. Fold the paper in half. Put the paper on the floor."		———	3
9. Ask the patient to read and obey the following command: "CLOSE YOUR EYES." (Write in large letters.)		———	1
10. Ask the patient to write a sentence of his or her choice. (The sentence should contain a subject and an object and should make sense. Ignore spelling errors when scoring.)		———	1
11. Ask the patient to copy the design shown. (Give one point if all sides and angles are preserved and if the intersecting sides form a quadrangle.)		———	1
		———	30
		(Total)	(Total)

[a]Scores of less than 20 suggest delirium or dementia (organic impairment) or, less commonly, depression or schizophrenia. Adapted with permission from Folstein MF, Folstein SE, McHugh PR: 'Mini-Mental State': A practical method for grading the cognitive state of patients for the clinician. *J Psychiatr Res* 1975; 12:189–196. Copyright 1975, Pergamon Press Inc.

Sharing bad news affects both the patient and the physician, albeit to a lesser degree. Mrs. Graves in Case 8-4, who was not expecting any bad news at all during her otherwise normal pregnancy, is likely to be quite unprepared emotionally and intellectually for the interaction about her test results. She will likely respond with disbelief, anger, shock, or denial. At some point, she will have questions about how the disease was transmitted to her, including questions about her husband and his sexual practices, and their other respective sexual partners. She will have questions regarding what this implies about her health, the health of her child, and the viability of her pregnancy. The physician will feel an urgency to talk about the need for medical follow-up and treatment, and will want especially to talk with the patient about how she can take good care of herself and her family during a stressful time. And yet these subjects cannot be discussed before the patient is ready to hear them and to accept the diagnosis. This process could take weeks, and the physician may feel impatient waiting for the patient to be ready to hear what needs to be done. In addition, timely intervention will help the child, even if the mother's condition cannot be changed. It is difficult for the physician both to be empathic, to stay with the patient in her "hell," and to be clear-sighted enough to move forward and help her get the treatment she and her child need.

Much research about sharing bad news acknowledges there is no one best way to deliver such information. However, research by Buckman (1992) and Maynard (1991) offers some guidelines: (1) assessing the recipient as much as possible to know prior to the delivery of bad news what preferences the patient might have, including setting and involvement of significant others or family members, (2) forecasting the bad news, by indicating that what is to follow is bad news, can help briefly prepare the patient for what he is about to hear and acknowledges the effect on the patient of what is about to be told, and (3) not overwhelming the patient with additional information, but rather waiting, silently, for the patient to respond and being patient with that reaction are important to the patient's feeling comfortable in expressing grief, anger, or in asking questions that are most central to him. Physicians often tend to overwhelm the patient with data, facts, and probabilities; while this information may be useful to the patient, even precious, it is often delivered in a manner that is more anxiety producing for the patient. If delivered too rapidly or too soon, it may be a way of the physician avoiding the anxiety associated with the patient's grief at hearing bad news.

DR. O'BRIEN: Ms. Graves, I need to talk with you about some bad news from the testing we did the other day.

MS. GRAVES: What is it? Is it my baby? What's wrong?

DR. O'BRIEN: No, it's not about your baby. I told you I was running some other tests, including a test for HIV. Your HIV test came back positive, indicating you have the virus that causes HIV disease or AIDS. (Pauses)

MS. GRAVES: Oh my God. I can't believe it. There's no way I could have AIDS! What about my baby?

DR. O'BRIEN: Your baby has approximately a 30% chance of having the virus. There are some treatments we should talk about which might help you and may prevent the development of the disease in your baby so she can not have the disease. What are you thinking right now?

MS. GRAVES: Well, I'm not thinking, I'm so scared, doctor. What can I do? (Begins crying)

DR. O'BRIEN: (Sits silently) Let's just sit for a while together.

CASE 8-5

Mrs. Coldwell is a 74-year-old woman who has been a patient in the practice for 4 years. She has CHF, impaired mobility from arthritis, and has frequently missed scheduled appointments. During her most recent physical examination 6 months ago, she had blood in her stool and was told to have a sigmoidoscopy or colonoscopy within the next month. She said she would schedule the appointment but since has only called for refills of her medication. Her primary physician sent her a certified letter indicating that she needed to come back for a follow-up visit. She told the nurse who called her that she was worried about not being able to pay for the test, and that her cousin who had the test was found to have cancer, followed by chemotherapy before she died.

PATIENTS WHO DON'T WANT TO FOLLOW A PLAN

Patients sometimes have reasons for not accepting medical advice or for not following it despite believing the advice to be useful. These reasons may be rational, such as disagreeing with a physician's assessment or diagnosis of a problem. Patients may be willing but unable to follow treatment recommendations because of lack of money or transportation. They may receive other advice from family or friends that is more influential. Each of these circumstances can challenge the physician, who may feel angry or powerless in the face of the patient's behavior. These feelings can result in a dismissal of the patient, either emotionally or in reality from the practice. The patient who decides that another form of treatment is better, who doesn't seem to trust the physician, may be responding to the physician's lack of clear explanation or to the physician's lack of understanding of the patient's belief system.

Mrs. Coldwell in Case 8-5 had several barriers to seeking treatment, including money for medical care, lack of insurance, and transportation difficulties, but most important was the difference between her goals and those of her physician. She was not certain that she wanted treatment even if she had cancer. Her physician felt obligated to educate her about the consequences of her thinking.

CASE 8-6

Ms. Russo is a 38-year-old woman who is a new patient to the practice. She has been treated for borderline hypothyroidism and hyperprolactinemia. She has been taking synthroid 0.1 mg po qd and bromocroptine 0.5 mg po bid. She is concerned because she had an unusually light period 2 weeks ago at the normal time, and yesterday began bleeding heavily and having severe cramps. She is angry because she called her gynecologist and could not get an appointment for 2 weeks. Today, before her appointment, she called and yelled at the front desk receptionist about how long it took her to answer the telephone.

PATIENTS WHO ARE ANGRY

The physician seeing Ms. Russo in Case 8-6 may fear opening the examination room door and facing Ms. Russo's anger. And it is quite likely that she will be angry for a few minutes. The wise physician will allow the patient to talk, and will just listen for the first few minutes, while the patient relates what's wrong. It will also be important to respond to her emotional expressions of fear, anger, or sadness, acknowledging these as normal and reasonable responses to what has happened to her. It will also be critical to let her complete as much of the story as she is willing to tell, to let her cool down, before moving to the underlying reason for the visit. It is important to not engage in problem solving at the content level about the other physician's office, or in detail about your office staff although feedback from patients is often useful information.

DR. JONAS: Ms. Russo, I'm Dr. Jonas. How are you?

MS. RUSSO: Not so great. I've been trying to get in and get some help about my bleeding, and getting through to my gyn and to your office has been ridiculous. What kind of offices do you run, anyway? You doctors must not really want to actually see patients, do you? I just can't believe you would let me keep on bleeding and not see me right away.

DR. JONAS: You felt you should be seen right away.

MS. RUSSO: I guess I really was worried.

DR. JONAS: Well, it sounds as though you've had quite an experience. I really do try to see patients and am glad you got in to see me today. Why don't you tell me more about your bleeding?

MS. RUSSO: Okay, well, it started 3 days ago . . . .

Dr. Jonas in Case 8-6 was wise to allow the patient to express her feelings without letting her "hook" him: He did not react with anger, as often is the most likely response, but rather was able to remember that the patient's anger is *her* feeling, and does not necessarily need to be his as well. The physician was able to reflect the patient's feelings using her words, a simple technique to indicate listening and attention to the patient's words.

CASE 8-7

Mr. Chester is a 70-year-old man who has been coming into the office for 6 years. During this time, he has been diagnosed with Alzheimer's disease, which has been progressing. He also has diabetes mellitus and lives alone. Despite his Alzheimer's disease, he has been able to care for himself and has been managing his insulin and his diet. A visiting nurse sees him twice a week. His children, who live out of town, visit each weekend and cook and clean for him. He came to the office today with a blood sugar of 750 mg/dl. The patient is sure that he took his insulin this morning, but cannot tell what day of the week it is.

WORKING WITH FAMILIES

As in Case 8-3, the physician in Case 8-7 needs to document the patient's mental status through a series of examinations. However, including the family as additional historians may offer fruitful data about the course of Mr. Chester's illness and help project the needs for additional care or treatment. A family meeting with the children and Mr. Chester may yield some useful discussion and a decision about how to care for Mr.

Chester in the future. The physician who wants to care for the patient must mobilize the entire family around a plan that they can all support. This mobilization entails asking who all of the relevant participants are and inviting them to join the meeting. It is important for the physician to greet each person and to ask each one to talk about what he wishes for the care of the patient. In addition, the physician may find himself involved in trying to negotiate differences among family members, and an important task is clarifying viewpoints for family members without taking sides in existing triangles in the family system.

DR. BRUNO: Thanks for coming today. Your father and I thought it would be good if we could all talk together about what's happening. Why don't we start with you, Mr. Chester; what are your concerns about how you're doing?

MR. CHESTER: Well, I sure hate getting sick enough to come to the hospital. But I ain't goin' to a nursing home either.

DAUGHTER: Dad, stop that. We aren't going to put you in a home . . .

SON: June, don't say that. Dad, we need to do whatever's best for you. We can't promise that you won't need to go to a nursing home; that's the doctor's decision.

DR. BRUNO: Well, actually, that's a decision we all will make together today. Mr. Chester, I know we've talked and you don't want to go to a nursing home. But as your doctor, I can't allow you to stay someplace where you're not safe. Lately, you have been sick more often, and I don't feel you can be safe if you live alone. So today we need to talk about having someone live with you in your home, or you living with one of your children, or your moving somewhere safer.

MR. CHESTER: Okay.

CASE 8-8

The last scheduled patient of the day in the clinic is a 25-year-old primagravida artist, Mrs. Munoz, who is 12 weeks into her pregnancy. She and her husband have come to the office for a regularly scheduled checkup. The nurse indicates that neither of the couple speaks English. They have brought the husband's 13-year-old sister along as a translator. This visit requires a pelvic examination, scheduling for the α-fetoprotein (AFP) test, and an ultrasound.

LANGUAGE OR COMMUNICATION BARRIERS

The usual difficulty of explaining a test and the potential results is exacerbated by the language barrier in Case 8-8. It is critical that the patient and her husband understand the reason for the test, and the limits of its interpretation. And yet, without a translation, the interactants may be reduced to communicating through hand gestures and broken phrases while conveying highly technical content. However, the inclusion of a 13-year-old relative as a translator can be difficult and even unacceptable in some cases. The inclusion of a younger relative as a translator is common, and yet it is unclear what issues can safely be addressed with a family member in the room. Discussion of sexual practices, including needs for an STD or HIV check, can become difficult at best. It may be questionable practice to perform a pelvic examination in the presence of a young girl, and yet to cut off communication during the examination can compromise patient care. It may be useful for the physician to include the translator as much as possible in the general history, and for more specific questions or difficult subjects to try to find a translator (or to have the practice use the ATT Language Line for translation) for a subsequent visit. Above all, recognition of the need for professional translation in critical circumstances may require ingenuity and creativity in a more remote medical setting.

CASE 8-9

A 36-year-old man, Mr. Thomas, is seeing Dr. Sonja Smyth for the first time. He is a healthy man who is requesting a preemployment physical. He has a family history of early MI (his father had an MI at 40) but is otherwise in good health.

DR. SMYTH: *Mr. Thomas, I'm Dr. Smyth. How are you today?*

MR. THOMAS: *Very well, thank you. Please call me Dave.*

DR. SMYTH: *Thank you Dave. I see you're here for a preemployment physical. Have you had any recent illnesses or problems you'd like to talk to me about?*

MR. THOMAS: *No, not really, I'm in good health. I'm excited about my new job, and just hope I can meet the right woman in this city . . .*

DR. SMYTH: *(noticing that Mr. Thomas is an exceptionally handsome man when smiling) Well, I hope so, too. Tell me more about your move here . . .*

PHYSICIAN FEELINGS FOR PATIENTS

The patient in Case 8-9 inspired some feelings in Dr. Smyth that are in conflict with her professional role. While sexual feelings are normal, and occur often in patient–physician encounters, they are not to be acted on. Yet many physicians report engaging in sexual relationships with patients, despite explicit prohibitions against such contact by the ethical standards of physicians (Gartrell, 1992). The wise physician will notice such feelings as they arise and will respond to set appropriate limits when necessary, deliberately steering the conversation onto professionally safer ground.

MR. THOMAS: . . . so I hope I can find the right woman here.

DR. SMYTH: I hope that happens for you, too. Tell me about what illnesses you have had in the past . . .

CASE 8-10

Laura Boaz, a 21-year-old college student, came to the physician for a checkup 6 months into her first pregnancy. She was very concerned about completing her education, and described herself as sure that she wanted to put the baby up for adoption. She had discussed this with her boyfriend, Mark, who was supportive of her desire to have the baby and to seek adoption arrangements. Neither Laura nor Mark had told their parents about the pregnancy. Despite the presence of two of Laura's sisters at college, Laura believed they hadn't noticed that she was pregnant.

Dr. Potter liked Laura. She and the patient had gone to the same Catholic high school; both of their families went to the same church. They were both the eldest daughters in working-class families, and over the course of the pregnancy shared stories of their families. Dr. Potter respected Laura's decision, and felt Laura was exceptionally mature in the manner she handled her feelings about the pregnancy and her family. After the delivery, Dr. Potter counseled Laura and was satisfied that her patient felt comfortable with the adoption, and was prepared to use abstinence or birth control to prevent another pregnancy. Dr. Potter was dismayed to see Laura on her schedule 8 months later for another prenatal visit, with a due date in 3 months.

WHY THE VISIT CAN GO TOO WELL

A sneaky aspect of countertransference can occur when patient and physician like each other and relate well: They can assume that they are too much alike, and the physician may not recognize signs of problems or difficulties the patient is not overtly sharing (Stein, 1985c). This blind spot can result in insufficient attention and discussion of areas of disagreement between patient and physician, with the result that issues may resurface. In particular, the physician in Case 8-10 felt disappointed with the patient (and ultimately with herself) for not working harder to probe Laura's true feelings and resolution of her problems.

CONCLUSION

This chapter has focused on the difficulties that may arise between patients and physicians in clinical conversations. Particular types of problems, including misunderstandings at the content level, differences in agendas or expectations, battles for control in the interview, and issues of countertransference, were identified. Specific skills for working with patients who are angry, who have a terminal illness, or who have been abused were identified.

Students who have difficult encounters with patients are encouraged to notice patterns in their encounters and to identify whether those patterns are the result of particular countertransferences or family interactions from the student's past. Ongoing consultation with peers, colleagues, or teachers concerning difficult relationships can be useful in identifying and changing patterns of interaction.

Noticing when conflicts occur between patients and physicians at the content level (such as disagreements or misunderstandings) and when they occur at the relational level (such as battles for control) can help the student determine when a conflict can easily be resolved.

CASES FOR DISCUSSION

CASE 1

You are a fourth-year medical student on call at midnight on the family practice service. You are asked by your supervising resident (who is in the ER) to do an admitting history and physical on a patient. You enter the room and introduce yourself as a fourth-year student working with the family practice team. The patient says, "Oh, dear, you're too young and cute to be a doctor! I can't wait until you examine me."

1. *What do you say next to the patient?*
2. *How do you structure the interview (physically, by seating, facial expression, and eye contact) and verbally (by telling the patient what you are going to do) to maintain good rapport with the patient?*
3. *How do your answers differ if the patient is:*

   a. *a 35-year-old woman who is very attractive*
   b. *a 22-year-old man who is very handsome*
   c. *a 76-year-old woman who is not very appealing*
   d. *an 87-year-old man who smells like alcohol*

CASE 2

Mr. Graves is a 74-year-old man with end-stage renal disease. He has survived many operations, daily dialysis, but his kidney failure is now untreatable. You are the third-year clerk on the renal service, and Mr. Graves pleads with you to be honest and tell him if he has a chance to live. His son, who is in the room, looks stricken, and tells his father, "Of course you'll be fine, dad. . . ."

1. *What do you say to Mr. Graves?*
2. *How can you respond to his fears and his son's false reassurance, without contradicting his son?*
3. *Who would you ask for help in working with the patient and his family?*

CASE 3

Ms. Cornell is a 27-year-old mother of four who has been seeing your preceptor in the family practice center for 5 years. She has been in good health, with some depression noted 2 years ago, which was successfully treated with medication. She is returning today for a Pap smear and routine annual examination. Your preceptor asks you to see the patient and take a history. When you enter the room, you notice that Ms. Cornell has bruises along her upper arm, and she looks tearful.

1. *How do you begin the interview?*
2. *How do you ask about the bruises?*
3. *Ms. Cornell says she is fine, but is still crying throughout the conversation. How do you reflect this observation to her?*

CASE 4

Tommy Capione is a 6-year-old boy who has been in good health until the past year. Since the beginning of first grade, he has visited the family practice center eight times for a variety of infections. His mother has brought him to the office because he is wheezing and sounds very congested. Tommy is lethargic and disoriented. You begin to suspect that this pattern of infections may be ominous and want to test Tommy for HIV.

1. *How do you begin to explain the need for an HIV test to Tommy and to Tommy's mother? Do you speak to them together or alone?*

2. *When she protests, saying there is no way for Tommy to have AIDS, how do you respond?*
3. *How do you suggest they discuss the need for the test with Tommy's father, who is at work during the appointment?*

CASE 5

Mrs. Pink is a 38-year-old woman who has been treated for clinical depression for the past 3 months. She has been on medication and in psychotherapy for problems with her marriage. Her husband is verbally abusive and dominates her. She has wanted to become pregnant, but he has forbidden her to try, saying that she is like a child already and is incapable of taking care of a child. Today, she has come to the office requesting a pregnancy test. The test is positive. She is convinced that the medication she is taking will harm her child and that she should terminate the pregnancy to avoid any further problems with her husband.

1. *What steps would the physician need to take to talk with the patient?*
2. *How should the physician respond to the patient's returning home to her husband after the visit?*
3. *Mr. Pink calls and demands the physician tell him whether his wife is pregnant or not. How should the physician respond?*

———— RECOMMENDED READINGS ————

Balint M: *The Doctor, His Patient, and the Illness.* New York, International Universities Press Inc, 1964.

Balint's classic work describes the therapeutic role of the physician's understanding of the patient as a "drug." This chapter is an excellent summary of the ways "difficult patients" ask for help from physicians, and how physicians can work with patient requests.

Brody H: *The Healer's Power.* New Haven, CT, Yale University Press, 1992.

Discusses the power of healing in the patient–physician relationship and the struggles of working ethically with difficult patients.

Candib L: *Medicine and the Family.* New York, Guilford Press, 1995.

This is a wonderful discussion of the feminist relational view of the patient–physician relationship. The reader will learn how to view relationships in the context of society.

Newell R: *Interview Skills for Nurses and Other Health Care Professionals.* London, Routledge & Kegan Paul, 1994.

This book uses a cognitive behavioral model for structuring work with patients, including specific skills for working with emotions, assessing the patient, and helping patients change behaviors.

Peterson M: *At Personal Risk: Boundary Violations in Professional–Client Relationships.* New York, WW Norton & Co Inc, 1992.

The author compares physicians, psychotherapists, and ministers in an analysis of "traps" in patient encounters that result in boundary violations, including sexual relations with patients/clients.

Stein H: *The Psychodynamics of Medical Practice.* Berkeley, University of California Press, 1985.

A useful introduction to the ideas in this chapter about relationships between patients and physicians.

CHAPTER 9

Clinical Decision-Making

Frank H. Lawler and Robert M. Hamm

CASE 9-1

Mrs. Jones is an 88-year-old demented nursing home resident who is admitted to the hospital one night with dehydration and a urinary tract infection that may have spread to her bloodstream. The resident on duty treats aggressively with IV fluids and also obtains a "do not resuscitate" (DNR) order. Mrs. Jones subsequently develops rales in her lungs that suggest heart failure. She also develops bradycardia down to about 45 beats per minute. Her systolic blood pressure drops to 60 mm Hg with the bradycardia. Mrs. Jones's condition is likely terminal but the bradycardia can be corrected with a transvenous pacemaker. The family is equivocal, suggesting that the physician do whatever can help. After a family conference and an ethics consultation, the physician decides that Mrs. Jones deserves a pacemaker. She arrests in the recovery room after the procedure and cannot be resuscitated.

——————— EDUCATIONAL OBJECTIVES ———————

On completion of this chapter, the student should be able to:

1. Appreciate the uncertainty inherent in medical practice
2. Describe the three basic concepts in the analysis of decisions: probability, utility, expected utility
3. Draw a decision tree for a medical problem and describe the reasoning used in its development
4. Describe the concept of cost-effectiveness
5. Demonstrate how to deal with patients around the issue of their preferences

6. Describe how physician and patient can discuss outcomes informally
7. Use simple techniques to produce a numerical measure of a patient's preference for a specific outcome

INTRODUCTION

Physicians make innumerable judgments and decisions in the care of their patients. These judgments include conclusions about the reliability of a patient's history, the severity of a physical finding, or the significance of a laboratory result, and choices about which diagnostic test to use, which treatments to prescribe, and the likelihood of a given therapeutic result.

A few decisions are made with minimal cognitive input from the patient. For instance, the patient in a coma or in the emergency department suffering from a gunshot wound to the chest has little to offer in the way of cooperative decision-making. However, most medical care involves making a decision with the patient. At a minimum the physician should educate the patient, solicit input and agreement, and confirm acceptance.

The standard model of how physicians think about what is ailing the patient is called the *hypothetico-deductive model*. A physician generates a list of potential diagnoses (hypotheses) from the chief complaint, and then seeks further information to substantiate or refute these hypotheses until some level of diagnostic surety is attained. This is the same process that a mechanic uses to diagnose and repair our cars.

Physicians judge the *probabilities* of their hypotheses informally, although there are formal rules about how the probability of the hypothesis should change as the physician gains information (e.g., Bayes theorem). Physicians form an instinctive probability regarding each hypothesized disease based on what they've been taught and their experience.

Because in most cases the physician already knows the diagnosis and merely confirms it, the hypothetico-deductive model is probably used in only a minority of patient–physician interactions. Unfortunately, the way that physicians decide about ordering lab work or therapeutic interventions doesn't always follow the logic of this model. Physicians tend to respond reflexively to patients, following well-learned scripts without much conscious deliberation (Abernathy & Hamm, 1995). For example, if meningitis is a strong possibility, a spinal tap is automatically performed, the patient is admitted to the hospital, and antibiotics are ordered. There may be very little conscious deliberation about the way to proceed in most clinical encounters. Actions flow spontaneously from the choice of diagnosis. As a result, tests or treatments are sometimes ordered that contribute little to the evaluation or confirmation of the disease hypotheses or to the treatment of the illness.

Sir Arthur Conan Doyle, a physician, loved to tell readers how Sherlock Holmes arrived at astounding conclusions from a few given facts. A similar reasoning process occurs for experienced physicians. Intermediate steps in thinking are performed subconsciously. When the rationale for decisions is brought into the conscious realm and explained, the conclusions usually make sense. The ability to manage most patients in this subconscious manner is what separates experienced clinicians from everybody else. The expert physicians "know the script" when others are at a loss about what to do next or even what to think next. Usually the script helps the physician move quickly to the right questions, although sometimes the reasoning may be inaccurate or inefficient. The beginning physician may know one script for lower respiratory infection and apply it to every patient with a cough, whereas the expert may know a dozen variants and be able to select the right one for almost every patient with a cough.

CASE 9-2

Dr. Melton is seeing a 10-year-old girl for the first time. The patient has a 3-month history of fevers and skin rashes. After an extensive history and physical examination he orders a complete blood count, a blood culture, and an antinuclear antibody test (ANA). At the follow-up visit a week later the blood count is normal, the blood culture is negative, and the ANA is positive at a high titer. He makes the diagnosis of juvenile rheumatoid arthritis and institutes appropriate therapy. Six months later the patient is doing well.

─── TESTING AND TREATMENT THRESHOLDS ───

Physicians have many adjectives for describing probability since they deal with it every day of their professional lives. Studies have shown, however, that what one physician means by "most likely" or "rarely" means an entirely different thing to another (Kong *et al.,* 1986; Hamm, 1991). To avoid communication gaps, therefore, it is more efficient to simply state the probability as a decimal number between 0 and 1 or as a percentage.

A graphic tool used in clinical decision-making for translating probabilities into action is the threshold diagram shown in Figure 9.1.

The estimate of the probability of a disease entity from the list of differential diagnoses can be placed on this diagram. As one proceeds through the *hypothetico-deductive model* more data are acquired that raise or lower that probability. As illustrated in Case 9-2, the physician finally moved from the "test" region into the "treat" region of the threshold model for the diagnosis of juvenile rheumatoid arthritis. This is the point at which the physician is *comfortable* enough with the probability of the diagnosis being correct that treatment is implemented.

It is easy to imagine how that threshold might change for different diseases. For example, a clinician may be only 50% certain that a 12-year-old has a streptococcal throat infection, but will treat her anyway (i.e., low risk from treatment), whereas a neurosurgeon may need to be close to 99% sure that a patient has a large cerebral artery aneurysm before performing therapeutic surgery (i.e., high risk from intervention, serious disease).

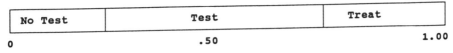

Figure 9.1. Threshold model of decision-making. Based on the physician's perception of the likelihood of a disease in a patient, the actions will follow according to this model.

CASE 9-3

A 55-year-old male presents to the emergency room with 45 minutes of severe, heavy substernal chest pain and mild diaphoresis. The physician, after getting the briefest history, estimates the probability of myocardial infarction at 75%. He asks for an electrocardiogram. It is absolutely normal. Is the probability of MI now 5%, 40%, or 70%? He looks up the sensitivity and specificity of an electrocardiogram (0.57 and 0.98, respectively) in Sox et al. (1988), and, using the Bayes' theorem, finds that it is now 43%.

As more evidence mounts that appears to rule out a given differential diagnosis, the probability that that disease is causing the problem falls farther to the left until it drops below the "no test/test threshold." This is the point of probability below which the clinician is *comfortable* that the patient does *not* have the disease. If this occurs, that particular diagnosis should be removed from the "list" of diseases under consideration for diagnosis.

Again, the no test/test threshold can be almost anywhere, depending on many factors, including the seriousness of the disease, the consequences of missing a diagnosis, or the risks, if any, associated with the treatment. For example, even if the probability the patient has hemorrhoids is 25%, the clinician may not test for it because treatment is not very satisfactory and the disease is benign. However, physicians routinely test for cervical cancer, which occurs with a probability of less than 1% in females of any age. This testing is done because the test is easy to do, and because of the potentially lethal nature of the disease and the serious ramifications of missing it.

The difficulty in dealing with probability lies in how clinicians *adjust* their probability estimates of disease when new information becomes available. Any new information (e.g., history, change in symptoms, physical examination findings, or test results) has the ability to change the probability that a specific disease is causing the patient's problems.

Sensitivity and specificity are measures of the accuracy of a test. Sensitivity tells us whether the test will detect disease in a population, and specificity tells us if a disease can be excluded in those without the disease. These two measures are characteristic for a given test and have no connection to how common the disease in question may be.

The usefulness of a test is called the predictive value. This concept means that performing a test will tell us whether the disease is present, or in mathematical terms, the change in probability that a disease is present after a test is performed. Predictive value links the sensitivity and specificity of a test with how common the disease is (prevalence). Predictive value can be positive (PV+), meaning the probability that the patient has the disease if the test is positive. Alternatively, negative predictive value (PV−) means the likelihood that the patient doesn't have the disease if the test is negative. Predictive values (positive or negative) can range from zero to 100%. Naturally, better tests have higher values.

How does one know if a disease is present or absent, given a specific test result? (That is, how do we generate predictive values?) There is a formal technique for calculating the change in probability that a disease is present, given a specific test result. To do this, however, one needs some estimate of the prevalence or prior probability of the disease in the patient to whom are applying the test. One can use published prevalence estimates (often difficult to find), or the physician can use an intuitive estimate of the probability that the patient has the disease. Sensitivity and specificity can be determined from published sources (e.g., Sox *et al.*, 1988). Once armed with prevalence (or pretest probability), sensitivity, and specificity, then predictive values can be calculated using the Bayes' theorem. The new, or posterior, probability can be compared with the prior probability to ascertain the value of the test. The formulas are:

Predictive value positive

$$= \frac{\text{sensitivity} \times \text{prevalence}}{[\text{sensitivity} \times \text{prevalence}] + [(1 - \text{specificity}) \times (1 - \text{prevalence})]}$$

Predictive value negative

$$= \frac{\text{specificity} \times (1 - \text{prevalence})}{[\text{specificity} \times (1 - \text{prevalence})] + [(1 - \text{sensitivity}) \times \text{prevalence}]}$$

Using these formulas we can quickly come up with predictive values. Remember, the predictive value negative is the probability a patient does *not* have a disease given a negative test; it is *not* the probability the patient *has* the disease given a negative test. The numbers from Case 9-3 are: sensitivity equals 0.57, specificity equals 0.98, and pretest probability (prevalence) equals 0.75. Because the test result is negative, we use the formula for negative predictive value. The result is $(0.98 \times 0.25)/[(0.98 \times 0.25) + (0.43 \times 0.75)]$, or 0.43. However, because of the serious nature of coronary artery disease and the medical and legal consequences of missing the diagnosis, the "no treat" threshold is probably less than 2%. Therefore, even with a negative ECG, we are still in the test portion of the threshold model and admit the man to the hospital for further testing over a period of time (usually 24 hours).

CASE 9-4

Dr. White receives a visit from a 48-year-old longtime patient. The man has abdominal pain, which he reports as tolerable but aggravating. Physical examination suggests fullness in the left upper quadrant. Dr. White orders a CT scan of the abdomen, which shows the left adrenal gland to be at the upper limits of normal size, but no specific abnormal findings are seen. The patient returns with continued pain. In spite of several normal laboratory tests, Dr. White remains concerned about adrenal disease because a relative of hers had adrenal disease that was missed 20 years ago. Dr. White decides to pursue the diagnosis with blood and urine tests and abdominal imaging studies.

———————— HEURISTICS ————————

The starting point for the initial probability estimate for a differential diagnosis hypothesis should be the overall *prevalence* of that condition, that is, the proportion of people in the general population who could be expected to have the condition at any one time. Certainly any historical or symptomatic clues from the patient may increase or decrease that baseline probability.

A *heuristic* is a term used for a shortcut or rule that physicians use in judging probability (Kahneman *et al.*, 1982). Heuristics are used often without our conscious knowledge and can have a significant impact on the validity of our conclusions. There is a long list of possible medically relevant heuristics. The three most important are: (1) the availability heuristic, (2) the representativeness heuristic, and (3) the anchoring and adjustment heuristic.

The availability shortcut occurs when we see a case that reminds us of an easily remembered similar case that was unusual. Case 9-4 demonstrates this heuristic; all subsequent tests were negative for adrenal disease. The anxiety of missing a rare disease may precipitate excessive testing. The unusual aspects of the case are what makes the case easy to remember. Another example is the clinician who orders CT scans of the head on all patients with severe headaches because he had one patient with severe headaches who later died of a brain tumor. That one bad outcome has artificially raised the clinician's perceived prevalence of brain tumors in patients with headache. The danger of the availability heuristic is that is can greatly inflate our probability estimates, and therefore decrease the accuracy of the data on which we base our decisions. It makes the "don't worry" zone in the threshold model nonexistent.

The representativeness heuristic states that we often assign a probability to a specific differential diagnosis based on how well the patient's findings match our idea of a "textbook" case. For example, if a clinician sees a woman with central obesity, fatigue, some facial whiskers, and mild hypertension, she may think that this patient has Cushing's disease. For her, each "characteristic" that this patient manifests raises the probability of Cushing's by an equal amount. She is forgetting, however, that Cushing's is fairly rare, and that each of these "signs" is also seen in a large number of people without the disease.

The third heuristic, known as the anchoring and adjustment heuristic, is relevant to the threshold model discussed previously. Basically, this heuristic says that we tend to "anchor" our probability early on, and often quite solidly. It is often difficult for physicians to "adjust" their probability estimates of disease up or down appropriately depending on the new information available. When not using quantitative data, it is almost impossible to adjust probability estimates accurately. Therefore, a clinician may estimate that a positive test does not push him over the "treat" threshold when in fact it should.

CASE 9-5

A 15-month-old child is brought to the emergency department by his 15-year-old mother. He is diagnosed as having an ear infection and mild dehydration. Although it is obvious to the ED personnel that the young mother loves her child dearly, they are concerned that because of family financial problems, transportation problems, and inadequate maternal parenting skills, the child should be admitted, even though such an admission is not medically necessary. After extended discussion and protests, the mother acquiesces to admission reluctantly.

PATIENT INVOLVEMENT IN DECISION-MAKING

A critical question in every clinical encounter is: How much does a physician need to explain her reasoning process in a given clinical situation? She must ascertain the level of involvement the patient desires and reconcile that preference with her desire to decrease the uncertainty of the case. Case 9-5 illustrates the difficulty in reconciling patient needs with family needs. Historically, physicians have had to give little explanation of their rationales and decisions. Increasingly the physician must consider: Does the patient want to be involved in the decision-making process? How much uncertainty is really involved? Does the physician's mental script for the disease automatically account for any inherent uncertainty in the case (Bergus *et al.*, 1995; Poses *et al.*, 1990)? Who will need an explanation: a consultant, an insurance company, the patient's family, an attorney?

Patients are asking to be more involved in clinical decision-making. Sometimes they will ask for tests, such as blood tests or radiographs, that may not be indicated in their particular circumstances. It is important for the physician to explain the types of tests available, the costs of the tests, and the possibility that tests will give false results, either false positive or false negative. Sometimes it is better not to test at all, since the gain in knowledge (the increase or decrease in probability of disease) is so small.

Patients hate surprises. Before a patient leaves the office or hospital, the physician has an obligation to explain, within reason, the possible outcomes. Intervention to the extent demonstrated in Case 9-5 is uncommon, but necessary. The risks and benefits of likely outcomes and patient (parent) preferences need to be balanced by the physician. Patients should be educated as to how to handle the possible outcomes and given instructions on unforeseen outcomes. A rote verbal explanation in the office is usually not very helpful. Prepared instruction sheets may be more useful. The physician may want to write instructions for the patient or family members to read later, particularly if the advice is complicated. Research is ongoing on formal programs to implement shared decision-making to improve patient participation and the quality of care (Kasper *et al.*, 1992).

CASE 9-6

As part of an annual physical examination a physician decides to order a multi-chemistry panel (Chem-25) on a patient. The liver enzymes come back slightly elevated. Because of the patient's occupation as a dental hygienist, the physician orders a hepatitis panel without consulting the patient. The results show that the patient is positive for hepatitis B surface antibody. The patient is laid off from her job and files for workers' compensation; she considers suing her employer as the source of her infection. Subsequent research shows that the first result was positive because of immunization during her training. She considers suing the physician for ordering the hepatitis profile without her consent.

———— PHYSICIAN DECISION-MAKING ————

Certain considerations affect the decisions to use certain tests. For example, a test may have a low return but be rather cheap, such as a urinalysis at every pediatric visit. A test may be extremely accurate but expensive, such as coronary angiography for chest pain. A test may be accurate and expensive but the disease under consideration may not be altered by therapy, such as a brain biopsy for Alzheimer's disease or culturing for viral identification in patients with a common cold. At times a second confirming test, with high specificity, will be required before initiation of expensive, painful, or irreversible therapies. For example, a Western blot test (sensitivity of 0.95, specificity of 0.995) is used to confirm a positive ELISA test for HIV disease (sensitivity of 0.9898, specificity of 0.98), before deciding that a person is infected with HIV.

Mold and Stein (1986) describe a cascade effect in medical care in which care of simple problems escalates into major, expensive, prolonged endeavors. In an effort to decrease diagnostic uncertainty, numerous unforeseen complications in the patient's care may result. The testing that occurred in Case 9-6 illustrates the potential downside of additional testing without additional patient input.

To what degree should physicians acknowledge uncertainty in diagnosis? Should a patient continue to see a physician who routinely confessed not knowing the reason for his symptoms? Would a patient prefer a physician who made diagnostic pronouncements with no history, no examination, and no laboratory testing? Would a patient prefer someone who would order tests, some unnecessary and expensive, indefinitely?

Physicians never know for sure whether their treatments will produce the desired effect. To what degree should physicians acknowledge uncertainty in the likelihood of a therapeutic outcome? Individual patients and physicians differ as to how much risk they can tolerate. Some people are willing to take a chance, despite a low probability of benefit; others will resist intervention, even when clearly beneficial.

Logically, treatment decisions are made with the probable consequences in mind: What will happen if the treatment is given? A decision about whether to operate for throat cancer is influenced not only by the probabilities (what is the chance the patient will die in the operating room? what is the probability that the patient will lose his voice?) but also by judgments of how good or bad the consequences are. Some people may tolerate the challenge of learning to communicate without a voice, while others may think it is completely unacceptable.

CASE 9-7

A teenager suffers severe head injuries in an automobile accident. The parents are torn between a choice of pursuing all available therapeutic avenues, even though likely futile, or looking to donate all suitable organs.

DIFFICULT DECISIONS

Should a physician assume that she knows what the patient wants? Should the patient have ultimate control over the decision-making process? Suppose orchiectomy for prostate cancer will prolong life 2 years on average; how much time is the average male willing to give up to retain his maleness?

There are cases where the physician may have more insight than a patient. When the stakes are high, as in paraplegia or quadriplegia, the patient may think that death is preferable to life, and the physician perhaps can't claim any special insight. Also, patients' preferences may change over time (Christensen-Szalanski, 1984). A patient's decision to forego resuscitation may be reversed as the likelihood of needing resuscitation increases. The parents in Case 9-7 have a difficult decision, and will need support and assistance from the physicians. Information from previous discussions with the victim expressing be useful.

There may be situations, especially elective procedures or childbirth, where a bad outcome may be particularly devastating and the patient may sue. How might the possibility of such an outcome affect the physician's decisions about whether to perform a procedure, say a cesarean section? Some tests have a known risk of complications. How paranoid or risk-averse should a physician be in weighing the benefits versus the risks of a test or procedure? Clinical decision-making may offer help in dealing with difficult decisions (Eddy, 1994).

CASE 9-8

A 76-year-old woman, previously in excellent health, comes to the hospital with shortness of breath. Evaluation leads to a diagnosis of mitral valve disease. The cardiothoracic surgeons suggest valve replacement. Although not as eager, the cardiologists also concur that valve replacement is probably the best chance for continued quantity and quality of life. As the physicians discuss the medical and surgical options, the patient says, "Stop right there. I'm not having surgery, no matter what any of you say." The patient is started on appropriate medicines.

—— ASSESSMENT OF PATIENT PREFERENCES ——

Some physicians, recognizing the difficulty of making appropriate decisions, have taken a formal approach to analyzing patient preferences regarding these difficult decisions. Physicians try to measure how bad each possible outcome would be for that particular patient, using a measure called "utility," which reflects the relative desirability of two or more options. If the utility of all possible consequences of a treatment can be measured, then one can get an overall measure of how good a particular treatment is. One calculates such an "expected utility" for each treatment option and picks the option with the highest expected utility. This approach can be used to analyze a number of medical decisions, such as whether to replace hip joints or accept the continued pain from arthritis.

The decision tree in Figure 9.2 shows a comparison between two treatments for a patient. Treatment A is successful 90% of the time and its outcome is measured as 95 on the utility scale (100 is best, 0 is worst, values set arbitrarily). When Treatment A fails, its outcome has a utility of 50. Treatment B is successful 70% of the time. Success with Treatment B has a utility of 98; failure with treatment B has a utility of 60.

Which treatment is better? Calculating the expected value gives an answer. To calculate the expected value, the utilities of each possible outcome are multiplied by the probability that the outcome would occur. For Treatment A the expected value is $0.9 \times 0.95 + (1-0.9) \times 50$ or 90.5. The expected value of Treatment B is $0.7 \times 98 + (1-0.7) \times 60$ or 86.6. If the tree and the numbers make sense to the physician and to the patient, then a higher utility could be expected if Treatment A is chosen.

The terms *utility* and *effectiveness* are sometimes used interchangeably. Utility refers to the subjective value of an outcome, whereas effectiveness refers to a more objective construct, such as years of life gained or days of hospitalization avoided.

194

CLINICAL
DECISION-
MAKING

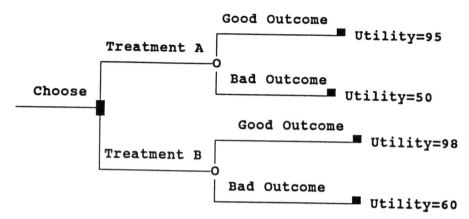

Figure 9.2. Decision tree with outcomes for two therapeutic choices.

Sometimes it is helpful to evaluate options in terms of how much it costs to attain an outcome. For example, clinicians in a managed care setting need to consider how best to spend their monthly capitation check to benefit their patients' health. The cost of each strategy can be included in the decision analysis. If we divide the cost of a treatment by the good that it produces, we produce a ratio, the cost–effectiveness ratio or cost–utility ratio. The ratios for the various strategies can be compared. A small favorable difference in utility may be overwhelmed by a large difference in cost. Smaller is better when comparing cost–effectiveness ratios. For example, it may be possible to gain more from a dollar spent on immunization, compared with a dollar spent on treating the disease the immunization might have prevented (Eddy, 1992a–c).

Cost–effectiveness ratios are important only when one strategy is favored in effectiveness and another is favored in cost. If one strategy is favored in both cost and effectiveness we are foolish to consider any other option. Although it may seem morbid, currently accepted values on human life range from $20,000 to $100,000 per year of life. An example would be a $7 million jury award for a birth injury where the infant might reasonably have expected 70 healthy years ($7 million divided by 70 equals $100,000 per year of life).

Numerical utilities and cost–effectiveness ratios are rarely formally assessed in clinical practice, although numerous examples exist in the literature (Krumholz *et al.*, 1993; Goldman *et al.*, 1993; Gray *et al.*, 1993; Siegel *et al.*, 1992). Instead, physicians rely on discussing the possible consequences with patients to get a sense of how the patient would react and which treatment option the patient would prefer. What patients want from medical care is a matter of some debate (Tsevat *et al.*, 1994).

CASE 9-9

An 80-year-old woman with severe hip arthritis sees her primary care physician for assistance. He tells her that she can continue on medications for another 8 years with about a 90% chance of ordinary function. Alternatively, hip replacement can return her to 100% function; however, because of perioperative mortality from complications such as development of blood clots, the average life expect-

ancy is only 7.5 years. Her physicians recommend hip replacement but she chooses medical therapy.

195

ASSESSMENT OF
PATIENT
PREFERENCES

In the research setting several techniques have been used to assess utilities. For example, if a treatment offers the possibility of a complete cure but a chance of death, as in lung cancer surgery, a patient might be asked to consider how much of his life expectancy he would sacrifice in order to change from his current imperfect health state to a perfect or improved health state. Would he be willing to die 2 years sooner than he would otherwise, if his remaining time could be in the good health state? This is called the *time trade-off* technique (Figure 9.3).

This method measures the utility of a health state using duration of life spent in that state. It assumes that patients would prefer to have a shorter life in a good health state, rather than a longer life in a bad health state. Case 9-9 illustrates that the patient's values don't always equal the physician's values.

The investigator should adjust the number of years lost, Y, until the patient is indifferent between living a shorter life in perfect health and a longer life in the imperfect health state. The patient is taken through a similar procedure for each health state that is a possible outcome of the decision. The difference in life expectancy in poor health compared with fewer years in perfect health when the patient shows no preference for either health state provides a measure of utility for the imperfect state of health. How much time is a person willing to trade for perfect health?

Another technique for assessing utilities is the *standard gamble*. A standard gamble involves asking whether a patient will take a sure loss (or gain) versus a chance of no loss (or gain) or a bigger loss (or gain). This method measures the utility of a health state using the probability of a "standard gamble" that the patient considers to be equally preferred to the health state. A standard gamble has a probability, P, of getting a very good state, such as perfect health, and the complementary probability, $1 - P$, of getting a very poor state. The patient is given a description of the state whose utility we want to measure, as well as descriptions of the very good health state and the very bad health state, and is asked to make the comparison shown in Figure 9.4.

The investigator adjusts the probability of the standard gamble, P, until the patient is indifferent between the sure option of living in the described health state and the gamble with a P probability of living in perfect health and a $1 - P$ chance of living in very bad health. One can go through a similar procedure for each health state that is a possible outcome of the decision. The question is how much risk the person is willing to take to achieve a better state of health. That is the measure of the utility of the current health state.

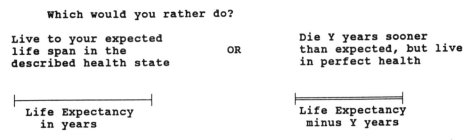

Figure 9.3. The time trade-off technique for assessing utility. How many years of poor health is equivalent to what quantity of perfect health?

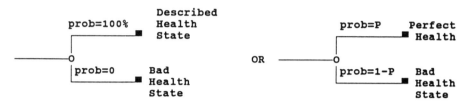

Which would you rather do?

Live to your expected life span in the described health state

OR

Take a gamble with a probability P of living to your expected life span in perfect health or a 1-P chance of living that long in very bad health

Figure 9.4. The standard gamble technique for assessing utility. A person can take a risk of trading years of poor health for a quantity of perfect health. How much risk is a measure of the utility of the imperfect health state.

Another use of the standard gamble technique is to measure a patient's feelings about taking risks. As an example, the patient might be asked to suppose there is a therapy for cancer that will definitely yield 3 years of life and there is a new, experimental therapy that is either immediately fatal or adds 6 years. The chance of surviving for 6 years with the new therapy is measured with a probability, P. Depending on the patient and the situation, some people take the sure gain and some take the gamble. Then the probability that the new therapy succeeds is systematically varied until a probability, P_E, is found at which the patient is indifferent between the treatment guaranteeing 3 years' survival and the treatment with a P_E chance at 6 years' survival. This number, P_E, can be used to express the patient's general attitude toward risk.

CASE 9-10

A urologist performs a transurethral resection of the prostate on an apparently healthy 70-year-old man. Postoperatively the patient does poorly, enters the intensive care unit, and succumbs within a week to previously undetected hypothyroidism. The urologist has never had a postoperative fatality before. The family is murmuring about suing. The urologist is torn between talking with the family or avoiding the family and calling his lawyer. He chooses to have a family conference, with the primary care physician in attendance. After extended discussion the family seems to understand the course of events and the patient's role in not seeking help for his minor symptoms of hypothyroidism.

—————— DEALING WITH UNCERTAINTY ——————

Because uncertainty is so common in patient care, physicians must learn to deal with it. What are the rational goals for a physician faced with uncertainty? We need to acknowledge either to ourselves, or to our patients, or both, that uncertainty exists. We need to help the patient and family to think about uncertainty and its implications for the future. We need to gather information, if possible, to decrease our own uncertainty.

There are several approaches physicians use to allay fear of uncertainty. Educating the patient and soliciting input may help attenuate anxiety and even clarify the situation. Talk *with* the family, not just *to* them. Discussion with clinical colleagues either formally or informally may also be useful. Young physicians may blame themselves for not studying hard enough; this is misguided and unproductive. There are circumstances that all of the study in the world would not have made clear. It is better to have good strategies for dealing with uncertainty.

It is hard for physicians to admit that they don't know everything; reaching the level of self-realization where one can acknowledge this fact and be comfortable with it is difficult. One approach that can help is to "triage" the uncertainty. One can rule out or address the lethal or serious diagnoses and consequences and then the uncertainty or ambiguity associated with the remainder of the diagnostic possibilities is more easily tolerated. Use of perspective may be helpful if it amounts to more than just rationalization. One doesn't want to get a reputation for always being uncertain, but patients and colleagues appreciate the humanity and humility of acknowledging that uncertainty exists.

Although it is not generally encouraged, sometimes it is better to act as if one is certain about one's decisions. As an example, a common finding on chemistry panels in active young men is an elevated creatine kinase. This finding has been noted frequently, but our literature search shows no reports on the prognostic significance of this finding. Patients seem to have no symptoms or complaints. At present, a justifiable routine may be to inform and reassure the patients, but not pursue further workup. As another example, the urine of a hospice patient with a short life span may turn up bacteria or crystals. The patient has minimal symptoms and the finding probably has no impact on quality or length of life. The physician may choose to make no report to the family.

Patients often express uncertainty when the physicians have no doubts. The principles that help physicians deal with uncertainty can also be helpful to patients. Communication is important, with lucid explanations at a level the patient can understand. The physician may be as uncertain about a given situation as the patient; this feeling by itself may be cause to reexamine the situation.

—————————— CONCLUSION ——————————

In this chapter we have discussed the threshold model of how physicians make decisions. We have also discussed the uncertainty in medical practice and some of the shortcuts that physicians use to deal with that uncertainty. The potential shortcomings of these shortcuts were addressed. Physician and patient input into decision-making is a complex area, as noted in several case studies. Two methods for assessment of patient preference, the time trade-off technique and the standard gamble, were illustrated.

In conclusion, physicians have enormous responsibility and make numerous complicated decisions daily with less than perfect data. Even so, most physicians are not overwhelmed or depressed and enjoy the challenges of medical practice and the rewards and satisfaction of helping people. Most clinical decisions are made easily, with a minimum of angst or regret.

———————— CASES FOR DISCUSSION ————————

CASE 1

Jane Doe is a third-year medical student on rotation at the VA hospital. She is assigned to work up a 35-year-old man with fatigue. After spending 3 hours on a history, physical examination, and reading in the medical library, she is confused and perplexed on what might be ailing this man. Her differential diagnosis ranges from AIDS to bacterial endocarditis to leukemia to toxic exposure in the Gulf War. She is afraid to let the resident or attending physicians know how uncertain she is, given the mass of data she has accumulated. She thinks that if she had just studied harder in pathophysiology, she would have known the diagnosis.

On rounds the next day she lets the resident present the patient. He has missed several pieces of information that are likely to be important. She adds the details without fanfare. The attending physician concurs that this case is especially difficult and details an extensive diagnostic workup to help sort out the differential diagnosis.

1. *Was her fear justified? Why or why not?*
2. *Why are students and residents afraid to express uncertainty?*
3. *How comfortable should medical professionals be with uncertainty? How should they deal with it?*

CASE 2

John Smith is a second-year medical student spending the summer on a rotation with the family physician in his hometown. A young man home for a family reunion comes in with sniffles and malaise for the past 2 weeks. After a brief examination the attending pronounces that the young man is suffering from allergies or a cold virus. Mr. Smith thinks that hepatitis or AIDS should be a diagnostic consideration.

1. *What should Mr. Smith do?*
2. *Should Mr. Smith discuss his hypotheses with the patient?*
3. *How much has the family physician allowed her past experience (called the availability heuristic) to affect her clinical judgment?*
4. *What should be done?*

CASE 3

Dr. Jim Hubbard is third-year resident moonlighting in a small hospital in rural Oklahoma. A 75-year-old man comes in complaining of diffuse chest pain after chopping wood. The man has never been in the hospital and takes no medications. Dr. Hubbard orders an electrocardiogram, which shows no acute changes. He diagnoses a muscle strain and sends the patient home on nonsteroidal anti-inflammatory medicine. The patient comes back by ambulance in 4 hours in full cardiac arrest and cannot be resuscitated.

1. *What should Dr. Hubbard tell the family?*
2. *How sure should a physician be that there is no heart attack before sending out someone complaining of chest pain?*
3. *If there was a mistake made, how should the physician address it? Should Dr. Hubbard notify his malpractice carrier?*

June Williams is a 30-year-old secretary for a construction company who presents at my office with a 3-month history of headaches. She is under a lot of stress. History and examination are normal except for a minimal inequality in pupil size, even though they react to light well and the funduscopic examination is completely normal. I think she probably has tension headaches, but she is concerned about a brain tumor. She has no insurance benefits, but I am also a little concerned, estimating the probability of serious disease at about 1%. She says that she wants a CT scan of her head. I send her to the local hospital, which will probably not get paid for the scan. The scan is normal and the anxiolytic medications I prescribed have helped a little, but not a lot.

1. *Am I reassured? Am I less uncertain?*

The headaches persist and over the next month seem to be getting worse. I debate over an MRI or a neurology consult, knowing that these will probably not be reimbursed. I explain the situation to Ms. Williams. She offers to borrow from her credit card to pay for a neurology consult. I acquiesce. She waits another 3 weeks to see the neurologist, who is surly, but does an extensive examination and finds no pathology. She says that an MRI might be useful, but would probably be superfluous. On the golf course the day after the visit she thanks me for the referral but teases me about my self-confidence. The patient is mad about the $200 evaluation that didn't reveal any new information.

1. *Am I reassured? Am I less uncertain?*
2. *What do I do next?*

Several weeks later the patient brings in her son for a preschool physical and says that the headaches disappeared after she switched jobs.

CASE 5

S. D., an 81-year-old man, goes to see his physician for health maintenance. S. D. is quite robust, golfing daily and traveling extensively. His physician finds a prostate nodule on rectal examination. The physician, thinking of the article by Mold et al. (1992), discusses the options with the patient. The patient has a high chance of having prostate cancer. Treatment for the cancer, if that is the problem, may result in impotence, incontinence, or surgical castration, without necessarily prolonging life. The physician calls for a conference with S. D.'s wife and children. His wife prefers not to deal with an incontinent old man and his children prefer to eradicate the cancer however possible.

1. *How would one evaluate the respective utilities?*
2. *Does cost–effectiveness have any role in the clinical decisions?*
3. *How should the physician proceed?*
4. *What would a simple decision tree look like?*

CASE 6

B. M. is a 21-year-old female with homozygous sickle-cell anemia and frequent hospitalizations for pain control. Keeping well informed about her disease, she realizes that a bone marrow transplant can cure her illness. She also realizes that there is a risk of dying of graft-versus-host disease. Her hematologist and family physician discuss the dilemma with her using a standard gamble technique (see Sox et al., 1988). She has a sure thing in not changing her current treatment, with a life expectancy of 20 pain-filled years. She can take the gamble with the bone-marrow transplant, with a small risk of death within 6 months or 40 to 60 years of good health.

1. *How would one draw the standard gamble diagram? (Hint: see Figure 9.4).*
2. *What is your advice to B. M.?*
3. *How would your views change if you knew that this procedure costs $100,000 and sickle cell is not an approved indication?*

―――――――――― **RECOMMENDED READINGS** ――――――――――

Abernathy CM, Hamm RM: *Surgical Intuition: What It Is and How to Get It*. Philadelphia, Hanley & Belfus, 1995.

This book covers the processes by which physicians solve problems, make diagnoses and decisions, create solutions, and think with visual images. The many exhibits make the presentation lively.

Bergus G, Cantor S (eds): *Primary Care: Clinics in Office Practice*. Philadelphia, WB Saunders Co, 1995.

This volume is an excellent overview of many of the aspects of formal clinical decision-making. It is targeted at an introductory level.

Sackett DL, Haynes RB, Guyatt GH, Tugwell P: *Clinical Epidemiology: A Basic Science for Clinical Medicine*. Boston, Little, Brown & Co, 1991.

A textbook designed to link epidemiology and clinical decision-making for practicing physicians. It is thorough, perhaps excessively, yet clear and entertaining.

Sox HC, Blatt MA, Higgins MC, Marton KI: *Medical Decision Making*. Boston, Butterworths, 1988.

The standard reference as an introductory text. It contains excellent diagrams and examples and is quite readable.

Weinstein MD, Fineberg HV: *Clinical Decision Analysis*. Philadelphia, WB Saunders Co, 1980.

Considered to be the comprehensive, authoritative reference. Read Sox *et al.* first.

CHAPTER 10

Patient Education

Ellen Beck

CASE 10-1

A mother brings her 14-year-old daughter to the office for a checkup. The daughter's grades have dropped at school, and she is frequently tired. The mother is concerned that something is going on, but whenever she asks her daughter, the girl slams the door and tells her mother to get out of her life.

The physician thanks the mother and explains that it is his practice to maintain his patients' confidentiality unless there is a serious medical condition that would be dangerous for them or others. He then asks the mother if she would mind leaving the room. He assures the patient that he is her physician and that unless there is something going on that is dangerous to herself or others, he will maintain confidentiality.

He takes her history. She has already completed a questionnaire about her life-style, habits, health concerns, and the like. At a certain point, he asks about her friends and directly about sexual activity, smoking, drugs, and alcohol. She tells him that she and her boyfriend have been "fooling around for a while" and that they use protection sometimes. She heard that the Pill gives you cancer; anyway, she states, "I'm not worried." She and the guys smoke sometimes, too. She mentions that she hasn't told her mother because she would be grounded, and her mother smokes and brings home guys too, and she is fine.

At present, this young woman has no medical diseases and no significant past medical history. On the other hand, she is at risk for several serious, potentially life-threatening conditions, including AIDS, hepatitis, other sexually transmitted diseases, and teenage pregnancy. If she continues to smoke, she is at risk for lung cancer, heart disease, chronic obstructive lung disease, and stroke. In this case, the physician's primary role is that of prevention and education.

────────── **EDUCATIONAL OBJECTIVES** ──────────

After completing this chapter, the student will:

1. Understand the importance of patient education and the role of the physician in patient education
2. Know ten basic principles of adult education
3. Know five barriers to effective patient education and a set of tools to overcome these barriers
4. Know the types of adjunctive tools used in the process of patient education
5. Know how to find additional resources in patient education
6. Be able to develop an approach and a basic patient education program for clinical problems

────────── **INTRODUCTION** ──────────

The word *doctor* comes from the Latin *docēre*, meaning "to teach." Physicians spend much of their time teaching. This may include explaining procedures or prescriptions, describing illnesses, showing links between life-style and illness, and giving patients tools to cope with chronic illness and pain. Medical training rarely involves courses or instruction in teaching skills, yet whether it is with patients or their families, students, or residents, teaching is a constant and integral role of the physician (Bates, 1988; Cantrell, 1973; Jason, 1989; Hitchcock *et al.*, 1980).

Everyone has experienced "good" and "bad" teachers. Characteristics of "bad" teachers may include: mumbles a lot, uses a lot of jargon, talks down to students, does not listen to the goals or needs of students, does not seem to care, is too critical or judgmental. "Good" teachers inspire, arouse curiosity, have good communication skills, show students respect, and make understanding easy and learning fun (see Table 10.1).

────────── **CASE 10-2** ──────────

A 35-year-old woman with four children comes to see Dr. Smith in a community clinic because she has been experiencing lower abdominal pain for about 1 month. After her last child 4 years ago, she had a tubal ligation and has not seen a

Table 10.1
A Good Teacher

Knows how it feels to be a learner
Shows respect
Can give positive reinforcement
Can give useful feedback
Does not intimidate
Creates an environment in which the student can say, "I don't know"
  or "I think I made a mistake"
Creates an enjoyable learning environment
Is knowledgeable on the subject
Knows his or her limits and can say, "I don't know"

---

physician since. She has always been healthy and has no physical complaints other than her pain. Her family history and past medical history are otherwise negative. She has no health insurance at this time. Dr. Smith offers her a Pap smear since it has been 4 years since her last one, and since Dr. Smith's clinic has a free Pap screening program as part of a Department of Public Health screening program. Dr. Smith also checks that she has no blood in her stools, diagnoses her pain as constipation, and gives her advice about treating constipation. She is also advised to return to the clinic if the pain gets worse or does not improve.

Two weeks later Dr. Smith receives a note that the patient's Pap result shows a cervical carcinoma in situ. *The clinic tries to call her, but she has no phone. Dr. Smith sends a letter to her last known address asking that she come back for further evaluation. Dr. Smith also asks the front office staff to let him know if she comes in again with her children and to schedule an appointment for her. He also puts a note on the children's charts. Three months later she comes in with her 5-year-old for the child's prekindergarten checkup, and she then schedules an appointment with Dr. Smith.*

Dr. Smith learned several lessons from this experience. He began asking the patients to call 1 month after the Pap to check the result, and began providing more information for the patient, including brochures in the patient's primary language. He also made sure that the clinic had an adequate Pap smear follow-up method for every patient (Schofield et al., *1994; White* et al., *1993; Paskett* et al., *1990).*

PATIENT EDUCATION: RESEARCH AND THEORY

The National Task Force on Training Family Physicians in Patient Education (1979) developed the following definition:

> Patient education is a process of influencing patient behavior, producing changes in knowledge, attitudes, and skills required to maintain or improve health. The process may begin with the imparting of factual information, but it also includes interpretation and integration of the information, in such a manner as to bring about attitudinal or behavioral changes which benefit the person's health status. Thus, patient education not only involves the world of medical scientific facts, but in its process it is also closely interwoven with psychology, sociology, behavioral science, and cultural anthropology.

Patient education is as old as the practice of medicine itself. In a modern translation of the Yellow Emperor's *Classic of Internal Medicine,* one of the oldest existing medical texts, the Yellow Emperor addressed T'ien Shih, the divinely inspired teacher, "I have heard that in ancient times the people lived to be over a hundred years, and yet they remained active. But nowadays people only reach half that age and yet become decrepit and failing. Is it that mankind if becoming negligent?"

Ch'i Po, the Emperor's physician, answered, "In the most ancient times the teachings of the sages were followed by those beneath them. They said that weakness and noxious influences and injurious winds should be avoided at specific times. . . : The ancient sages instructed those who were not yet ill" (Veith, 1972).

In 1931, Kress published a pamphlet entitled "The Cigarette as a Physician Sees It." He advised the physician to be a role model, counselor, and source of support to help patients stop smoking.

Patient education is an important therapeutic modality. It has been demonstrated to improve health outcomes as measured by decreases in risk behaviors, risk factors, need for medication, duration of treatment, and hospital stays (Haynes *et al.*, 1979; Logsdon & Rosen, 1984; Mullen *et al.*, 1985; Pederson, 1982; Holme *et al.*, 1985; Levine *et al.*, 1979; Stamler *et al.*, 1980; Kaplan & Stamier, 1983; National Task Force on Training Family Physicians in Patient Education, 1979; Morisky *et al.*, 1983; Spiegel *et al.*, 1989; Lindeman, 1971; Egbert *et al.*, 1964; Ornish, 1993).

Research demonstrating the effectiveness of patient education has been reported in many medical settings. Morisky *et al.* (1983) studied the effectiveness of three health education interventions in a group of urban poor hypertensive patients over 5 years. The overall mortality of the experimental groups decreased 57.3% as compared with the control group, while the hypertension-related mortality rate was down 53.2% in the same groups. Rose and Hamilton (1978) designed a randomized controlled trial on the effect of advice to quit smoking on middle-aged men. After 3 years they found a 36% abstinence rate in the intervention group, those who had received strong advice from their physician to stop smoking, as compared with 14% in the control group. The Oslo study was a 5-year primary prevention trial designed to study the effect of advice about diet to reduce cholesterol. Cholesterol fell by about 10% in the intervention group, leading to an overall 35% difference in coronary heart disease risk between groups (Holme *et al.*, 1985).

Ornish (1993) studied men with known heart disease. Patients participated in a program combining life-style suggestions, dietary recommendations, exercise, and meditation. His study demonstrated angiographic improvement in these patients' coronary artery disease. Spiegel *et al.* (1989) studied women with metastatic breast cancer. Subjects in the intervention group participated in an ongoing support group and learned techniques of autogenic therapy, self-hypnosis, and other self-help techniques. Overall mortality and morbidity were decreased for the women in the experimental group as compared with a control group.

A study conducted in Harlem with elderly black women who were attending a public hospital medical clinic found that the major reasons these women had not sought Pap smears or mammograms were that a physician had not recommended them or that the women did not know that they needed them. One of the authors' main conclusions was that patient education could enhance the use of early cancer detection procedures in this age group (Mandelblatt *et al.*, 1992).

A study of elderly Hispanic women residing in Los Angeles demonstrated that recency of screening, including Pap smears and mammograms, was linked to media-based health information, a different patient education format. The authors recommend that cancer prevention programs should use the Spanish language media to reach a wider Hispanic audience, especially for those patients who are monolingual (Ruiz *et al.*, 1992).

These studies demonstrate that various modalities of patient education can lead to behavior change that in turn leads to risk factor reduction or alteration in the course of a disease leading to improved prognosis and outcomes. Recent research has shown that brochures in a physician's office are insufficient to lead to behavior change (Mead *et al.*, 1995).

Past research demonstrates that an individualized approach to patient education is far more effective than a routine strategy. Lorish *et al.* (1985) studied the effect of an individualized versus a routine program in teaching patients with rheumatoid arthritis how to better care for their illness. Those patients who received the individualized program demonstrated a 100% greater learning gain than those who were given a routine program.

Adult education theory espouses several core principles for both the student and the educator. Wilkerson *et al.* (1990) describe adult learners as: a rich resource for teaching one another, more autonomous learners, and wanting to apply their new learning immediately. Teachers who utilize adult learning principles will: treat the learner as a peer, communicate in a respectful way, listen well, be open to and welcome questions, expect skepticism, be comfortable with saying "I don't know," involve the learner in the process, be relevant, and know or have access to the "data."

"Empowerment" is a central aspect of patient education. To empower a patient is to ask the following question in every situation: "How can I create an environment in which the patient, family, or community can take maximum charge of their lives and achieve health and well-being?"

If patient education is perceived as "creating an environment conducive to learning" or "creating an environment in which the patient can take charge of his health," physicians start to see their role differently (Table 10.2). The most important step is to establish trust. Without trust, the patient will not accept the physician's advice. Physicians establish trust by being courteous, respectful, consistent, honest, and relevant. They utilize "good" communication skills and demonstrate caring, compassion, and empathy. How the information is communicated may range from an oral explanation by the physician, a written pamphlet given to the patient, a videotape playing in the waiting room, a questionnaire for patients to complete, or an invitation to attend a lecture or join a support group.

Physicians must see each moment with patients as a possible "teachable moment." Patient education is integrated into all aspects of a physician's practice, whether it is calling back a young mother to reassure her about her child's fever or explaining to a worried wife in the emergency room that her husband had a heart attack.

CASE 10-3

Mr. H. is a 25-year-old white male police officer who comes in for a work physical.

Table 10.2
Patient Education as Empowerment

Instead of giving a lecture on a subject such as diabetes mellitus to the patient, the physician might think of "education" in terms of the following steps:
1. Establish trust
2. Elicit the patient's interest or motivation
3. Communicate information
4. Assess that the information has been received
5. Explore barriers and questions
6. Develop a shared plan and "homework"
7. Arrange for follow-up

CASE 10-4

Mrs. Y. is a 22-year-old Hispanic woman who recently had her first child. She is breast-feeding and is concerned about "not having enough milk." She also wants to know what she can do to not become pregnant again.

CASE 10-5

Mr. T. is a 45-year-old executive who comes to the office for a checkup. On history, Mr. T. indicates that his father died of a heart attack at age 50. The patient is a smoker. His blood pressure is 170/100 mm Hg.

BARRIERS TO EFFECTIVE
PATIENT EDUCATION

Patient education is based on a model of communication that comprises three basic components: the sender, the message, and the receiver. Each of these components functions within a larger environment. Breakdown of effective patient communication can occur at any point for a number of reasons (see Figure 10.1).

THE SENDER

In order to be effective, the sender of the message must become aware of her own assumptions and prejudices. She must let go of stereotypes, belief systems, and prior judgments and be willing to believe and communicate that behavior change is possible and within the capacity of the patient.

For example, if a physician's stereotype of Mr. H. in Case 10-3 is the "tough, macho police officer," this may discourage the physician from asking certain questions because included in this simple typecasting is a whole set of beliefs and assumptions. The physician may be unlikely to ask the officer if he is gay and then fail to ask him about certain risk factors for HIV or about his sexual behavior.

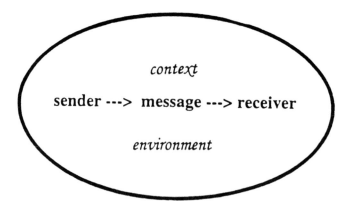

Figure 10.1. Barriers to effective patient education can occur at any point in the system.

In Case 10-4, if the physician allows his own beliefs about breast-feeding to dictate his practice, he may not refer Mrs. Y. to a lactation consultant, or if she is ambivalent, he may encourage her to switch to bottle feeding.

In Case 10-5, if a physician believes that Mr. T. will never take the time to stop smoking, she may not encourage it. On the other hand, a physician may be more willing to work with such patients as Mr. T., because of his socioeconomic status, nagging him so much that eventually he refuses all medical care.

Another barrier at the sender level is jargon or medical terminology. Using words that patients may not know or using a language in which the patient is not fluent inhibits the message from being communicated accurately. In large urban areas translators may be available, but some women may not be willing to give their history via a male translator, especially if it is related to gynecologic illness. Educational materials should be available in a number of languages, which will help overcome the language barrier.

THE MESSAGE

The message itself may be problematic. If it is confusing or garbled, the message will be hard to understand. Recently, the author asked a patient if she was planning to have more children. The patient said, "No." When the patient was asked what she was planning to use for contraception, she answered, "The injection," meaning medroxyprogesterone acetate (Depo-Provera or DMPA) injections, which are normally given every 3 months. The physician then asked, "When are you due for your next injection?" The patient replied, "In about a year and a half." A little surprised, the physician asked why she thought it would work for 18 months when usually it is given every 3 months. The patient answered, "The pamphlet I read said that the woman remains infertile for up to 18 months." The information provided to help women understand the possible side effects of the Depo-Provera injection had led the patient to think that the injection was effective for 18 months instead of 3 months. This experience reinforces the importance both of developing patient education materials that communicate the message well and of the physician verifying that the message has been clearly understood.

The actual content of the message is important. It should be accurate, phrased in a positive manner, practical, and achievable. Ideally, it should also be realistic and affordable. If the message is too frightening, it may not be effective; in fact, it may have the opposite result. If the behavior that needs to be changed, e.g., smoking, is one of the ways a specific patient deals with anxiety, then a strong fear-evoking message may make the patient more anxious and lead to an increase in the very behavior the patient is trying to stop. The physician must create a balance in the message, tuning it to the individual patient and illness. Leventhal (1965) found that smokers who had watched a film of a lung cancer operation were less likely to get a chest X ray than those smokers who did not view the film. He hypothesized that "the message" led to an increase in fear that interfered with the goal.

CASE 10-6

An elderly Guatemalan woman is brought to the emergency room with an arrhythmia (irregular heartbeat), vomiting, and a complaint of "everything looks yellow." She was discharged from the hospital 2 weeks before after an episode of pneumonia and congestive heart failure and is on several medications, including an antibiotic, furosemide, digitalis, and lisinopril. Blood tests indicate that she is experiencing digitalis toxicity.

Additional blood tests show that there is no change in her kidney or liver function. Further history reveals that she has mixed up the antibiotics and the digitalis because both pills are round and peach colored. She had been taking the digitalis four times a day instead of once a day and the antibiotics once a day rather than four times a day.

The resident who took care of her during her last admission is surprised. He remembers explaining carefully to the patient in Spanish how to take her medication and wrote it down for her as well. The resident, however, was not aware that his patient was illiterate. She had tried to be cooperative but she could neither read his note nor the medication bottles. Furthermore, even though he had also provided the explanation orally, the information he had given her was too much to remember.

After being treated successfully for digoxin toxicity, she was discharged from the hospital. She went home with a pill dispenser that holds the right number of pills for each day of the week. A home nurse will visit her weekly to help set up the pill dispenser and to ascertain that she is taking them correctly. A neighbor has also offered to help.

THE RECEIVER

Barriers to the receipt of the message may occur because of the context in which the message is received, including culture, language, literacy, and ethical concerns. Other issues such as possible side effects, denial, disinterest, or a belief that one can't change may also affect the receipt of the message. For example, smokers are sometimes reluctant to stop smoking because they are concerned they will gain weight. A Catholic couple may be interested in natural family planning for child spacing but may feel uncomfortable if the physician describes it as a form of contraception. To be effective, the communication has to be consistent with the patient's frame of reference, it has to have meaning and importance to the individual, and it must be acceptable within their belief and value system.

A young father may begin to face his problem with alcohol when his physician suggests that he might want to change his alcohol intake for his son, to set a good example. Another father might start to adjust his diet to reduce his cholesterol when he realizes that he would like to be present for his son's college graduation. A woman may decide to have a mammogram because her friend was just diagnosed with breast cancer. A teenager decides to take diabetes medication because he has just met "the girl of his dreams." Each person has different issues that motivate, that give her life meaning and importance. Ideally, of course, people should take care of themselves because it is good to be healthy and responsible for one's health, but often the things that truly motivate are more subtle.

One of the most important patient education tasks is to help the patient realize he can take charge of his life, that he can change. Sometimes this requires an exploration of the patient's inner dialogue. If the patient is convinced that he is unable to change and continually gives himself internal messages that attempting to change is hopeless, it is unlikely that he will be able to alter his behavior. If, however, he realizes that he is impeding himself via his internal messages, he may learn to change his inner dialogue. He could say I *can* change instead of I can't. To achieve this the patient has to realize that the inner voice is his own, not his parents' or teachers', and therefore capable of change. Also, some of our behaviors that are hardest to change are those learned at an early age, that were perceived by the individual as essential for survival, e.g., a young man grows up in a violent family and decides at an early age that he will stay calm at all costs. Later on in life, he smokes cigarettes, drinks, and smokes marijuana to stay calm. With the help of a physician or counselor, he may begin to realize that the very behaviors that helped him stay calm at all costs when he was younger are now a disservice to him, and he may choose to change, to learn new ways, and remain well.

CASE 10-7

A 2-year-old child is brought to her physician by her parents for a checkup. She is well, and had a normal birth and delivery. Her past medical history is negative except for a frightening near-drowning accident that occurred several months ago. The child has been active and well since the accident.

PATIENT EDUCATION THROUGHOUT THE LIFE CYCLE

Depending on the individual's age, the approach to patient education will differ. Case 10-7 and the following cases will illustrate this approach. Each case example represents a common problem at a different stage of the life cycle. Principles of patient education regarding the specific problem presented, including several pertinent references and resource recommendations, are also presented.

In the early life of children, as in Case 10-7, it is the parent rather than the child who is the primary focus of education. As part of the checkup of young children, there are a number of principles of anticipatory guidance at each stage of the life cycle.

Child safety is an important part of parent education activity for physicians. Questions must be specific and teaching practical. Questions can be prefaced with a statement about the importance of child safety. Rather than a desire to interrogate, the physician may state that she simply has a few practical suggestions. Examples of questions are: Do you have a pool? Please describe the gate. Is it always locked? Where do you keep your household cleaning products? If your child wanted to reach them, how would he do it? At the end of the visit, the physician can offer the parents a checklist of home safety features that they can complete and bring back at their next visit.

In Case 10-7, it is also important to explore the parents' feelings about the accident, including whether they are experiencing guilt or fear and how they're coping with these feelings. The physician has an important role to play in helping the family accept themselves, forgive themselves, and practice prevention without overprotection.

CASE 10-8

A 14-year-old girl comes into the ER in coma. Her Medic-Alert bracelet indicates that she is Chris R. with insulin-dependent diabetes mellitus. She is diagnosed and receives appropriate treatment for diabetic ketoacidosis.

It is several days later. She tells you that the last thing she remembers is that she went to a party, had a few drinks, and decided to go away for a weekend with some of her friends.

Certain chronic illnesses, such as diabetes mellitus and cystic fibrosis, require a great deal of self-discipline, attention, and individual responsibility. For the adolescent this can be very difficult. The road to adulthood is difficult enough without having to deal with a life-threatening illness. A need to rebel, a desire to be "one of the guys," a desire to live as if the disease doesn't exist, a wish as simple as wanting to eat whatever you feel like eating, all of these desires may lead to life-threatening situations for the diabetic teenager. Clearly, patient education in this population is as much about teaching individual responsibility and the tasks of adulthood as it is about the techniques and skills of disease management. Establishing trust can also be difficult in this population. Confidentiality is an important issue to them. The teenager needs to feel that the physician is *his* doctor, not his parents'.

In practice, the physician must establish ground rules regarding confidentiality, trust, and behavior. Consider asking the parent to leave the room during examinations. Nourish maturity. Suggest that the patient be a camp counselor or mentor for a child with the same illness. Suggest workshops that maximize personal growth. Involve him in case management, offer choices regarding treatment modalities, and make sure he knows outcomes of risk behaviors. Be straightforward in addressing possible "trouble spots."

Regular summer camps may not be willing to accept children with serious illnesses or children with chronic illnesses and parents may be reluctant to send their children to these settings. To address this problem, many communities have developed week-long summer camps for children with specific illnesses, such as diabetes mellitus, cystic fibrosis, and cancer. These experiences can be memorable and encouraging for children.

Finally, referral to a health educator, a diabetes treatment program, and the American Diabetes Association may help the family access nutritional, educational, and support services. In these situations, the patient must feel that the physician is still his doctor, but that other resources may be of help too.

CASE 10-9

A 17-year-old male comes to your office because for 3 days he has had a whitish discharge from his penis. He has never had this problem before and he wants it fixed. After diagnosing and treating the patient's sexually transmitted infection the physician explore the patient's sexual activity, whether the patient is using any form of contraception, and why or why not. The patient states the following, "Well, I like to hang out with the guys. Sometimes we pick up girls and you know, just take it from there. Sometimes you do it, and sometimes you don't. Sometimes they're using something to protect themselves, sometimes they're not. It's up to them, I figure, in terms of getting knocked up. As for me, sometimes I use a rubber and sometimes I don't. I don't like 'em, it don't feel the same, but some girls, from some neighborhoods, I figure, maybe I should, but lots of time I don't have one or I figure she's OK. I don't need it, and man, it's worked. This is the first time I ever got the clap and with this stuff I know I'll be OK."

The physician then asks the patient if he want to keep having sex this frequently, or does he do it just because the guys think it is cool? Then the physician discusses the possible consequences of the patient's behavior, focusing particularly on the risks and long-term outcomes to the patient and his partners. They discuss HIV disease, hepatitis, gonorrhea, syphilis, and pregnancy. The physician clarifies that HIV does not pick neighborhoods; it hangs out everywhere.

The young person coming for a checkup may not perceive the need for patient education related to his sexual behavior or other aspects of his life-style. The physician must establish trust and comfortably ask direct questions related to the patient's sexual behavior. Possible questions are: What is your sexual preference? When you have intercourse, what form of contraception/disease prevention do you use?

In practice, the physician should be direct and practical. Remind the patients of risk factors for HIV and other sexually transmitted diseases. Talk about responsibility. Show the patient how to use different forms of contraception. Listen to the patient's honest concerns. Think of practical ways to help, such as recommending that the patient carry a condom with him. Be careful of your own prejudices and judgments. Advising abstinence may or may not be useful in a sexually active male with multiple partners. Resources the physician can offer include free condoms, pamphlets, posters in your office, and reading material.

CASE 10-10

Mr. and Mrs. Morris bring their son Larry to your office. Larry was recently diagnosed with asthma. His parents are worried about him, and are quite protective. Larry sits quietly in a corner of the office.

——— PATIENT EDUCATION RESOURCES ———

In Case 10-10 both Larry and his parents are learners. There is much to learn about illness and approaches to management. Most important, perhaps, is the goal of helping the child feel healthy and independent and helping the parents learn to "empower" the child.

Teaching Larry to use inhalers appropriately is important and should be practiced and demonstrated in front of the physician; techniques to avoid allergens should be discussed, and stress management techniques such as relaxation therapy, self-hypnosis, and visualization should be suggested. Including Larry in the stress management discussion is important. Asking him to draw how he feels about the illness, or to draw the illness itself, or his family may help to initiate contact between the physician and the child.

The physician can also recommend resources including books about and for children with asthma such as *Luke has Asthma, Too* by Alison Rogers (1987) and *Teaching Myself about Asthma* by Kay Tiernan. For Larry's parents the physician can recommend support groups such as the American Lung Association and the Asthma and Allergy Foundation.

Books like *Children with Asthma: A Manual for Parents* by T. F. Plaut, M.D., and newsletters such as "The MA Report" by Mothers of Asthmatics, Inc. are also helpful.

Many organizations exist to offer support and educate individuals and families dealing with health problems and chronic illness. These organizations often develop educational materials for use by physicians and patients. For example, the American Cancer Society, in addition to developing pamphlets, produces teaching aids such as plastic breast models, which are pieces of foam shaped like breasts with small harder nodular pieces of foam hidden within, to help patients learn breast self-examination. Lists of self-help organizations with addresses and phone numbers should be available in the physician's office (see Recommended Readings).

There are many ways physicians can use patient education materials in their office practice. Educational videotapes and reading material can be available in the waiting room. Computer programs exist that provide individualized patient education material. Educational materials may vary from a current list of times and locations of local Alcoholics Anonymous and Narcotics Anonymous meetings to a printout of practical steps to manage fever in infancy. Age, language, and literacy level must be considered in choice of reading material; e.g., a young man waiting for a sports physical might pick up *Focus on Steroids, A Drug-Alert Book* by Katherine S. Talmadge (1991).

CONCLUSION

The foundations of patient education are those qualities that form the basis of a good physician–patient relationship, a good knowledge base, compassion, conscientiousness, and a knowledge of one's own limits. The physician who can empower, who can truly create an environment in which her patient can take charge of his life and achieve well-being, is practicing the art of patient education.

In the practice of patient education, the provision of knowledge is not enough. To transform an attitude, one must provide knowledge as well as experience. To effectively communicate, one must enter the frame of reference of the other, establish trust, consider the stage of the life cycle, and be aware of cultural differences.

Effective patient education addresses possible obstacles at the level of the sender, the message, and the receiver, always in the context of the larger environment. Patient education should be individualized and not punitive. Resources, including audiovisual material, support groups, and other organizations, should all be utilized.

Often as the physician proceeds on her own life path, life experiences lead her to become more effective at patient education. Confronting life experiences, learning the skills of personal growth, facing mental and physical illness in loved ones, and understanding limitations—these experiences teach compassion and humility and increase empathy. It is often too easy to judge patients, whether the patient is a smoker, an alcoholic, overweight, or depressed. Often the best patient education tools a physician can offer are those she has learned in her own times of difficulty. The most effective patient education is a partnership, for the illness or problem belongs to the individual and it is ultimately the individual who must change his behavior. The physician's role is to teach, guide, and empower and to remain as an ongoing source of support and guidance for the patient as he continues on his journey through life.

CASES FOR DISCUSSION

CASE 1

A 13-year-old obese girl comes in with her mother for a checkup. Other than her obesity she is a healthy, average student. She has always been healthy. Her physical shows that she is 4'8" and weighs 140. Her mother says that her daughter is lonely and has few friends.

1. *After ruling out medical problems as the cause of her obesity, what are the educational issues here?*
2. *What are possible barriers?*
3. *What kind of approach will help this young person?*
4. *Design a patient education plan for this patient.*
5. *What kind of follow-up should be used to determine the effectiveness of the physician intervention?*

CASE 2

An 18-year-old sexually active male has had a whitish penile discharge for the last week.

1. *What patient education issues may need to be addressed?*
2. *What additional history questions will help you to focus the patient education issues?*
3. *How would you address the patient education issues in this young man and what would you advise him?*

CASE 3

A 40-year-old black female visits you because of a cough. She has felt ill for several days, has a runny nose and headache, and is coughing up yellow sputum. In addition to her current problem, she has smoked a pack a day for the last 20 years. For the last 2 years, she has frequently coughed up sputum in the morning. You decide to spend some time counseling her about smoking cessation.

1. *What would be the initial approach to this patient? How could the message be successfully communicated?*
2. *What might be possible barriers? What would be the steps in helping her stop smoking?*
3. *Initially she is reluctant and says she has tried to quit many times before. How could her reluctance be addressed?*
4. *She eventually agrees to try, knowing how important it is to do so. What will be the steps in her antismoking program and what would be your plan for follow-up?*

CASE 4

A 50-year-old business executive comes to your office for a checkup. His father died of a heart attack at age 60. His mother is 75 and healthy. He has never been seriously ill except for recurrent low back pain that acts up whenever he does heavy lifting or strenuous exercise. He works long hours and in his spare time enjoys being at home with his family. His history and functional assessment are *completely negative. Results of his physical examination are normal except for a blood pressure of 160/100 mm Hg. The only abnormality in a panel of laboratory tests is his total cholesterol, which is 300 mg/dl (normal <200 mg/dl). A lipid profile confirms an elevated LDL and lowered HDL.*

1. *Which of this man's current problems might benefit from patient education?*
2. *What patient education recommendations would you give him?*
3. *How would you follow him?*
4. *How might you involve his family?*

CASE 5

A 70-year-old woman is diagnosed with breast cancer. The surgeon recommends mastectomy. Several years later, she develops bone metastases. The oncologist recommends chemotherapy. The patient doesn't respond to the chemotherapy, and within a year is nearing death.

1. *At each stage of her illness, what are important patient education issues that need to be addressed?*
2. *How would you explain do-not-resuscitate orders, living wills, and durable power of attorney?*
3. *Would you discuss hospice? If so, how?*
4. *How would you advise the family?*

—————— RECOMMENDED READINGS ——————

ASTHMA

Weinstein A: *A Useful Guide to Self-Management of Asthma and Allergies for Patients and Families.* New York, McGraw–Hill Book Co, 1987.

Explains the condition and management of special situations, such as out-of-control asthma and other special problems.

CANCER

Keogh C: *The Complete Book of Cancer Prevention.* Prevention Magazine Health Books, Emmanus, Penn, Rodale Press Inc, 1988.

A listing of prevention approaches for 20 common cancers, including listing fears, facts, and practical techniques (e.g., breast self-examination) followed by general discussion of nutrition, life-styles, possible carcinogens, skin protection, and approaches to treatment problems at home and what to expect at the physician's.

CHILD HEALTH

Cunningham N: *The Columbia University College of Physicians and Surgeons Complete Guide to Early Child Care.* New York, Crown Publishers Inc, 1990.

Describes development and explains medical conditions and prevention.

HEART DISEASE

Ornish D: Can lifestyle changes reverse coronary heart disease? *World Rev Nutr Diet* 72: 38–48, 1993.

A description of a life-style program, including meditation, exercise, and nutritional and dietary changes that led to angiographically proven improvement in coronary artery disease.

Legato M, Coleman C: *The Female Heart*. New York, Simon & Schuster Inc, 1991.

A book about heart disease and prevention from the female perspective. Most of the cardiac research has been on helping and understanding men with heart disease; this book is about and for women who have or are at risk for heart disease.

MEDICAL TESTS

Sobel D, Ferguson T: *The People's Book of Medical Tests*. New York, Summit Books, 1985.

A review of lab, radiology, and other medical tests presented in layman's language, so that individuals can understand the indications, risks, costs, and procedures involved in medical testing. It is the authors' hope that this knowledge will lead to more informed choices.

MIND BODY MEDICINE

Shealy CN, Myss CM: *The Creation of Health: Merging Traditional Medicine with Intuitive Diagnosis*. Walpole, NH, Stillpoint Publishing, 1988.

An excellent text on merging traditional medicine with intuitive diagnosis, organized by medical problem.

NUTRITION

Herbert V: *The Mount Sinai School of Medicine Complete Book of Nutrition*. New York, St. Martin's Press Inc, 1990.

A book addressing nutritional requirements and approaches for a variety of health and medical situations.

PARENTING

Albert L, Popkin M: *Quality Parenting*. New York, Random House, Ballantine Books Inc, 1987.

Practical advice on parenting issues and challenges. How to transform the everyday moments we spend with our children into special meaningful time.

PATIENT EDUCATION

Society of Teachers of Family Medicine. *Patient Education. A Handbook for Teachers*. Report of the National Task Force on Training Family Physicians in Patient Education. Washington, DC, December 1979.

Review of principles and practice in patient education, excellent lists of resources, bibliography, checklist for assessing patient education materials and practical skills.

PREGNANCY

Samuels M, Samuels N: *The Well Pregnancy Book*. New York, Summit Books, 1986.

A practical adjunct to childbirth classes. This book contains practical advice, as well as an extensive bibliography. These authors have also written *The Well Baby Book* and *The Well Child Book*.

SELF-CARE

Vickery DM, Fries JF: *Take Care of Yourself—Complete Guide to Medical Self Care*. Reading, Mass, Addison–Wesley Publishing Co Inc, 1993.

Discussion of prevention, choosing a doctor, a listing of common medical problems with practical charts.

SKIN DISEASE

Grossbart TA, Sherman C: *Skin Deep, A Mind–Body Program for Healing Skin*. New York, William Morrow & Co Inc, 1986.

Description of a mind/body approach to skin diseases at Harvard Medical School. Practical suggestions that can be integrated with medical practice.

SMOKING

The National Cancer Institute with cooperation from The American Cancer Society and Doctors Ought to Care (DOC). *Target Intervention—How to Help Your Patients Stop Smoking*. San Francisco, 1988.

An excellent manual for healthcare providers to help their patients stop smoking.

TRAVEL MEDICINE

Forgery W: *Traveler's Medical Resources*. Merrillville, Ind, ICS Books Inc, 1990.

A guide to health and safety worldwide.

CHAPTER 11

Negotiation with Patients

Jeannette E. South-Paul

CASE 11-1

A 49-year-old woman presents to the emergency room with multiple rib fractures and a displaced, pathologic, subtrochanteric fracture of the left hip. She is 4 years post right radical mastectomy for breast cancer. She is in severe pain and wants treatment. On obtaining a history, completing a physical examination, and obtaining radiographs of the affected areas, the patient notes that she is a Jehovah's Witness and will not allow blood transfusions. She notes that if family or friends see her receiving a transfusion, they will think she has betrayed her faith.

EDUCATIONAL OBJECTIVES

By the end of this chapter you will be able to:

1. Define what is meant by "negotiating" in the clinical setting
2. Describe the differences between "soft" and "hard" negotiating
3. Define positional bargaining and describe its advantages and disadvantages
4. Define principled negotiation and describe its advantages and disadvantages
5. Describe the physician's role as patient advocate
6. Describe the framework of the clinician–patient relationship needed for successful negotiation to take place
7. Describe how cultural differences can influence clinician–patient negotiations
8. Describe the LEARN model for multicultural interactions
9. Describe ways to avoid negotiation by improving the communication with patients

217

INTRODUCTION

Case 11-1 illustrates a difficult situation that requires that the physician establish a rapport with the patient before attempting to address the dilemmas. Recognizing the situations in which negotiation must occur is the first step toward becoming comfortable and effective in negotiating.

The first step is the gathering of historical information from the patient in a non-threatening manner. If the patient first began experiencing symptoms several days or even weeks before presenting, the clinician has an opportunity to ask the patient why she didn't seek care earlier. This allows the patient to describe her concerns and fears. On revealing her Jehovah's Witness faith, the clinician can encourage the patient to describe the specific medical guidelines or restrictions under which she is bound. This provides actual information about the issues that may conflict with more traditional biomedical guidelines for her problem. Questions about family and support systems will provide information regarding her special needs. The patient can be asked whether she wishes to make decisions by herself or with the assistance of someone else. If yes, who? It is always helpful and important to clarify those whom the patient considers her family. Lastly, she should be queried regarding her fears about hospitalization. Is she afraid of surgery, or is the possibility of transfusion her only concern? This line of questioning can be interwoven with the other, more traditional, questions that are usually included in the history-taking process.

Whenever there is interaction between individuals there is the possibility of disagreement. The quality of the communication that takes place during the interaction is dependent on many factors, such as willingness to listen to the other person, understanding of the issues presented, availability of time for adequate problem solving, and a sincere desire to reach agreement. This is no less true when considering interactions between clinicians and patients, which are critically dependent on whether effective communication occurs. When effective communication occurs, the clinician understands the patient's wishes and needs and the patient understands the clinician's assessment and recommendations. When the patient's wishes appear unrealistic, the clinician is challenged to extend and expand his communication to reach understanding and agreement. When reaching agreement becomes difficult, but both parties wish to accomplish a mutually agreeable objective, negotiation becomes the logical next step.

Negotiation is a term used predominantly in the business sector. Thus, it requires clarification if it is to be used in reference to the clinician–patient encounter. When negotiation is being considered in the business arena, two or more parties have usually approached a situation with different goals and have been unable to reach agreement. In contrast, when speaking of interactions related to the therapeutic relationship, the goals of both clinician and patient are similar and usually involve restoring the patient to a state of health. Should negotiation truly be necessary in this setting, one of two situations is present: (1) The patient is faced with a complex set of decisions potentially resulting in significant loss, e.g., disability, surgery, or (2) there has been serious compromise to the clinician–patient relationship. At this point, the clinician must assess the patient's needs, ensure the patient's understanding of the situation, and reach agreement. So whenever the term *negotiation* is used in this setting, the hope is that it is occurring in a framework of good communication. Tact and wisdom are then the tools needed to elicit information, concerns, and feelings so that the best outcomes for both patient and clinician are possible.

*Two clinicians have recently completed training and are considering going into
practice together. They have no established patient base, but wish to arrange
office space in a building near what will be their primary referral hospital.
Clinician A wants to hire his wife as office manager to take care of all of the
business headaches of the practice. His goal is to become financially productive as
soon as possible. Clinician B feels that they should manage the money themselves,
be financially conservative, and initially employ the minimum number of staff.*

BUSINESS MODEL OF NEGOTIATION

All clinicians evaluating patients are taught to use a methodical, well-recognized
approach. In such a fashion, young clinicians are told that they will be less likely to miss
important information, and thus less likely to make a wrong diagnosis. The same can be
said about the process of negotiation. To be effective, negotiation must also proceed
through a series of logical steps.

One of two negotiating styles is typically chosen. The style of *soft* negotiation is one
that seeks to avoid conflict and concedes easily. Compromises are offered up front in an
attempt to reach an amicable solution quickly. However, the soft negotiator often feels
shortchanged in the end. In contradistinction to soft negotiation, the goal of *hard* negotiation is to win and to hold out as long as possible. As a result, this rigid, aggressive style
often harms chances of future collaboration.

Usually negotiators use their respective approaches to engage in *positional bargaining*. This method depends on successively choosing and giving up a series of positions.
Advantages of this technique are that (1) it is easy and requires little preparation, (2) it is
universally understood, and (3) it can give one the opportunity to observe or listen to the
opponent, getting to know him better. The dilemma is that the more one defends the
position chosen, the more committed one must be, and, therefore, the less flexible one can
be or the less able to compromise. Positional bargaining (1) can produce unwise agree-
ments, (2) is inefficient, (3) is a method that endangers an ongoing relationship, and (4) is
difficult to manage when more than two parties are involved (Fisher *et al.*, 1991).

A different method that has been offered by those at the Harvard Negotiation Project
is that of *principled negotiation*. This method, also called *negotiation on the merits*, allows
decision on an issue on the basis of merit rather than through a haggling process of what
each side will or will not do. The dilemma comes when deciding who determines the
merits of an issue. In business, parties present data to suggest the number of people being
affected and the costs of each decision to provide a framework for the negotiations. This
method suggests that each party look for mutual gains. The goal is to obtain what you feel
you are entitled to and still maintain a clear-cut and defensible approach. It is based on
establishing and working with four elements: people, interests, options, and criteria. One
must separate the people from the problem. The interests of each side must be identified in
terms of needs, desires, and concerns. One must characterize options that can be mutually
beneficial. Finally, the outcome is based on objective criteria.

In Case 11-2, if Clinician B is a soft negotiator, he will raise his concerns about
employing Clinician A's spouse with him, suggesting that they should save money when
initially establishing themselves. He leaves an obvious opening for Clinician A to suggest

an alternative to saving money so that his wife can still be hired. If Clinician B is a hard negotiator, he will probably note up front that there should be a rule prohibiting the hiring of relatives in the practice.

The positional bargaining approach could involve setting down guidelines about how much to spend on staff salaries at the beginning of the discussion and progress with a series of discussions about how much to spend on each employee and the possible returns on each of these staff expenditures. Principled negotiation involves objectively laying out the advantages and disadvantages of hiring an office manager separately from any discussion of personalities, then assessing the merits of employing family members as a separate issue to facilitate an efficient, honest discussion prior to reaching a decision.

The implication is that one negotiates in order to obtain an outcome that would not otherwise be possible. To be fully prepared, one must consider the situation when negotiation is not possible, described by Fisher and Ury (1991) as the BATNA, the *best alternative to negotiated agreement*. BATNA is the standard against which any negotiated agreement is measured. It serves as a guide for preventing one from accepting an undesirable agreement. If one has not thought of a BATNA, there is the insecurity of not knowing what target to aim for or not recognizing your bottom line. There is the risk of being too optimistic and thinking alternatives exist that do not. Likewise, one may be too pessimistic of the consequences of failed negotiations.

In contrast to the business arena, when dealing with patients, the patient is the party who ultimately decides the merits of any suggested therapy, what risks are considered acceptable, and how much the projected outcome is worth. In effect, the clinician works for and is an advocate of the patient. It is the responsibility of the clinician to find and describe a BATNA for any recommended therapy in the event that the patient finds the first recommendation unacceptable. Thus, clinicians are challenged to focus on the patient's needs and wants, since clinicians exist because of patients and in order to meet the patient's needs.

Unfortunately, the clinician–patient decision-making process has become more complex in recent years with the increase of the third-party payment industry. A third party now has to be considered when making decisions about the outcome of medical care. At one time, the clinician diagnosed or evaluated the complaint and made recommendations regarding treatment. The patient sought further clarification, contemplated the information received, perhaps discussed the options with family, and made a decision regarding therapy. The contracts held by most managed care organizations now limit the type of diagnostic testing that can be reimbursed, often require the patient to be evaluated by another clinician to render a second opinion, and usually involve administrative personnel when deciding what therapies can be reimbursed. Reimbursement thus impacts compliance with medical recommendations. Negotiations between clinician and insurance entity or between patient and insurance entity have become relatively common in order to achieve optimal patient care.

Elements from the business approach can be used in the framework of Case 11-1. The clinician must initially assess the medical problem presented without unduly focusing on the patient's religious beliefs. Factors of religion, family, and social situation must then be defined and integrated into the total assessment. The clinician must then uncover and understand the patient's interests, that is, what does the patient really want? Is pain control without intervention the uppermost desire? Is definitive treatment more important? Does the patient desire strict adherence to religious guidelines or are other options acceptable? If so, is she willing to accept the possibility of poor surgical outcome or completely losing the option of surgical intervention? Once the patient's desires and the clinician's perceptions and assessment are defined, the clinician must present as complete a list of options as possible, including all of the risks as well as the benefits. Recognizing each of these criteria, both patient and clinician negotiate to reach a mutually acceptable plan.

CASE 11-3

A 72-year-old woman with poorly controlled hypertension, multiple drug sensitivities, degenerative arthritis, and cataracts lives 45 miles from your office. Because she doesn't drive, her husband must take her to all of her appointments. He has non-insulin-dependent, insulin-requiring diabetes mellitus, coronary artery disease, and peripheral vascular disease. She has maintained better blood pressure control since being followed at your clinic, but now has access to an urgent care center that recently opened 10 miles from her house. She is worried about her husband's health and wishes he didn't have to drive so far to obtain her care. She now asks her physician's advice regarding where to continue her care.

NEGOTIATING CARE IN THE
HEALTHCARE SYSTEM

In considering Case 11-3, it is clear that the patient is faced with multiple decisions. These decisions are not always obvious to the casual observer, however. Thus, it is useful to systematically assess each interaction to improve the chance of recognizing and addressing all of the decisions that can be negotiated.

An initial question to ask the patient is where she prefers receiving care. If she notes no preference between the continuity clinic and the urgent care center, you might suggest allowing her husband to decide since he is providing the transportation. If she has a distinct preference for maintaining the current clinician–patient relationship, she should be queried about whether her major concern is occupying her husband's time or negatively impacting on his health. Then it would be appropriate to offer to discuss the issue with both members of the couple. That discussion should be prefaced with a general summary of her medical problems and prognoses. Other issues to explore with both patient and spouse would be their preference of inpatient facility should the patient require hospitalization. This choice may also influence selection of primary care provider.

A targeted discussion between patient and primary care provider may assist the patient in recognizing the importance of feeling comfortable with a provider and how this impacts on compliance. By helping her to see the many issues that impact on her care, the patient can confront the issues that she may find unacceptable and incorporate them in her decision-making.

The nature of the clinician–patient interaction affects the patient's decision-making. This interaction, typically called the doctor–patient relationship, has been described as a contractual model where there is a nonlegalistic statement of general obligation and benefits for both parties (Brody, 1981). The decision-making responsibility is shared between physician and patient in acknowledgment of the patient's right to control the significant decisions in his own life. The patient recognizes that the physician has the requisite skills to make the technical decisions needed to implement that general goal to which the patient has agreed. However, the patient expects that the physician will take no major action without allowing the patient to make the decision, while not expecting to be consulted on all of the technical details. Likewise, the physician retains the right not to enter into the contract, or to end the contract if the implementation of the patient's wishes would violate the physician's own moral values. When the clinician–patient relationship operates within these guidelines, negotiation is rarely necessary.

One of the issues that greatly affects the decision-making process is the patients' personal needs, as in Case 11-3. Is she struggling to pay her rent and, thus, has little extra to fund expensive trips to a clinic or new medications? Is she the primary caretaker for her grandchildren and, therefore, unable to leave them to come a long distance for appointments? Does resolution of such issues supersede medical concerns in the patient's mind? The clinician may need to enlist the assistance of community or social services to address basic needs before the patient can focus on herself.

In addition to the status of the patient's needs, the significance of cultural elements must also be recognized in order to avoid noncompliance, misunderstandings, and simultaneous care-seeking from multiple practitioners without coordination. Patients' expectations of the healthcare system and the culture of the healthcare system vary from one country to another and between cultural groups. Generally, in U.S. society today, there is the expectation among patients that almost any medical miracle is possible, given the right institution and enough money. This societal expectation affects the individual demands patients make on clinicians.

Furthermore, the medical anthropologist and psychiatrist Arthur Kleinman describes the significance of the culture of the medical establishment itself. The factors judged most important to the delivery of good care and the priority each is given differ between patients and the medical establishment. At a Veterans Affairs hospital, priority for care is assigned based on the relationship of the patient's condition to military service. Emergency room providers prioritize patients according to how life threatening the presenting condition is rather than how uncomfortable the patient feels. Patients do not always understand or agree with these decisions.

Therefore, it is important to know the culture of the system in which the clinician is operating and the cultural affiliations of the patient. Does the patient in Case 11-3 feel equally comfortable receiving care from either facility? Is there a general feeling in the community that one facility prefers not to treat poor patients, or minority patients, or patients from a religion different than that of the sponsors of the hospital, or patients who use traditional healers?

Patients from other cultures often have lower expectations for cure, especially by Western medical therapies. They would rather use traditional or herbal remedies. When patients choose a healthcare provider, do they feel comfortable sharing their beliefs about alternative therapies, or are such therapies used in parallel without the practitioner of either being aware of the other? A nonthreatening approach to eliciting this information is incorporating a statement such as this: "Many of us were raised using home remedies for common ailments. Do you recall any you used?"

Thus, there are numerous elements required for successfully obtaining healthcare in any system. Few patients are aware of all of these elements. However, it is incumbent on the primary care provider to anticipate the existence of these elements, discuss them with patients, and then assist patients in making choices regarding their own care that are influenced by these issues.

Dr. H. is providing maternity care for a 30-year-old woman who is in her second trimester of pregnancy and whose 2-year-old daughter has Down's syndrome, congenital heart disease, and failure to thrive. Dr. H. is also providing routine pediatric care for the woman's 4-year-old son. The daughter's cardiologist wants to see her biweekly to monitor her growth. The mother is finding it difficult to keep these multiple appointments and asks Dr. H.'s advice regarding how to better coordinate her family's care.

SITUATIONS REQUIRING NEGOTIATION

Case 11-4 illustrates a family requiring access into the healthcare system for multiple conditions. Each family member has particular needs that cannot be delayed indefinitely without undesirable consequences. The first step is to determine the specific medical and healthcare needs of individual family members and who can adequately provide that care. This assessment includes determining where the family is currently receiving care. The mother can receive maternity care from a family physician, an obstetrician, or a nurse midwife. The 4-year-old can receive well-child care from a family physician, a pediatrician, a nurse practitioner, or a physician's assistant. The 2-year-old has several problems requiring the input of a pediatric cardiologist as well as the primary care clinician.

Established clinician–patient and clinician–family relationships must be considered when problem solving. One clear goal is the necessity for ensuring regular care-seeking because of the nature of the conditions being followed. Clinician–patient relationships and arrangement of appointments must support and encourage the understanding of and compliance with support and encourage the understanding of and compliance with recommended therapies. The fewer the number of providers prescribing medications and treatments minimizes the possibility of misunderstanding and confusion. Furthermore, the patient has one person with whom questions regarding therapy can be clarified.

When there is more than one serious condition present, there may be more than one healthcare provider, most of whom are strong-willed, vying for control of the patient's care. Providers are challenged to negotiate among themselves regarding who maintains the primary liaison between nurses, therapists, or even family members about specific problems. The fewer people talking with the family, the less potential for confusion exists. However, this necessitates forethought among clinicians, including planning, collaboration regarding results, and the negotiation of agreement regarding the plan or changes to a previous plan.

One of the greatest challenges in this situation is the challenge of the egos of the clinicians involved. The primary care provider has often been involved the longest with the family and likely will be involved for the longest period following the acute crisis or hospitalization. By virtue of the scope of clinician expertise and length of the relationship, the clinician may be better able to recognize medical issues or social needs of the family. In contrast, if the patient needs to be hospitalized, the consultant may be better able to provide specialized care for the patient and expects to be in charge. How does the primary care provider retain a place at the negotiating table in order to provide valuable input into the case?

At this point, negotiation between healthcare providers becomes crucial. The first, and arguably the most important, step is for the primary care clinician to be present and available as part of the acute care team. The clinician should make frequent visits to the hospitalized patient and receive updates from consultants, patients, and nursing staff. He will often make the first step in introducing himself to the consultant and establishing his desired level of involvement. Second, there should be an understanding between the patient, family, and primary care clinician that the clinician wishes to remain involved with the patient's care during the crisis and continues to serve as the patient's primary advocate. If the patient and family have questions or clarifications regarding information received from the inpatient team, or merely want a second opinion from a professional who knows them better, they are likely to approach their primary care clinician. Third, the primary care provider should be available and integral to any search for additional consultants or for discharge planning. By adopting this approach, the primary care provider will retain that role, provide the maximal support for the patient, and improve the overall quality and continuity of care.

Once a family member requires inpatient admission, the stage and the players change for them as well. Outpatient providers may not be the admitting clinicians. Therapies that were the patient's responsibility in the outpatient setting often automatically become the responsibility of inpatient clinicians, many times without clarifying with the patient what changes are being made. Roles and responsibilities, therefore, shift on admission and again on discharge from the hospital. If hospitalization occurs for a condition resulting in a disability, outpatient self-care and rehabilitation must now be arranged. Tasks that were cheerfully performed for the patient while in the hospital suddenly become the responsibility of the patient or the family at home (Doyle & Stern, 1992; Roberts & Krouse, 1990). Furthermore, when the family in question is also poor, or from a traditionally underserved community, questions arise as to ease of access for referrals and affordability of certain therapies. In addition, the underserved or disenfranchised are often easily intimidated by large institutions or limited by language barriers and thus may be inhibited from follow-up.

Negotiation with other clinicians is most important when done on behalf of a child. Who is a part of the discussion and who makes decisions depend on the age and mental competence of the child, the presence of relatives, and the understanding, ability, or willingness of the family to make decisions. There must be agreement between family and clinicians regarding who is the primary spokesperson for the child and the frequency of communication to update them on progress and the therapeutic plan.

The primary care clinician in Case 11-4 may suggest to the cardiologist that they alternate the biweekly evaluation for failure to thrive so that one visit can be combined with one of the mother's prenatal care appointments. Then, by frequent phone communication and sharing of medical records, both primary care clinician and consultant can keep abreast of the 2-year-old's problems while decreasing the appointment time required of the mother.

CASE 11-5

Mrs. K. seeks prenatal care from Dr. P. in the middle of the second trimester. She notes her reluctance to come earlier because she has been pregnant before, had an arduous labor, and eventually required a cesarean section, and feels that physicians do not listen to patients as they should. During the next 3 months Mrs. K. misses several appointments completely and is more than an hour late for the others. At 38 weeks' gestation, during a regular prenatal visit, Mrs. K. announces that she will not allow Dr. P., or anyone else, to do a pelvic examination on her in the clinic. She does not see the need for such an examination until labor begins and does not want to be a guinea pig on whom clinicians can practice.

--------- **PROBLEM SOLVING** ---------

IMPROVING COMMUNICATION SKILLS

As noted at the beginning of this chapter, the quality of communication directly affects the success of each clinician–patient interaction. Careful attention to asking open-ended questions, maintaining good listening skills, allowing time for discussion, and recognizing clues that indicate additional areas for evaluation promote good communication. Only when efforts to expand and improve communication have failed is it necessary to consider negotiation.

Mrs. K. obviously has some major concerns that are impacting on the level and extent of care she is willing to accept. Dr. P. must augment the questions used at the standard prenatal visit to explore Mrs. K.'s unwillingness to be examined. Questions such as "Do you understand the type of information that can be obtained from a third-trimester pelvic examination? Is there something in particular that frightens you about the examination? Did you have a previous negative experience during a similar examination?" can open the door for Mrs. K. to reveal her fears. She may disclose events that indicate previous or current abuse or a negative interaction in this clinic or with a previous provider. She may choose to have someone with her to provide support during the examination—spouse, mother, or friend. Only by opening the door for increased communication will the clinician be able to determine whether there is agreement on the need to negotiate.

DEVELOPING NEGOTIATION SKILLS

In order to develop the skills of effective negotiation, one must understand that negotiations require that two or more parties come together, with all parties wanting something. Therefore, the first step in the process is identifying the needs of each party. The more basic the need, the more likely the party will be willing to negotiate. How successful the negotiation is becomes a function of whether the issue really is negotiable, whether the parties involved are willing to give and take, and if there is some trust between the parties. If meeting the patient's needs is not the preeminent goal, the clinician must reflect on her motivation or lack thereof with regards to the patient. Alternatively, the clinician may feel that the patient has a hidden agenda that must be elicited in order to establish an ethical, honest relationship.

Certain skills are necessary to negotiate effectively. Kelly has defined these skills as technical, human, and conceptual (Kelly in Glanville & Tiller, 1990). The technical skills are speaking, writing, listening, and demonstrating. These skills are integral to the tactics used to assist parties in arriving at mutually agreeable settlements. Human skills, according to Kelly, include empathy, building of trust, interviewing, communicating, sensing, and anticipating. Empathy is crucial to the understanding of the physician–patient relationship (Brock & Salinsky, 1993). Mastery of empathetic skills can be difficult, but often improves with training. Keen conceptual skills allow the negotiator to help gather and interpret information to shape strategies (Kelly in Glanville & Tiller, 1990).

ADEQUATE PREPARATION FOR NEGOTIATION

The patient and the clinician begin a relationship from a different perspective and, thus, approach problem solving differently. The first step in preparing to negotiate is to use the technical skills described earlier to gather as much pertinent information as possible. The clinician seeks details regarding the patient's illness, family values and dynamics, current occupation and how they and their families have been affected by the illness, particular avocations that have been affected, and what the patient's expectations of the interaction with the clinician are. Likewise, the patient must seek information. The patient should ascertain the clinician's expertise and comfort level with the illness, the level of involvement desired by the clinician, and the threshold for referral.

The second step involves the human skills described by Kelly and is identification of questions and concerns of the patient and the family. When the concerns are not verbalized, misunderstandings are common. The patient or the family may not appear satisfied, but want to be asked before revealing the etiology of their dissatisfaction. These concerns may not be revealed unless there is an atmosphere of empathy, trust, like values, and caring.

The third step involves the conceptual skills noted earlier and is an open discussion of the clinician's recommendations and any other options that may be suggested by family and friends. This step requires frequent pauses to clarify details of the recommendations and consistent encouragement to discuss all concerns. Hopefully, this discussion will lead to an understanding of the problems and issues that have been under discussion so that strategies may be defined for resolution in a win–win fashion.

REALITY NEGOTIATION

When a patient has experienced a physical loss accompanied by loss of hope, depression, or the onset of disability, the discussion that ensues has been termed *reality negotiation*. In reality negotiation, the patient is called on to judge the accuracy and importance of information gathered from the environment (Ersek, 1992). When a patient has experienced a major illness, such as a cerebrovascular accident or a devastating accident, and becomes disabled, the clinician or therapist working most closely with the patient must assess where the patient is in terms of understanding the new limitation (the patient's view) and begin working from that point. Early assessment of the patient's view includes a determination of the patient's strengths and supports. Does the patient rely heavily on religious faith, personal fortitude, spouse, family, or friends for strength?

When a patient's recognition of limitations or disabilities is substantially different from that of the therapist, reality negotiation is crucial. The clinician must respect the patient's vision for the future without undermining expectations of the patient's capabilities in order to construct a reasonable rehabilitation regimen. The honesty and accuracy of the plan become crucial not only to how the patient approaches the necessary rehabilitative tasks, but also to how the clinician interacts with the patient, immediate family members, and loved ones.

When the healthcare provider is a majority individual and represents a majority institution providing care for a patient from a different culture, special skills and understanding are required to maximize the effectiveness of communication. Patients are a product of their own culture. What is often forgotten is that the same is true for healthcare providers. When the backgrounds of provider and patient are significantly different, conflict is a distinct possibility and the ability to negotiate is hampered. If the clinician recognizes and values these differences, she can allow extra time for discussion and clarification. Conflict should not be a given, but anticipated and avoided when possible.

It may be necessary with such patients to begin discussion of any problem with a description of the relevant points of the case from a medical perspective in simple, direct terms, understandable to the patient. The practitioner should then query the patient regarding his belief system and how it interfaces with biomedicine. In negotiating treatment options with patients, practitioners should generally seek to preserve helpful beliefs and practices, accommodate patient beliefs that are neither helpful nor harmful from the viewpoint of Western medicine, and repattern harmful beliefs or practices.

Many of the beliefs and practices of non-Western systems have proven to be efficacious when studied by Western medicine, e.g., acupuncture. Medications commonly used today, such as digoxin and quinine, were originally herbal medicines used by traditional healers (Jackson, 1993). Although the process of eliciting traditional health beliefs and negotiating treatment plans is time-consuming and sometimes difficult, practitioners must be open-minded, flexible, creative, and persistent. The results can justify the time and energy expended because fewer patients are likely to be dissatisfied and drop out of care if their beliefs are taken into account. Only by knowing about these other providers or beliefs can the primary care clinician be aware of the patient's condition, can she anticipate potential interactions, or be able to negotiate compliance with patient and alternative provider.

Vander Zanden (1983) identified four common patterns of minority reactions to those who are perceived as controlling resources: acceptance, aggression, avoidance, and assimilation. These patterns have usually been described in populations traditionally considered minority, but can also be observed in those who are economically disadvantaged or medically underserved. The acceptance pattern is often observed in the attitudes of blacks in the rural southern United States (Vander Zanden, 1983). This was a common pattern of survival for blacks during slavery and can still be observed today. An aggressive pattern is one in which the minority-group member strikes out by engaging in hostile acts against those in control. For example, blacks have been socialized to hide the hostilities that are common reactions to frustration, but if levels of frustration rise too high, the acceptance pattern is superseded and violence can result (Vander Zanden, 1983). With avoidance, minority-group members may try to escape from situations where they might experience prejudice and discrimination. This type of response often prevents the disadvantaged from seeking assistance. Finally, with assimilation, minority-group members may attempt to become socially and culturally fused within the dominant group. U.S. blacks have experienced greater problems with assimilation than other minority groups (Glanville & Tiller, 1990).

Vander Zanden's model only describes the patient perspective, however. As mentioned above, the background and environment of the clinician also impact on the interaction and can affect the negotiation process. The problems that arise from focusing on the patient perspective only are graphically illustrated by Swartz in a description of the political organization of health and mental health care in South Africa (Swartz, 1991). Although the maldistribution of resources by race is well known, little attention has been given to the impact of the negotiation of power in the clinical setting. Swartz focuses on interactions in ward rounds on the "Black side" of a South African psychiatric hospital.

CASE 11-6

A white clinician in South Africa interviewed a black female patient who speaks good English:

CLINICIAN: *You have bad dreams.*
PATIENT: *I do not have dreams.*
CLINICIAN: *You are troubled by your bad dreams.*
PATIENT: *I do not have bad dreams.*
CLINICIAN: *You have bad dreams about your son.*
PATIENT: *(Quickly and apparently angrily) I do not have any dreams.*

[After the patient left, the clinician shrugged and stated that the patient's quick denial that she was having bad dreams confirmed that she was indeed having such dreams (Swartz, 1991).]

In Case 11-6, the brevity of the interaction, the structure of the communication in that the clinician is making statements rather than querying the patient, and the clinician's predilection for making a judgment without gathering additional information indicate his reliance on preconceived concepts of disease, devaluing her input rather than exploring the reasons why the patient presented and her view of illness. The propensity of individual clinicians to reproduce aspects of apartheid practice in their individual patient interactions directly impacts on the atmosphere of the clinical encounter, what is heard during the history taking, what diagnosis is chosen, and how therapy is prescribed.

Cross-cultural encounters between healthcare providers and patients are now routine. They pose dilemmas for all aspects of clinical interactions. When describing the effect of these interactions on consultations involving ethical issues, Orr notes four elements that are essential for successful resolution of problems: (1) communicate effectively, allowing more time, and not making assumptions, (2) learn and understand cultural differences, (3) identify the cross-cultural conflicts, and (4) compromise through showing respect for beliefs that differ from yours (Orr *et al.*, 1995). A mnemonic that has been developed to assist clinicians in multicultural interactions is LEARN (Berlin & Fowkes, 1983):

Listen with sympathy and understanding
Explain your perceptions
Acknowledge differences
Recommend treatment
Negotiate agreement

CONCLUSION

As healthcare continues a transition from an "illness focus" to a "wellness focus," the challenge becomes how to modify old methods of clinician–patient interactions. The paternalistic approach of the biomedical model is changing. Rather than the emphasis being on maintaining as much control as possible over patients, it has become clear that therapies must be more patient centered. When the overcontrolling approach to psychiatric care was evaluated, it was found to be linked to increased violence, prolonged hospitalization, and increased use of resources (Johnson & Morrison, 1993). Rather than controlling our patients, the clinician's goal should be to maximize communication and support patient involvement in decision-making. When problems arise, negotiation should be considered as an option whenever possible. This paradigm shift must be modeled by the healthcare leadership in order for it to be incorporated into everyday practice.

Thus, successful clinician–patient encounters depend on clear and sensitive communication between all parties involved, often including family and friends. Only when the goals of clinician and patient seem at odds or are not understood is negotiation considered. The negotiation style selected by the clinician will affect the time needed to complete the process, the status of the relationship between the parties involved at the end of the process, and prospects for success. Attention to cultural influences on the presenting complaint and the clinician–patient interaction is a given and should be explored.

CASES FOR DISCUSSION

CASE 1

A 26-year-old G2P1 at 20 weeks' gestation presents for her first prenatal visit, wants you to take care of her, but insists on using herbal preparations provided by her grandmother rather than prenatal vitamins and iron, and doesn't want an IV or monitoring during labor.

1. *What is the first step in negotiating the patient's preferences in this case?*
2. *Should you invite the grandmother to prenatal visits and during labor if during your initial discussions you learn that the grandmother is the one who feels strongly about the daughter's choices?*
3. *Is it important to know what the grandmother thinks of the principles of Western medicine and your practice?*
4. *Who are the other significant people in the patient's life? How involved are they in her care?*

CASE 2

A 19-year-old college student is financing his education on a track scholarship, has been training for the Boston Marathon, and presents with a tibial stress fracture. He doesn't want to stop training.

1. *What is the student's purpose in desiring to run the Boston Marathon? Is he doing it to please his buddies, someone else, or himself?*

2. *Does he realize the complications of stress fractures that can arise if he continues to train?*
3. *What other options for financing his college education does he have if he is unable to fulfill the requirements of his athletic scholarship?*

CASE 3

An 11-year-old boy complaining of right lower quadrant pain, fever, and anorexia is brought to your office by his parents. You are concerned that he may have an acute appendicitis and inform his parents of the need for exploratory surgery. They prefer to take him home and pray about his condition.

1. *What is the parents' understanding of the nature of appendicitis?*
2. *What is the parents' understanding of the risks of laparotomy versus observation?*
3. *Are the parents willing to pray at the hospital while the child is being observed rather than taking him away?*

CASE 4

A 55-year-old podiatrist presents with transient ischemic attacks and is found to be in atrial fibrillation of unknown duration. Anticoagulant therapy is recommended, but the patient prefers naturopathic therapy.

1. *Why doesn't the patient want to take the anticoagulant?*
2. *What is the nature of the alternative therapy the patient prefers?*
3. *Does the patient understand the natural history of atrial fibrillation when anticoagulation is not used?*
4. *Would a second opinion be persuasive for the patient?*

CASE 5

A 70-year-old woman has been under the care of Dr. S. for several years, being seen primarily for annual examinations and refills of verapamil and digoxin to maintain control of supraventricular tachycardia. She presents acutely for evaluation of a cough without associated pain. The evaluation reveals a renal cell carcinoma metastatic to the liver and lungs. The oncology consultant finds the patient ineligible for all of the open chemotherapy protocols to treat this cancer. The family seeks evaluation at a national center that presents a treatment that offers a 10% chance of tumor regression. The family is leaning strongly toward this therapy and seeks your advice.

1. *What are the patient's immediate and short-term expectations?*
2. *What do the patient and family understand regarding tumor regression?*
3. *Have the patient and family asked about and understand the side effects of the therapy?*
4. *What are the patient's fears? the family's fears?*

RECOMMENDED READINGS

Brody H: *The Healer's Power.* New Haven, CT, Yale University Press, 1992.

> The author, a physician with a doctorate in philosophy, examines the physician's stance on authority with regard to patient rights. The book is organized into three areas: medical ethics, physician–patient relations, and power.

Fisher R, Ury W, Patton B: *Getting to Yes: Negotiating Agreement Without Giving In,* ed 2. New York, Penguin Books, 1991.

Negotiation takes place on a daily basis, but is not always easy or done well. This book is about the method of principled negotiation. The first chapter describes problems that arise in using the standard strategies of positional bargaining. The next four chapters lay out the four principles of the method. The last three chapters answer the questions most commonly asked about the method: What if the other side is more powerful? What if they will not play along? And what if they use dirty tricks?

Helman CG: *Culture, Health, and Illness: An Introduction for Health Professionals.* London, Butterworth–Heinemann Ltd, 1994.

This book provides an overview of culture to health and illness—spanning the self-contained "specialities" of cross-cultural psychiatry, nutritional anthropology, AIDS research, and international health aid. A range of case histories from different parts of the world are used to illustrate some of the major global health problems now faced and the pressing need for primary healthcare in many poorer countries.

Johnson RA: *Negotiation Basics: Concepts, Skills, and Exercises.* Beverly Hills, CA, Sage Publications Inc, 1993.

This book is designed to demonstrate how negotiation works, to outline options and procedures for negotiation preparation, to identify the common negotiating problems and deficiencies, and to show how skill building can be integrated into preparation for negotiation. In an effort to help students learn and experience negotiations from both a theoretical and a practical perspective, each chapter explores and discusses a major negotiation concept; the concept is then linked to a related skill necessary for negotiating success. Broad guidelines for applying the skills and concepts are integrated into the text. Then exercises drawn from everyday negotiating problems are furnished to simulate the experiences related to the topic.

Kleinman A: *Patients and Healers in the Context of Culture.* Berkeley, University of California Press, 1980.

This book presents a theoretical framework for studying the relationship between medicine, psychiatry, and culture. It discusses the critical role of social science (especially anthropology and cross-cultural studies) in clinical medicine and psychiatry and encourages study of clinical problems by anthropologists and other investigators involved in cross-cultural research. The approach is interdisciplinary and includes ideas, methods, problem-frames, and solution-frames from social science and clinical science.

Vander Zanden JW: *American Minority Relations,* ed 4. New York, Alfred A Knopf Inc, 1983.

This book presents a sociological approach to our current minority groups and distinguishing features of who they are and how they interact with other community members. Definitions and descriptions of terms such as *prejudice, stereotypes,* and *discrimination* are discussed.

CHAPTER 12

Managing Chronic Illness

John S. Rolland

CASE 12-1

Janice, a married woman in her 30s with two small children, received the most up-to-date medical treatment and expert surgical interventions during her 4-year bout with cancer. Six months after her physician pronounced her cured, Janice and her husband Sam separated. A prolonged emotional and financially draining divorce and custody battle ensued. Sam drank heavily and became verbally abusive. Both children developed behavioral problems at home and at school that required crisis intervention, bringing this disintegrating family to treatment for the first time.

———————— EDUCATIONAL OBJECTIVES ————————

1. Describe a comprehensive family systems model for assessment and clinical intervention with families facing chronic illness and disability
2. Describe the psychosocial demands of illness based on the pattern of: onset, course, outcome, incapacitation, and level of uncertainty
3. Describe the crisis, chronic, and terminal phases of illness, the transitions between phases, and the psychosocial developmental tasks associated with each phase
4. Discuss the interface of illness, individual, and family life cycles; multigenerational legacies of illness and loss; and how these relate to coping and adaptation to chronic illness
5. Describe how health belief systems will affect a patient's or family's response to illness

—————— **INTRODUCTION** ——————

This chapter provides a family systems-oriented model for patients with chronic and life-threatening illness and disability. At the heart of systems thinking is the focus on *interaction*. With physical disorders, particularly chronic disease, the focus is the interaction of a disease with an individual, family, and other biopsychosocial systems (Engel, 1977, 1980). The Family Systems–Illness Model presented in this chapter places the family as its central reference point (Rolland, 1994). This choice is made with the recognition that the family is a system influenced heavily by a range of social, economic, institutional, and political forces in the larger environment.

This chapter presents this clinical model to provide a pragmatic way of thinking about family coping and adaptation to chronic conditions. This discussion will highlight the interactive processes between the psychosocial demands of different chronic disorders over time and key components of family functioning. Beginning with the expected psychosocial demands of a disorder through its various phases, this chapter will cover family systems dynamics that emphasize: (1) multigenerational patterns, (2) family and individual life cycles, (3) family belief systems (including those associated with culture, ethnicity, and gender), and (4) family factors that facilitate or impede the relationships between patient, family, and health professionals (Rolland, 1984, 1987a,b, 1990, 1994). Figure 12.1 depicts one useful way to represent the interface between illness and family.

CASE 12-2

Dan and Kathy are a young dual-career couple with two children, aged 3 and 1, living in a large metropolitan area. Kathy had a 2-week history of intermittent double vision, fatigue, and mild numbness and a "heavy feeling" in both legs.

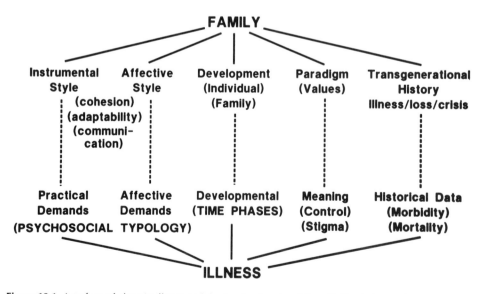

Figure 12.1. Interface of chronic illness and the family. Reprinted from Rolland JS: Family systems and chronic illness: A typological model. *J Psychother Fam* 3(3):143–168, 1987.

With persistent symptoms, her internist referred her to a neurologist, who after a quick workup informed the couple that Kathy has multiple sclerosis. Her symptoms respond well to a brief course of steroids. The neurologist has explained the treatment approach to her disease, informed her that the disease is very unpredictable, describing the range of possible complications, and instructed her to contact him immediately if symptoms return.

Dan, Kathy, and their extended families are terrified. Kathy wonders if her illness will destroy her budding career as a real estate broker, while Dan feels maybe he should take a second job to ensure an adequate income for the family. The couple wonders whether they should cancel their plans to have more children and move out of their recently purchased first home, a three-story old Victorian. Kathy feels insecure about her ability to be an adequate mother if her condition worsens. Her parents feel the couple should move back to their small hometown to be close to their large extended families. Neither Dan nor Kathy has ever lived with a chronic disorder and their parents are in good health. To them, the psychosocial implications of multiple sclerosis are akin to being suddenly transported to a foreign country and living under a permanent, amorphous, and unpredictable "dark cloud."

PSYCHOSOCIAL TYPOLOGY AND TIME PHASES OF ILLNESS

In order to think in a truly interactive or systemic manner about the interface of the illness and the individual or the illness and the family, one needs a way of describing illness itself in systems terms and a schema that recasts the myriad of biological diseases in psychosocial terms over time. Such a schema must simultaneously remain relevant to the interactions between the psychosocial and biological worlds and provide a common language that transforms or reclassifies our usual medical terminology.

There have been two major impediments to progress in this area. First, insufficient attention has been given to the areas of diversity and commonality inherent in different chronic disorders. Second, there has been a glossing over of the qualitative and quantitative differences regarding how various diseases are manifest over the course of an illness. Chronic conditions need to be conceptualized in a manner that organizes these similarities and differences over the disease course so that the type and degree of demands relevant to clinical practice are highlighted in a more useful way.

The psychosocial importance of different time phases of an illness is not well understood. Clinicians often become involved in the care of an individual or family coping with a chronic illness at different points in the "illness life cycle." Understanding the evolution of a long-term illness is hindered because clinicians rarely follow the family through the complete life history of a disease.

Only a few clinical studies have addressed the importance of broad time phases of illness. One example has been studies that examine the adaptive versus harmful role of denial, loosely defined as one's attempts to negate the existence of a problem, at different points of the disease course. For parents of a child with leukemia, denial may enable them adaptively to perform necessary duties during earlier phases of the illness, but might lead to devastating consequences for the family if maintained during the terminal phase.

Likewise, denial may be functional for recovery on a coronary care unit after a myocardial infarction, but harmful if this translates into ignoring medical advice vis-à-vis diet, exercise, and work stress over the long term.

The problems of illness variability and time phases are addressed on two separate dimensions: (1) Chronic illnesses are grouped according to key biological similarities and differences that dictate significantly distinct psychosocial demands for the ill individual and her family, and (2) the prime developmental time phases in the natural evolution of chronic disease are identified.

PSYCHOSOCIAL TYPOLOGY

The goal of the psychosocial typology presented here is to create clinically meaningful and useful categories with similar psychosocial demands for a wide array of chronic disorders across the entire life span; it is not intended for traditional medical treatment or prognostic purposes, but for examining the relationship between family or individual dynamics and chronic disease. This typology conceptualizes broad distinctions of the pattern of (1) onset, (2) course, (3) outcome, (4) type and degree of incapacitation, and (5) degree of uncertainty. These categories are hypothesized to be the most psychosocially significant for a wide range of illnesses and disabilities. Although each variable is actually a continuum, it will be described here in a categorical manner by the selection of key anchor points along the continuum.

Onset

Illnesses can divided into those that have either an acute onset, such as strokes, or a gradual onset, such as Parkinson's disease. Although the total amount of family adaptation might be the same for both types of illness, for acute-onset illnesses these affective and practical changes are compressed into a short time, requiring of the family more rapid mobilization of crisis management skills. Families able to tolerate highly charged affective states, exchange clearly defined roles flexibly, problem-solve efficiently, and utilize outside resources will have an advantage in managing acute-onset illnesses. The rate of family change required to cope with gradual-onset diseases allows for a more protracted period of adjustment.

Course

The course of chronic diseases can take three general forms: progressive, constant, or relapsing/episodic. A *progressive* disease (e.g., Alzheimer's disease, emphysema) is one that is continually or generally symptomatic and progresses in severity. The individual and family are faced with the effects of a perpetually symptomatic family member, where disability increases in a stepwise or progressive fashion. This means that a family must live with the prospect of continual role change and adaptation as the disease progresses. Periods of relief from the demands of the illness tend to be minimal. Increasing strain on family caretakers is caused by both exhaustion and the continual addition of new caretaking tasks over time.

A *constant*-course illness is one where, typically, an initial event occurs after which the biological course stabilizes. A single-episode myocardial infarction or spinal cord injury are two examples. Typically, after an initial period of recovery, the chronic phase is characterized by some clear-cut deficit or residual functional limitation. Recurrences can occur, but the individual or family is faced with a semipermanent change that is stable and predictable over a considerable time span. The potential for family exhaustion exists without the strain of new role demands over time.

A *relapsing* or *episodic* course in illnesses like ulcerative colitis and asthma is distinguished by the alternation of stable periods of varying length, characterized by a low level or absence of symptoms, with periods of flare-up or exacerbation. Strain on the family system is caused by both the frequency of transitions between crisis and noncrisis and the ongoing uncertainty of *when* a recurrence will occur. This requires a family flexibility for alternation between two forms of family organization. Also, the wide psychological discrepancy between periods of normalcy versus illness is a particularly taxing feature unique to relapsing diseases.

Outcome

The extent to which a chronic illness is a likely cause of death and the degree to which it can shorten one's life span are critical features with profound psychosocial impact. The most crucial factor is the *initial expectation* of whether a disease is a likely cause of death. On one end of the continuum are illnesses that do not typically affect the life span, such as lumbosacral disk disease or arthritis. At the other extreme are illnesses that are clearly progressive and usually fatal, such as metastatic cancer or AIDS. There is also an intermediate more unpredictable category, including both illnesses that shorten the life span such as cardiovascular disease, and those with the possibility of sudden death, such as hemophilia. Perhaps the major difference between these kinds of outcomes is the degree to which the family experiences anticipatory grief and its pervasive effects on family life.

When loss is less imminent or certain an outcome, illnesses that may shorten life or cause sudden death provide a fertile ground for idiosyncratic family interpretations (Rolland, 1990). The "it could happen" nature of these illnesses creates a nidus for both overprotection by the family and powerful secondary gains for the ill member. This is particularly relevant to childhood illnesses such as hemophilia, juvenile-onset diabetes mellitus, and asthma (Herz 1989; Minuchin *et al.*, 1975, 1978).

Incapacitation

Incapacitation can result from impairment of cognition (e.g., Alzheimer's disease), sensation (e.g., blindness), movement (e.g., stroke with paralysis, multiple sclerosis), energy production (e.g., cardiovascular disease), and disfiguring diseases (e.g., severe burns) associated with social stigma (e.g., AIDS).

The extent, kind, and timing of incapacitation imply sharp differences in the degree of stress facing a family. For instance, the combined cognitive and motor deficits of a person with a stroke necessitate greater family role reallocation than a spinal cord-injured person who retains his cognitive abilities. For some illnesses, like stroke, incapacitation is often worst at the time of onset and would magnify family coping issues related to onset, expected course, and outcome. For progressive diseases, like Alzheimer's disease, disability looms as an increasing problem in later phases of the illness, allowing a family more time to prepare for anticipated changes. It provides an opportunity for the ill member to participate in disease-related family planning.

By combining the kinds of onset, course, outcome, and incapacitation into a grid format we generate a typology with 32 potential psychosocial types of illness. This grid is shown in Table 12.1.

Table 12.1
Categorization of Chronic Illnesses by Psychosocial Type[a]

	Incapacitating[b]		Nonincapacitating[b]	
	Acute	Gradual	Acute	Gradual
Fatal				
Progressive		Lung cancer with CNS metastases AIDS Bone marrow failure Amyotrophic lateral sclerosis	Acute leukemia Pancreatic cancer Metastatic breast cancer Lung cancer Liver cancer Incurable cancers in remission	Cystic fibrosis*
Relapsing				
Shortened life span, possibly fatal				
Progressive		Emphysema Alzheimer's disease Multi-infarct dementia Multiple sclerosis (late) Chronic alcoholism Huntington's chorea Scleroderma		Juvenile diabetes* Malignant hypertension Insulin-dependent adult-onset diabetes

Course				
Relapsing	Angina	Early multiple sclerosis; Episodic alcoholism; PKU and other congenital errors of metabolism	Sickle-cell disease*; Hemophilia; Mild myocardial infarction; Cardiac arrhythmia	Systemic lupus erythematosus*; Hemodialysis-treated renal failure; Hodgkin's disease
Constant	Stroke; Moderate/severe myocardial infarction			Non-insulin-dependent adult-onset diabetes
Nonfatal — Progressive		Parkinson's disease; Rheumatoid arthritis; Osteoarthritis		
Nonfatal — Relapsing	Lumbosacral disk disorder		Kidney stones; Gout; Migraine; Seasonal allergy; Asthma; Epilepsy	Peptic ulcer; Ulcerative colitis; Chronic bronchitis; Irritable bowel syndrome; Psoriasis
Nonfatal — Constant	Congenital malformations; Spinal cord injury; Acute blindness; Acute deafness; Survived severe trauma and burns; Posthypoxic syndrome	Nonprogressive mental retardation; Cerebral palsy	Benign arrhythmia; Congenital heart disease	Malabsorption syndromes; Hyper-/hypothyroidism; Pernicious anemia; Controlled hypertension; Controlled glaucoma

[a]Modified from Rolland JS: Toward a psychosocial typology of chronic and life-threatening illness. *Fam Sys Med* 2:245–263, 1984 Reprinted with permission of Family Process Inc.

[b]Asterisks indicate early.

Uncertainty

The predictability of an illness and the degree of uncertainty about the specific way or rate at which it unfolds overlay and color the other attributes: onset, course, outcome, and incapacitation. For illness with highly unpredictable courses, such as multiple sclerosis, family coping and adaptation, especially future planning, are hindered by anticipatory anxiety and ambiguity about what they will actually have to deal with. Families unable to put long-term uncertainty into perspective are at high risk for exhaustion and dysfunction.

The complexity, frequency, and efficacy of a treatment regimen, the amount of home- versus hospital-based care required because of the disease, and the frequency and intensity of symptoms vary widely across illnesses, with important implications for individual and family adaptation. Some regimens require significant financial resources and caregiving time and energy (e.g., home kidney dialysis, cystic fibrosis). Treatments least likely to be adhered to are those that have a high impact on life-styles, are difficult to accomplish, and have minimal effects on the level of symptoms or prognosis (Strauss, 1975). Although they reduce time-consuming dependence on medical centers, home-based treatments place heavier responsibility on patient and family. Therefore, the degree of family emotional support, role flexibility, effective problem solving, and communication in relation to these treatment factors will be crucial predictors of long-term treatment compliance.

It is important to consider the likelihood and severity of disease-related crises and associated family anxiety (Strauss, 1975). A clinician should assess the family's understanding about the possibility, frequency, and lethality of a medical crisis. How congruent is the family's understanding with that of the medical team? Are their expectations catastrophic or do they minimize real dangers? Are there clear warning signs that the patient or family can recognize? Can a medical crisis be prevented or mitigated by detection of early warning signs or institution of prompt treatment? When a patient or family heed the early warning signs of a diabetes insulin reaction or asthma attack, a full-blown crisis can usually be averted. How complex are the rescue operations? Do they require simple measures carried out at home (e.g., medication, bed rest) or do they necessitate outside assistance or hospitalization? How long can crises last before a family can resume "day to day" functioning? It is essential to ask a family about its planning for such crises and the extent and accuracy of their medical knowledge. How clearly has leadership, role reallocation, emotional support, and use of resources outside the family been formulated? If an illness began with an acute crisis (e.g., stroke), then assessment of that event provides useful information as to how that family handles *unexpected* crises. Evaluating the overall viability of the family's crisis planning is crucial.

TIME PHASES OF ILLNESS

In this psychosocial schema of chronic diseases, the developmental time phases of illness are a second dimension. The concept of time phases provides a way for the clinician to think longitudinally and to reach a fuller understanding of chronic illness as an ongoing process with landmarks, transitions, and changing demands. Each phase has its own unique psychosocial developmental tasks that require significantly different strengths, attitudes, or changes from a family. To capture the core psychosocial themes in the natural history of chronic disease, three major phases can be described: (1) crisis, (2) chronic, and (3) terminal. The relationship between a more detailed chronic disease time line and one grouped into broad time phases is diagrammed in Figure 12.2.

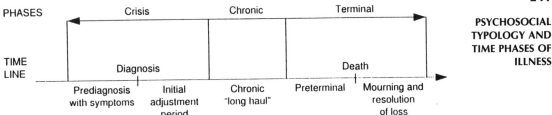

Figure 12.2. Time line and phases of illness. Reprinted from Rolland JS: Toward a psychosocial typology of chronic and life-threatening illness. *Fam Systems Medicine* 2:245–262, 1984.

The Crisis Phase

The crisis phase includes any symptomatic period before diagnosis and the initial period of readjustment and coping after the problem has been clarified through a diagnosis and initial treatment plan. This period holds a number of key tasks for the ill member and family. Moos (1984) describes certain universal practical illness-related tasks, including: (1) learning to deal with pain, incapacitation, or other illness-related symptoms, (2) learning to deal with the hospital environment and any disease-related treatment procedures, and (3) establishing and maintaining workable relationships with the healthcare team. In addition, there are critical tasks of a more general, sometimes existential nature. The family needs to: (1) create a meaning for the illness event that maximizes a preservation of a sense of mastery and competency, (2) grieve for the loss of the preillness family identity, (3) gradually accept the illness as permanent while maintaining a sense of continuity between their past and future, (4) pull together to undergo short-term crisis reorganization, and (5) in the face of uncertainty, develop a system flexibility toward future goals.

During this initial crisis period, providers have enormous influence over a family's sense of competence and the methods devised to accomplish these developmental tasks. The initial meetings and advice given by providers at the time of diagnosis can be thought of as a "framing event." Because families are so vulnerable at this point, clinicians need to be extremely sensitive in their interactions with family members. Who is included or excluded (e.g., patient) from a discussion can be interpreted by the family as a message of how a family should plan their communication for the duration of the illness. One family, accustomed to open, frank discussion, described how the physician came to the mother's hospital room and took the family members to a separate room to inform them that the mother had cancer and discuss the diagnosis. At this vulnerable moment, the family felt that they were being instructed implicitly to exclude the mother in any discussion of her cancer. Providers who in some fashion blame the patient, a family member, or the whole family for an illness (e.g., delay in seeking an appointment, negligence by parents, poor health habits) or distance themselves from a family may undercut a family's attempt to sustain a sense of competence.

The Chronic Phase

The chronic phase, whether long or short, is the time span between the initial diagnosis and readjustment period and the third phase when issues of death and terminal illness predominate. This era can be marked by constancy, progression, or episodic change. Thus, its meaning cannot be grasped by simply knowing the biological behavior of an illness. Rather, it has been referred to as "the long haul," or "day-to-day living with chronic illness" phase. Often the individual and family have come to grips psychologically or organizationally with the permanent changes presented by a chronic illness and have devised an ongoing modus operandi. The ability of the family to maintain the semblance of a normal life under the "abnormal" presence of a chronic illness and heightened uncertainty is a key task of this period. If the illness is fatal, this is a time of "living in limbo." For certain highly debilitating but not clearly fatal illnesses, such as a massive stroke or dementia, the family can become saddled with an exhausting problem "without end." Paradoxically, a family's hope to resume a "normal" life cycle might only be realized after the death of their ill member. This highlights another crucial task of this phase: the maintenance of maximal autonomy for *all* family members.

For long-term disorders, customary patterns of intimacy for couples become skewed by discrepancies between the ill member and well spouse/caregiver. Emotions often remain underground and contribute to "survivor guilt." As one young husband lamented about his wife's cancer, "It was hard enough 2 years ago to absorb that, even if Ann was cured, her radiation treatment would make pregnancy impossible. Now I find it unbearable that her continued slow, losing battle with cancer makes it impossible to go for our dreams like other couples our age." Psychoeducational family interventions that normalize such emotions related to threatened loss can help prevent cycles of blame, shame, and guilt. Also, when physicians inquire about and validate the psychosocial burden of caregivers, especially well spouses, they help prevent the physical burden of the patient from becoming the only currency in family relationships. This approach facilitates families seeing a chronic disorder as a "we" problem rather than solely the domain of the patient, a major contributor to dysfunctional family dynamics when living with serious illness or disability.

Medical care for chronic illnesses is often provided in specialty clinics, where patients and families dealing with similar disorders may develop significant relationships, even in the clinic waiting area. Progression, relapse, or death of another patient can trigger fears of "Will I (we) be next" and deflate family morale. It is useful for clinicians to inquire about such contacts and offer family consultations.

The Terminal Phase

The last phase is the *terminal* period including the preterminal stage of an illness in which the inevitability of death becomes apparent and predominates family life. It encompasses the periods of mourning, bereavement, and resolution of loss (Walsh & McGoldrick, 1991). This phase is distinguished by the predominance of issues surrounding separation, death, grief, resolution of mourning, and resumption of "normal" family life beyond the loss. Clinicians should keep in mind recent evidence (Wortman & Silver, 1989) that supports a much broader range of nonpathological grief reactions, somewhat tempering how we use traditional stage theories of loss (Kubler-Ross, 1969).

The transition to this phase is fraught with possibilities for blame, shame, and guilt. The family may blame the medical team for failing to provide a cure, especially if physicians had earlier given an overly optimistic prognosis. The patient and family members may blame themselves or one another for having lost "the battle." This is particularly true of families guided by a strong sense of personal responsibility and control.

As families enter this phase, one of the key tasks is a shift in their anticipation of the possibility of a terminal phase to its probability, and finally its inevitability. Clinicians can function as a guide for families, helping them gently relinquish their hopes for cure, initiate a humane plan for palliative care, and instill hope in developing a pathway for the experience of death. Clinicians should expect intense grieving related to giving up the often protracted struggle to overcome the disease. This is distinct from the experience of anticipatory grief, where family members prepare for the loss of a loved one. Mastery in the chronic phase, which emphasized maintaining autonomy within the constraints of the disorder, must now be redefined in terms of a process of preparing emotionally and practically for death. Similar to the initial crisis phase, families generally need to accept more intense involvement by health professionals. However, the role of the professional and medical technology is geared more toward caregiving, providing physical and emotional comfort, than medical stabilization and improvement. In this sense, families need not only to reinclude health providers more, but also to see their role differently. Clearly, this change of roles is often more challenging for the healthcare team than for the family, because of strong beliefs about professional success being equated with life not death.

For the terminally ill member, the most important needs are controlling pain and suffering, preserving dignity and self-worth, and receiving love and affection from family and friends. When families are coping with anticipatory loss in the final phase of an illness, the *quality* as much as the quantity of time becomes a priority. Clinicians need to explore a family's fears about the process of dying and about the loss itself. Anticipation of a family member's increasing pain or suffering is often of greater concern that death. This is especially common in long-standing progressive diseases, in which the anticipation of death has been rehearsed many times. Early reassurance about effective means of pain control and informed discussion with the family concerning the ill member's wishes about lifesaving measures can alleviate a major source of anguish. Families face a number of practical tasks in the terminal phase. As distinguished from sharing emotions, families need to decide when and who to tell about the transition. If they have not decided beforehand, the patient together with key family members need to decide about such things as: the redefinition of family roles in this final stage of an illness; a living will; the extent of medical efforts desired; who has power of attorney if the patient is not competent to make sound decisions; preferences about dying at home, in the hospital, or at hospice; and wishes about a funeral and memorial service.

Transition Periods

Critical transition periods link the three time phases. Carter and McGoldrick (1989) and Levinson (1978, 1986) have clarified the importance of transition periods in the family and adult life cycle literature. Transitions in the illness life cycle are times when families reevaluate the appropriateness of their previous life structure in the face of new illness-related developmental demands. Unfinished business from the previous phase can complicate or block movement through the transitions. Families can become permanently frozen in an adaptive structure that has outlived its utility (Penn, 1983). For example, the usefulness of pulling together in the crisis period can become a maladaptive and stifling prison for all family members in the chronic phase. Enmeshed families would have difficulty negotiating this delicate transition.

The interaction of the time phases and typology of illness provide a framework for a chronic disease psychosocial developmental model that resembles models for human development. The time phases (crisis, chronic, and terminal) can be considered broad developmental periods in the natural history of chronic disease. Each period has certain basic tasks independent of the type of illness. Each "type" of illness has specific supplementary tasks. The basic tasks of the three illness time phases and transitions recapitulate in many respects the unfolding of human development. For example, the crisis phase is similar in certain fundamental ways to the era of childhood and adolescence. Child development involves a prolonged period during which the child learns the fundamentals of life as parents temper other developmental plans (e.g., career) to accommodate raising children. In an analogous way, the crisis phase is a period of socialization to the basics of living with chronic disease, when other life plans are frequently put on hold by the family to accommodate to the illness. Just as the transition from adolescence to adulthood is marked by the relinquishing of a moratorium in order to assume adult identity and responsibilities, the transition to the chronic phase of illness emphasizes autonomy and the creation of a viable ongoing life given the realities of the illness. In the transition to the chronic phase, a "hold" or moratorium on other developmental tasks that served to protect the initial period of socialization/adaptation to life with chronic disease is reevaluated. The separate developmental tasks of "living with chronic illness" and "living out the other parts of one's life" must be brought together.

The typology and phases of illness can be combined so that each "psychosocial type" of illness can be thought about in relation to each of the time phases. The addition of a family systems model creates a three-dimensional model (Figure 12.3). Psychosocial illness types, illness time phases, and components of family systems variables constitute the three dimensions. This model allows consideration of the importance of strengths and weaknesses in various components of family functioning in relation to different disease types and at different illness phases.

CLINICAL IMPLICATIONS

By facilitating a clinician's grasp of chronic illness and disability in psychosocial terms, this model provides a framework for assessment and clinical intervention with

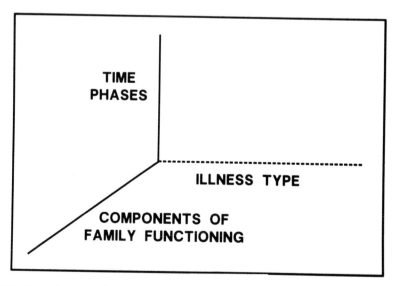

Figure 12.3. Three-dimensional model: illness type, time phase, family functioning. Reprinted from Rolland JS: Chronic illness and the life cycle: A conceptual framework. *Fam Process* 26(2):203–221, 1987.

affected families. The clinician can think with greater clarity and focus. Attention to features of onset, course, outcome, and incapacitation provide markers that focus a clinician's questioning of a family. For instance, acute-onset illnesses demand high levels of adaptability, problem solving, role reallocation, and balanced cohesion. A high degree of family enmeshment might make a family less likely to be able to cope with these demands. Forethought on this issue would cue a clinician toward a more appropriate family evaluation.

The time line of an illness delineates psychosocial developmental stages of an illness, each phase with its own unique developmental tasks. It is important for families to solve phase-related tasks within the time limits set by the duration of each successive developmental phase of an illness. The failure to resolve issues in this sequential manner can jeopardize the total coping process of the family. Therefore, attention to time allows the clinician to assess a family's strengths and vulnerabilities in relation to the present and future phases of the illness.

The model clarifies treatment planning. Taken together the typology and time phases provide a context to integrate other aspects of a comprehensive assessment. Awareness of the components of family functioning most relevant to particular types or phases of an illness guides goal setting. Sharing this information with the family and deciding on specific goals will provide a better sense of control and realistic hope to the family. This knowledge educates the family about warning signs that should alert them to call on a family therapist at appropriate times for brief goal-oriented treatment.

CASE 12-3

Joe, his wife Ann, and their three teenage children presented for a family evaluation 10 months after Joe's diagnosis with moderate–severe asthma. Joe, aged 44, had been successfully employed for many years as a spray painter. Apparently, exposure to a new chemical triggered the onset of asthmatic attacks that necessitated hospitalization and occupational disability. Although somewhat improved, he continued to have persistent and moderate respiratory symptoms. Initially, his physicians had predicted that improvement would occur, but remained noncommittal as to the level of chronicity. Continued breathing difficulties contributed to increased symptoms of depression, uncharacteristic temperamental outbursts, alcohol abuse, family discord, and finally admission to an alcohol detox unit.

In my initial assessment, after discharge to outpatient psychiatric treatment, I inquired as to their prior illness experience. This was the nuclear family's first encounter with chronic illness, and their families of origin had limited experience. Ann's father had died 7 years earlier of a sudden and unexpected heart attack. Joe's brother had died in an accidental drowning. Neither had experience with disease as an ongoing process. Joe had assumed that improvement meant "cure." In addition, Joe had a history of alcoholism that had been in complete remission for 20 years. Illness for both had meant either death or recovery. The physician/family system was not attuned to the hidden risks for this family coping with the transition from the crisis to chronic phase of his asthma, the juncture where the permanency of the disease needed to be addressed.

MULTIGENERATIONAL HISTORY OF
ILLNESS, LOSS, AND CRISIS

Many systems-oriented practitioners have emphasized that a family's present behavior cannot be adequately comprehended apart from its history (Boszormenyi-Nagy & Spark, 1973; Bowen, 1978; Carter & McGoldrick, 1989; Framo, 1976; Walsh & McGoldrick, 1991). Historical questioning is a way to track key events and transitions to gain an understanding of a family's organizational shifts and coping strategies *as a system* in response to past stressors. This is not a cause-and-effect model, but reflects a belief that such a historical search may help explain the family's current style of coping and adaptation. A historical systemic perspective involves more than simply deciphering how a family organized itself around past stressors; it also tracks the evolution of family adaptation over time. Patterns of adaptation, replications, discontinuities, shifts in relationships (e.g., alliances, triangles, cutoffs), and sense of competence are important considerations. These patterns are transmitted across generations as family myths, taboos, catastrophic expectations, and belief systems (Walsh & McGoldrick, 1991). By gathering this information a clinician can create a family genogram (McGoldrick & Gerson, 1985). A chronic illness-oriented genogram focuses on how a family organized itself as an evolving system specifically around previous illnesses and unexpected crises in the current and previous generations. A central goal is to bring to light the adults' "learned differences around illness" (Penn, 1983).

The psychosocial types and phases of illness are useful concepts in the family evaluation. Although a family may have certain standard ways of coping with any illness, there may be critical differences in their style and success in adaptation to different "types" of diseases. A family may show a disparity in their level of coping with one disease versus another, disregarding differences in demands. If the clinician inquires about different types of illnesses (e.g., relapsing versus progressive, life-threatening versus non-life-threatening), she will make better use of historical data. For instance, a family may have consistently organized successfully when faced with illnesses that were not life-threatening, but reeled under the weight of the mother's metastatic breast cancer. Such a family might be particularly vulnerable if another life-threatening illness were to occur. Another family may have experienced only non-life-threatening illnesses and be uninformed about how to cope with the uncertainties particular to life-threatening diseases. Cognizance of these facts will draw attention to areas of strength and vulnerability for a family facing cancer or any life-threatening illness. In Case 12-3, I learned critical family background information, which if it had been incorporated into the initial treatment plan might have averted a family crisis, relapse of alcohol abuse, and hospitalization.

Tracking a family's coping capabilities in the crisis, chronic, and terminal phases of previous chronic illnesses highlights complications in adaptation related to different points in the "illness life cycle." A family may have adapted well in the crisis phase of living with a spinal cord injury, but failed to navigate the transition to a family organization consistent with long-haul adaptation. A rigidly enmeshed family may have become frozen in a crisis structure and been unable to deal appropriately with issues of maximizing individual and collective autonomy in the chronic phase. Another family with a member with chronic kidney failure may have functioned very well in handling the practicalities of home dialysis. However, in the terminal phase their limitations around affective expression may have left a legacy of unresolved grief. A history of phase-specific difficulties can

247

MULTI-
GENERATIONAL
HISTORY OF
ILLNESS, LOSS,
AND CRISIS

alert a clinician to potential vulnerable periods for a family over the course of the current chronic illness. The following case illustrates the interplay of problems coping with a current illness, fueled by unresolved issues related to a particular type or phase of disease in one's family of origin.

CASE 12-4

Mary, her husband Bill, and their son Jim sought treatment 4 months after Mary had sustained a serious concussion in a life-threatening head-on auto collision caused by the driver of the other vehicle. For several months, there was some concern by the medical team that she might have suffered a cerebral hemorrhage. Ultimately, it was clarified that this had not occurred. Over this time, Mary became increasingly depressed and, despite strong reassurance, continued to believe she had a life-threatening condition and would die from a brain hemorrhage.

In the initial evaluation, she revealed that she was experiencing vivid dreams of meeting her deceased father. Apparently her father, with whom she had been extremely close, had died of a cerebral hemorrhage after a 4-year history of a progressive debilitating brain tumor, marked by progressive and uncontrolled epileptic seizures. Mary, 14 at the time, was the "baby" in the family, her two siblings being much older. The family had shielded her from his illness, culminating in her mother's decision that she not attend either the wake or the funeral. This event galvanized her position as the "child in need of protection"—a dynamic that carried over into her marriage. Despite her hurt, anger, and lack of acceptance of the death, she had avoided dealing with her feelings with her mother for over 20 years. Other family history revealed that her maternal grandfather had died when her mother was 7 years old. She had had to endure an open casket wake at home. This traumatic experience was a major factor in her mother's attempt to protect her daughter from the same kind of memory.

Mary's own life-threatening head injury had triggered a catastrophic reaction and dramatic resurfacing of previous losses involving similar types of illness and injury. Therapy focused on a series of tasks and rituals that involved her initiating conversations with her mother and visits to her father's grave.

The family's history of coping with crises in general, especially unanticipated ones, should be explored. Illnesses with acute onset (e.g., heart attack), moderate–severe sudden incapacitation (e.g., stroke), or rapid relapse (e.g., ulcerative colitis, diabetic insulin reaction, disk disease) demand in various ways rapid crisis mobilization skills. In these situations the family needs to reorganize quickly and efficiently, shifting from its usual organization to a crisis structure. Other illnesses can create a crisis because of the continual demand for family stamina (e.g., spinal cord injury, rheumatoid arthritis, emphysema). The family history of coping with moderate–severe ongoing stressors is a good predictor of adjustment to these types of illness.

For any significant chronic illness in either adult's family of origin, a clinician should try to get a picture of how those families organized to handle the range of disease-related affective and practical tasks. Also, it is important to find out what role each played in handling these emotional or practical tasks. Whether the parents (as children) were given too much responsibility (parentified) or shielded from involvement is of particular note. What did they learn from those experiences that influences how they think about the current illness? Whether they have emerged with a strong sense of competence or failure is essential information. In one particular case involving a family with three generations of hemophilia transmitted through the mother's side, the father had been shielded from the knowledge that his older brother who died in adolescence had had a terminal form of kidney disease. Also, this man had not been allowed to attend his brother's funeral. From that trauma he made a strong commitment to openness about disease-related issues with his two sons with hemophilia and his daughters who were genetic carriers.

By collecting such information about each adult's family of origin, one can anticipate areas of conflict and consensus. Unresolved issues related to illness and loss can remain dormant in a marriage, and suddenly reemerge triggered by a chronic illness in the current nuclear family (Penn, 1983; Walker, 1983). Penn describes how particular coalitions that emerge in the context of a chronic illness are replications of those that existed in each adult's family of origin. The following case is prototypical:

> If a mother has been the long-time rescuer of her mother from a tyrannical husband, and then in her own family bears a son with hemophilia, she will become his rescuer, often against his father. In this manner she continues to rescue her mother but, oddly enough, now from her husband rather than from her own father. . . . In this family with a hemophiliac son, the father's father had been ill for a long period and had received all the mother's attention. In his present family, this father, though outwardly objecting to the coalition between his wife and son, honored that relationship, as if he hoped it would make up for the one he had once forfeited with his own mother. The coalition in the nuclear family looks open and adaptational (mother and son), but is fueled by coalitions in the past (mother with her mother, and father with his mother). (Penn, 1983)

The reenactment of previous system configurations around illness can occur largely as an unconscious, automatic process. Further, the dysfunctional complementarity can emerge *de novo* specifically within the context of a chronic disease. On detailed inquiry, couples frequently reveal a tacit unspoken understanding that if an illness occurred they would reorganize to reenact "unfinished business" from their families of origin. Typically, the role chosen represents a repetition or opposite of a role played by themselves or the same sex parent. A clinician needs to maintain some distinction between functional family process with and without chronic disease. For families that present in this manner, placing a primary therapeutic emphasis on the resolution of family-of-origin issues might be the best approach to prevent or rectify an unhealthy triangle.

Families, like those just described, with encapsulated illness "time bombs" need to be distinguished from families with more pervasive, long-standing dysfunctional patterns where illnesses can become embedded in a web of preexisting fused family transactions. In the traditional sense of "psychosomatic," this kind of severely dysfunctional family displays a greater level of baseline reactivity such that when an illness enters their system, this reactivity gets expressed somatically through a poor medical course or treatment noncompliance. These families lack the foundation of a functional nonillness system. The initial focus of therapeutic intervention may need to be targeted more on pragmatic immediate help rather than family-of-origin work, with more limited therapeutic aims.

A third group of symptomatic families facing chronic disease are those without significant intra- or intergenerational family dysfunctional patterns. Any family may falter in the face of multiple superimposed disease and nondisease stressors that impact in a relatively short time. With progressive, incapacitating diseases or the concurrence of illness in several family members, a pragmatic approach that focuses on expanded or creative use of supports and resources outside the family is most productive.

THE ILLNESS, INDIVIDUAL, AND FAMILY LIFE CYCLES

To place the unfolding of chronic disease into a developmental context, it is crucial to understand the intertwining of three evolutionary threads: the illness, individual, and family life cycles. The psychosocial typology and phases of illness offer a language to characterize diseases in psychosocial and longitudinal terms, each illness having particular patterns and expected developmental life course. Since an illness *is* part of an individual, it is essential to think simultaneously about the interaction of individual and family development.

The *life cycle* is a central concept for both family and individual development. Life cycle means there is a basic sequence and unfolding of the life course within which individual, family, or illness uniqueness occurs. A second key concept is the human *life structure*. Levinson (1978) described life structure to mean the design of a person's life at any given point in the life cycle. This design is made up of an individual's various commitments (e.g., work, family, religious affiliation, hobbies) and the relative importance of each commitment. The life structure mediates transactions between the individual, the family, and the environment. Although Levinson described the individual adult male life cycle, his concepts can be applied to the family as a unit.

Illness, individual, and family development have in common the notion of periods or phases marked by different developmental tasks. For instance, a major task of early adulthood is to separate from one's family of origin and establish an independent life structure. Levinson (1978) has described five major eras in individual life structure development: childhood and adolescence, early, middle, and late adulthood, and late, late adulthood. Each lasts approximately 20 years.

Levinson noted that these life cycle eras are linked by the alternation of *life structure-building/maintaining (stable) and life structure-changing (transitional) periods*, each lasting roughly 5 to 7 years, during which certain developmental tasks are addressed independently of marker events. The primary goal of a structure-building/maintaining period is to form a life structure and enrich life within it based on the key choices an individual and family has made during the preceding transition period. In a transition period one weighs different possibilities for personal and family life, eventually deciding on and drawing up the blueprints for the next phase.

The delineation of separate periods derives from a set of developmental tasks associated with each. Transition periods are potentially the most vulnerable because previous individual, family, and illness life structures are reappraised in the face of new developmental tasks that may require major, discontinuous change rather than minor alterations.

The concept of phases in the family life cycle is particularly useful to the task of integrating illness, individual, and family development. Family life cycle theory has tended to divide development into stages demarcated by nodal events such as marriage or birth of a first child. Carter and McGoldrick (1989) have delineated the following six family life cycle stages: (1) the unattached young adult, (2) the newly married couple, (3) the family with young children, (4) the family with adolescents, (5) launching children and moving on, and (6) the family in later life. Combrinck-Graham (1985) proposes a family life spiral model in which the entire three-generational family system oscillates through time between periods of high family cohesion (centripetal) and periods of relatively lower family cohesion (centrifugal). These periods coincide with oscillations between family developmental tasks that require intense bonding or high cohesion, such as early child rearing, and tasks that emphasize personal identity and autonomy, such as adolescence. During a higher-cohesion period, both the individual member's and family unit's life structure emphasize internal family life. External boundaries around the family are tightened while personal boundaries between members are somewhat diffused to enhance family teamwork. In the transition to a lower-cohesion period, the family life structure shifts to accommodate goals that emphasize an individual family member's life outside the family. The external family boundary is loosened while separateness between some family members increases.

Several key life cycle concepts provide a foundation for understanding the experience of chronic disorders. The life cycle contains alternating transition and life structure-building/maintaining periods. Further, particular periods can be characterized as requiring either higher or lower cohesion in order to meet psychosocial demands (Figure 12.4).

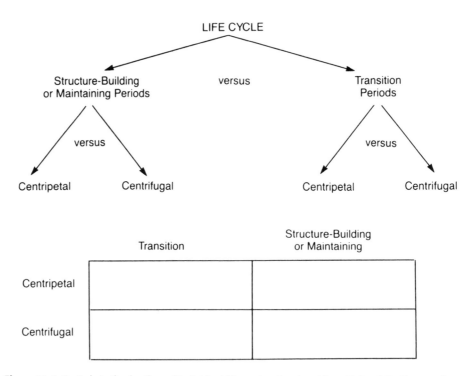

Figure 12.4. Periods in the family and individual life cycles. Reprinted from Rolland JS: Chronic illness and the life cycle: A conceptual framework. *Fam Process* 26(2):203–221, 1987.

Tom and his wife Sally presented for treatment 6 months after Tom had sustained a severe burn injury to both hands that required skin grafting. A year of recuperation was necessary before Tom would be able to return to his job, which required physical labor and full use of his hands. Prior to the injury, his wife had been at home full time raising their two children, aged 3 and 5. Although Tom was temporarily handicapped in terms of his career, he was physically fit to assume the role of house husband. Initially, both Tom and Sally remained at home using his disability income to "get by." When Sally expressed an interest in finding a job to relieve financial pressures, Tom resisted and marital strain caused by his injury flared into dysfunctional conflict.

Sufficient resources were available in the system to accommodate the illness and ongoing child-rearing tasks. Their definition of marriage lacked the necessary role flexibility to master the problem. Treatment focused on rethinking his masculine and monolithic definition of "family provider," a definition that had, in fact, emerged in full force during this higher cohesion phase of the family life cycle.

INTEGRATING INDIVIDUAL, FAMILY, AND ILLNESS DEVELOPMENT

A basic question is: What is the fit between the practical and emotional demands of a condition and family and individual developmental tasks and life structures at a particular point in time? How will this fit change as the course of the illness unfolds in relation to the family life cycle and the development of each family member? In general, chronic conditions tend to push individual and family developmental processes toward increased cohesion and transition.

The idea of degrees of cohesion is useful in linking the illness life course to individual and family life cycles. Analogous to the addition of a new family member, the occurrence of chronic illness or disability sets in motion a high-cohesion period of family socialization to illness. Symptoms, loss of function, the demands of shifting to new illness-related practical and affective roles, and the fear of loss through death all refocus a family inward.

Periods of Higher and Lower Cohesion

If the onset of an illness coincides with a lower-cohesion period for the family, it can derail the family from its natural momentum. If a young adult becomes ill, she may need to return to the family of origin for disease-related caretaking. Each member's autonomy and individuation are at risk. The young adult's ability to establish a life away from home is threatened either temporarily or permanently. Both parents may have to relinquish interests outside the family. Family dynamics as well as disease severity will influence whether the family's reversion to a high-cohesion life structure is a temporary detour within their general movement outward, or a permanent reversal. A highly cohesive or enmeshed family frequently faces the transition to a more autonomous period with trepidation. A chronic illness provides a sanctioned reason to return to the "safety" of the prior high-cohesion period. For some family members, the giving up of the building of a new life structure already in progress can be more devastating than when the family is still in an earlier phase with more preliminary future plans. An analogy would be the difference between a couple discovering that they do not have enough money to build a house versus being forced to abandon their building project with the foundation already completed.

Disease onset that coincides with a high-cohesion period in the family life cycle (e.g., early child rearing) can have several important consequences. At a minimum, it can foster a prolongation of this period. At worst, the family can become permanently stuck at this phase of development, when the inward pull of the illness and the phase of the life cycle coincide. The risk here is their tendency to amplify one another. For families that function marginally before an illness onset, this kind of mutual reinforcement can trigger a runaway process leading to overt family dysfunction. Minuchin and colleagues' (1975, 1978) research of "psychosomatic" families has documented this process in several common childhood illnesses.

When a parent develops a chronic disease during a higher-cohesion child-rearing phase of development, a family's ability to stay on course is severely taxed. The impact of the illness is like the addition of a new infant member with "special needs" competing for potentially scarce family resources. In psychosocially milder diseases, efficient role reallocation may suffice to keep family development on course, as in Case 12-5.

If the disease affecting a parent is more debilitating (e.g., traumatic brain injury, cervical spinal cord injury), its impact on the child-rearing family is twofold. A "new" family member is added, a parent is "lost," and the semblence of a single-parent family with an added child is created. For acute-onset illnesses, when both events occur simultaneously, family resources may be inadequate to meet the combined child-rearing and caretaking demands. This situation is ripe for the emergence of a parentified child or the reenlistment into active parenting of a grandparent. These forms of family adaptation are not inherently dysfunctional. A clinician needs to assess these structural realignments. Are certain individuals assigned rigid caretaking roles, or are they flexible and shared? Are caretaking roles viewed flexibly from a developmental vantage point? For an adolescent caretaker, this means the family being mindful of the approaching developmental transition to an independent life separate from the family. For grandparent caretakers, it means sensitivity to their increasing physical limitations or need to assist their own spouse.

The need for family cohesion varies enormously in different types and phases of illness. The tendency for a disease to pull a family inward increases with the level of incapacitation or risk of death. Progressive diseases over time inherently require more cohesion than constant-course illnesses. The ongoing addition of new demands as an illness progresses keeps a family's energy focused inward. After a modus operandi has been forged, a constant-course disease (excluding those with severe incapacitation) permits a family to get back on track developmentally. The added inward pull exerted by a progressive disease increases the risk of reversing normal family disengagement or freezing a family into a permanently fused state.

CASE 12-6

Mr. L., aged 54, had become increasingly depressed as a result of severe and progressive complications of his adult-onset diabetes mellitus that had emerged over the past 5 years. These complications included a leg amputation and renal failure that recently required instituting home dialysis on a four times a day basis. For 20 years, Mr. L. had had an uncomplicated constant course, allowing him to lead a full active life. An excellent athlete, he engaged in a number of recreational group sports. Short- and long-term family planning had never focused around his illness. This optimistic attitude was reinforced by the fact that two people in Mrs. L's family of origin had had diabetes mellitus without complications. Their only child, a son aged 26, had uneventfully left home after high school and had recently married. Mr. and Mrs. L. had a stable marriage, where both maintained many outside independent interests. In short, the family had moved smoothly through the transition to a more centrifugal phase of the family's life cycle.

His disease's transformation to a progressive course coupled with the incapacitating and life-shortening nature of his complications had reversed the normal process of family disengagement. His wife took a second job, which necessitated her quitting her hobbies and civic involvements. Their son and his wife moved back home to help his mother take care of his father and the house. Mr. L., disabled from work and his athletic social network, felt a burden to everyone and blocked in his own midlife development.

The essential goal of family treatment in developmental terms centered around reversing some of the system's centripetal overreaction back to a more realistic balance. For Mr. L., this meant a reworking of his life structure to accommodate his real limitations while maximizing a return to his more independent style. For Mrs. L. and her son, this meant developing realistic expectations for Mr. L. and reestablishing key aspects of their autonomy within an illness/family system.

Relapsing illnesses alternate between periods of drawing a family inward and periods of release from the immediate demands of disease. However, the on-call state of preparedness dictated by many such illnesses keeps some part of the family in a centripetal mode despite medically asymptomatic periods, hindering the natural flow between phases of the family life cycle.

One way to think about the phases of illness is that they represent to the family a progression from a crisis phase requiring high cohesion to a chronic phase demanding less cohesion. The terminal phase, if it occurs, forces most families back into being more inwardly focused and cohesive. The so-called "illness life structure," developed by a family to accommodate each phase in the illness life cycle, is colored by the inherent inward pull of each time phase. For example, in a family where illness onset has coincided with a lower-cohesion phase of development, the transition to the chronic phase permits a family to resume more of its momentum.

Transition and Stable Periods

Clinicians need to be mindful of the timing of the onset of a chronic illness, with individual/family transition and life structure-building/maintaining periods of development. All *transitions* involve the basic processes of endings and beginnings, generating an undercurrent of preoccupation with death and finiteness (Levinson, 1978). Chronic and life-threatening illness precipitates the loss of the preillness identity of the family. It forces the family into a transition in which one of the family's main tasks is to accommodate the anticipation of further loss and possibly untimely death. When the onset of a chronic illness coincides with a transition in the individual or family life cycle, issues related to previous, current, and anticipated loss will be likely magnified. Transition periods are often characterized by upheaval, rethinking of prior commitments, and openness to change. As a result, those times hold a greater risk for the illness to become unnecessarily embedded or inappropriately ignored in planning for the next developmental period. During a transition period, the very process of loosening prior commitments creates a context for emergence of family rules regarding loyalty through sacrifice and caretaking. Indecision about one's future can be "resolved" by excessive focus on a family member's physical problems. This focus can be a major precursor of family dysfunction in the context of chronic disease. By adopting a longitudinal developmental perspective, a clinician will stay attuned to future transitions and their overlap.

An example can highlight the importance of the illness in relation to future developmental transitions. Imagine a family in which the father, a carpenter and primary financial provider, develops multiple sclerosis. At first, his level of impairment is mild and stabilized, allowing him to continue part-time work. Because their children are all teenagers, his wife is able to undertake part-time work to help maintain financial stability. The oldest son, aged 15, seems relatively unaffected. Two years later, father experiences a rapid progression of his illness leaving him totally disabled. His son, now 17, has dreams of going away to college to prepare for a career in science. The specter of financial hardship and the perceived need for a "man in the family" creates a serious dilemma of choice for the son and the family. In this case there is a fundamental clash between developmental issues of separation/individuation and the ongoing demands of progressive chronic disability on the family. This vignette demonstrates the potential clash between simultaneous transition periods: the illness transition to a more incapacitating and progressive course, the adolescent son's transition to early adulthood, and the family's transition from the "living with teenagers" to "launching young adults" stage. Also, this example illustrates the significance of the type of illness. A less incapacitating or a relapsing illness (as opposed to a progressive or constant-course disease) might interfere less with this young man's separation from his family. If his father had an intermittently incapacitating illness, like disk disease, the son might have moved out but tailored his choices to remain nearby and thus available during acute flare-ups.

Illness onset may cause a different kind of disruption if it coincides with a *life structure-building/maintaining period* in individual or family development. These periods are characterized by the living out of choices made during the preceding transition period. Relative to transition periods, family members try to protect their and the family unit's current life structure. Diseases with only a mild level of psychosocial severity (e.g., nonfatal, none/mild incapacitation, nonprogressive) may require some revision of individual/family life structure, but not a radical restructuring that would necessitate a return to a transitional phase of development. A chronic illness with a critical threshold of psychosocial severity will demand the reestablishment of a transitional form of life, at a time when individual/family inertia is to preserve the momentum of a stable period. An individual's or family's level of adaptability is a prime factor determining the successful navigation of this kind of crisis. In this context, family adaptability involves the ability to transform its entire life structure to a prolonged transitional state.

For instance, in the previous example, father's multiple sclerosis rapidly progressed while the oldest son was in a transition period in his own development. The nature of the strain in developmental terms would be quite different if his father's disease progression had occurred when this young man was 26, had already left home, finished college, secured a first job, married, and had a child. In the latter scenario, the oldest son's life structure is in a centripetal, structure-maintaining period within his newly formed nuclear family. To fully accommodate the needs of his family of origin would require a monumental shift of his developmental priorities. When this illness crisis coincided with a developmental transition period (age 17), although a dilemma of choice existed, the son was available and less fettered by commitments in progress. Later, at age 26, he has made commitments and is in the process of living them out with his newly formed family. To serve the demands of an illness transition, the son might need to shift his previously stable life structure back to a transitional state. And, the shift would happen "out of phase" with the flow of his individual and nuclear family's development. One way to resolve this dilemma of divided loyalties might be the merging of the two households.

This discussion raises several key clinical points. From a systems viewpoint, at the time of a chronic illness diagnosis it is important to know the phase of the family life cycle and the stage of individual development of all family members, not just the ill member. This is important information for several reasons. First, chronic disease in one family member can profoundly affect developmental goals of another member. For instance, a disabled infant can be a serious roadblock to a mother's mastery of child rearing, or a life-threatening illness in a young adult can interfere with the spouse's readiness to become a parent. Second, family members frequently do not adapt equally to chronic illness. Each member's ability to adapt and the rate at which they do so is related to the individual's own developmental stage and role in the family. The oldest son in the previous example illustrates this point.

There exists a normative and nonnormative timing of chronic illness in the life cycle. Coping with chronic illness and death are considered normally anticipated tasks in late adulthood. On the other hand, illnesses and losses that occur earlier are "out of phase" and tend to be developmentally more disruptive (Herz, 1989; Neugarten, 1976). As untimely events, chronic diseases can severely disrupt the usual sense of continuity and rhythm of the life cycle. The timing in the life cycle of an unexpected event, like a chronic illness, will shape the form of adaptation and the event's influence on subsequent development (Levinson, 1978).

The notion of "out of phase" illnesses can be conceptualized in a more refined way. First, since serious diseases demand higher family cohesion, they can be more disruptive to families in a lower-cohesion phase of development. Second, the onset of chronic disease tends to create a period of transition, the length or intensity of which depends on the psychosocial type and phase of the illness. This forced transition is particularly "out of phase" if it coincides with a life structure-building/maintaining period in the individual's or family's life cycle. Third, if the particular illness is progressive, relapsing, increasingly incapacitating, or life-threatening, then the phases in the unfolding of the disease will be punctuated by numerous transitions. Under these conditions a family will need to more frequently alter their illness life structure to accommodate the shifting and often increasing demands of the disease. This level of demand and uncertainty keeps the illness in the forefront of a family's consciousness, constantly impinging on their attempts to get back "in phase" developmentally. Finally, the transition from the crisis to the chronic phase of the illness life cycle is often the key juncture where the intensity of the family's socialization to living with chronic disease can be relaxed. In this sense, it offers a "window of opportunity" for the family to recover its developmental course.

Chronic diseases that occur for adults in the child-rearing period can be most devastating because of their potential impact on family financial and child-rearing responsibilities (Herz, 1989). Again, the actual impact will depend on the "type" of illness and preillness family roles. Families governed by rigid gender-defined roles as to who should be the primary financial provider and caretaker of children will potentially have the greatest problems with adjustment and need to be coached toward a more flexible view about role interchange.

In the face of chronic disease, an overarching goal is for a family to deal with the developmental demands presented by the illness without family members completely sacrificing their own or the family's development as a system. Therefore, it is vital to ask about what life plans had to be canceled, postponed, or altered as a result of the diagnosis. It is useful to know whose plans are most and least affected. By asking a family when and under what conditions they will resume plans, put on hold or address future developmental tasks, a clinician can anticipate developmental crises related to "independence from" versus "subjugation to" the chronic illness. Family members can be helped to resume their life plans, at least to some extent, by helping them resolve feelings of guilt, overresponsibility, and hopelessness and find resources internal and external to the family for more freedom, both to pursue their own goals and to provide needed care for the ill member.

CASE 12-7

Lucy and Tom G., a young couple, have a child Susan, aged 5, who is terminally ill with leukemia. The pediatric oncologist offers the parents the choice between an experimental treatment with a low probability of success or halting treatment.

Tom's position is "Let's stop; enough is enough." Lucy, on the other hand, feels, "We must continue; we can't let her die." The couple cannot reach an agreement, and the physician is immobilized. He requests a psychiatric consultation for the couple.

When the consultant asks, "What is your explanation of how your daughter got leukemia?" the critical story emerges. Tom basically sees it as bad luck. Lucy, however, has a very different belief. During her pregnancy with Susan, Lucy's father had a heart attack and died several months later from a second episode. Lucy experienced this as a time of great stress and grief, which she feels adversely affected the intrauterine life of Susan. After Susan's birth, by normal delivery, Lucy was still mourning the loss of her father, and feels that this affected the quality of her bonding with Susan and led to a hidden depression in her infant. Further, Lucy had read research linking depression with lowering of the effectiveness of the immune system, which could, in turn, decrease normal surveillance and clearing of cancer cells from the body. She believes this combination of factors caused her child's cancer, and that if she had been a more competent mother, this never would have happened. Lucy said she had never told this story to anyone, because no one had ever asked, and she was very ashamed. She had hoped for a cure so that the whole issue could be resolved. She cannot accept stopping treatment because, to her, it means that Susan's death will be her fault.

HEALTH/ILLNESS BELIEF SYSTEMS

Each of us as an individual and as a part of larger systems adopts a value orientation, belief system, or philosophy that shapes our patterns of behavior toward the common problems of daily life in society (Kluckhohn, 1960). Beliefs provide coherence to family life, facilitating continuity between past, present, and future and a way to approach new and ambiguous situations. Depending on which system we are speaking of, this phenomenon can be labeled as values, culture, religion, belief system, worldview, or family paradigm.

Reiss (1981) has shown that families as a unit develop paradigms for how the world operates. One component of the family's overall construction of reality is their set of health/illness beliefs that will determine how they interpret illness events and guide their health-seeking behavior (Rolland, 1987b). Although individual family members can hold different beliefs, the values held by the family unit may be the most significant.

At the time of a medical diagnosis a primary developmental task for the family is to create a meaning for the illness that preserves a sense of competency and mastery in the context of partial loss, possible further physical compromise, or death. Since serious illness is often experienced as a betrayal of our fundamental trust in our bodies and belief in our invulnerability and immortality (Kleinman, 1988), the creation of an empowering narrative can be a formidable task. Family health beliefs help us grapple with these existential dilemmas of our fear of death, attempts to sustain our denial of death, and attempts to reassert control over unjust suffering and untimely death. At a practical level, belief systems serve as a cognitive map guiding decisions and action.

In the initial crisis phase, it is useful for clinicians to inquire about key beliefs that shape families' illness narratives and coping strategies. This means gaining an understanding of a family's overall belief system, of family beliefs brought into play by the strains of a serious health problem, and the meanings associated with the condition itself. A thorough assessment includes tracking beliefs about: (1) normality, (2) mind–body relationship, control, and mastery, (3) meanings attached by a family, ethnic group, religion, or the wider culture to symptoms (e.g., chronic pain), types of illness (e.g., life-threatening disorders), or specific diseases (e.g., AIDS), (4) assumptions about what caused an illness and what will influence its course and outcome, (5) multigenerational factors that have shaped a family's health beliefs, and (6) anticipated nodal points in illness, individual, and family life cycles when health beliefs will be strained or need to shift. Second, a clinician needs to assess the fit of health beliefs within the family and its various subsystems (e.g., spouse, parental, extended family) as well as between the family and the healthcare system and wider culture.

BELIEFS ABOUT NORMALITY

A family's beliefs about what is normal or abnormal and the importance they place on conformity and excellence in relation to the average family have far-reaching implications for adaptation to chronic disorders (Rolland, 1994; Walsh, 1993). Families with values that allow having a "problem" without self-denigration have a distinct advantage in utilizing outside help and maintaining a positive identity in the face of chronic conditions. Help seeking that is defined as weak and shameful undercuts this kind of resilience. Essentially, in situations of chronic disorders where problems are to be expected and the use of professionals and outside resources are necessary, a belief that pathologizes this normative process adds insult to injury.

Two excellent questions to elicit beliefs about how families define normality are, "How do you think other *normal, average* families would deal with a similar situation to yours?" And, "How would a *healthy* family cope with your situation?" The first question gives a good indication of whether family members have a sense of the range of possible experiences and what is typical. Do they make their comparisons in relation to situations that really have similar psychosocial demands, or are they making unrealistic or unfair ones? A family dealing with the initial phase of a traumatic brain-injured member could do themselves a disservice by comparing their coping ability and strategies with a family facing a seizure disorder. The second question invites a family to share their views about what is healthy or optimal. Like couples that unrealistically describe optimal relationships as problem-free, without conflict or suffering, often families facing chronic disorders have a narrow, romanticized version of healthy adaptation that is unrealistic and leaves them feeling deficient.

Families with strong beliefs in high achievement and perfectionism tend to equate normality with optimal. They tend to define normality or successful family functioning in terms of ideal or "problem-free" characteristics. Families that define normality in this way are prone to apply standards in a situation of illness where the *kind* of control they are accustomed to is impossible. Particularly with "off-time" conditions that occur early in the life cycle, there are additional pressures to keep up with normative socially expectable developmental milestones of age peers or other young couples. The fact that life cycle goals may take longer or need revision requires a flexible belief about what is normal and healthy. This lack of a comparison group is one reason why self-help groups and networks can be so useful to families dealing with off-time conditions. It provides a normalizing context.

Successful coping and adaptation are enhanced when a family believes in a biopsychosocial frame for illness that normalizes a psychosomatic interaction. This highlights the importance of the initial "framing event" and whether professionals actively normalize a psychosomatic interplay, thereby helping to counteract pathologizing family and cultural beliefs. A physician might say, in a hypothetical situation, to a family facing asthma, "Many families notice that asthma is affected by stressful times, but fear that I would view that as a definite sign of psychiatric problems. I want you to know that asthma normally gets worse during the inevitable strains that arise in family life. It is important that you keep me informed about major family stresses so that I can decide with you whether adjusting Susan's medication or finding better ways to reduce stress will be the best approach." This promotes a positive attitude toward the potential role of psychosocial factors in influencing disease course and the quality of life. Rather than a shameful liability, a family can approach a psychosomatic interplay as an opportunity to make a difference and increase their sense of control.

MIND–BODY RELATIONSHIPS

The concept of mind–body relationship has been the subject of discourse and debate for millenia. The term *mind–body relationship* has come to represent several related but distinct beliefs that are important to differentiate.

First, there is one assumption that the mind and body are separate worlds and that what goes on in each can interactively affect the other. There is tremendous diversity about how this distinction is seen, if at all, and the degree to which the interaction is seen as equal or more a one-way street. Until recently, traditional Western medicine has tended to minimize the potential impact of the mind on the body.

Second, we need to distinguish beliefs about the mind as a logical, thinking process that can determine *actions* that may help in healing the body (e.g., seeking medical care, changing diet or activity patterns), versus the mind as a source of thought or energy that can directly impact body physiology. The latter includes beliefs about the importance of emotional states such as positive attitude, love, anger, humor, or depression on maintaining physical health and promoting or interfering with healing of the body from disease. It includes beliefs about the mind as the locus of responsibility and the role of willpower in affecting the body. Healing practices such as meditation or guided imagery are based on beliefs about the importance of the mind.

Traditional mental health theories and research endeavors have been pathology-based, tending to emphasize character traits or emotional states that affect body chemistry adversely. From this perspective, emotions can affect the body negatively, but possible positive influences of healthy attitudes have been neglected. We need to be aware of our own belief biases, often promoted in our professional training, which is typically based on the study of pathology, disease, or dysfunction.

More recently, the public has been increasingly drawn to popular literature citing the importance of positive attitudes in healing. These practitioners emphasize the unity of mind and body rather than as distinct worlds. In turn, they describe healing as a state of being, rather than in strictly biological terms. We need to be particularly mindful that families may have more exposure to these positive possibilities, while our own professional thinking remains antiquated and skewed to a more exclusive view of a mind–body relationship that is pathology-based. The danger lies in not inquiring about family beliefs that are more health-promoting. Or worse, based on our own rigid mind-set, which we defend on the basis of the lack of "hard research data," we may communicate to a family our lack of interest in these ideas or even dismiss them as unscientific and unworthy. In the process, we can undermine a possible powerful source of healing, shame a family, and undermine a mutual workable alliance necessary for any effective treatment.

Third, we need to understand beliefs about "mind" that extend beyond the individual to include family, community, or a higher spiritual force. To what extent do family members see the locus of energy that can both harm the body and heal it as residing in these other parts of the larger ecosystem? Anthropologists have found tremendous diversity in the role of family, community, God, or nature as a source of healing. Such beliefs are typically expressed in the form of rituals. In our society, a family's religious community will often organize a prayer service to promote healing for an ill member.

Clinician understanding of family members' beliefs about mind–body relationships provides a foundation for joining with a family and tailoring biopsychosocial treatment strategies more sensitively (Griffith & Griffith, 1994). Areas of strength and vulnerability can be identified, and ways of including the family in a complementary fashion with other treatments can be suggested.

THE FAMILY'S SENSE OF MASTERY OVER AN ILLNESS

It is critical to determine how a family defines mastery or control in general and how it transposes that definition to situations of illness. Mastery is similar to the concept of health locus of control (Lefcourt, 1982), which can be defined as the belief an individual or family has about their influence over the course/outcome of an illness. It is critical to distinguish whether a family's belief system is based on the premise of internal control, external control by chance, or external control by powerful others.

An internal locus-of-control orientation means that there is a belief that an individual/family can affect the outcome of a situation. Families with such a belief about their health will endorse such statements as, "I am directly responsible for my health" or "If I become sick, I have the power to make myself well again."

An external orientation entails a belief that outcomes are not contingent on the individual's or family's behavior. Families that view illness in terms of chance will agree with such statements as, "Luck plays a big part in determining how soon my family member will recover from an illness," or "When I become ill it's a matter of fate."

Individuals who see health control as in the hands of powerful others will see health professionals, God, or sometimes "powerful" family members, rather than themselves, as exerting control over their bodies. They will endorse statements such as, "Regarding my health, I can only do what my doctor tells me to do," or "My family has a lot to do with my becoming sick or staying healthy."

A family may adhere to a different set of values concerning control when dealing with a *biological* process as opposed to other day-to-day types of problem solving. Therefore, it is important to assess a family's basic value system first, and then, with increasing specificity, to assess notions about control for illnesses in general, chronic and life-threatening illness, and finally the specific disease facing the family. A family guided normally by an internal locus of control may switch to an external viewpoint when a member develops any chronic illness, or perhaps only in the case of a life-threatening disease. Such a change might occur in a family with a strong need to remain in accord with society's values, a particular ethnic background, or a specific cross-generational experience with life-threatening diseases. One can inquire as to whether a family has any particular beliefs surrounding specific types of illnesses. Regardless of the actual severity in a particular instance, cancer may be equated with "death" or "no control" because of medical statistics, cultural myth, or prior family history. For many, certain types of heart disease with a similar life expectancy as certain forms of cancer could be seen as more manageable because of prevailing cultural beliefs. Imagine a family traditionally guided by a strong sense of personal control. If the paternal grandfather, the powerful patriarch of the family, died at midlife because of a rapidly progressive and painful form of cancer, the family may develop an encapsulated exception to their views about control that is specific for cancer or generalized to include all life-threatening illnesses.

A family's value orientation about mastery strongly affects the nature of its relationship to an illness and to the healthcare system. A family's beliefs about control are a predictor of certain health behaviors, particularly treatment compliance, and suggest the family's preferences about participation in their family member's treatment and healing. In my experience, families that view disease course/outcome as a matter of chance tend to establish marginal relationships with health professionals largely because their belief system minimizes the importance of their own or a health professional's relationship to a disease process. Just as any psychotherapeutic relationship depends on a shared belief system about what is therapeutic, a fit between the patient, his family, and the healthcare team in terms of these fundamental values is essential. Families that express feelings of being misunderstood by health professionals are often referring directly or indirectly to a lack of joining at this basic value level.

Variations in a family's beliefs about mastery can occur dependent on the time phase of the illness. For some illnesses, the crisis phase involves a lot of involvement outside the family. For instance, the crisis phase after a stroke may begin with an intensive care unit and months of extended care at a rehabilitation facility. This kind of protracted care outside the family's direct control may be stressful for a family that prefers to tackle its own problems with a minimum of outside leadership. For this family, the patient's return home may increase the workload but allow members to reestablish more fully their values concerning control. A family guided more by a preference for external control by experts will have greater difficulty when their family member returns home. For this family, leaving the rehabilitation hospital may be the most difficult time, because it means the loss of their locus of competency, the professionals caring for them. Health providers' cognizance about this basic difference in belief about control can guide a psychosocial treatment plan tailored to each family's needs.

In the terminal phase of an illness a family may feel least in control of the biological course of the disease and the decision-making regarding the overall care of their ill member. Families with a strong need to sustain their centrality may need to assert themselves more vigorously with health providers. Effective decision-making regarding the extent of heroic medical efforts or whether a patient will die at home, an institution, or hospice requires an effective family–provider relationship that respects the family's basic beliefs.

THE FAMILY'S BELIEFS ABOUT THE CAUSE OF AN ILLNESS

When a significant health problem arises, all of us wonder "Why me (or us)?" and "Why now?" As illustrated poignantly in Case 12-7, we construct an explanation or narrative that helps organize our experience. The context within which an illness event occurs is a very powerful organizer and mirror of a family's belief system. The limits of current medical knowledge mean tremendous uncertainties persist about the relative importance of a myriad of factors in the onset of disease, and this allows individuals and families to develop highly idiosyncratic ideas about what caused their family member's illness.

A family's beliefs about the etiology of an illness need to be assessed separately from its beliefs about what can affect the outcome. One way to gather this information is to ask *each* family member for his or her explanation of the existence of the disease. Responses will reflect a combination of the current level of medical knowledge about the particular disease in concert with family mythology.

Negative myths may include punishment for prior misdeeds (e.g., an affair), blame of a particular family member ("Your drinking made me sick"), a sense of injustice ("Why am I being punished? I have been a good person"), genetics (e.g., cancer runs on one side of the family), negligence by the patient or parents (e.g., sudden infant death syndrome), or bad luck. Asking this question can function as an effective family Rorschach, bringing to light unresolved family conflicts.

Attributions about the cause of an illness that invoke blame, shame, or guilt are particularly important to uncover. Beliefs of this nature make it extremely difficult for a family to establish functional coping and adaptation to an illness. In the context of a life-threatening illness the blamed family member is held accountable for potential murder if the patient dies. Decisions about treatment can become confounded and filled with tension. A mother who feels blamed by her husband for their son's leukemia may be less able to accept stopping a low-probability experimental treatment than the angry, blaming husband. A husband who believes his drinking caused his wife's coronary and subsequent death may have a pathological grief reaction and may increase his drinking to mask his profound guilt.

In my clinical experience, families with the strongest, at times extreme, beliefs about personal responsibility and those with the most severely dysfunctional patterns will be those most likely to attribute the cause of an illness to a psychosocial factor. For high internal locus-of-control families, an ethos of personal responsibility guides all facets of life, including the etiology of an illness. For these families, a relative lack of acknowledgment of "outrageous fortune" as a factor in illness events can create for these families a nidus for blame, shame, and guilt. For highly dysfunctional families, characterized by unresolved conflicts and intense blaming, attributions of what or who is responsible for an illness often become ammunition in long-term family power struggles.

It is difficult to characterize an "ideal" family health belief about mastery or control. On one hand, a major thesis of systems-oriented medicine is that there is always an interplay between disease and other levels of system. On the other hand, illnesses and phases in the course of disease may vary considerably in their responsiveness to psychosocial factors versus their inherent nature. Distinctions need to be made between a family's beliefs about their overall participation in a long-term disease process, their beliefs about their ability to control the biological unfolding of an illness, and the flexibility with which a family can apply these beliefs. Optimal family narratives respect the limits of scientific knowledge, affirm basic competency, and promote the flexible use of multiple biological and psychosocial healing strategies.

A family's belief in their participation in the total illness process can be thought of as independent from whether a disease is stable, improving, or in a terminal phase. Sometimes, mastery and the attempt to control biological process coincide. A family coping with a member who has cancer in remission may tailor its behavior to help maintain health. This might include changes in family roles, communication, diet, exercise, and balance between work and recreation. Suppose the ill family member loses remission and vigorous efforts to reestablish a remission fail. As the family enters the terminal phase of the illness, participation as an expression of mastery must now be transposed for a successful process of letting go.

The difference between a family experiencing a loss with a sense of competency versus profound failure is intimately connected to this kind of flexible use of their belief system. For instance, it can be helpful if clinicians recognize that the death of a patient, whose long debilitating illness has heavily burdened others, can be a matter of relief as well as sadness to some or all family members. Since a sense of relief over death goes against most conventions in our society, it can trigger massive guilt reactions that may be expressed tangentially through such symptoms as depression and negative family interactions. Clinicians will need to help family members accept, with a minimum of guilt and defensiveness, the naturalness of ambivalent feeling they may have for their deceased member.

Thus, flexibility within the family and the health-provider system may be the key variable in optimal family functioning. Families can view mastery in a rigid, circumscribed way that views biological outcome as the sole determinant of success, or families can define control in a more "holistic" sense where involvement and participation in the overall process is the main criterion defining success. This is analogous to the distinction between "healing the system" and curing "the disease." Healing the system may influence the course or outcome of an illness, but disease outcome is not necessary to a family feeling successful. This flexible definition of mastery permits the quality of relations within the family or between the family and health providers to become more central to criteria of success. It permits the health provider's competence to be viewed from both a technical and a caregiving perspective (Reiss & Kaplan De-Nour, 1989) that is not linked only to the biological course of the disorder.

As family illness beliefs are articulated, a clinician should inquire about the degree of family consensus or congruence among members concerning a particular value, such as health locus of control. This is important because it is a common, but unfortunate, error to regard "the family" as a monolithic unit that feels, thinks, believes, and behaves as an undifferentiated whole.

In assessing the family's level of agreement, one should learn about the family's general tolerance for differences. Is the family rule "We must agree on all/some values" or are diversity and different viewpoints acceptable? Further, clinicians should determine whether the family policy about consensus is adhered to in relation to prevailing cultural or societal beliefs. Can the family hold values that differ from the wider culture? The family's general rule has multiple determinants that include cultural norms, historical context (era of "family consensus" versus each member "doing his/her own thing"), and the beliefs of the adults' families of origin.

A family's rules about consensus can have profound implications for permissible options when a family faces chronic illness. If consensus is the rule, then individual differentiation implies deviance. If the guiding principle is "We can hold different viewpoints," then diversity is allowed. When working with illness-related values in a family where consensus is the rule, attention to the entire family is mandatory. One treatment goal can be to help families negotiate their differences and support the separate identity, needs, and goals of each member. In a family where diversity is permitted there may be greater latitude to work on certain disease-related psychosocial issues with the ill member alone or with other family members without mobilizing family resistance.

Next, it is important to look into the *actual* level of agreement with regard to illness values both within the family and between the family and medical system. How congruent are the family's basic beliefs about control with their illness value system? A family that is uniformly external will generally adapt best if psychosocial interventions are tailored to that fact. On the other hand, a family that generally adheres to an internal locus of control but feels the opposite with a particular disease may, through exploration of underlying issues, be able to change its beliefs about illness. It is critical to keep in mind that beliefs about control refer to a family's beliefs about the importance of their *participation in the total illness process* rather than just their beliefs about a disease's curability.

It is important to analyze differences among family members in terms of illness values. Disparities in two- and three-person relationships involving the ill member are particularly significant. Consider a common situation in which there is a long-standing loyalty conflict for a man caught between his spouse and his mother. Both women vie for his devotion, while he is unable to define boundaries between his family of origin and nuclear family. This dysfunctional triangle may have smoldered for years in a precarious balance when the man develops a slowly progressive and debilitating illness such as multiple sclerosis. If the man and his mother share a strong sense of internal control while his spouse grew up in a family that saw chronic illness as a matter of fate, an unbalancing of this triangle is likely to occur. The smoldering mother–son coalition now reemerges in full force fueled by shared basic beliefs concerning mastery, while the marital couple is driven apart.

The different ethnic backgrounds of the adults in a family may be a primary reason for the kind of discrepancies about illness beliefs that emerge at the time of a major illness (McGoldrick *et al.*, 1982). Differences may occur in such areas as the definition of the appropriate "sick role" for the patient; the kind and degree of open communication about the disease; who should be included in the illness caretaking system (e.g., extended family, friends, professionals); and the kind of rituals viewed as normative at different stages of an illness (e.g., hospital bedside vigils, healing and funeral rituals) (Imber-Black, 1991; Wolin & Bennett, 1984). In families of mixed ethnic heritage, clinicians should assess these areas for consensus, disagreement, and negotiation.

It is common for differences in beliefs or attitudes between family members to erupt at major transition points in the treatment or disease course. For instance, in situations of severe disability or terminal illness, one member may want the patient to return home while another prefers extended hospitalization or transfer to an extended care facility. Since the chief task of patient caretaking is usually assigned to the wife/mother, she is the one most apt to bear the chief burdens in this regard. If this family also operates under the constraint of traditional role assignments where the wife/mother defers to her spouse as the family decision maker, she may not make her true feelings known and may become the "family martyr," taking on the home nursing tasks without overt disagreement at the time critical decisions are made with health professionals. Clinicians can be misled by a family that presents this kind of united front. A careful and perceptive assessment can help avert the long-term consequences to such a family of role overload, resentment, and deteriorating family relationships.

It is essential to assess the fit between the belief systems of the family and the healthcare team. The same questions asked of the family are relevant to the medical team. What is the attitude of the healthcare team about their and the family's ability to influence the course/outcome of the disease? How does the heath team see the balance between their versus the family's participation in the treatment and control of the disease? If basic differences in beliefs about health locus of control exist, it is critical to assess how to reconcile these differences. Because of the tendency of most health facilities to disempower individuals and thereby foster dependence, utmost sensitivity to family values is needed to create a therapeutic system. Many breakdowns in relationships between "noncompliant" or marginal patients and their healthcare providers are related to lack of agreement at this basic level.

The relative need for consensus will vary according to the illness phase (Reiss & Kaplan DeNour, 1989). One point where a good fit of values is usually needed is during the initial crisis period when health providers engage in much high-technology medicine and rapid decision-making and exchange of information, especially if life-threatening circumstances prevail. Teamwork is particularly important. Illnesses characterized by recurrent crises or key transitions have nodal points of stress where consensus will again become important.

One major transition is the often murky junction between the chronic and terminal phases of an illness. The attitudes and behaviors of the medical team can have a major influence in either facilitating or hindering this process for a family. A medical team that maintains heroic efforts to control the terminal phase of an illness can convey confusing messages. Families may not know how to interpret continued lifesaving efforts. Is there still real hope that should be taken by families as a message to redouble their faith in and support of medical improvement? Do the physicians feel bound to a technological imperative that requires them to exhaust *all* possibilities at their disposal, regardless of the odds of success? Often physicians feel committed to this course for ethical reasons, a "leave no stone unturned" philosophy, or because of fears concerning legal liability. Is the medical team having its own difficulties letting go? Strong relationships with certain patients can be fueled by identifications with losses, often unresolved, in health providers' own lives.

Healthcare professionals and institutions can collude in a pervasive societal wish to deny death as a natural process truly beyond technological control (Becker, 1973). Endless treatment can represent the medical team's inability to separate a general value placed on controlling diseases from their beliefs about participation (separate from cure) in a patient's total care. Professionals need to closely examine their own motives for treatments geared toward cure rather than palliation, particularly when a patient may be entering a terminal phase. Professionals' self-examination needs to be done in concert with a careful understanding of the family's belief system.

Because information about and linkage to community resources and services is frequently valuable, the clinician must assess how family health beliefs influence their overall illness behavior within a community (Mechanic, 1978). Clinicians need to know the availability of and access to community resources relevant to the management of long-term illnesses. This includes a range of primary, secondary, and tertiary medical, rehabilitation, respite, transportation, housing, institutional, and financial entitlement services. Also, it includes potential psychosocial support from friends, neighbors, and self-help groups, and religious, ethnic, cultural, or other group affiliations. On the family side, one must inquire about a family's prior experience using such resources. Have these experiences been affirming or alienating? To what extent is the family adequately informed about potential outside sources of help? Ignorance may reflect family isolation from the community as a result of such things as geographical distance in a rural setting, lack of education (e.g., literacy), language barrier, poverty, race, and ethnic or religious distinctions from the wider culture. On the other side, a family's willingness to use outside resources may be limited by ethnic/cultural values, certain family dynamics, and their own illness paradigms.

For example, rigidly enmeshed families tend to view the world as dangerous and threatening to their fragile sense of autonomy. Individual autonomy is sacrificed to keep the family system intact. Their beliefs about control will need to be defined within a framework of family exclusiveness that minimizes the role of outsiders. The occurrence of a chronic illness presents a powerful dilemma for these families. The illness may necessitate frequent excursions beyond the family borders or require the inclusion of outside professionals for disease management. Any hope of establishing a viable family–healthcare team relationship depends on exquisite sensitivity to this interplay of dysfunctional family dynamics and their belief system.

CONCLUSION

This chapter has described a three-dimensional model for looking at the impact of chronic illness on families. On the first dimension, psychosocial "types" of illnesses are created based on combinations of four components: onset, course, outcome, and degree of incapacitation. The second dimension distinguishes three phases in the life history of chronic disease: crisis, chronic, and terminal. The third dimension includes various universal and illness-specific components of family functioning. Particular attention was given to the family health beliefs, multigenerational history of illness, loss, and crisis, and the interface of the individual and family life cycles with chronic disease. This three-dimensional model provides a framework for effective clinical intervention that takes into account the important interactions between illness, individual patients, and their families.

—————— CASES FOR DISCUSSION ——————

CASE 1

Tom and Sally, a young, successful dual-career couple in their early 30s, have been married for 4 years, when Tom, who has had a lifelong mild case of hemophilia, contracts AIDS from a contaminated blood factor infusion he required after a heated discussion with his wife during which he had punched a wall. Tom, who has an intense belief in personal control and overcoming adversity, decides that he will cure himself within a year. He had always maintained excellent control of his hemophilia, which he inherited through his mother's side of the family.

Past family history is significant. Tom's mother decided to divorce his father when Tom was 5 years old. Subsequently, his father's business failed, and he committed suicide when Tom was a teenager. Tom's mother sees her son as the shining star of the family, who unlike his derided father will be a big success in life. Sally was an only child; her mother had left Sally's father when Sally was a teenager. Her father was described as nice but ineffectual; he had a series of psychiatric hospitalizations for depression. Sally had tried to help her father, but felt unsuccessful. Sally sees in Tom the strong-willed, successful man, who unlike her father had mastered chronic illness (hemophilia).

1. *Given the family histories, what do you see as the major psychosocial risks for Tom and Sally and their marriage? What if Tom becomes terminally ill, develops a dementia, and cannot be managed at home? What are the possible issues of blame, shame, and guilt? Who else in the extended family might be at risk, and why?*
2. *Given Tom's beliefs about control and mastery, what are the psychosocial risks given the lethality of his disease? Would you try to intervene and how?*
3. *Discuss the possible strains on Tom, Sally, and the marriage of an "off-time" terminal illness.*
4. *What dysfunctional skews could develop between Tom and Sally in their roles as patient and well spouse/caregiver?*
5. *How are the psychosocial demands of hemophilia and AIDS similar and different?*

CASE 2

You are called by the head nurse for the ICU to intervene with a patient and his mother who were disrupting the unit because the mother insists on staying at her son's bedside. The ICU's customary rules limit family visits to 10 minutes. The patient, Stavros, aged 42, had been admitted with symptoms of intractable angina. He is first-generation Greek American, married for 15 years to Dana, who is from a Scandinavian background. A long-standing smoldering triangular conflict has existed for the couple in terms of Stavros's divided loyalties between his strong relationship to his family of origin, particularly his mother, and his spouse. On admission, his mother began a 24-hour vigil by her son's hospital bed. Dana greatly resents her mother-in-law's seemingly intrusive behavior. Stavros's mother is critical of what she perceives as Dana's emotional coldness and relative lack of concern. Stavros feels caught between his warring mother and wife and complains of increased symptoms.

1. *Thinking in terms of different ethnic traditions of the family members, including your own, how would you react to this case? Thinking systemically, how would you approach a consultation with the patient/family?*
2. *Thinking in terms of the intersection of three distinct belief systems—your work setting (hospital and ICU), yourself as a physician, and your personal cultural/ethnic/family*

values—how might these affect your strategy with this case? What biases might interfere with your effectiveness? How could you avoid taking sides?

267

**CASES FOR
DISCUSSION**

CASE 3

Mrs. L. tells you that she is concerned that her daughter Janice, aged 5, has been compulsively masturbating for the past 3 months, and that this is an indication of sexual abuse. When the child assessment reveals no evidence of abuse, you inquire about other recent stressful events in the family. Only at that point does the mother reveal that her husband had a subtotal gastrectomy 9 months ago because of stomach cancer, and that 3 months earlier he had been rehospitalized for further tests that proved inconclusive. When Mrs. L. is asked what the children have been told, she reports that, after her husband's surgery, they had told the children only that, "Daddy had a tummy ache, so the doctors removed Daddy's stomach so he'd feel better." Mrs. L. reveals that she herself worries constantly about her husband's condition, but that he won't come in and won't discuss it, stating that after the surgery, "He was adamant that he did not want ever to talk about it. He went back to work almost immediately, and insisted that everything is fine." Asked if this medical crisis had had any impact on the children, especially Janice, she replies, "Well, she doesn't tell me about any worries. But now that you ask, at dinner every night, when we say grace, Janice prays out loud for Daddy's stomach. But no one in the family comments on this."

1. *Thinking in terms of healthy family communication in the face of threatened loss, how would you intervene in this case? Who would you try to convene and why?*
2. *In what ways would you handle communication with children differently than with the couple?*
3. *How would you view the husband's personal decision to minimize his problem and keep it private in the context of other symptomatic family members?*

CASE 4

Mr. and Mrs. S., both in their early 70s, live alone in their home of 40 years. Mrs. S. has had congestive heart failure for 5 years and more recently a progressive dementia caused by a series of minor strokes. A recent exacerbation of her condition has led to a hospitalization. The family physician feels the couple have reached their limits and has suggested a nursing home placement for Mrs. S. The family includes three adult children, Ann, Joe, and Beth. All live far away, are married and raising children. Ann has come to visit her parents during her mother's hospitalization. Family history is significant in that when Mr. and Mrs. S. had their first child, Ann, Mrs. S.'s aging mother, who also had advanced heart disease, had been living with them for several years. At the time, Mr. S. felt that her mother should enter a home while Mrs. S. was strongly opposed. Eventually, Mrs. S. deferred to her husband's wishes. Her mother went to a nearby nursing home and died within a year. Mrs. S. feels the placement hastened her mother's demise and continues to blame her husband for forcing this "cruel decision." The family is in a stalemate about the current dilemma. Mr. S. and Ann are strongly opposed, while Joe and Beth, feel the physician's suggestion is correct and necessary.

1. *How is the multigenerational story of Mrs. S.'s mother critical to understanding this case? How might it affect each family member's feelings about placing Mrs. S. in a nursing home?*
2. *Would you have a family meeting? How would you decide whether to include Mrs. S.? What about Joe and Beth, who are not in town?*
3. *How are gender norms a factor in this case? How might you address them with this family?*

4. *How are life cycle issues (e.g., couple in later life, adult children in child-rearing phase with aging parents) pertinent, and how would you make them part of the consultative process?*

5. *What do you see as the choices for this family? How would you explore them in a collaborative manner?*

CASE 5

Bill, a highly competent first-year pediatric resident, sought brief therapy complaining of intense feelings of guilt and anger toward his mentally retarded brother and his parents, which had surfaced a few months after starting his residency. During the initial visit he exclaimed, "No matter what I do, I never feel I can do enough to make everyone happy." Bill grew up in a working-class family as the oldest son, and the first of his family with a college education. He was the family "success story." His family situation was compounded by his father's seeing the disabled son as a source of shame. Bill was aware that his choice to become a pediatrician was motivated partly by his deep desire to overcome his feelings of well-sibling survivor guilt by helping other children with chronic disorders.

1. *Using this vignette as a stimulus, consider your own multigenerational family history regarding illness and loss. Is there an illness story that stands out? How were you involved? How has this experience affected you, in particular your choice to become a health professional? Are there aspects of this experience that are a source of strength? Any that are a source of fear or vulnerability? In what clinical situations do you think this experience might come to the fore, and in what ways?*

—————— RECOMMENDED READINGS ——————

Families, Systems, and Health: The Journal of Collaborative Family Health Care (formerly *Family Systems Medicine*).

> This is the only journal that is interdisciplinary and devoted to the area of families and health, with a particular focus on models of collaboration. Topics include family or systems approaches to chronic and life-threatening illness. Formats include: review articles, clinical research, theory, commentary, and dialogue. For subscription information contact: *Families, Systems and Health* Subscription Department, P.O. Box 460, Vernon, NJ 07462.

McDaniel S, Hepworth J, Doherty W (eds): *Medical Family Therapy: A Biopsychosocial Approach to Families with Health Problems.* New York, Basic Books Inc, 1992.

> This book does an excellent job of describing the various uses and roles for family consultation and therapy in a variety of healthcare contexts and medical situations.

Rolland JS: *Families, Illness, and Disability: An Integrative Treatment Model.* New York, Basic Books Inc, 1994.

> Rich with practical clinical detail, this book provides a much fuller description of the Family Systems–Illness Model outlined in this chapter. Includes separate chapters on assessment and treatment issues for families, couples, and common personal issues and strains for clinicians working with chronic and life-threatening illness. Nominated by American Medical Writers Association as Book of the Year.

CHAPTER 13

Counseling and Behavioral Change

Larry B. Mauksch

CASE 13-1

Dr. Jacobson entered the room of his patient, Mr. Lawford. During the last 2 years Mr. Lawford gained 20 pounds and had rising blood pressure. Dr. Jacobson was concerned about these changes and wanted to help his patient address them before more serious health problems emerged. Dr. Jacobson expressed curiosity about Mr. Lawford's day-to-day activities. Mr. Lawford described working long hours with burgeoning responsibilities in recent years. He used to exercise at least four times a week and now was lucky to exercise once on the weekend. Neither of his parents exercised and both of them had been overweight. His father worked hard as a plumber, retired 5 years ago, and died 1 year later at 67 of a heart attack. Although Mr. Lawford acknowledged his weight gain, decreased exercise, and stress at work, he was not concerned about his health.

—————— EDUCATIONAL OBJECTIVES ——————

By the end of this chapter the learner should be able to:

1. Define the basic attributes of the effective physician-counselor
2. Describe one model of change, namely, *motivational interviewing*
3. Define the contextual factors affecting patient behavior
4. Describe why physicians and mental health professionals benefit from working together

5. Demonstrate the use of questioning to determine the patient's readiness for change
6. Perform reflective listening
7. Demonstrate establishing focus in counseling
8. Define the BATHE model of counseling
9. Demonstrate interview skills to assess relationships within the patient's family
10. Demonstrate skills for working with mental health professionals

---

INTRODUCTION

In Case 13-1 Dr. Jacobson is faced with a challenge. What skills will be useful in helping his patient? Whose responsibility is it to muster the motivation to change, the physician's or the patient's? Most people go to their physician first for help with mental health and life-style concerns (Schurman *et al.*, 1985). Requests for help sometimes come disguised as complaints about physical ails. Physicians who work effectively with these patients are sometimes said to practice "the art of medicine." The use of the term *art* gives the medical trainee a mixed message. Artists have innate talent. This leaves students wondering if they will be fortunate to manifest this talent. An alternative perspective to the "art of medicine" view is a skill-based perspective.

The skills and knowledge described in this chapter are useful to physicians, irrespective of the setting, medical discipline, or length of time spent with patients. Although psychiatrists and primary care physicians may employ these skills more often than others, all physicians are confronted with patients who are noncompliant or fearful or simply need support in dealing with health problems. Physicians who master these skills promote healing in their patients.

Mastering psychosocial skills has practical value beyond enhancing the quality of care. At least half of high users of medical services have psychiatric diagnoses (Katon *et al.*, 1992). Neglecting the mental health of these patients usually means spending more dollars on duplicated and overdone medical assessments, unnecessary procedures, and hospital admissions. As this country moves rapidly into a capitated healthcare system, the large volume of dollars spent on unnecessary medical service comes from physicians' pockets. Frustration in dealing with complicated patients who are high users of medical service can sour medical practice. Physician job satisfaction is compromised by fears of malpractice litigation. Moreover, the strongest hedge against malpractice litigation is the formation of a strong physician–patient relationship (Beckman *et al.*, 1994). The integration of counseling skills into the physician's repertoire promotes better care for patients, cost savings, and greater physician job satisfaction.

BEHAVIORAL CHANGE AND THE PHYSICIAN-COUNSELOR

Mental health professionals have their version of the light bulb joke. Namely, how many psychotherapists does it take to change a light bulb? Answer: Only one, *but* the light bulb must want to change.

To many people around the world, Western physicians have the reputation of being miracle workers. However, it is easy to lose sight of the role patients play in the process of change. While we focus on the dramatic effects of new surgeries or medications, we forget that for each medical success there is a patient who has consented to treatment and followed a prescribed protocol. Transplant surgeons have learned to consult mental health professionals to assess and prepare patients for difficult surgeries (Leedham *et al.*, 1995). They recognize that the patient is an essential part of the team. In less dramatic circumstances the same is true. The best diagnostician and medical therapist is ineffectual without a patient who believes in the treatment and is willing to participate in therapy. Hypertension, often called "the silent killer," is a good example. While it is easy to diagnose and treat most cases of hypertension, only half the people treated will follow a physician's advice after 1 year (Clark, 1991). Those who aspire to help people make changes in their lives should be on guard for those patients who believe that physicians can do it all. During their training, psychotherapists are taught that the patient's motivation to change should equal or surpass the psychotherapist's desire for change. When physicians believe they "can do it all" they exhaust themselves and eventually resent their patients.

Why do people change? Attempts to answer this question have filled volumes over centuries. While no easy answer exists, we do know that certain ingredients increase the likelihood of change. First, people have to identify a reason to change. Simply doing something different because one is told what to do does not motivate most people to change. Reasons to change come in different forms. Sometimes a major life event like marriage, birth, or death alters one's perspective. A major illness affecting an individual or a significant other may prompt change. Sometimes new information, like the connection between smoking and cancer, creates the incentive to change.

Second, people have to believe in their capacity to change. While many people know why they ought to change, they may lack the confidence to proceed. "I think I can, I think I can," the words of *The Little Engine That Could*, is an example of one storyteller's appreciation of this principle. Contemplating how to instill confidence in patients desiring to change leads to a third essential ingredient. Change is facilitated by supportive networks of family, friends, and, hopefully, healthcare providers.

Attributes of the effective (physician) counselor are described in texts spanning all of the helping and healthcare professions (Patterson, 1986; Wilson *et al.*, 1991). These attributes help create a relationship in which the patient can feel safe. Interpersonal safety, the sense that one will be cared for and not judged, is an essential prerequisite for the exploration of feelings and ideas about which one feels vulnerable. These attributes include:

- A respectful and nonjudgmental presence
- Accurate empathy
- Skillful listening
- A belief in the patient's capacity to change and grow
- Willingness to find a way to like the patient

A professional stance that is helpful to patients but protects providers from becoming overly responsible for creating change is *curiosity*. It is hard to be curious and authoritarian at the same time. When a patient is approached by a physician who is genuinely curious, the patient is more likely to feel cared for and willing to be vulnerable. Patients who have curious physicians begin to be curious about themselves, their beliefs and behaviors. Genuine curiosity expressed by the physician, not to be confused with coercion, is unlikely to compromise the patient's sense of autonomy.

Physicians who skillfully counsel their patients have an ability to measure a patient's readiness for change. Offering interventions requiring motivational levels higher than the patient possesses runs the risk of alienating the patient, creating guilt, inadequacy, and even resentment. The physician confronted with a patient who stumbled after being forced down the path to change may be left feeling disappointed and deflated in her attempts to provide assistance.

CASE 13-1 (*continued*)

Dr. Jacobson is confronted with a difficult situation. Mr. Lawford has a paternal history of heart disease and appears to be using his father as a model for his behavior. The weight gain, decreased exercise, rising blood pressure, and increased work stress combined with a family history devoid of health-conscious role models suggests that Mr. Lawford's health is at significant risk. However, he reveals no sign of concern.

Dr. Jacobson expressed awareness that things must be stressful for his patient. He then asked what Mr. Lawford's workday was like. Mr. Lawford rarely took time for lunch or other breaks. He "ate on the run" and frequently went to the company store for snacks. In response to Dr. Jacobson's appreciation of the hurried work pace, Mr. Lawford noted that he felt out of control. He had never considered how eating and rushing were linked. Dr. Jacobson shared the idea that his patient's behavior seemed similar to what his father had done. This comparison interested Mr. Lawford, who then pondered the comparison and expressed concern about the long-term implications of continuing this pattern. As time was limited, Dr. Jacobson ended the interview with a request for a follow-up appointment in 2 weeks. He expressed appreciation to Mr. Lawford for talking with him.

At their next meeting, Dr. Jacobson asked Mr. Lawford about the good things and less good things of his eating and exercise patterns. Mr. Lawford noted that the major advantage of decreased exercise and missing lunch was increased time for work. After a long pause, he also questioned this advantage. When Dr. Jacobson acknowledged this confusion, Mr. Lawford admitted that he didn't always work in the most creative or efficient fashion. He added that he realized that his behaviors were not healthy. Dr. Jacobson asked for clarification. With obvious sadness, Mr. Lawford admitted that he did not want his life cut short as happened to his farther. His father had been gone a lot during his childhood and adolescent years. He expressed grief about the death of his father and fear that he might miss time with his family.

At this point Dr. Jacobson summarized their discussion and again expressed appreciation and empathy to Mr. Lawford. Dr. Jacobson asked Mr. Lawford if he wanted help adjusting his life-style to promote a healthier and longer life. Mr. Lawford said yes and agreed to return in 2 weeks to make specific plans for change.

ASSESSING READINESS FOR CHANGE AS A GUIDE FOR TREATMENT

The Transtheoretical Model of change describes stages of readiness for people in a variety of clinical situations, including smoking, alcohol abuse, drug abuse, weight gain,

273

ASSESSING
READINESS FOR
CHANGE AS A
GUIDE FOR
TREATMENT

Table 13.1
The Transtheoretical Model of Change

Precontemplation:	Not thinking about behavior change
Contemplation:	Considering the possibility and value of change *but* feeling ambivalence that includes consideration of the disadvantages of change
Preparation:	A commitment to change exists and the effort is imminent
Action:	A plan to change is implemented
Maintenance:	Sustained change, usually lasting longer than 6 months
Relapse:	Return to an old behavior pattern

exercise avoidance, safe sex/condom use, and sunscreen use (Prochaska *et al.*, 1994). Developed in the early 1980s by Prochaska and DiClemente (Prochaska & DiClemente, 1982), this model has six stages (see Table 13.1).

Rather than thinking of readiness for change as occurring in discrete stages, Miller and Rollnick (1991) suggest it be viewed on a continuum. They have developed a progression of strategic questions. These questions serve two functions. First, they are tools to assess the patient's degree of readiness. Second, they are designed to gently motivate the patient to move to states of greater readiness. They name their approach *motivational interviewing*. The value of these strategies is drawn from five foundational concepts that are a unique and creative synthesis of useful approaches transcending a variety of counseling protocols (see Table 13.2). Combined, these general principles promote respectful ways to help people help themselves. Successfully translating this approach into action requires training and practice. Physicians who use this approach become skilled at gauging a patient's readiness for change. All too often, providers push for change before the patient is ready.

What should the physician do when she is concerned about an aspect of the patient's life, e.g., smoking, exercise, relationship conflict, drug use? Miller and Rollnick's (1991) progression of questions includes the following approaches. A curious question about how the patient's life-style, health, and daily activities involve the behavior in question will

Table 13.2
General Principles of Motivational Interviewing

1. *Express empathy.* The empathic physician conveys acceptance of the patient, making it easier for the patient to feel safe in experimenting with change.
2. *Develop discrepancy.* Physicians help patients contrast where they are and where they want to be. This process is done in a respectful, curious, and patient fashion. It is the patient who must make the comparisons and acknowledge discrepancies between current patterns and long-term goals. Physicians often make the mistake of doing this for patients, which easily results in creating guilt and alienation.
3. *Avoid argumentation.* Motivational interviewing uses "soft confrontation" through curious inquiry about the patient's decision to maintain behaviors that compromise health. However, the physician should avoid trying to convince the patient that he or she has a problem. Coercion creates resistance and defensiveness.
4. *Roll with resistance.* Remember that the decision to change is made by the patient. Hesitance is normal and predictable and exists for a reason. Its purpose should be explored and respected. Often the acceptance and examination of resistance reveals a new understanding of the world. This perceptual shift may decrease resistance.
5. *Support self-efficacy.* The physician must believe in the patient's capacity to change. This belief fosters confidence in the patient's ability to cope with the challenges of change. The physician empowers the patient through supportive, encouraging, and tolerant responses.

offer a glimpse of readiness. "Tell me about your day-to-day activities. How does smoking fit in?" Those who acknowledge ambivalence may be able to compare what Miller and Rollnick call "the good things and the less good things" about the behavior in question. "What are some good things about smoking and some not so good things about smoking?" Patients who are able to discriminate the benefits from the deficits of a behavior may be ready to receive some information. This should be confirmed first: "Would you like some information about the effect of smoking on health?" For patients who are clearly ready to discuss the problematic aspects of a behavior, ask about their concerns. "What concerns do you have about smoking?" When concerns are expressed, the final step before creating a plan is to ask, "You sound concerned about the effect of smoking on your health. What do you want to do next?" At this point you will hear a commitment to change or more ambivalence. Sorting through ambivalence is necessary, predictable, and normal, although time-consuming. The patient who is encouraged to examine his goals in contrast to current behaviors will fare better than the patient who is pressured to change.

The continuing saga of Mr. Lawford in Case 13-1 illustrates several ingredients of a successful counseling encounter beginning with curious, empathic, and reflective listening. Dr. Jacobson's pace and choice of questions combined with skillful listening demonstrate his effort to assess the patient's readiness for change. He trusted that helping his patient carefully examine his decisions in the context of their long-term implications would foster a reevaluation of his behaviors. Once Mr. Lawford acknowledged clear concern about the future, a contract for change could be negotiated.

CASE 13-2

Dr. Fred Richard entered the room of his next patient, Ms. Laura Thompson.

DR. R: *Hello, Laura, how are you doing? How can I help you today?*

MS. T: *(Looking up briefly, smiles, then eyes drift to the floor) Well . . . OK. I want to try to quit. But I'm afraid I'll fail again.*
(Ms. Thompson had tried to quit smoking on three occasions, each effort lasting at least 6 months but never longer than a year. The most recent relapse occurred a few months ago.)

DR. R: *Quitting has been hard for you. (Noting to himself that she seems subdued)*

MS. T: *Yeah, there is always something that gets in the way.*

DR. R: *Something that gets in the way . . . I'm not sure I understand.*

MS. T: *Sooner or later something gets to me . . . and I get stressed out.*

DR. R: *So something in your life gets hard, and that makes staying away from cigarettes a challenge.*

COUNSELING SKILLS

REFLECTIVE LISTENING

The most important counseling skill to learn is often simply described in one word—listening. If we expand the name of this skill by calling it *reflective* listening, the core listening behaviors become more explicit. The skilled listener incorporates four skills, which can be remembered with the acronym LUCE (listen, understand, clarify, energy).

Listen. The skilled practitioner conveys interest and understanding with nonverbal behaviors such as eye contact, head nodding, and a focused body position. Many behaviors are destructive to listening such as looking around the room, standing for long periods of time, folding arms, and clock watching.

Understand. Paraphrasing the speaker conveys an understanding of what is heard or perceived, as Dr. R. demonstrated in Case 13-2. This is the heart of reflection. True understanding builds compassion. Another benefit of reflection is overlooked by many. *Reflected statements force the speaker to listen to himself.* People who seek professional help are frequently stuck in efforts to solve a problem. They go over and over the same ideas, not progressing beyond an invisible barrier. Hearing the sequences of one's own thought forces the speaker to evaluate his reasoning and feelings. The famous "pregnant pause" often occurs after sensitive, accurate reflections. Comfort with silence, at least 5 seconds, is crucial to this process. The patient feels compelled to carry ideas and questions to more evolved states. To beginners, offering reflections and tolerating silence is awkward and slow. Many trainees admit feeling guilty for charging patients for reflective listening. "I didn't do anything" is the frequent novice report.

Two dynamics may interfere with reflective listening, namely, listener disagreement and mixed messages. Efforts to show understanding may be more difficult if the speaker's message conflicts with the listener's beliefs. Remember that understanding is not synonymous with agreement.

The listener should reflect back to the speaker verbal and nonverbal messages. Sometimes verbal and nonverbal messages are incongruent. For example, while frowning, a patient may report feeling "great." Conversely, a patient may describe life as "awful" while wearing a smile. In these situations it is wise to reflect the painful portion of the message. If incongruent messages persist, try reflecting both the verbal and nonverbal messages and then acknowledge confusion. Incongruent communication patterns are often born in families where the honest expression of feelings or ideas is discouraged.

Clarify. When the message is unclear or confusing, it is best to ask for clarification. The listener may experience feeling lost, not being able to trace the speaker's progression of reasoning. Confusion may be caused by the speaker switching topics, going on tangents, or lapsing into stories where the meaning is not apparent. Novice physicians will assume that the confusion is the result of a lapse in their own concentration. Most of the time this is not the case. The listener's need for clarification may come from the speaker making a "leap" in reasoning. The novice listener may assume an understanding of the reasoning leap. Whether correct or not, the listener may unwittingly perpetuate dysfunctional thought patterns if clarification is not requested. Whatever the cause, trust yourself. Your confusion is usually diagnostic of confusion within the speaker.

Energy. The effective listener puts energy into the relationship. Therapeutic listening is not a passive process. The listener should track the speaker's thought patterns and emotions. Empathy and compassion require energy. It takes energy to monitor one's own emotions, and keep them separate from the experience of the speaker. While listening requires the expenditure of energy, it need not be draining. Experienced healthcare providers regularly leave therapeutic interactions feeling energized. The patient feels an enhanced sense of responsibility and motivation. Helping another person help herself is an honor with its own rewards.

The interview between Dr. Richard and Ms. Thompson, the woman who wants to stop smoking but noted that "sooner or later something gets to me" causing a relapse, continues:

DR. R: *Something gets to you . . . ?*

MS. T: *I don't enjoy my work. It's boring and I don't feel valued. I want to get a new job but don't ever seem to do anything about it. The money is too important.*

DR. R: *So your job is not satisfying but it's been hard to look for something else. Anything else?*

MS. T: *My husband and I don't get along. Also, I worry about my daughter. She has a boyfriend who mistreats her.*

DR. R: *You and your husband have some difficulties and you are troubled about your daughter. That sounds like two concerns.*

MS. T: *Yeah, my husband smokes more than I do.*

DR. R: *I see. Is this a separate concern from you and your husband not getting along? Or is this part of what makes it hard for the two of you?*

MS. T: *Well, we fight about other things too. He won't clean up his mess and won't do the laundry. I end up doing too much work.*

DR. R: *It sounds like you and your husband are having a hard time for several reasons. Outside of your marriage, your concerns at work, and worries about your daughter, does anything else concern you?*

MS. T: *I wish we made more money, but we get by. It is hard to save and I am tired of living from month to month.*

DR. R: *I see. Anything else?*

MS. T: *Not that I can think of.*

DR. R: *That is a lot of stuff to be thinking about, to have going around and around in your head.*

MS. T: *Sometimes I just feel worn down and it is just too much.*

DR. R: *I suggest that we make a list of all your concerns. Maybe if you didn't think about them together, but in separate parts, things might be easier to handle. After you chip away at the parts, one at a time, it might be easier to work on stopping the smoking. How does that sound?*

MS. T: *OK, that makes sense.*

ESTABLISHING FOCUS

Eugene Gendlin, Ph.D., proposes that identifying a focus is at the heart of psychological change (Gendlin, 1981). Establishing focus accomplishes several things. The inability to define discrete, manageable problem areas is characteristic of many who are depressed and anxious. People jump from issue to issue, avoiding a commitment to solving any one problem. When counseling bogs down or goes around in circles, a common cause is a lack of focus. In these situations, the counselor may be drawn into the patient's nonfocusing patterns. Defining a focus makes the counseling process more satisfying for patient and provider. Satisfaction comes, in part, because defining a focus provides direction including setting a goal for treatment. The pursuit of a mutually agreeable and definable goal promotes responsibility in the patient and instills hope in the provider and the patient. Possessing hope means one is oriented toward the future instead of dwelling in the past, blaming others for one's difficulties. Finally, defining focus enhances efficiency and therefore helps control cost.

Case 13-2, which might appear complicated, portrays a common human feature. People desiring to change must address multiple layers of an issue that intersect in a unique way. When these layers are dissected and then individually addressed, change will flow more easily. The inexperienced clinician will focus only on the first identified problem (smoking, drinking, exercise avoidance) and not recognize and address other unresolved issues that block change of the identified behavior. When uncovered, these newer issues become, for a time, the focus of treatment. For Ms. Thompson in Case 13-2, communication skills in the relationship with her husband became the focus.

Eight useful skills needed to establish focus in counseling are:

1. *Make a list.* Before delving into any one problem area, make a list of all concerns you can elicit from the patient. This means *never* accepting the first answer when inquiring about a patient's concerns. Many people need to be convinced that their physician is genuinely interested in their feelings and concerns. Issues that come out on the second, third, or fourth request ("anything else?") are often associated with more pain and confusion than initially evident. After each request for a new item, wait 4 or 5 seconds. This skill is useful for physicians in all facets of practice. It helps avoid the dreaded statement, "Doctor, by the way, there is one other thing" as you have your hand on the doorknob, about to leave the room.

2. *Place the development of the physician–patient relationship above the need to establish focus.* People need to be heard. At times, usually during a crisis or early in the formation of the physician–patient relationship, it is wise to delay the pursuit of focus. When the patient expresses a lot of emotion or describes a traumatic event, it is best to do one thing—listen. People wishing to change have the need to tell their stories. The patient's story will include many of the issues later organized in a list of concerns. The perceptive physician will be patient and curious, internally making a list of the concerns a patient expresses as his story unfolds. Being patient, allowing the patient to be understood, remembering LUCE, builds trust. The patient will be better able to focus once his story has been told.

3. *Ask the patient to prioritize the list.* Once you are satisfied that the patient has no more concerns to list, (a) review the entire list of concerns, (b) let the patient know that each concern deserves attention and, if the list is too long, determine which issue to address first, and (c) if the patient is able to see links, themes, or patterns that transcend issues on the list, acknowledge these and then ask, "Where is the best place to start?" Sometimes the patterns or themes will become a new area of focus. For example, a patient may complain of problems in relationships at work and then at home. After separating and prioritizing these problems, it may become apparent that the patient lacks conflict negotiation skills and even avoids conflict. Two new items on the list may be learning conflict management skills and examination of how conflict was handled in the family of origin.

4. *Express your concerns about particular issues.* Sometimes you may have a concern that the patient does not list or has placed at a low priority. For example, if your concern is about domestic violence, substance abuse, suicidal thought, or chest pain, you are ethically and legally obliged to pursue these problems. In these situations it is *always* important to acknowledge the patient's priorities before expressing your concerns. A common provider mistake is to assert one's own priorities over the patient's. This "pro-

vider-centered" approach risks missing the area of greatest concern to the patient. The patient may feel discounted or misunderstood. In such cases, the patient is less likely to follow through with plans that are imposed. The physician, not understanding the dynamics, then labels the patient "noncompliant." If you feel that you know what the "real problem" is, but it is not a life-or-death issue, wait for a timely opportunity to express your idea. You may find that your chief concern is, after all, not as important as that which the patient has identified.

5. *Incorporate the patient's way of thinking (belief system) and language into your interview.* Western medicine and psychology have their own language and collection of theories that may not fit for the patient. Starting the counseling process using the patient's language and "explanatory model" is respectful and essential in forming what psychotherapists call a therapeutic alliance (Like & Steiner, 1986). Maintain a curious stance.

6. *When possible, place problems in an interpersonal context.* A large proportion of behavioral and psychological problems are connected to relationship dynamics. Three common relational arenas are (a) the family of origin, (b) the nuclear family, or (c) the school or work setting. Change, dysfunction, or loss in relationships are causes underlying much of the depression and anxiety in patients. Treatment design should consider the perspectives and life experiences of others whose behavior has an impact on your patient. When possible, include important people in counseling sessions (see Chapter 6, "Family Systems," in *Fundamentals of Clinical Practice*).

7. *Seek confirmation and commitment.* When the list appears complete and is prioritized and when the necessary negotiations have occurred, describe the list to the patient to check for accuracy. If the patient confirms your understanding, then request a commitment from the patient to work on the top identified problem. It is easy to assume that when a list of concerns is developed and prioritized, the patient is ready to work on the top item. As noted earlier, many people experience ambivalence during the contemplation phase of change.

8. *Regularly request evaluation of the counseling process.* After the work on an identified area of concern has begun, ask the patient about two issues, namely, (a) is the counseling helpful? and (b) are you addressing the most important issue? Remember that the physician–patient relationship is hierarchical. As a physician you have more power and are less vulnerable. Patients may not feel comfortable expressing displeasure with the process, yet they may have valuable suggestions about how you can help them. As your discussion progresses, the patient may feel finished with an identified topic. Your experience may be boredom or loss of focus. Ask if the identified topic still feels relevant. This provides the patient with the opportunity to reevaluate her own priority of issues.

THE BATHE APPROACH

BATHE is an acronym for five approaches that rely on listening and establishing focus as a foundation. Psychologist Marion R. Stuart, Ph.D., and family physician Joseph A. Lieberman, M.D., have developed BATHE to help physicians "structure effective and efficient psychotherapeutic interventions" (Stuart & Lieberman, 1993). The acronym is a clever mnemonic because it conjures up images of immersing the patient in a cleansing process. The questions included in the BATHE approach may be used to start visits and in response to a patient's request for help. Here we examine what constitutes "BATHEing" a patient.

B reminds you to examine the *background* of the patient. Stuart and Lieberman suggest using the question, "What is going on in your life?" This question begins to establish a focus by asking the patient to describe important life events. Gaining insight into current and past life experiences is essential to understanding and placing the patient's response in an appropriate context.

A reminds you to attend to the *affect* of the patient. Stuart and Lieberman recommend asking, "How do you feel about what is going on?" Helping patients identify and describe feelings is as central to counseling as balance is to riding a bicycle. Left unexpressed, feelings that build up create anxiety and depression. Stored emotions are eventually expressed in some fashion, but often in a way that is out of control. These out-of-control expressions of emotion can erode self-esteem or damage relationships, worsening the patient's situation.

Many people do not use a "feeling language." Words such as *sad, lonely, scared, inadequate,* and *disappointed* are not evident in the way they describe troubles. Even in response to a direct question about feelings, many will answer with a statement about how they *think.* Consistently asking "How are you feeling?" or "How is this for you?" will help them learn to identify and express their feelings. Sometimes even asking about specific feelings is necessary because it teaches a vocabulary of feelings. An empathic reflection ("You were sad when your friend left") or an empathic inquiry ("I imagine you were sad when your friend left?") helps patients name their feelings.

T reminds you to ask what most *troubles* the patient. Asking "What about this situation troubles you the most?" will help establish focus. As discussed earlier, it is important to help patients name as many life concerns as possible. Grouping related issues and prioritizing them comes next.

H reminds you to ask how the patient is *handling* the problem. The answer to this question provides information about what has and has not worked to solve the problem. Common areas to address to improve "handling" problems include: family relationships, thought patterns, educational issues, and underappreciated strengths and successes. These areas will be discussed next.

Family Relationships

Patients may have difficulty in managing relationships. Helping patients learn communication and negotiation skills is helpful (see Chapter 11). Patients may not recognize that their emotional pain extends from relationship dynamics in nuclear families or families of origin. The patient may be assuming disproportional responsibility for family problems. Others in the family may have unappreciated painful feelings. In these cases, including spouses, parents, and children in counseling is a productive and efficient means of facilitating change (McDaniel *et al.,* 1990).

Thought Patterns

It is prudent to assess the thought patterns of patients. People who experience anxiety or depression often create self defeating ("I'm not smart enough"), self-deprecating ("I'm not attractive"), and catastrophic ("I'll get fired") thoughts. In a parallel manner, these patients imagine that they are seen in a negative way by others ("He doesn't think I am capable" or "She doesn't care how I feel"). Dysfunctional family patterns are often the source of these negative thoughts. Negative thoughts create emotional pain. Helping patients become aware of their negative thoughts, learn ways to stop creating them, and replace them with self-accepting thoughts decreases emotional pain. This approach, named *cognitive therapy*, is effective in the treatment of depression and anxiety (Burns, 1980).

Educational Issues

Education helps motivated patients who lack the knowledge about how to handle stressful life circumstances. For example, physicians can teach parenting skills to struggling parents, communication skills to couples, or even basic financial management skills.

Underappreciated Strengths and Successes

Patients may not recognize their own strengths and successes. Dwelling on failures and hopelessness can take on a life of its own. Pessimistic views of the world may become self-fulfilling prophecies. In the last 15 years, psychotherapists have emphasized "solution-oriented" approaches (Berg, 1994). In essence, counselors help patients find "exceptions" to their failures. Examining the characteristics of these unusual successes and expanding their use is the strategy of counseling.

E reminds you that the expression of *empathy* validates the patient's feelings. Empathy is the oxygen of counseling. If it is not present, the counseling effort will suffocate.

CASE 13-3

Mr. Oakly developed a bleeding ulcer. In addition to direct medical management, his physician, Dr. Claren, thought it wise to learn about her patient's world. Mr. Oakly worked as a supervisor in a software company. He viewed his job as difficult because his supervisees needed to be "checked on constantly." Now, at age 45, Mr. Oakly was in his second marriage, in which he had his third child, 10-year-old Mark, and was the primary parent for his children from the first marriage, 17-year-old Craig and 16-year-old Julie. Julie had struggled through high school, failing a few courses, and had begun experimenting with alcohol. He and his second wife, Tricia, had developed marital problems and blamed their difficulties on Julie. Mr. Oakly admitted that it was hard to trust Tricia as a parent for his children, particularly his daughter. However, he did describe Tricia as a competent, loving person.

Mr. Oakly was the oldest child in a family where his father was absent much of the time. His mother was depressed during much of his childhood and drank alcohol excessively. He raised his two younger siblings. As an adult he was married at 24 and divorced at 30. He left his wife, Nancy, who abused alcohol and drugs and did not care for their two children.

Through asking questions about Mr. Oakly's relationships and life events, Dr. Claren constructed a genogram (Figure 13.1), a map of Mr. Oakly's relational world. In studying his family history, it became apparent to Mr. Oakly that he had difficulty trusting the work of others, particularly women, because of his experiences in his family of origin and his marriage. At work his supervisees felt that he "hovered" too much. Tricia complained about his interference in the

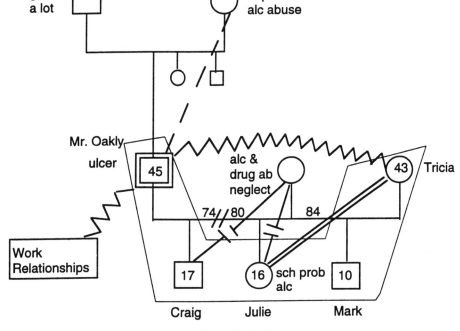

Figure 13.1. The Oakly family genogram.

relationship between she and Julie. Julie needed a supportive connection with an adult female. Mr. Oakly agreed to a meet with his wife and physician. Dr. Claren helped Mrs. Oakly express her frustration and concerns. During subsequent meetings that first included Julie and then all three children, the family acknowledged their love and concern for Mr. Oakly, but described him as "too controlling." He agreed to "pull back" and be more supportive of his wife's role in the family and more trusting of his children.

One year later Mr. Oakly was symptom-free. His daughter was doing better in her last year of high school. Mr. Oakly took his lessons from home into work. He felt relief in pulling back from hovering over his supervisees.

UNDERSTANDING PATIENTS
IN LARGER CONTEXTS

The biopsychosocial model (Engel, 1980) is a problem-solving method useful for many of the challenges in clinical medicine. This model, which is based in systems theory, served as the framework for Dr. Claren in helping Mr. Oakly and his family. While it is beyond the scope of this chapter to describe the biopsychosocial model and systems theory in detail, a few applications will be provided:

1. *If 2 + 2 ≠ 4, examine the patient in her surrounding contexts.* There are two

common examples of "things not adding up": (a) when symptoms persist after treatment is administered or (b) when the cause of symptoms is not apparent or does not make sense. Examples of surrounding contexts are: a marital or couple's relationship, the nuclear family, the family of origin, the work setting, the community, the culture. A large proportion, if not all, of human experience and human behavior is influenced by relationships in one of these domains. In Case 13-3, Mr. Oakly's family of origin and marital experience made it difficult for him to rely on women and to trust his supervisees.

2. *Look for circles and tree branches.* A patient's symptom can be seen as (a) part of a circular chain of events that go around and around or (b) created by several, seemingly independent causes converging to produce symptoms. Mr. Oakly's family contains an example of "circular causation." He interfered with the relationship between his wife and daughter. The absence of a female parent figure contributed to his daughter's behavioral and school problems. Mr. Oakly's effort to solve his daughter's problem created tension between him and his daughter and between him and his wife. Several sources of stress converging to create or inflame a symptom creates a tree branch design. This is known as multicausality. A combination of stresses, work difficulties, conflict with his daughter, conflict with his wife, worry about his daughter, in Mr. Oakly's life contributed to his ulcer symptoms.

3. *Families need effective leadership.* Systems need a hierarchical organization for optimal function. As a cell needs a nucleus, so does a family need effective parents. When parents are ineffective, absent, abusive or in conflict with one another, children often exhibit behavioral or emotional problems, e.g., school difficulties, fighting, stealing, withdrawal, disobedience, or physical symptoms, e.g., headaches, stomachaches, chronic illness, instability. Julie's symptoms are related to insufficient connections to a female parent and to conflict between her parents.

Using systems thinking to solve problems means looking for the interrelatedness of things. Two skills are helpful in making systemic assessments and initiating treatment: (a) asking relationship questions and (b) constructing a genogram.

RELATIONSHIP QUESTIONS

A relationship question asks the interviewee to think abut relationships and begins the process of examining a problem in context. A relationship question is created to test a hypothesis. For example, in knowing of Julie's problems in Case 13-3, Dr. Claren reasoned that relationships in her life may be troublesome. Dr. Claren was also curious about connections between Mr. Oakly's symptoms and his daughter's difficulties. A series of questions designed to assess the Oakly family might include: "Mr. Oakly, how are things between you and your daughter?"; "What is the relationship like between your wife and Julie?" Sometimes it is helpful to compare perspectives on a relationship. Noting differences can stimulate change. "How does Julie feel about Tricia as a stepmother?" "How is it for Tricia to be a stepparent for Julie?" "What has the relationship been like between Julie and her biological mother, Nancy?" The answers to these questions might reveal Julie's need for a female parent figure. It is useful to ask questions that include three parties. For example, "Mr. Oakly, how do you feel about Tricia as a parent for Julie?" Then, "How does Tricia feel when you prevent her from parenting Julie?"

These questions are particularly helpful to physicians who usually see only one person in a family but need to know about the perspectives of others. The use of these questions extends beyond family problems. Family beliefs and support, or lack thereof, have enormous influence on the course of chronic illnesses. For example, after suggesting dietary changes to an overweight man with hypertension, like Mr. Lawford in Case 13-1, it would be wise to ask, "How will it be for your wife to change her cooking?"

In summary, relationship questions are constructed in the following way: (1) They extend from the clinician's curiosity about the connection between relationship and symptoms. (2) Two or more people are included in each question. The person to whom the question is asked is not always the focus of the question. That is, you may ask one person about the relationship between two or more others. (3) Questions may also be constructed to compare perspectives between people. This is done by first asking for one person's perspective on a relationship and then asking for another person's perspective on the same relationship.

USING A GENOGRAM

Over the last 15 years the genogram has emerged as a versatile, efficient method for storing family information (McGoldrick & Gerson, 1985). In fact, a genogram, introduced in Chapter 6, "Family Systems" in *Fundamentals of Clinical Practice*, is more than just a record keeping device. Its maplike format forces the clinician and patient to view problems in context, essentially, to think systemically. Genograms help clinicians develop hypotheses that, in turn, guide treatment efforts.

The genogram is an adaptation of the pedigree or family tree used in genetics. In addition to basic family structure, it includes information about age, marital status, major illnesses, life events, and important relationships.

When familiar with genogram symbols, this format (see Figure 13.1) conveys a lot of information about Mr. Oakly and his family in Case 13-3. The jagged line between Mr. Oakly and Tricia and between Mr. Oakly and his work describes a conflictual relationship. The dashed line between Mr. Oakly and his mother describes a distant relationship. The lines between Craig, Julie, and their mother denote a "cut-off" relationship. The double line between Julie and Tricia describes a close relationship. The line surrounding Mr. Oakly, the children, and Tricia denotes the people living together with Mr. Oakly. This genogram displays the combination of stresses in the various relationships in Mr. Oakly's world. Imagine knowing nothing about Mr. Oakly before seeing this genogram. If you were told that Mr. Oakly suffered from a stress-related disorder, e.g., irritable bowel, hypertension, an ulcer, what would your reaction be? For most of us, possible causes jump off the page after viewing Mr. Oakly in this network of his relationships.

Genograms also describe pregnancies, including history of termination, miscarriage, or stillbirth, overclose relationships, major life events, religious information, and significant relationships with friends. The minimal time necessary to complete a detailed genogram is 12 to 15 minutes and revisions occur during subsequent visits. When physicians construct a genogram, patients feel cared for and understood. While it may not be practical to draw a genogram during every patient visit, there are certain times when it pays to do so. These times include the following situations:

1. When symptoms persist despite expected resolution
2. When symptoms do not make sense
3. When a severe or chronic illness is diagnosed
4. When there are psychosocial problems

CASE 13-4

Dr. Michaels finished performing the fourth termination of pregnancy for his patient, Ms. Stanley. During the procedure she was very tearful. In his office, after the procedure, they talked. In the back of Dr. Michaels's mind were Ms. Stanley's frequent visits to his office. Her life seemed to be in constant chaos. She described feeling overwhelmed in the last 6 months. Dr. Michaels asked if she would consider seeing a counselor. Ms. Stanley was afraid to talk with someone about her problems because she feared "falling apart" and being diagnosed as "crazy." Her family didn't believe in seeing "head doctors." Dr. Michaels explained that he worked with a family counselor, Mr. Phillips. He assured Ms. Stanley that she was not crazy nor would counseling make her crazy. He described the counseling process and the personal characteristics of Mr. Phillips. Ms. Stanley was assured that he (Dr. Michaels) would stay involved in her care. She agreed to meet the counselor. A few minutes later, Mr. Phillips was introduced to Ms. Stanley. Dr. Michaels summarized his concerns about Ms. Stanley to Mr. Phillips while Ms. Stanley listened. They made an initial follow-up appointment.

Six months later, Ms. Stanley had seen Mr. Phillips ten times and sorted out many of her issues. Her father had sexualized their relationship. He was gone from the home for long periods of time during her early childhood. When her parents divorced, he rarely saw the children, often not showing up when he promised to visit. As a teenager and young adult, Ms. Stanley had a series of relationships with abusive men. Therapy helped to build her self-esteem and become more selective in choosing men. Medical utilization decreased. Regular communications between Dr. Michaels and Mr. Phillips improved care and saved money. When Ms. Stanley spoke about physical problems to Mr. Phillips, he discussed these with Dr. Michaels, often saving unnecessary tests and visits. Each member of this treatment triangle regularly received input from two others, creating an atmosphere of stability and increased quality of care.

COLLABORATION BETWEEN —— NONPSYCHIATRIC PHYSICIANS AND —— MENTAL HEALTH PROFESSIONALS

There are several reasons why mental health professionals and medical providers should work together. Yet, significant barriers prevent collaboration between these two professional worlds.

Why should mental health providers and medical providers work together? The majority of mental health problems present first in the general medical arena. The highest healthcare users have a complicated mix of medical and psychosocial problems (Katon *et al.*, 1992). For a variety of reasons, most patients resist referrals "away" from their physician. However, when patients are referred to a mental health provider in the same clinic, referrals are more likely to be accepted. Mental health consultation and treatment improves quality of care and, if administered in limited doses, decreases overall healthcare costs (Mumford *et al.*, 1984). Beyond quality and cost savings, professional rewards are notable. Working in an interdisciplinary team provides a support and educational network.

How can the chasm between mental health and medicine be so great when there are so many reasons to work together? Seventeenth century Cartesian thought, often described as "mind–body dualism," has persisted in its influence (McDaniel, 1995). Despite what we know about the myriad of interactions between the mind and the body, healthcare systems still function as if these connections did not exist. Insurance benefits for mental health do not equal medical benefits, creating financial barriers to treatment (Glenn, 1987). Members of each profession have maintained derogatory stereotypes of one another. Mental heath care has always had stigma attached to it. Patients may not have family support for seeing a psychotherapist. Many patients somatize their psychological pain and reject the notion that psychosocial help is relevant. For these reasons and more it is hard to bring mental health and medicine together.

In the last 15 years a variety of books, articles, journals, and conferences have explored collaboration. Primary care training in family medicine, general internal medicine, and pediatrics includes behavioral science curricula. The vast majority of family medicine residencies have behavioral science faculty who help create collaborative practice models in training. The influx of managed care demands that professionals from all healthcare disciplines collaborate. The new catchphrase, "integrated care," expresses the need for professionals to educate one another and to avoid duplication of services. Because the majority of medical visits involve a psychosocial component, integrated care should include mental health professionals. Listed below are a few guidelines for collaboration:

1. *Arrange to have interdisciplinary teams working together in the same setting.* Working in the same setting ensures a level of communication between professionals that is otherwise impossible to maintain, as demonstrated in Case 13-4. This communication creates better care, saves money, and ensures interdisciplinary education.
2. *Let your patients know that you work as a part of a team.* Patients appreciate when providers communicate with each other to coordinate care.
3. *Work to develop relationships with collaborators.* Ongoing collaboration means ongoing work. This work includes respectful and open communication. Develop mechanisms that facilitate communication such as shared charts, interdisciplinary conferences, and office designs that create proximity instead of distance.
4. *Establish a shared purpose or vision for collaboration.* Ask yourself, "Why am I collaborating?" Ask your colleague, "Why is collaboration important to you?" Sharing these reasons strengthens relationships.
5. *Be suspicious of your feelings of distrust of another provider.* Complicated patients often deal with the world in a black-and-white way. They split relationships into "good guys" and "bad guys." This behavior, which is usually habitual, can create conflict between team members. In these situations it makes sense to communicate directly with other providers and avoid solely communicating through the patient.

CONCLUSION

In this chapter we have examined counseling and behavioral change. Effective counseling means mastering skills like empathic listening, reflective listening, and intentional curiosity. These are summarized in the acronym LUCE. Helping patients establish and maintain a focus in counseling creates an efficient and productive process. A useful way to organize a counseling approach is via BATHE, wherein reflection and focus are core components. Respecting individual, family, and cultural beliefs is critical in building respect and creating viable treatment plans. In the course of helping patients change behavior, it is essential to assess readiness for change. This assessment helps create realistic expectations of the patient, reducing "noncompliance" problems and physician–patient conflicts. Effective counseling requires an ability to monitor the physician–patient relationship. It is essential to examine the patient in the context of important relationships, including the family of origin, the nuclear family, and the school and work setting. Relationship questioning and genograms are two useful tools for assessing relationships. The physician counselor must become an expert in relationships.

Physicians of the twenty-first century, along with other healthcare providers, will work in interdisciplinary teams. These teams can provide better care, save money, and create work atmospheres that maintain vitality and prevent provider burnout. In this regard, it is important to develop collaborative relationships with mental health professionals.

CASES FOR DISCUSSION

CASE 1

Mr. Anderson asked his physician, Dr. Maxwell, for help with recurrent sleep difficulties. He finds it hard to get to sleep. Once he falls asleep he stays asleep until 9:00 or 10:00 AM. Mr. Anderson, who is unemployed, spends much of his days sitting around. He naps frequently, watches TV, and rarely goes to bed before midnight. He drinks beer most evenings. His wife works a swing shift.

Following a series of questions in an interview directed by Dr. Maxwell, Mr. Anderson is told not to nap during the day and to cut down on his drinking. Three weeks later, Mr. Anderson returns, still complaining about sleep difficulty. He is still drinking most evenings and naps most days. He says, "Doc, it was hard to do those things you suggested."

1. *What approach would you use in working with this patient?*
2. *What are the disadvantages to being directive and prescriptive early on in treatment?*
3. *How would you assess this patient's stage of readiness?*
4. *What else might you want to know about the patient's family?*

CASE 2

A colleague asks you for some advice. He wants to learn counseling skills and has found a patient with whom he wants to work. However, he feels overwhelmed. During the first visit, his patient, a 35-year-old married mother of two boys, aged 2 and 4, noted the following concerns: parenting difficulties with the 2-year-old, some symptoms of depression including lethargy, sleep disturbance, weight gain, and dysphoria. She also noted a lack of sexual interest from her husband, and some questions about her dormant professional life.

1. *Is this an appropriate patient for your physician colleague to counsel?*
2. *If so, what advice would you offer in response to your colleague's feelings of being overwhelmed? If not, how should the physician handle the next visit?*
3. *Would you refer this patient to a mental health professional?*

CASE 3

Mr. and Ms. Foreman come to you with concerns about their 12-year-old daughter, Rachel. One evening last week, after asking her to help clean the dinner table, she exploded. Loud objections and obscenities shocked the parents. Similar outbursts have occurred four or five times in the last year. Ms. Foreman and her husband appear to disagree about how to handle these situations, but both express concern and some anger about their daughter's behavior. Mr. Foreman notes that when he was a child his parents would never have tolerated such behavior. "I would have felt someone's hand," he said. "That kind of discipline doesn't work," fired back Ms. Foreman.

The Foremans are a family of six. The oldest child is a 15-year-old boy. Rachel is the next oldest, with younger sisters aged 9 and 7. Ms. Foreman doesn't work outside of the home, but is very involved in community activities related to their children's interests. Mr. Foreman works long hours as a civil engineer and has to travel frequently. The Foremans report having had similar difficulties with their oldest child when he was about 13.

1. *Construct a genogram and consider what information is missing.*
2. *What hypotheses can you formulate about this family's difficulties?*
3. *What relationship questions would you want to ask to test your hypotheses?*

CASE 4

A 35-year-old patient, Mr. Rosner, has made several visits to you in the last 6 months. He has multiple physical complaints, most of which are unresponsive to your suggested treatments. You know that last year his wife was diagnosed with ovarian cancer. He has been assuming the bulk of family responsibilities, cleaning, paying bills, parenting. On today's visit he tells you about a series of anxiety attacks in the last few weeks. To calm himself down and help him sleep he is drinking one or two glasses of wine each night.

In the past you have suggested that Mr. Rosner consider counseling. He has never received this suggestion with much enthusiasm. Since his last visit, your practice has expanded to include a medical family therapist.

1. *What hypotheses do you have about the cause of Mr. Rosner's symptoms?*
2. *To determine the effect of his behavior on the family, what relationship questions would you construct?*
3. *You decide that it would be helpful to share this case with your new family therapist colleague, but feel leery about suggesting the referral because of Mr. Rosner's prior disinterest in counseling. How would you approach this referral with Mr. Rosner? Would you consult with the family therapist first?*

CASE 5

You receive a call from Dr. Reed, a local psychologist, about Richard McClure, a 14-year-old patient of yours. Richard was referred by a school counselor to Dr. Reed for behavior problems and suspicion of drug abuse. Dr. Reed has just completed his first visit with Richard and would like to learn about his family from your experience working with them.

You know that Mr. McClure, Richard's father, has a history of alcohol abuse. He has had two marital separations and 1 year ago you prescribed an antidepressant for Mrs. McClure. You suspect that there are multiple family problems. Despite having concern about this family, you feel ineffective, indeed powerless, in your efforts to treat or refer them.

Now Dr. Reed is on the phone. You have three patients waiting and are 30 minutes behind, but you want to talk about your experience with this family and to learn from Dr. Reed how to help the McClures and others like them.

1. *What information do you share with Dr. Reed?*
2. *How can you arrange to keep in touch with him to learn about working with multiple-problem families?*
3. *What services can you offer to augment Dr. Reed's treatment effort?*

RECOMMENDED READINGS

Gendlin ET: *Focusing.* New York, Bantam Books, Inc, 1981.

> Focusing describes a simple, efficient counseling approach. It is an elegant way of helping patients define the sources and relative importance of stress. It is particularly helpful to patients making connections between body and mind. The book offers a concise description and includes a useful "handbook" section.

McDaniel S, Campbell T, Seaburn D: *Family-Oriented Primary Care: A Manual for Medical Providers.* New York, Springer-Verlag, 1990.

> This book is a well-written, practical guidebook for primary care physicians. The authors all work in family medicine, one physician trained in family therapy and two family therapists. Each chapter has a clear focus, providing practical guidelines for dealing with common problems in a family context, e.g., marital problems, depression, death and dying, and somatization. Each chapter ends with an outline summarizing clinical suggestions. This book is required reading for all of my family medicine residents.

Miller W, Rollnick S (eds): *Motivational Interviewing: Preparing People to Change Addictive Behavior.* New York, Guilford Press, 1991.

> This is an edited book with contributions from many experts in behavioral change and addictions. Some chapters are addressed specifically to physicians. For any physician who wishes to develop skills in working with life-style behaviors that jeopardize health, this text is one of the best available.

Stuart M, Lieberman J: *The Fifteen Minute Hour: Applied Psychotherapy for the Primary Care Physician,* ed 2. New York, Praeger Publishers, 1993.

> These authors developed the BATHE acronym from their experiences as a family physician (Lieberman) and psychologist-medical educator (Stuart). It is a well-written, practical introduction to psychotherapy for primary care physicians. It is an excellent library addition for any nonpsychiatric physician wishing to develop psychotherapeutic skills.

CHAPTER 14

Functional Assessment

Kathleen R. Farrell

CASE 14-1

Mr. Smith, an 82-year-old man with a history of dementia, hypertension, and osteoarthritis, visited the physician's office because of Mrs. Smith's concerns that her husband "hadn't been himself" lately. Questioning by the physician revealed that the patient had strained his back 2 weeks earlier while helping his wife move a table. When prompted, the patient complained of back pain, and Mrs. Smith reported that her husband now spent most of his time lying on a couch. His appetite diminished, he slept fitfully, and he had worsening constipation. Mrs. Smith needed to help her spouse with bathing and dressing. Two days before the visit, she borrowed a neighbor's cane for her spouse because he appeared unsteady when walking. Being frail herself, Mrs. Smith worried about her own health and inability to continue caring for her husband. She asked the physician if her husband needed placement in a nursing home.

On examination, Mr. Smith had marked kyphosis and point tenderness at the L1 and L2 spine levels. His gait was hesitant and unsteady. He held the borrowed cane incorrectly as he walked, and the physician observed that it was incorrectly adjusted for Mr. Smith's height. A rectal examination showed a large amount of hard stool in the rectal vault. Lumbar spine X rays revealed diffuse osteopenia with a new compression fracture at L1 and old fractures at T10 and L4.

Mr. Smith had become deconditioned and fecally impacted from back pain and inactivity. The physician prescribed analgesics for pain control and laxatives for the impaction. A social worker arranged for a home health aide to help Mr. Smith bathe, and a physical therapist organized an exercise program for him. A month later, Mr. Smith had minimal back pain and normal bowel movements. He displayed increased strength, endurance, and appetite. He walked independently with a pistol-grip cane correctly adjusted for his height.

———————— **EDUCATIONAL OBJECTIVES** ————————

On completion of this chapter, students should be able to:

1. Contrast the traditional medical model with the functional model
2. List five characteristics of geriatric patients that affect function
3. Define and list the components of functional assessment
4. List the Activities of Daily Living
5. List the Instrumental Activities of Daily Living
6. Describe the components of mobility
7. Describe the indications for and the correct use of common ambulatory devices
8. Describe how to evaluate gait and balance
9. Define comprehensive geriatric assessment
10. List five benefits of comprehensive geriatric assessment

———————— **INTRODUCTION** ————————

Case 14-1 illustrates a common situation that physicians encounter when treating older adults, namely, a patient who presents with multiple—and often ill-defined—problems. Rather than describing specific signs or symptoms, the patient or caregiver describes problems that reflect functional limitations. In Mr. Smith's case, he could no longer bathe, dress, or walk without help.

Many adults find functional limitations that affect their ability to perform previously habitual activities more bothersome than the disease or illness that caused those limitations. Their inability to perform ordinary activities, which they previously took for granted, translates into a loss of function and a loss of independence. Physicians play an important role in helping adults of all ages to adapt and cope with debilitating conditions. This chapter will describe how to recognize and successfully treat patients with functional problems. It will also describe instruments and techniques useful for evaluating functional skills, such as self-care and mobility. Although the chapter will focus on older adults, many of the functional principles and instruments its discusses can also apply to younger adults. Everyone has functional concerns and needs.

What is function? In the simplest sense, function is the ability to perform a given activity or role. Patients with normal function can dress and bathe themselves, drive, and use the telephone. Function becomes a concern to people when they lose it. Loss of function can be defined at more than one level (World Health Organization, 1980), as follows:

1. *Diseases,* such as diabetes or hypertension, cause loss of function via pathology at the cellular or molecular level. A person is often unaware of a disease at this stage.
2. *Impairments,* such as renal insufficiency or atherosclerosis, cause loss of function at the organ level. With an impairment, a person may develop signs or symptoms of the disease, but still can perform daily activities.
3. *Disabilities,* also called functional limitations, cause loss of physical function at the person level. With a disability, a person is aware of physical limitations while

performing activities. A person with hemiplegia from a stroke who can no longer walk or a person with blindness from diabetic retinopathy who can no longer drive are two examples of disability. Loss of function in this chapter will generally refer to disabilities, that is, loss of physical function.

4. *Handicaps* cause loss of function at the societal level by preventing a person from fulfilling expected roles. Handicaps are reversible problems if society addresses them. A blind person can travel independently if public signs are displayed in Braille. A paraplegic can work if wheelchair access is provided at the workplace.

Loss of function can occur at any or all of these levels, and it is often the first indication of disease or illness in an elderly patient. Even small changes in function can profoundly affect that person's independence and self-respect. Older people, when asked what they fear most, often respond "loss of independence," which may mean being unable to perform or enjoy everyday activities, needing help from others, or requiring nursing home placement—a common fear of many elderly patients.

In Case 14-1, Mrs. Smith and her husband shared these concerns. Mr. Smith had a functional decline that caused his wife to assume more of his care. Her presenting complaints focused on her husband's inability to perform physical activities such as bathing and dressing. Pain and deconditioning caused difficulty with self-care (a disability); compression fractures (an impairment) caused pain; osteoporosis (a disease) caused the compression fractures.

The traditional medical model focuses on disease, which presents as a single problem or as a well-defined constellation of signs and symptoms. Signs, such as melenic stools and skin pallor, direct the patient's workup toward causes of gastrointestinal blood loss. Symptoms, such as shortness of breath or chest pain, elicit a prompt search for cardiovascular or pulmonary disease. The medical model of disease works well for acute, reversible conditions, such as infections or metabolic abnormalities. It does not always work well for older adults or for younger adults with many disabilities.

Thus, the functional model, in addition to diagnosing and treating disease, incorporates *functional assessment* into the evaluation and treatment of a patient's health problems. Functional assessment, the systematic evaluation of a person's abilities, is useful in identifying the causes of functional decline and targeting goals for recovery. The standard history and physical, designed to diagnose disease, provides a general sense of patients' health; but it overlooks function, since patients with long problem lists may be functionally independent while those with short problem lists may be completely dependent on others. Measurement of physical skills complements the history and physical. In its strictest sense, functional assessment evaluates a person's physical abilities, e.g., self-care, household skills, and mobility.

The functional model is particularly useful to physicians caring for older adults, since such patients have unique characteristics and problems. For one, elderly patients often present with *nonspecific complaints*, such as weakness, falling, or "just not feeling well." In Mr. Smith's case, his wife's concern that "he wasn't himself" became more meaningful in the context of his functional decline. Older patients also present with *multiple problems*. Sorting through these problems, especially if complex, poses a challenge to physicians.

On the other hand, some older patients *underreport health problems* because they believe that these problems are a normal part of aging. Many older adults and their families accept without question that forgetfulness, incontinence, and hearing or visual impairment are the inevitable consequences of aging. Physicians are also susceptible to this bias, termed *ageism*, leading them to delete evaluations and treatments that could benefit older patients.

Atypical presentation of illness is another characteristic of older adults' health problems. For example, a patient with a urinary tract infection may present with confusion or falls instead of the classic dysuria or urinary frequency. Similarly, a patient who presents with weight loss may have an underlying depression rather than cancer. Even when an older patient's problem is well-defined, the problem is likely to have *multiple causes*. An older patient who falls probably has several contributing factors to the falls. Poor vision, side effects from medications, muscle weakness, and a cluttered house could all be cofactors.

Finally, older patients often have *chronic problems*, and these may require more attention than their acute problems. Most older persons have at least one chronic condition and many have several conditions. Of the ten most common chronic conditions reported by adults over age 65, half are problems with physical function: arthritis, hearing impairment, cataracts, visual impairment, and orthopedic impairments (Schick & Schick, 1994). Seeing, hearing, and walking are abilities most people take for granted—until lost.

In an acute model of care, illness occurs episodically, and treatment is cure-driven. Adults of all ages may suffer loss of function after an illness or injury. A person's independence and sense of well-being depend on his or her ability to adapt or cope with loss of function. For older adults or disabled younger adults, where a chronic model of care predominates, illness may be progressive or permanent, and treatment is restorative to whatever extent possible.

CASE 14-2

Mrs. Wilson, an 85-year-old widow, slipped on a patch of ice one winter day while getting her mail and fell. A neighbor heard her calls for help and found Mrs. Wilson complaining of right hip and thigh pain. She was taken to a nearby emergency room, diagnosed with a right hip fracture, and taken to surgery that evening to stabilize the fracture. Mrs. Wilson developed a postoperative confusion that slowly cleared. She also developed diarrhea from an antibiotic-associated colitis. Seven days after admission, Mrs. Wilson remained weak and required help with most of her self-care, including bathing, dressing, and toileting. She was also incontinent of urine and walked only with the help of two people.

Her physician consulted the rehabilitative services, including physical therapy, occupational therapy, and social work. The physical therapist worked with Mrs. Wilson every day to increase her bed and chair mobility and provided a front-wheel walker for support. The occupational therapist learned that Mrs. Wilson could dress herself when given a reacher to grab her clothes and a long-handled shoehorn to put on her shoes. The social worker contacted a nearby niece who was willing to help her aunt with errands on her return home. A short-term stay at a nearby nursing home was arranged for Mrs. Wilson to complete her rehabilitation.

Three weeks later, Mrs. Wilson returned home. She walked up to 50 feet at a time with a front-wheel walker. Home adaptive equipment, including a tub trans-

fer bench and raised toilet seat, were provided to make bathing and toileting easier for her. Meals-on-Wheels came daily.

293

ASSESSMENT OF
PHYSICAL
FUNCTION

——— ASSESSMENT OF PHYSICAL FUNCTION ———

ACTIVITIES OF DAILY LIVING

Case 14-2 illustrates another common situation, namely, a patient who suffers a functional decline during hospitalization. Functional assessment allows healthcare providers to recognize loss of function. Elderly patients, particularly if frail or lacking social support, may not fully recover from an illness or injury unless prompt interventions are taken to reverse the causes of decline.

Two categories of physical skills have been defined to provide physicians with a broader view of a person's capabilities. The first category, Activities of Daily Living (ADLs), are basic self-care skills that people of all ages and cultures habitually perform: feeding, walking, toileting, dressing, grooming, and bathing. Continence of bowel and bladder, while not functional activities in the same sense, are usually included as ADLs, since social independence requires both. Katz originally defined and measured these abilities after observing that elderly patients on rehabilitation units needed to perform certain physical activities before regaining their independence (Katz *et al.*, 1963). The Katz ADL scale, shown in Table 14.1, remains one of the most commonly used functional assessment instruments.

The Katz ADL scale measures independence in six physical skills: feeding, continence, transfer (the ability to get in and out of bed or chairs), toileting, dressing, and bathing. Independence with each skill usually means that a person can perform it without help from another person. A person who loses function usually loses physical skills in a predictable order: first bathing, then dressing, then toileting, followed by transferring,

Table 14.1
Basic Activities of Daily Living (ADLs)[a]

Activity	Independent	
Bathing (sponge bath, tub bath, or shower): receives either no assistance or assistance in bathing only one part of the body	Yes	No
Dressing: gets clothes and dresses without any assistance except for tying shoes	Yes	No
Toileting: goes to toilet room, uses toilet, arranges clothes, and returns without any assistance (may use cane or walker for support, and may use bedpan or urinal at night)	Yes	No
Transferring: moves in and out of bed and chair without assistance (may use cane or walker)	Yes	No
Continence: controls bowel and bladder completely by self (without occasional "accidents")	Yes	No
Feeding: feeds self without assistance (except for help with cutting meat or buttering bread)	Yes	No
Total ADL score = number of "yes" answers, out of possible 6.		

[a]Modified from Katz S, Ford AB, Moskowitz RW, Jackson BA, Jaffe MW: Studies of illness in the aged: The index of ADL: a standardized measure of biological and psychosocial function. *JAMA* 185:914–919, 1963. Copyright by The Gerontological Society of America. Reprinted with permission.

continence, and feeding. A person who regains function often recovers those same abilities in reverse order: first feeding, then continence, then transfer, and so on. Katz arranged the elements of the scale to show the typical progression in loss or recovery of these skills. Sociologists have speculated that this sequence of skills parallels the development of self-care skills during childhood—and perhaps their emergence in primitive man (Katz *et al.*, 1963).

The Katz ADL scale has been shown to be valid, reliable, and easy to administer. Its major drawback, as with many assessment instruments, is its inability to detect small changes in function that may over time reflect a large loss of function. The Katz ADL scale nevertheless remains a useful tool for assessing physical function. Other ADL instruments are available (Applegate *et al.*, 1990), which vary in length and in the skills assessed (e.g., walking, climbing stairs, and grooming). Such instruments are clinically useful because they provide a practical way to obtain information about a person's abilities.

During her hospitalization, Mrs. Wilson, in Case 14-2, lost several key ADLs, and her functional decline resulted in loss of independence. Addressing these functional deficits was as important to her recovery as treating her medical–surgical problems. A rehabilitative approach was used. *Rehabilitation* is the restoration of function following disease, illness, or injury. Geriatrics emphasizes a rehabilitative approach since maintaining function and preventing its loss are key to an older patient's health and well-being.

INSTRUMENTAL ACTIVITIES OF DAILY LIVING

The second category of functional skills, the Instrumental Activities of Daily Living (IADLs), comprise a more complex set of skills: shopping, preparing food, keeping house, using transportation, and handling finances. As with the ADLs, everyone needs IADLs to live independently in a community. The Lawton–Brody IADL scale, shown in Table 14.2, is one of the earliest IADL instruments (Lawton & Brody, 1969). Adults vary in level of independence with IADLs just as with ADLs. Their functional level measured with IADLs often determines whether a person can continue to live in the community. Mrs. Wilson, for instance, would have been unable to return home without help from her niece and community services.

Capability versus performance is an issue when assessing ADLs and IADLs. A good rule of thumb is "Say do, can do, do do." That is, patients sometimes *say* they can perform an activity whether they can or not; patients *can* perform an activity but choose not to for whatever reason; and patients may actually *do* the activity that they say they do. Similarly, patients who are in denial about illness or who have cognitive impairment often overestimate their physical abilities, while patients who lack motivation or who are depressed often underestimate them.

Cultural biases also complicate the accurate assessment of IADLs. For example, many older men have never cooked or kept house, but these same men might be able to perform such activities if the need arose. Their lack of actual performance does not necessarily mean they are incapable of those activities.

Most functional assessments are obtained directly from the patient or from the patient's family or caregivers. While direct observation of a patient's physical performance is the most objective and accurate way to assess a patient, such observations are often impractical, especially with IADLs. Hence, most functional evaluations come from patient or family reports and limited observations. Patients tend to report their own

Table 14.2
Instrumental Activities of Daily Living Scale (IADLs)[a]

Ability to use telephone

Operates telephone on own initiative; looks up and dials numbers, etc.   1

Dials a few well-known numbers.   1

Answers telephone but does not dial.   1

Does not use telephone at all.   0

Shopping

Takes care of all shopping needs independently.   1

Shops independently for small purchases.   0

Needs to be accompanied on any shopping trip.   0

Completely unable to shop.   0

Food preparation

Plans, prepares, and serves adequate meals independently.   1

Prepares adequate meals if supplied with ingredients.   0

Heats and serves prepared meals or prepares meals but does not maintain adequate diet.   0

Needs to have meals prepared and served.   0

Housekeeping

Maintains house alone or with occasional assistance (e.g., heavy work, domestic help).   1

Performs light daily tasks such as dish washing, bed making.   1

Performs light daily tasks but cannot maintain acceptable level of cleanliness.   1

Needs help with all home-maintenance tasks.   1

Does not participate in any housekeeping tasks.   0

Laundry

Does personal laundry completely.   1

Launders small items, rinses stockings, etc.   1

All laundry must be done by others.   0

Mode of transportation

Travels independently on public transportation or drives own car.   1

Arranges own travel via taxi but does not otherwise use public transportation.   1

Travels on public transportation when initiated or accompanied by another.   1

Travel limited to taxi or automobile with assistance of another.   0

Does not travel at all.   0

Responsibility for own medications

Is responsible for taking medication in correct dosages at correct time.   1

Takes responsibililty if medication is prepared in advance in separate dosages.   0

Is not capable of dispensing own medication.   0

Ability to handle finances

Manages financial matters independently (budgets, writes checks, pays rent and bills, goes to bank), collects and keeps track of income.   1

Manages day-to-day purchases but needs help with banking, major purchases, etc.   1

Incapable of handling money.   0

Score = _____ points out of a possible 8

[a]From Lawton MP, Brody EM: Assessment of older people: Self-maintaining and instrumental activities of daily living. *Gerontologist* 9:179–186, 1969. Copyright by The Gerontological Society of America. Reprinted with permission.

abilities at higher levels than nurses do, while families tend to report patient's abilities at lower levels than the nurses do (Rubenstein *et al.*, 1984).

Physicians should routinely ask patients about their function. Ask for a description of their daily routine. Ask how or if the presenting problem affects that routine. Find out what activities are no longer performed compared with a year ago. Ask how the patient performs the stated activity. Sometimes, such open-ended questions yield surprising information. For example, one gentleman, who asserted that he bathed independently, did so only by using his cane as a hook on the bathroom doorknob to get in and out of the tub!

During the interview, observe what the patient does for herself. Does a family member answer questions for the patient? Can the patient state what medications are taken? Is help needed to sit on the examination table? Does the patient have difficulty unbuttoning a shirt or releasing a belt? Questions and observations such as these provide clues about a patient's function.

Two common causes of functional decline in hospitalized patients are *deconditioning* and *iatrogenesis*. Deconditioning refers to the physiological changes that occur with prolonged bed rest or inactivity (Vorhies & Riley, 1993). Such changes can develop quickly, in a matter of days, and affect almost every organ system in the body. Early signs and symptoms of deconditioning include shortness of breath with minimal exertion, a resting heart rate elevated above the patient's baseline, orthostasis, decreased endurance, and decreased muscle strength. Muscle strength may decline as much as 1.3 to 3.0% per day of bed rest in adults of all ages (Hoenig & Rubenstein, 1991). Such losses in an older patient—whose physical reserve is already at a low threshold—may markedly slow the rate of recovery.

Iatrogenesis—complications resulting from medical care—is a serious problem for older hospitalized adults. Iatrogenesis takes many forms: deconditioning from enforced bed rest, pressure ulcers from poor skin care, nosocomial infections, malnutrition, incontinence, and adverse effects from almost any medication. Medications alone account for nearly half of all iatrogenic problems (Gorbien *et al.*, 1992).

Mrs. Wilson suffered both deconditioning and iatrogensis while in the hospital. Her deconditioning, while a natural consequence of a broken hip, might have been lessened by more aggressive postoperative mobilization. Her confusion, a common complication after hip fractures, probably had multiple causes: side effects from medications (anesthetics, analgesics, sedatives), an unfamiliar hospital environment, and an infection (colitis). Her original injury interacted with the subsequent problems to produce a functional decline.

CASE 14-3 (Part 1)

Mr. Warren, a 75-year-old retired automobile mechanic, came to the physician's office because of falls. The patient could not recall the details, but Mrs. Warren counted four falls in the previous 3 months. She suspected there had been others as well. Two occurred while her husband was getting up to void at night. After one of those falls, he required treatment in an emergency room for a scalp laceration. Mr. Warren's medications included hydrochlorothiazide and enalapril for hypertension, a nitroglycerin patch for stable angina, and triazolam for insomnia.

———— ASSESSMENT OF MOBILITY ————

Falls are a classic presentation of functional decline in older adults. At least one-third of all community-dwelling older adults—and one-half of those institutionalized—fall each year (Tinetti & Speechley, 1989). Some falls, for example Mrs. Wilson's, result in serious injury. Most do not, but even these can have serious consequences. Older patients who have fallen may develop a fear of falling, which leads to decreased activity, followed by deconditioning and eventually immobility.

Falls indicate a problem with mobility, defined as the ability to maneuver throughout the environment. Mobility is an important functional skill that interacts with ADLs and IADLs. Lack of mobility compromises a patient's function and independence and often is the determining factor for nursing home placement. Physicians treating elderly patients therefore should routinely evaluate their mobility. Areas of interest include gait, balance, and range of motion in the upper and lower extremities.

As illustrated in Case 14-3, the first step to successfully evaluating falls is to obtain a description of the event(s). Many older patients do not recall the details surrounding a fall. Therefore, witnesses are invaluable sources for confirming particulars of the event: how the patient fell, whether there was loss of consciousness or incontinence of bowel or bladder, or if hazards, such as throw rugs or poor lighting, were present.

Since falls are a common nonspecific presentation of underlying illness, the clinician also should inquire about signs and symptoms of acute illness, e.g., infection or heart disease. The review of systems should focus on potential sensory or neuromuscular deficits that might interfere with mobility. Questions about vision, hearing, joint pain, balance, strength, and sensation provide important information.

Lastly, a careful review of the patient's medications, both prescription and over the counter, is critical. Certain classes of medications, including antihypertensives and sedatives, as well as the total number of medications, increase the risk of falls (Tinetti & Speechley, 1989).

After completing the history, the physical examination should include the musculoskeletal and neurologic systems. The musculoskeletal examination focuses on range of motion in the upper and lower extremities, joint deformities, and pain in these areas. Simple exercises, such as asking patients to put both hands behind their head or to touch their toes with the opposite hand, mimic the types of movements needed when putting on a shirt or shoes. Picking up a pen from the table mimics the use of eating utensils. Simply observing the patient taking off a coat, buttoning it, or reaching for a glass gives almost as much information about range of motion as formal testing.

The standard neurologic examination, originally designed to localize neurologic lesions, is an important part of the examination but provides limited information about function. The abnormalities detected by a neurologic examination don't necessarily correlate with those detected by a mobility evaluation. Tinetti and Ginter (1988) showed that the neuromuscular abnormalities detected on a standard neurologic examination in older patients did not predict who had difficulty getting in and out of a chair.

Assessment of mobility includes analysis of a patient's gait and balance. At least 15% of patients over age 60 have an abnormal gait (Sudarsky, 1990), and gait disturbances are a known risk factor for falls. The normal gait cycle has three phases: stance, swing, and double-limb support. The stance phase, which occupies about 60 to 65% of the gait cycle, beings when the right heel contacts a surface. It ends when the right toe leaves that surface. The swing phase, occupying about 15 to 20% of the cycle, begins when the right toe leaves a surface and lasts until the right heel again contacts that surface. The double-limb support phase, the part of the cycle when both feet are on the ground, is about 20 to 25% of total cycle time (Sudarsky, 1990).

Many diseases produce characteristic gait patterns that physicians can learn to recognize. Cerebellar disease produces a wide-based stance and ataxia (an unsteady and wandering path). Stroke patients often circumduct (swing outward) the affected leg and have

Table 14.3

Tinetti Balance and Gait Evaluation[a]

BALANCE

Instructions: Subject is seated in hard, armless chair. The following maneuvers are tested.

1. Sitting balance

    Leans or slides in chair   = 0

    Steady, safe   = 1

2. Arises

    Unable without help   = 0

    Able, but uses arms to help   = 1

    Able without use of arms   = 2

3. Attempts to arise

    Unable without help   = 0

    Able, but requires more than one attempt   = 1

    Able to arise with one attempt   = 2

4. Immediate standing balance (first 5 seconds)

    Unsteady (staggers, moves feet, marked trunk sway)   = 0

    Steady, but uses walker or cane or grabs other objects for support   = 1

    Steady without walker or cane or other support   = 2

5. Standing balance

    Unsteady   = 0

    Steady, but wide stance (medial heels more than 4 inches apart), or uses

    cane, walker, or other support   = 1

    Narrow stance without support   = 2

6. Nudge (subject at maximum position with feet as close together as possible, examiner pushes
   lightly on subject's sternum with palm of hand three times)

    Begins to fall   = 0

    Staggers, grabs, but catches self   = 1

    Steady   = 2

7. Eyes closed (at maximum position #6)

    Unsteady   = 0

    Steady   = 1

8. Turning 360°

    Discontinuous steps   = 0

    Continuous steps   = 1

    Unsteady (grabs, staggers)   = 0

    Steady   = 1

9. Sitting down

    Unsafe (misjudged distance, falls into chair)   = 0

    Uses arms or not a smooth motion   = 1

    Safe, smooth motion   = 2

Balance score= ___/16

minimal flexion at the hip and knee during the swing phase. Patients with dementia may have difficulty initiating steps and shuffle as they walk. Older patients, even in the absence of pathology, develop a characteristic gait pattern. Step length is decreased, stride is broader-based, and velocity is decreased.

CASE 14-3 (Part 2)

Mr. Warren was orthostatic on physical examination with a blood pressure of 152/82 mm Hg and a pulse of 78 while sitting and a blood pressure of 128/64 mm Hg and a pulse of 82 after standing 1 minute. He had a mild resting tremor in his

Table 14.3
(Continued)

GAIT

Instructions: Subject stands with examiner, walks down hallway or across room, first at "usual" pace,
then back at "rapid, but safe" pace (using usual walking aid such as cane, walker).

10. Initiation of gait (immediately after told to "go")
    - Any hesitancy or multiple attempts to start = 0
    - No hesitancy = 1
11. Step length and height
    - A. Right swing foot
        - Does not pass left stance foot with step = 0
        - Passes left stance foot = 1
        - Right foot does not clear floor completely with step = 0
        - Right foot completely clears floor = 1
    - B. Left swing foot
        - Does not pass right stance foot with step = 0
        - Passes right stance foot = 1
        - Left foot does not clear floor completely with step = 0
        - Left foot completely clears floor = 1
12. Step symmetry
    - Right and left step length not equal (estimate) = 0
    - Right and left step length appear equal = 1
13. Step continuity
    - Stopping or discontinuity between steps = 0
    - Steps appear continuous = 1
14. Path (estimated in relation to floor tiles, 12 inch diameter. Observe excursion of one foot over about 10 feet of the course.)
    - Marked deviation = 0
    - Mild/moderate deviation or uses walking aid = 1
    - Straight without walking aid = 2
15. Trunk
    - Marked sway or uses walking aid = 0
    - No sway but flexion of knees or back or spreads arms out while walking = 1
    - No sway, no flexion, no use of arms, and no walking aid = 2
16. Walking stance
    - Heels apart = 0
    - Heels almost touching while walking = 1

Gait score:———/12
Total score:———/28

*a*From Tinetti ME: Performance-oriented assessment of mobility problems in elderly patients. *JAGS* 34:119–126, 1986.
Permission obtained from author.

right hand and cogwheel rigidity in both arms. It took him three attempts to rise from the chair, and he became unsteady after a few minutes. His step length, step height, and arm swing were decreased symmetrically, and he displayed a flexed posture in the trunk and extremities. Initiation of gait was delayed, but when achieved, his gait speed accelerated. Questioning by the physician revealed that Mr. Warren had had the tremor at least a year, and that it took him longer to dress and bathe.

Mr. Warren was diagnosed with Parkinson's disease. His falls were attributed to several causes: orthostasis from medications and from probable underlying autonomic insufficiently (a common problem with Parkinson's patients), deconditioning from chronic immobility, and sedation from the hypnotic, triazolam.

He received a trial of carbidopa/levodopa, which improved his bradykinesia and ability to dress. Hydrochlorothiazide was discontinued. His blood pressure remained well controlled on enalapril alone. The triazolam was discontinued after the physician reviewed sleep hygiene techniques with him and his wife. Lastly, a physical therapist provided a front-wheel walker and a home exercise program to improve strength and endurance. Mr. Warren's orthostasis improved. Six months later, his wife reported only one fall.

Assessing Mr. Warren's mobility helped the physician to determine the causes for his falls. His gait provided an important clue for the diagnosis of Parkinson's disease. Gait analysis is easily accomplished, once a clinician recognizes the elements of normal and abnormal gait. The Performance-Oriented Assessment of Mobility, often called the Tinetti Balance and Gait Evaluation, is a standardized clinical instrument used to analyze mobility of older patients (Tinetti, 1986). This instrument, shown in Table 14.3, divides the components of mobility into a detailed list of observations about balance and gait.

To evaluate balance, first observe how patients sit in a chair. Patients with large strokes, for example, often have poor sitting balance and lean toward the affected side. Next, ask the patients to stand without using the hands as support. The need for multiple attempts or for the use of the arms to rise from sitting is typical in patients with lower extremity weakness, osteoarthritis of the hips or knees, and deconditioning. Likewise, falling into the chair when sitting suggests similar problems or poor vision. On standing, observe immediate (first 5 seconds) and delayed (after about 1 minute) standing balance. Unsteadiness could be from orthostasis, cerebellar disease, or weakness. Asking patients to stand with their eyes closed tests dependency on sensory input from proprioception and vision.

Important observations while patients walk include step length and height. Normal step length is at least the length of the patient's foot, and normal step height is 1 to 2 inches above the floor. The heel of the swing foot usually clears the opposite foot by 1 to 2 inches. Observe how quickly a patient initiates walking. Mr. Parker, like many Parkinson patients, had difficulty initiating walking but accelerated once started (called *festination*). An erratic gait path and excessive truncal sway suggest cerebellar dysfunction.

The Tinetti Balance and Gait Evaluation takes only a few minutes to complete once the physician is familiar with the tool. Scoring of the instrument has been useful primarily in research settings. Clinicians find the Tinetti Evaluation useful because it teaches them to observe the subtleties of gait and balance and because it provides a practical and objective way to evaluate mobility.

A shorter version of the test, called "the get-up and go test" (Mathias *et al.*, 1986), is a quick screen for gait and balance. To perform the test, instruct the patient to stand up from a chair without using his hands, walk 15 meters, turn around, and return. Before the patient sits down, perform the "nudge test." Ask the patient to close his eyes, then gently but firmly push on the patient's sternum, taking care to guard against a fall. Finally, ask the patient to sit down, again without using the hands. The "nudge test" evaluates a patient's righting reflexes, i.e., the ability to adjust the body's posture to changes in the environment. A patient with a positive "nudge" is unable to correct his posture without falling.

Sometimes even informal observations are helpful in evaluating mobility. When circumstances allow, watch the patient walk in or out of the examination room. At those times, patients are likely to perform in their usual manner. Is there unsteadiness? Does a family member or nurse need to help? Does the patient use an assistive device, such as a cane or walker? Is it used correctly? These observations provide information that is often unavailable in the examination room.

AMBULATORY DEVICES

Older patients who need ambulatory devices often use them incorrectly. Physicians should know which ambulatory devices help patients with poor mobility. They should also know how to use these devices correctly. The decision about the correct device and its use should be made in conjunction with physical therapists, however, who have expertise in treating mobility problems.

Canes, which can support up to 25% of a person's weight, are a good choice for older adults with unilateral weakness or pain while walking. Stroke patients with normal balance or those with hip osteoarthritis often benefit. When a patient uses a cane, make sure it is correctly adjusted for the patient's height. Look for a 20 to 30° angle at the elbow. The patient should hold the cane on the unaffected side, which decreases stance time and shifts weight away from the affected side. For example, Mrs. Wilson, who had a right hip fracture, should hold her cane in the left hand. To use it correctly, she should step forward simultaneously with her right leg and the cane in her left hand, then she should step forward with her unaffected left leg.

Walkers, which can support up to 50% of a person's weight, are better for patients with poor balance or general weakness. Demented patients, who have difficulty learning or remembering new information (e.g., how to properly use a cane), may be good candidates for walkers. Pickup walkers are useful to patients with poor endurance, such as those with chronic obstructive pulmonary disease or congestive heart failure. Pickup walkers require adequate balance and upper extremity strength, however. Front-wheel walkers offer more stability to patients with balance deficits, since this type of walker forces the patient's center of gravity forward into the walker. Parkinson patients, like Mr. Warren, tend to be retropulsive, i.e., to fall backwards. A standard pickup walker might exaggerate retropulsion and increase Mr. Warren's fall risk, whereas a front-wheel walker would offer more stability.

Wheelchairs provide mobility for patients who need postural support, or who have severe weakness. They provide patients who have progressive diseases, such as multiple sclerosis or amyotrophic lateral sclerosis, with mobility that they would not have otherwise. Safely transferring in and out of the wheelchair is a prerequisite for its use. When prescribing wheelchairs, always collaborate with physical therapists who have the expertise to recommend the right model and to teach its correct use.

Knowing the basics of ambulatory devices, especially canes and walkers, enables physicians to promote mobility and function for their patients.

CASE 14-4 (Part 1)

Mrs. Goldendale, a 91-year-old lady, came to the physician's office with her son, Steve, because of weight loss. He had observed a loss of almost 10 pounds over the preceding 8 months; his mother now weighed 78 pounds. She had a remote history of peptic ulcer disease, but denied gastrointestinal complaints. Her son observed that she needed frequent encouragement to eat and that she complained of back and right hip pain, which was relieved by an anti-inflammatory medication. Mrs. Goldendale had lived with her children over the past 3 years because of their concerns about her forgetfulness. Prior physicians attributed the memory loss to "old timer's disease."

Steve's brother and sister-in-law were recently frustrated when his mother left a bathroom faucet running and flooded the upstairs, causing considerable damage. He and his brother worried about their mother's health and disagreed about the need for nursing home placement. Until 2 months ago, Mrs. Goldendale had been independent with all ADLs; she now needed prompting to bathe and dress.

Physical examination revealed a petite and cachectic elderly woman who was disoriented to the date. She nodded to questions and allowed her son to answer most of them. Mrs. Goldendale had marked kyphosis and a limp while walking. She became unsteady while turning around; her "nudge test" was positive. The physician recognized that Mrs. Goldendale had many problems: weight loss, forgetfulness, and a functional decline. The physician also wondered if she would need nursing home placement. Since Mrs. Goldendale lived far away, the physician recommended admission to a nearby Geriatric Assessment and Rehabilitation Unit (GARU) to sort out the problems.

—— COMPREHENSIVE GERIATRIC ASSESSMENT ——

When patients like Mrs. Goldendale come to the office, their problems often cover many domains—medical, cognitive, affective, functional, social, economic, and environmental—that interact with one another to affect function. A multidisciplinary evaluation called Comprehensive Geriatric Assessment (CGA) assists healthcare professionals in developing diagnostic and treatment plans that improve an older patient's function. CGA is useful to patients who have well-defined rehabilitation needs, e.g., strokes or hip fractures. It is also useful for frail patients who have less well-defined problems or who have multiple problems, as in Case 14-4.

CGA is often provided on dedicated inpatient units that organize healthcare professionals from many disciplines into a team. The interdisciplinary team meets regularly to discuss and coordinate patient care. A physician, nurse, and social worker usually make up the core team, but other health professionals (including physical and occupational therapists, dietitians, speech pathologists, and pharmacists) participate as needed.

The frail population, meaning those with functional limitations, benefit most from such evaluations, since this population is most likely to have complex medical and psychosocial problems. Multiple randomized controlled trials (Rubenstein, 1987; Stuck *et al.*, 1993) show that CGA helps older patients by improving diagnostic accuracy, function, and affect, while decreasing mortality and medication use. CGA also reduces nursing home placement, hospital admissions, and healthcare costs. Patients most likely to benefit from CGA are those with recent functional declines, good social support, and relatively good cognition. CGA has occurred mostly on GARUs, but multidisciplinary evaluations can also be performed in outpatient or home settings.

Mrs. Goldendale's physician needed to evaluate more than the weight loss *per se*. Her problems extend into other areas of function that could affect her medical condition, including self-care, mobility, cognition, affect, and sensory evaluation.

On arriving at the GARU, team members evaluated Mrs. Goldendale. The medical workup uncovered an iron-deficiency anemia that was eventually attributed to severe gastritis from nonsteroidal anti-inflammatory drugs. For pain control, the physicians prescribed scheduled acetaminophen and a heating pad. They removed impacted cerumen from her ears. Her hearing improved and she began to answer questions rather than simply nod as she'd so frequently done before. An audiologist found Mrs. Goldendale had a moderate hearing loss and recommended hearing aides.

The geropsychiatrist interviewed Mrs. Goldendale. She expressed feelings of helplessness and hopelessness. She admitted that she had never really gotten over her husband's death 5 years earlier and that while living with her sons was helpful, their interests overshadowed hers. Mental status testing showed intact concentration and mild short-term memory loss. She was diagnosed with clinical depression and eventually with a mild underlying dementia.

Her physician began a trial of antidepressant medication. Her physical therapist prescribed a front-wheel walker for her unsteadiness as well as an exercise program. Her occupational therapist recommended installing grab bars and a tub transfer bench in the home to help her bathe safely. Lastly, the social worker suggested that Mrs. Goldendale attend a local senior center to increase her socialization.

Three years later, Mrs. Goldendale was still living with her children and was independent with her ADLs.

Good cognitive and affective function are critical to a patient's health. Normal motor skills and endurance are not enough to permit normal function. Physicians should screen for cognitive impairment and affective disturbances when evaluating patients with a functional decline.

Patients with cognitive impairment often present with forgetfulness, commonly caused by dementia. Both long-term memory (over years) and short-term memory (over hours or days) can be tested with simple questions. Long-term memory can be tested by asking for a birth date, place of birth, number of children, or date of retirement. Few patients forget these milestones unless cognitive problems are present. Short-term memory can be tested by asking the patient to repeat three common objects immediately, then at 5 minutes. Patients with intact memory should be able to name the objects. If the person is hesitant to do this, ask less-threatening questions. What did they have for breakfast that morning? What is their current address? Can they give directions to their home? If their answers can be verified, an inability to answer questions about everyday life may uncover memory problems.

The Mini-Mental State Examination (MMSE) is a reliable and easily administered screening test for cognitive impairment (Folstein *et al.*, 1975). It was originally designed to assess the severity of cognitive impairment and to monitor cognitive changes over time. As shown in Table 14.4, the MMSE contains 30 items that test orientation, memory, concentration, and language abilities. Once learned, it takes about 5 to 10 minutes to complete.

When administering the examination, keep several techniques in mind. Some authorities recommend that when asking for the county and floor in the orientation section, the

Table 14.4
Mini-Mental State Examination (MMSE)[a]

Questions	Points
1. What is the: Year? Season? Date? Day? Month?	5
2. Where are we: State? County? Town or city? Hospital? Floor?	5
3. Name three objects (Apple, Penny, Table), taking one second to say each. Then ask the patient to tell you the three. Repeat the answers until the patient learns all three.	3
4. Serial sevens. Subtract 7 from 100. Then subtract 7 from that number, etc. Stop after five answers. Alternative: spell WORLD backward.	5
5. Ask for the names of the three objects learned in #3.	3
6. Point to a pencil and watch. Have the patient name them as you point.	1
7. Have the patient repeat "No ifs, ands, or buts."	3
8. Have the patient follow a three-stage command: "Take the paper in your right hand. Fold the paper in half. Put the paper on the floor."	3
9. Have the patient read and obey the following: "CLOSE YOUR EYES." (Write it in large letters.)	1
10. Have the patient write a sentence of his or her own choice.	1
11. Have the patient copy the following design (overlapping pentagons).	1

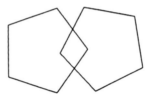

Assess level of consciousness along a continuum:
Alert—Drowsy—Stupor—Coma

Total Score = ___/30

[a]From Folstein MF, Folstein SE, McHugh PR: Mini-mental state: A practical method for grading the cognitive state of patients for the clinician. *J Psychiatr Res* 12:189–198, 1975. Used with permission from MF Folstein.

examiner may substitute the county and street, respectively, where the person lives (Tombaugh & McIntyre, 1992). In the registration section, the score is based on the first trial, although it may be necessary for the patient to repeat the three items several times to learn them for later recall. The examiner should confirm that the patient can correctly spell WORLD forward, before asking to spell it backward. Lastly, while WORLD backward and Serial 7s are both tests of concentration, they are not equivalent in difficulty. It is usually best to first ask the patient to spell WORLD backward before performing serial 7s. Count the highest of the two scores.

Commonly used cut off scores for the MMSE are: no cognitive impairment = 24 to 30; mild cognitive impairment = 18 to 23; and severe cognitive impairment = 0 to 17. These scores should always be interpreted with caution. Studies have shown that age, poor fluency in English, and less than an eighth-grade education may produce low scores in patients who do not have true cognitive impairment (Tombaugh & McIntyre, 1992). Nevertheless, the MMSE is a valuable screening tool that can alert physicians to underlying cognitive problems in patients. The physician can subsequently determine the need for further mental status evaluation.

Physicians should also screen for affective or mood disturbances such as depression. Serious depressive symptoms affect more than 10% of older community-dwelling adults.

Clinical depression is common in older hospitalized patients (10 to 15%), and even more common in patients with underlying cognitive impairment, e.g., dementia or Parkinson's disease (20 to 40%) (Blazer, 1989). Asking the patient "Do you often feel sad or depressed?" introduces further questions about depression.

The Geriatric Depression Scale (GDS) (Yesavage *et al.*, 1983), a 30-item questionnaire designed to help clinicians detect depressive symptoms in older adults, has been validated in both community-dwelling and hospital populations (Koenig *et al.*, 1988). An example of the GDS is shown in Table 14.5.

The GDS can be self-administered or administered by a physician, nurse, or family member. Score one point for each depressed answer. The higher the score, the more likely the patient is depressed. Various cutoff scores have been suggested for the GDS. A score of greater than 11 was found to provide a sensitivity of 92% and specificity of 89% in older hospitalized patients (Koenig *et al.*, 1988) and a sensitivity of 84% and specificity of

Table 14.5
Geriatric Depression Scale (GDS)[a]

Choose the best answer for how you felt this past week.

*	Are you basically satisfied with your life?	Yes	No
	Have you dropped many of your activities and interests?	Yes	No
	Do you feel that your life is empty?	Yes	No
	Do you often get bored?	Yes	No
*	Are you hopeful about the future?	Yes	No
	Are you bothered by thoughts you can't get out of your head?	Yes	No
*	Are you in good spirits most of the time?	Yes	No
	Are you afraid that something bad is going to happen to you?	Yes	No
*	Do you feel happy most of the time?	Yes	No
	Do you often feel helpless?	Yes	No
	Do you often get restless and fidgety?	Yes	No
	Do you prefer to stay at home, rather than going out and doing new things?	Yes	No
	Do you frequently worry about the future?	Yes	No
	Do you feel you have more problems with memory than most?	Yes	No
*	Do you think it is wonderful to be alive now?	Yes	No
	Do you often feel downhearted and blue?	Yes	No
	Do you feel pretty worthless the way you are now?	Yes	No
	Do you worry a lot about the past?	Yes	No
*	Do you find life very exciting?	Yes	No
	Is it hard for you to get started on new projects?	Yes	No
*	Do you feel full of energy?	Yes	No
	Do you think that your situation is hopeless?	Yes	No
	Do you think that most people are better off than you are?	Yes	No
	Do you frequently get upset over little things?	Yes	No
	Do you frequently feel like crying?	Yes	No
	Do you have trouble concentrating?	Yes	No
*	Do you enjoy getting up in the morning?	Yes	No
	Do you prefer to avoid social gatherings?	Yes	No
*	Is it easy for you to make decisions?	Yes	No
*	Is your mind as clear as it used to be?	Yes	No
*	Appropriate (nondepressed) answers = yes, all others, no	Score = number of "depressed" answers		

[a]From Yesavage JA, Brink TL, Rose RL, Lum O, Huang V, Adey M, Leirer VO: Development and validation of a geriatric depression screening scale: A preliminary report. *J Psychiatr Res* 17:37–49, 1983. Reprinted with permission from JA Yesavage.

95% in community-dwelling adults (Yesavage *et al.*, 1983). Many other instruments for assessing cognition and mood disturbances are available (Applegate *et al.*, 1990). These instruments, including the MMSE and the GDS, do not replace a physician's clinical judgment about a patient's condition, but may confirm a diagnosis or catch previously unsuspected cognitive and affective disturbances.

Other important functional abilities to screen are hearing and vision (Lachs *et al.*, 1990), since many older adults have trouble with these senses. Their inability to see or hear can profoundly impair function. To screen vision, ask the patient to read the letters of a Snellen chart at 14 inches while wearing corrective lenses. If the chart is unavailable, ask the patient to read a few sentences from a magazine or newspaper.

To screen hearing, use the "whisper test." The physician stands behind the patient, and while covering one of the patient's ears, asks the patient to repeat numbers whispered by the physician. Another screen is the "rub test," performed by rubbing the thumb and index fingers together near one of the patient's ears and asking if the patient heard the sound. One of the most important services a physician can perform is to remove cerumen occluding the external auditory canals, a simple solution to an often-overlooked problem.

These screening tests do not replace the more detailed examinations of specialists, but they remind physicians that older patients often have vision and hearing impairments. Physicians should have a low threshold for referring patients with these problems.

Mrs. Goldendale had multiple problems, some with multiple causes. Weight loss occurred from gastritis, chronic pain, and depression. Her cognitive impairments occurred from depression, dementia, and hearing loss. These problems were interrelated and produced her functional decline.

CONCLUSION

Evaluating and treating patients with multiple medical and functional problems challenges even the most experienced physicians. While cures may be impossible, improvement in physical, cognitive, and affective function is often possible. The Report of the Society of General Internal Medicine Task Force on Health Assessment (Rubenstein *et al.*, 1988) recommended that physicians learn to incorporate a functional approach toward older patients. For all patients over age 65, the task force suggested a targeted clinical interview and examination that focuses on physical function, assessment of the person's IADLs, and a screen for depression. For all patients over age 75 (or over age 65 with clinical indications), the task force recommended also assessing ADLs and cognition.

Healthcare providers, in all disciplines, are treating larger numbers of geriatric patients. This trend will continue because the percentage of adults over age 65 will almost double from 12.5% to 21% of the total U.S. population by 2030. Furthermore, the oldest old—those over age 85 and even over age 100—are the fastest-growing segments of the population (Schick & Schick, 1994). Levels of disability, rates of hospitalization, and healthcare costs all rise with age. As healthcare providers become increasingly aware of this rapidly growing population, effective models of management that include functional assessment will help physicians to successfully treat older adults as well as younger adults with disabilities.

Adults of all ages may have healthcare needs that do not fit into the traditional medical model of disease. Their concerns often extend to losses of function that require a different approach that complements the traditional model. Physicians who treat these patients can incorporate functional assessment into their daily practice through simple tools and techniques. Assessing ADLs, IADLs, and mobility provides useful information that cannot be obtained from the standard history and physical. Evaluating cognition, affect, and sensory impairments contributes to a more thorough evaluation. Many patients often need and benefit from the functional approach.

——— CASES FOR DISCUSSION ———

CASE 1

Mrs. Morgan, a 69-year-old semiretired teacher with a history of diabetes mellitus, hypertension, and macular degeneration, lived with her spouse and son in their ranch-style home. While she was preparing breakfast one morning for her family, slurred speech and right-sided weakness developed. She was taken to a nearby hospital and admitted with a new left cerebrovascular accident. Her neurologic symptoms progressed over the next 24 hours, leaving her with a dense right hemiparalysis.

During hospitalization, Mrs. Morgan required many medications for labile hypertension, antibiotics for an aspiration pneumonia, and tube feedings for a severe dysphagia. Twelve days poststroke, Mrs. Morgan showed some signs of neurologic recovery: improved swallowing and increased motor tone and strength in her right side. However, she displayed a moderately severe expressive aphasia, marked right hemiparesis, and urinary incontinence. She appeared to be uncooperative with the staff and required full assistance with all of her ADLs.

1. *List Mrs. Morgan's problems, both medical and functional. What problems would you want to prevent?*
2. *What healthcare providers should help with Mrs. Morgan's recovery?*
3. *Why might Mrs. Morgan be uncooperative with the hospital staff?*
4. *What factors make Mrs. Morgan a good or bad candidate for comprehensive geriatric assessment?*

CASE 2

Pete, a 51-year-old construction foreman, suffered severe crush injuries to both legs after a building collapse. Despite aggressive medical management after his rescue, he eventually required bilateral above-the-knee amputation of both legs. You have treated him in the past for hypertension and hyperlipidemia. On several occasions, you've recommended that he stop smoking cigarettes.

1. *What would you predict are Pete's functional limitations? How would you direct his rehabilitation to prevent further disabilities and handicaps?*
2. *Six weeks after the accident, Pete remains dependent on caregivers for dressing, transfers, and toileting. How would you evaluate his lack of progress?*
3. *Pete's wife visits him sporadically. On several occasions, the rehabilitation staff has commented on her reluctance to discuss discharge plans. What healthcare providers need to be involved at this point? What are their roles?*

CASE 3

Vera Olson, a 76-year-old retired clerical worker, comes to your office with many concerns: fatigue, dizziness, insomnia, constipation, and back pain. None of these symptoms are new, but she feels that previous physicians have not really "listened" to her. Her medical history includes emphysema, hypertension, osteoporosis, and peptic ulcer disease. Current medications are triamcinolone and albuterol metered-dose inhalers, propranolol, conjugated estrogen, calcium supplements, vitamin D, cimetidine, and diphenhydramine.

1. *How would you approach this patient, who presents with so many complaints?*
2. *What other information would you want to obtain from Miss Olson?*
3. *What instruments would be useful in sorting out Miss Olson's concerns?*

CASE 4

You have followed the Brown family in your practice for 12 years. David, 18 years old and the eldest of the four Brown children, is 2 weeks away from high school graduation when he suffers multiple injuries in a motor vehicle accident, including a lacerated spleen, rib fractures, and an incomplete spinal cord injury at the C7 level.

After almost 3 weeks in the intensive care unit, David is transferred to the medicine ward. On physical examination, David has resolving ecchymoses around the head and trunk. His abdomen has an intact laparotomy incision that is healing well. A Foley catheter is in place. Neurologically, motor strength in the upper extremities is 3/5 and in the lower extremities 1/5. He has mild flexion contractures of the elbows and wrists. Sensation to pinprick is intact at C7 and inferior.

Now that David's condition has stabilized, he and his family wonder what's next. Although David will continue to work with the rehabilitation team, he and his family still consider you his physician. They assume you will continue to follow David throughout his recovery.

1. *How would you begin to evaluate David's functional abilities? What are his current functional limitations, in terms of diseases, impairments, and disabilities?*
2. *How do David's functional limitations differ from those of an older adult?*
3. *What is your role in David's recovery?*
4. *Before the accident, David had lined up a summer job with plans to enroll that fall at a nearby community college. He now wants to know when he will be "a normal person again." What would you say?*

CASE 5

Mrs. Montimore, a 79-year-old widow, is brought to your office by her daughter, Beth, who is worried about her mother. Since her husband's death 2 years ago, Mrs. Montimore has continued to live in her two-story home. Although she denies any falls, Beth is certain of falls. One month ago, Beth noticed bruises on her mother's right arm and leg.

Beth also feels that her mother's memory is not as sharp as it once was. Mrs. Montimore used to attend a garden club every week, but now rarely leaves her home. Over the past 6 months, Beth has brought over prepared meals regularly and has also cleaned her mother's home to help out. Mrs. Montimore has a history of hypertension, diabetes mellitus, and glaucoma. When you ask what medications she is taking, she replies that she left them at home, but takes them just as the bottles direct her to.

1. *What further information do you want about Mrs. Montimore's function? How much is she really doing for herself?*
2. *What could be the causes of her functional decline?*
3. *What evaluations would you want to perform?*
4. *Beth is concerned that her mother may be unable to stay in her home much longer. All of her other children live far away, and Beth feels that the burden of care will rest on her. What could you do to help the daughter with her mother's care?*

RECOMMENDED READINGS

DeLisa JA (ed): *Rehabilitation Medicine, Principles and Practice.* Philadelphia, JB Lippincott Co, 1988.

This text provides a comprehensive reference for rehabilitation at all ages. It discusses general principles, including functional outcomes, diagnosis and management of common problems (such as contractures and neurogenic bowel and bladder), and specific disorders (such as spinal cord injuries and multiple sclerosis). A busy clinician can look up answers to rehabilitative questions with ease from the detailed index.

Kemp B, Brummel-Smith K, Ramsdell J (eds): *Geriatric Rehabilitation.* Boston, College-Hill Press, 1990.

This text provides a comprehensive overview of geriatric rehabilitation. It discusses the general aspects of rehabilitation such as functional assessment and organization of rehabilitation programs. It also discusses specific disabling conditions, such as stroke, emphysema, and arthritis. Several chapters delve into the psychosocial aspects of geriatric medicine.

Whittle MW: *Gait Analysis, An Introduction.* London, Butterworth–Heinemann Ltd, 1991.

A detailed and readable text about analysis of gait and balance. The book begins with a concise review of the anatomy, physiology, and biomechanics of gait. It then discusses the characteristics of normal and pathological gaits and suggests ways to apply gait analysis to clinical practice. Diagrams provide good visualization of the author's descriptions.

CHAPTER 15

Health Promotion and Disease Prevention

Larry L. Dickey

CASE 15-1

John T. is a 25-year-old patient who is seen by you because of pain in his right hand after bending a finger playing basketball. You diagnose mild soft tissue injury and suggest that he treat it with ice, ibuprofen, and rest. He also brings up that he would like his cholesterol tested because he "wants to live to be 100." Further discussion reveals that he has no medical or family history factors that would put him at risk for coronary artery disease. You have only 5 minutes left before you will need to go to see a patient in the hospital. Rather than order a cholesterol test, you decide to use the time to talk with John and discover that he drinks six beers daily, has had two serious traffic accidents in the last 2 years, and has had unprotected sex with five different partners in the last year. You advise him to not worry about a cholesterol test despite recommendations he has seen on television, but instead to eat a low-fat, low-cholesterol diet, limit his alcohol intake to two drinks per day, wear seatbelts, and use condoms with every sexual partner. He declines an HIV test. All of this makes you 5 minutes late getting to the hospital.

——————— EDUCATIONAL OBJECTIVES ———————

At the completion of this chapter students will be able to:

- Appreciate the importance of health promotion and disease prevention

- Describe the basic principles of performing the four types of clinical preventive services: counseling, screening testing and examination, immunization, and chemoprophylaxis
- Describe how guidelines for clinical preventive medicine are formulated by major authorities
- Formulate a protocol of preventive medicine procedures for your "own" practice
- Demonstrate the use of basic office resources for efficiently performing health promotion and disease prevention

INTRODUCTION

Preventive care is no longer as simple as the annual physical, having been replaced by an array of screening tests and other procedures that have different periodicities depending on patient age, sex, and risk factors. Case 15-1 illustrates many of the practical challenges facing clinicians today: how to decide on the most effective health promotion and disease prevention interventions in the context of differing recommendations from major authorities, pressure from a motivated but often poorly informed public, and time and economic constraints.

This chapter will give the student some of the basic knowledge and tools needed to begin coping with these challenges. It should be read with attention to detail while keeping in mind that the content of preventive care, like acute care, will change and grow as the knowledge base increases in future years. As you progress in your future training there will be many factors that may serve to convince you that preventive care isn't important. For the time being at least, suspend judgment on that issue and attempt to understand the sound scientific principles that underpin the field.

You should consider the cases described carefully, because they have been chosen to accurately reflect what you will see in everyday practice, particularly in a primary care field. Preventive care will probably consume a large portion of your future professional life, in some case as much as 50% or more. Patients like these will enter your office or clinic every day. The pattern of care you begin to develop today will likely persist throughout your career.

CASE 15-2

Roger J. is a 53-year-old businessman who was referred to you by his previous physician in his former city of residence. His presenting complaint is "high blood pressure" controlled with medication. You note that he is 50 pounds overweight, and on questioning discover that 50% of the calories in his diet come from fat. You also determine that physical activity for him is limited to bowling one night per week and an occasional walk with the family dog. You prescribe a diet that has only 30% of calories from fat and suggest that he increase his physical activity by briskly walking 2 miles every other night. Over the course of the next 6 months he tries to follow your instructions and loses 20 pounds. His blood pressure decreases and you tell him that if he continues to lose weight and exercise, he may be ready to discontinue his blood pressure medication.

Table 15.1 lists the leading causes of death in the United States for all ages in 1990 (National Center for Health Statistics, 1993). These leading causes are familiar to most health professionals and perhaps would more appropriately be called the proximal causes of death, the diagnoses entered onto death certificates. In reality, the underlying causes of death, the factors that eventually (but not finally) lead to death, may be more important. McGinnis and Foege (1993) published a list of what they called the "actual causes of death in the United States in 1990" (see Table 15.2). Using a complex methodology, they separated out the contributions of various nongenetic ("external") risk factors for mortality. Even when using the most conservative estimates they demonstrated that half of all deaths could be attributed to only nine causes, all of which are modifiable or preventable to some extent.

Most of these "actual causes" are the result of social and personal behaviors, e.g., smoking, substance abuse, unhealthy nutrition, and physical and sexual activity patterns. Although responsibility for their modification resides largely in the realms of personal responsibility and public policy, there is much that providers can do to help stem the tide of preventable and premature death. Clinicians are firsthand witnesses of the destructive effects of unhealthy behaviors and remain a trusted source of health-related information for most patients. Most Americans see a physician multiple times during each year—the average number of visits to a physician in 1993 was 6.0 (National Center for Health Statistics, 1995)—often when they are ill and most receptive to medical and life-style interventions.

The range of preventive interventions that a clinician can deliver can be divided into four basic types:

- Counseling
- Screening tests and examinations
- Immunizations
- Chemoprophylaxis

Table 15.1
Leading Causes of Death, United States, 1990[a]

Cause	Number
Heart disease	720,000
Cancer	505,000
Cerebrovascular disease	144,000
Accidents	92,000
Chronic obstructive pulmonary disease	87,000
Pneumonia and influenza	80,000
Diabetes mellitus	48,000
Suicide	31,000
Chronic liver disease and cirrhosis	26,000
Human immunodeficiency virus	25,000
	2,148,000

[a]Source: National Center for Health Statistics. *Advance Report of Final Mortality, 1990.* Hyattsville, Md, US Department of Health and Human Services, 1993. Monthly Vital Statistics Report, Vol. 41, No. 7.

Table 15.2
Actual Causes of Death in the United States in 1990[a]

Cause	Deaths	
	Estimated no.[b]	% of total deaths
Tobacco	400,000	19
Diet/activity patterns	300,000	14
Alcohol	100,000	5
Microbial agents	90,000	4
Toxic agents	60,000	3
Firearms	35,000	2
Sexual behavior	30,000	1
Motor vehicles	25,000	1
Illicit drug use	20,000	<1
	1,060,000	50

[a]Source: McGinnis JM, Foege WH: *JAMA* 270:2207–2212, 1993.
[b]Composite approximation drawn from studies that use different approaches to derive estimates, ranging from actual counts (e.g., firearms) to population attributable risk calculations (e.g., tobacco). Numbers over 100,000 rounded to the nearest 100,000; over 50,000 rounded to the nearest 10,000; below 50,000, rounded to the nearest 5000.

COUNSELING

Counseling can take many forms but usually consists of the clinician speaking directly with the patient about a health problem or health-related behavior, as in Case 15-2. Pamphlets and other printed media are useful adjuncts to verbal counseling, but by themselves are generally not sufficient to influence patient behavior significantly (Mead *et al.*, 1995; Kottke *et al.*, 1988). Recently, electronic media, such as interactive video disks, have been developed to help patients share in difficult medical decision-making processes (Kasper *et al.*, 1992). However, such tools remain experimental and in-person counseling remains the most trusted modality.

Patient counseling is an area of medicine that remains almost as much of an art as a science. However, some basic guidelines have been delineated, such as those published by the U.S. Preventive Services Task Force (1989) (see Table 15.3). These principles, while clear and comprehensive, require explanation and expansion. Principle 1, of course, applies to all clinical encounters, not only counseling or preventive interventions. Principle 2 addresses the fact that almost all patients have some health issues for which they could benefit from advice and guidance. Since many patients don't spontaneously volunteer problems and concerns, these must be assessed through actively soliciting information from patients. This can be either in person or through brief written questionnaires. Principle 3 is important because cognitive understanding of the relationship of behavior and health seems to be a necessary, although not usually sufficient, prerequisite to change.

Principles 4 to 6 address the importance of active patient involvement and commitment. Counseling provided to patients in only one form and on only one occasion tends to quickly lose effectiveness. For this reason it is important to use different strategies, Principle 7, and follow-up interventions, Principle 9, to reinforce the message and progress. Many patients can benefit from the concrete reinforcements of behavior modifica-

Table 15.3
USPSTF Principles of Patient Education and Counseling[a]

1. Develop a therapeutic alliance
2. Counsel all patients
3. Ensure that patients understand the relationship between behavior and health
4. Work with patients to assess barriers to behavior change
5. Gain commitment from patients to change
6. Involve patients in selecting risk factors to change
7. Use a combination of strategies
8. Design a behavior modification plan
9. Monitor progress through follow-up contact
10. Involve office staff

[a]Source: U.S. Preventive Services Task Force. Recommendations for patient education and counseling, in *Guide to Clinical Preventive Services*. Baltimore, Williams & Wilkins Co, 1989.

tion techniques. Involvement of office staff, Principle 10, can be crucial, since they often have more time and training for counseling and follow-up than do busy clinicians.

Personal experiences teach us that behavior and life-style changes are not quick or linear (see Chapter 13, "Counseling and Behavioral Change"). Small improvements are usually followed by relapses, hopefully smaller than the improvements. The work of Prochaska and colleagues has delineated six "stages of change" that are useful for clinicians. These stages are: precontemplation, contemplation, preparation, action, maintenance, and termination (Prochaska *et al.*, 1994). During precontemplation, people are in denial and have not yet recognized the problem behavior. During the contemplation stage they have acknowledged the problem and during the preparation stage have begun to plan concrete steps for dealing with it. During the action stage they actively carry out changes in behavior and during the maintenance stage endeavor to prevent relapses and consolidate gains. In the termination stage the temptation to relapse is no longer present and the problem is no longer active. Progress between stages can take months or years and the entire process a lifetime, with numerous episodes of relapse. Patience and persistence are vital.

Perhaps the most useful contribution of Prochaska's work is the identification of the types of interventions that are likely to be effective at each stage (see Table 15.4). Too much clinician effort is expended providing interventions that are either too advanced or too basic for the patient's stage of change. For example, establishing a behavior modification plan for a patient in the precontemplation or contemplation stages probably will fail; providing consciousness-raising information to a patient in the action stage will be of little use when what is really needed is supportive relationships and concrete rewards.

How effective is patient counseling for behavior change and is it really worth the effort? Data obtained from smoking cessation projects are helpful in answering this question. As a result of counseling by physicians, about 5% of smokers will quit for at least 6 months (Kottke *et al.*, 1988). It has been estimated that if all providers counseled their smoking patients to quit, the national smoking quit rate would almost double (U.S. Public Health Service, 1991). While 5% effectiveness may not seem like much to the individual clinician, for society as a whole and for individuals saved from fatal illnesses, this level of effectiveness may be highly significant. When considering the impact of counseling interventions, it is useful to keep in mind McGinnis and Foege's actual causes of mortality (Table 15.2) and the great burden of suffering ultimately brought on by

Table 15.4
Stages of Change in Which Particular Change Processes Are Most Useful[a,b]

Precontemplation	Contemplation	Preparation	Action	Maintenance
Consciousness-raising ----------------------------------→				
Social liberation--→				
	Emotional arousal ----------------------------→			
	Self-reevaluation ----------------------------→			
		Commitment ---→		
			Reward----------→	
			Countering ---------------------→	
			Environmental control ---------→	
			Helping relationships-----------→	

[a]From Prochaska JO, Norcross JC, DiClemente CC: *Changing for Good.* New York, William Morrow & Co, 1994. Used with permission of the publisher. Copyright 1994.

[b]Examples of change processes: consciousness-raising—education; social liberation—activities of advocacy groups; emotional arousal—fear, anger, or other strong emotions; self-reevaluation—thoughtful reassessment of personal situation and characteristics; commitment—promises to self and others to change; reward—emotional, material, or health gain from change; countering—substituting a healthy behavior for an unhealthy one; environmental control—changing surroundings to support and maintain change; helping relationships—supportive friends and family.

unhealthy behaviors. From this perspective, counseling interventions may be the most important services clinicians provide.

For many providers the most basic challenge is providing not the most effective counseling, but any counseling at all. A recent survey of health plan subscribers in California found that on average only 20% of counseling topics recommended by the U.S. Preventive Services Task Force had been discussed with patients by providers during the preceding 3 years (Pacific Business Group on Health, 1993). Low rates of counseling have also been found in studies of patient charts and clinician self-reports, less than 50% for most counseling areas (Lewis, 1988). Although very basic interventions can be effective (such as advising a patient to quit smoking), these are not consistently provided. For counseling interventions perhaps the first rule of practice should be: Above all, say something—regardless of how basic.

CASE 15-3

Mrs. Johnson is a 55-year-old woman who had a routine screening mammogram in July of 1994 that was read as negative for abnormality. In August of 1994 she noticed a small lump in her right breast but was not alarmed because of her recent negative mammogram. In October 1994 she saw her physician for treatment of a sprained ankle and mentioned the small lump. He quickly performed a breast examination but wasn't able to feel the lump clearly. He told her that he wasn't concerned because of her recent negative mammogram. He advised her to get another annual mammogram in July of 1995. This mammogram clearly revealed breast cancer and a subsequent bone scan revealed widespread metastases.

Mr. Jones is a 55-year-old white man who had prostate-specific antigen (PSA) testing at the suggestion of his physician as part of an annual checkup. Mr. Jones was without symptoms of prostate cancer, but very alarmed when his test results were elevated at 5 ng/ml. He had a good friend who died of prostate cancer at the age of 60. He was so distressed, in fact, that he was unable to work for 2 weeks while waiting for an appointment with the urologist. A needle biopsy was performed, the pathology report for which was "benign hypertrophy." Mr. Jones developed a mild prostate infection after the biopsy that was successfully treated with antibiotics. During this treatment he took off another 2 days of work. During the course of his workup and treatment he was passed over for a promotion in favor of a younger employee. Mr. Jones subsequently felt that he had been misled by his physicians since he had not been told that most men of his age and race with a PSA level of 5 ng/ml do not have prostate cancer.

SCREENING TESTS AND EXAMINATIONS

Screening tests, such as mammograms and PSA tests, are intended to detect a disease at an early, asymptomatic stage when it can be cured or effectively treated. Several criteria for judging the value of screening tests have been proposed. Those of Frame and Carlson (1975) are presented in Table 15.5.

Principles 1 to 4 can be briefly summarized: Screening is not worthwhile (and may cause more harm than good) if the condition cannot be treated more effectively as a result of early detection. Principles 5 and 6 touch on the increasingly important issue of cost, both for the individual patient and for society. In general, screening tests do not save society money, although they do save years of life. For example, mammography has been found to cost $20,000 to $50,000 for each year of life saved. Although this may seem high, it compared favorably with the cost-effectiveness of many treatment interventions, such as the treatment of mild hypertension with medications or the treatment of angina with coronary artery bypass surgery, $32,600 and $62,900, respectively, per year of life saved (Mushlin & Fintor, 1992).

Table 15.5
Judging the Value of Screening Tests in Medical Practice[a]

1. The condition must have a significant effect on the quality and quantity of life.
2. Acceptable methods of treatment must be available.
3. The condition must have an asymptomatic period during which detection and treatment significantly reduce morbidity and mortality.
4. Treatment in the asymptomatic phase must yield a therapeutic result superior to that obtained by delaying treatment until symptoms appear.
5. Tests that are acceptable to patients must be available, at a reasonable cost, to detect the condition in the asymptomatic period.
6. The incidence of the condition must be sufficient to justify the cost of screening.

[a]From Frame PS, Carlson SJ: A critical review of periodic health screening using specific screening criteria. *J Fam Pract* 2:29–36, 1975. Copyright 1975. Reprinted by permission of Appleton & Lange Inc.

The U.S. Preventive Services Task Force (1989) has employed an additional criterion for judging the worth of a screening test: "The test must be able to detect the target condition . . . with sufficient accuracy to avoid producing large numbers of false-positive and false-negative results."

To appreciate the importance of this criterion, it is necessary to understand the concepts of sensitivity and specificity, previously addressed in Chapter 4, "Appropriate Use of Laboratory Tests." Recall that sensitivity is the ability of a test to detect the presence of the target condition. With a sensitivity of 80%, 20% of patients who have the target condition will not be detected, a false negative. Specificity is the ability of a test to correctly identify those without a condition as not having the condition. Thus, with a specificity of 80%, 20% of patients without the condition will be falsely identified as having the condition, a false positive. As the incidence of a condition in the population declines, the proportion of people screened who do not have the condition will increase and, as a consequence, the proportion of people wrongly identified as having the condition will increase.

Since most routine screening tests have limited sensitivity, usually less than 90%, a negative test result does not ensure that the disease is absent. For example, 10% of breast cancers will not be identified by mammography. Screening tests may thus lead to an unjustified sense of security for both clinicians and patients. Significant symptoms and signs must not be overlooked, as in Case 15-3, despite negative screening test results.

It is important for the clinician and the patient to keep in mind that, because of the low incidence of most diseases targeted for screening and the limited specificity of most screening tests, usually less than 90%, patients identified as having a disease by routine screening often do not have the disease. For example, the specificity of a PSA test with a cutoff of 4 ng/ml is only about 30%. Up to 70% of men, such as Mr. Jones in Case 15-4, identified as positive by PSA screening do not have prostate cancer. Thus, a false-positive screening test can result in unnecessary anxiety, cost, and iatrogenic side effects from procedures performed, e.g., needle biopsy of the prostate, to work up falsely positive test results. When targeting asymptomatic individuals for screening tests and other preventive services, clinicians should keep in mind the ancient precept, "primum non nocere"—above all do no harm.

Cases 15-3 and 15-4 demonstrate the importance of clearly educating patients about the capabilities and limitations of screening tests both before they are performed and after results are returned. Some authorities have even proposed that this education be part of a formalized informed consent process for screening tests (Lee, 1993).

IMMUNIZATION

Immunizations are the prototypical clinical preventive service, with a distinguished history spanning from the first use of cowpox vaccine in the 1700s to the first complete eradication of an infectious disease, smallpox, in the 1970s. Immunizations are probably the easiest, most effective type of preventive service to administer, but are often overlooked by clinicians. It is important for clinicians to understand some basic facts about the effectiveness and administration of immunizations.

Immunizations need not totally prevent clinical disease in order to be effective. For example, influenza immunization of the elderly is only 30 to 40% effective at preventing clinical illness in the elderly, but 70 to 90% effective at preventing death from influenza in the elderly. Immunizations also need not confer immunity on 100% of recipients or be given to every member of the population to be effective. In fact, much of the value of immunizations is in the induction of "herd immunity," which protects all members of the population by limiting exposure and transmission. When a clinician immunizes a child against an infectious disease, protection is also provided to other children who have not been immunized or who have not responded to the vaccine.

Adults, like children, need to receive immunizations. This fact is surprisingly frequently overlooked. Immunization rates for adults are in the 20% (pneumococcus) to 40% (influenza) range. Conversely, some children and younger adults need immunizations routinely reserved for older adults, i.e., pneumococcus and influenza. In general, patients of any age with chronic respiratory or cardiovascular diseases, diabetes, or immunosuppression need these immunizations. Recipients need not be totally clinically well in order to receive routine vaccinations. Misconceptions regarding this point result in many missed opportunities for immunization. Clinicians should be aware of the true contraindications and relative contraindications for immunizations, especially since one of the main opportunities to immunize patients is when they are seen for treatment of an illness of some type.

CHEMOPROPHYLAXIS

Chemoprophylaxis is the use of a chemical, usually a drug or medication, to prevent the development of disease. Despite numerous theories and trials, there are currently only two chemoprophylactic agents widely endorsed for use with asymptomatic, low-risk populations: fluoride supplementation to prevent dental caries in children living in areas with low amounts of fluoride in the drinking water and folate supplementation for women of childbearing age to help prevent neural tube disorders in their offspring. For adults, the two most widely used agents are aspirin, for the prevention of heart disease in middle-aged men, and estrogen, for the prevention of osteoporosis and heart disease in postmenopausal women. All chemoprophylactic agents have potential side effects that can make their use problematic. Fluoride can lead to mottled teeth, folate supplementation can mask vitamin B_{12} deficiencies, aspirin may cause hemorrhagic stroke and gastrointestinal bleeding, and estrogen may increase the risks for breast cancer and uterine cancer.

Clinicians should carefully weigh the potential benefits and harms of each agent in light of each patient's medical characteristics and personal desires. Because the trade-off of potential benefits against side effects is often close, patient participation in decision-making is vital. For this reason, most major authorities have classified the provision of chemoprophylaxis in the general category of health counseling.

CASE 15-5

Dr. T. graduated from a good medical school and a good residency program in internal medicine. On finishing his training he established a successful practice in a medium-sized, midwest city. Dr. T. liked to approach the preventive care of his patients as he did their acute care, by relying on his excellent clinical judgment. Mr. J. was a 55-year-old man whom Dr. T. saw for a checkup once in 1990. Results of his examination and cholesterol and fecal occult blood tests ordered at this visit were normal. Mr. J. was not seen again until 1995, when he came into Dr. T.'s office complaining of rectal bleeding. Subsequent tests revealed metasta-

tic colon cancer. Dr. T. told Mr. J. that it was too bad that he had not come back to see him earlier, because he might have ordered a fecal occult blood test or screening sigmoidoscopy examination that might have discovered the cancer earlier. Mr. J. said that he did not know that he should have come back earlier because Dr. T. had not told him to and that, in any case, he expected Dr. T. to notify him of any need for preventive care, as does his dentist. Now Mr. J.'s lawyer wants to know what schedule of preventive care Dr. T. follows and what system he has to make sure that patients receive it.

CASE 15-6

Ms. T. is a 25-year-old woman who comes to Dr. J. for a routine checkup. Dr. J. knows that based on her age and gender she will definitely need Pap smears every 1 to 3 years, blood pressure, height, and weight measurements every 1 to 2 years, tetanus–diphtheria immunizations every 10 years, periodic counseling on nutrition, including folate supplementation, and counseling on physical activity. In order to assess her need for other preventive care interventions, Dr. J. asks her about a number of different aspects of her life and history. Based on the following information about Ms. T., he orders additional types of preventive care (in parentheses): she is a Native American who has spent much of her life living on a reservation (plasma glucose and tuberculosis screening), her mother died of heart disease at age 54 (cholesterol screening), she has had moderate asthma for 10 years (influenza and pneumococcal immunization), she works as a pottery maker (lead screening for her children), she is monogamously married with two young children but has had multiple male partners in the past (HIV screening), and drinks about 20 beers per week (alcohol abuse counseling).

ESTABLISHING A PREVENTIVE CARE PROTOCOL

One of the most basic tasks facing any primary care clinician is to decide on the types and frequencies of preventive services to be routinely provided to patients. Surprisingly, many clinicians never get around to doing this in any formal fashion. This results in confusion for clinicians, staff, and patients, which in turn probably contributes to poor performance rates. This is unnecessary since a number of major authorities, including all four major primary care physician organizations, have recently issued comprehensive schedules for preventive care that can serve as templates for clinicians to follow (American Academy of Family Physicians, 1994; American Academy of Pediatrics, 1995; American College of Obstetricians and Gynecologists, 1993; Eddy, 1992d; American College of Physicians Task Force on Adult Immunization and Infectious Disease Society of America, 1994).

There is a considerable amount of consensus among authorities (see Figures 15.1 and 15.2 adapted from tables published by the U.S. Public Health Service in the *Clinician's Handbook of Preventive Services*) (U.S. Department of Health and Human Services, 1994). In these charts, dark bars denote preventive services recommended by every major authority for asymptomatic patients, while the light bars denote preventive services recommended

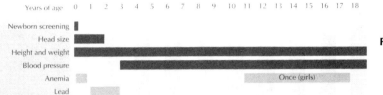

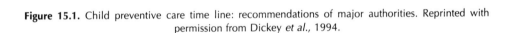

Figure 15.1. Child preventive care time line: recommendations of major authorities. Reprinted with permission from Dickey *et al.*, 1994.

by only some major authorities. It is reasonable that every clinician include the preventive services denoted by dark bars in any preventive care protocol for his or her practice.

The next step is to address the preventive services for which there is some disagreement among major authorities (light bars in Figures 15.1 and 15.2). In order to do this it is useful to have some basic knowledge about the major authorities and how their recommendations for preventive care are formulated. It is also wise to keep in mind that, from a medicolegal standpoint, there are no clear right or wrong answers for these gray areas.

ASSESSING THE AUTHORITIES AND THE EVIDENCE

The first attempts to bring order to the expanding area of clinical prevention in the United States were made by individual experts, such as Frame and Carlson (1975) and Breslow and Sommers (1977) in the late 1970s. Soon voluntary organizations, such as the American Cancer Society (1980), professional societies, such as the American College of Physicians (1981), and governmental agencies, such as the National Cancer Institute (1987), became active in the field. All of these authorities used somewhat different methodologies and often reached different conclusions. To help resolve the confusion, in 1984 the U.S. Public Health Service convened the U.S. Preventive Services Task Force (USPSTF). This group was composed of health professionals with expertise in assessing scientific and epidemiologic evidence. The USPSTF's comprehensive recommendations were issued in 1989 and 1996 in the *Guide to Clinical Preventive Services* (U.S. Preventive Services Task Force, 1989, 1996).

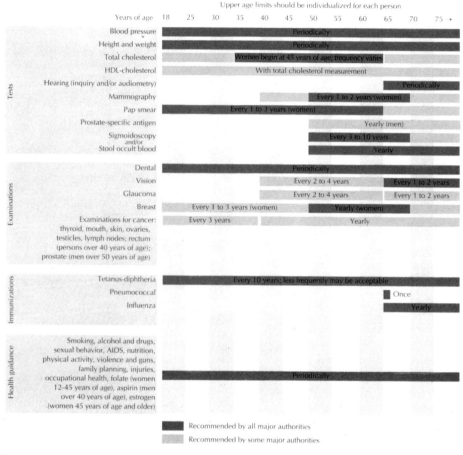

Figure 15.2. Adult preventive care time line: recommendations of major authorities. Reprinted with permission from Dickey *et al.*, 1994.

The USPSTF was the first U.S. body to employ a well-defined, explicit methodology for assessing scientific evidence and reporting recommendations. This methodology, which was largely adopted from the Canadian Task Force on the Periodic Health Examination (1979), emphasized carefully grading the quality of scientific evidence (see Table 15.6), with evidence from randomized controlled trials receiving the most weight and that from expert opinions receiving the least. In general, only preventive services supported by evidence in the top two categories, and occasionally reaching down to the third category, were recommended. The USPSTF has also emphasized the importance of actual health outcomes, as opposed to intermediate outcomes, such as service delivery, in formulating its recommendations. As a consequence, the USPSTF recommendations are among the most conservative, but scientifically respected, of any issued by a U.S. group.

The controversy regarding recommendations for mammography screening of women less than 50 years of age demonstrates how the USPSTF methodology differs from that of some other authorities. The American Cancer Society recommends routine mammography for all women beginning at age 40 (American Cancer Society, 1992), a position also

Table 15.6
USPSTF Rating System for Quality of Scientific Evidence[a]

I:	Evidence obtained from at least one properly designed randomized controlled trial
II-1:	Evidence obtained from well-designed controlled trials without randomization
II-2:	Evidence obtained from well-designed cohort or case–control analytic studies, perferably from more than one center or research group
II-3:	Evidence obtained from multiple time series with or without the intervention, or dramatic results in uncontrolled experiments (such as the results of the introduction of penicillin treatment in the 1940s)
III:	Opinions of respected authorities, based on clinical experience, descriptive studies, or reports of expert committees

[a]From U.S. Preventive Services Task Force. Task force ratings, in *Guide to Clinical Preventive Services.* Baltimore, Williams & Wilkins Co, 1989, p 388.

supported by the National Cancer Institute until 1994. This position is largely based on evidence that mammography can successfully detect cancer at an early stage in women of this age. Large trials, however have failed to demonstrate that mammography in women younger than 50, unlike that in women 50 or older, leads to a reduction in mortality (Tabar *et al.,* 1985; Verbeek *et al.,* 1984; A. B. Miller *et al.,* 1992). Lacking data to support this important health outcome, the USPSTF and some other authorities have not recommended beginning routine mammography before age 50.

Proponents of early mammography have argued that it is logical that early detection and treatment of breast cancer will lead to improved survival for younger women, as it has for older women, and that studies have failed to detect this effect because of defects in their designs. Proponents also argue that even if mammography does not lead to improved mortality for younger women, it may lead to improved quality of life. Opponents counter that breast cancer may be a biologically different, more aggressive disease in women younger than 50 such that early detection has no effect on mortality and that quality-of-life outcomes cannot be quantitatively assessed.

Large healthcare purchasers and insurers are increasingly refusing to provide services that have not been demonstrated in well-designed studies to result in improved health outcomes. As a result, an increasing number of insurers and healthcare purchasers have endorsed the preventive care recommendations of the USPSTF and other "evidence-based" groups over those based on expert opinion. Because the lack of insurance coverage can be a major barrier to obtaining preventive care, it is reasonable for the clinician to consider the realities of insurance coverage and availability of free or subsidized screening facilities in the community in determining a preventive care protocol for his or her practice.

Primary care clinicians face a dilemma when considering the preventive care recommendations of subspecialty societies. Primary care clinicians frequently defer to the judgment of subspecialists on treatment issues. Should not these same subspecialists also be the most reliable source of information on screening issues as well? Unfortunately, subspecialty training does not usually provide any expertise in epidemiology, public health, cost–effectiveness analysis, or other areas of central importance in determining population-based guidelines. On the contrary, subspecialists may be so invested professionally and financially in studying or treating a particular organ or disease that they don't understand or value these wider issues.

CONSIDERING RISK FACTORS

Most patients are at increased risk for preventable disease because of factors in one or more of the following categories: ethnic/geographic origin, family history, personal medical history, occupational/recreational history, sexual history, substance abuse history, and social/living situation. The major risk factors for each of these categories that have been described by major authorities, the relevant diseases, and the potentially effective preventive services have been compiled in Table 15.7. In treating large numbers of patients with pertinent risk factors, it may be advisable to include the relevant preventive services in the routine preventive care protocol for all patients. For example, a clinician who treats many migrant farm workers may choose to perform routine tuberculosis screening on all patients.

Information about the risk factor profile of a community or population can be obtained by consulting state and local public health officials. Information about the risk factors of individual patients must, in general, be obtained from the patient. In this task the use of brief questionnaires, either at the first or subsequent visits, can be very valuable. Recently, testing has begun on electronic tools for soliciting and analyzing patient risk factor information (Roizen *et al.*, 1992). Such tools, when fully developed and widely available, should make the complex task of tailoring preventive care to the patient much easier.

IMPLEMENTING HEALTH PROMOTION
AND DISEASE PREVENTION

Having decided on a preventive care protocol, the clinician has taken the first, most essential step toward making health promotion and disease prevention a prominent part of practice. There are, however, many steps left to be taken. The most mundane, but nonetheless critical, is instituting an office system to carry out the protocol.

It should be clear to the reader that modern health promotion and disease prevention practice is very complex, consisting of an array of immunizations, chemoprophylaxis, screening tests, and counseling interventions that need to be tailored to age, sex, and risk factor characteristics of patients. Keeping track of these for any one patient can be a chore, for an entire practice it can be an overwhelming task. To cope with this the assistance of office systems and nursing and office staff is essential.

The most important office system component is a tracking device of some type. Such a device can be as simple as a paper flow sheet/checklist in patient charts, or as sophisticated as a completely electronic medical record. A survey of primary care physicians in 1992 revealed that approximately 75% reported using a paper flow sheet/checklist of some type, while only 15% reported using a computerized tracking system, but only 1% used a computerized tracking system without also using a paper flow sheet/checklist (*Preventive Care Survey,* Dickey & Kamerow, 1996). Of those using a paper flow sheet/checklist, according to other studies, probably less than 50% actually enter data onto them consistently (Prislin *et al.*, 1986; Belcher, 1990).

The act of having to enter data twice, once onto flow sheets and again into patient progress notes, has undoubtedly been a major burden for many busy practitioners. Poor design and lack of standardization may also be barriers to flow sheet/checklist use. To address this the U.S. Public Health Service has published flow sheet templates as part of the Put Prevention Into Practice campaign (see Figure 15.3) (Dickey & Kamerow, 1994).

Table 15.7
Summary Table of Risk Factors, Diseases, and Preventive Services[a]

325

ESTABLISHING A
PREVENTIVE CARE
PROTOCOL

Risk factor	Disease(s)	Preventive service(s)
Ethnic and geographic origin		
Asian, African, Mediterranean, Caribbean, Latin American	Hemoglobinopathies	Sickledex test and/or hemoglobin electrophoresis
Native American, Hispanic, African American (adults)	Diabetes mellitus	Plasma glucose test
Native American, foreign-born from countries with high TB prevalence (i.e., Africa, Asia, Latin America)	Tuberculosis	Tuberculosis skin test
African American (adults ≥ age 40)	Glaucoma	Comprehensive eye exam
Family history		
Iron-deficit mother (infant)	Anemia	Hemoglobin/hematocrit test
Sibling treated for lead poisoning (child)	Lead poisoning	Lead test
Parent cholesterol level ≥240 mg/dl, parent or grandparent ≤55 had myocardial infarction, angina pectoris, peripheral vascular disease, sudden cardiac death, coronary artery bypass or angioplasty (child ≥ age 2)	Hypercholesterolemia	Total cholesterol test
Breast cancer in first-degree relative (women ≥ age 35)	Breast cancer	Mammography
Colon cancer in first-degree relative	Colon cancer, familial polyposis, cancer family syndrome	Digital rectal exam, fecal occult blood, sigmoidoscopy, colonscopy, or barium enema
Prostate cancer (men ≥ age 40)	Prostate cancer	Digital rectal exam, prostate-specific antigen test
Skin cancer (adults)	Skin cancer	Skin exam
Diabetes mellitus in first-degree relative	Diabetes mellitus	Plasma glucose test
Personal medical history		
Low birth weight, prematurity (infant)	Anemia	Hemoglobin/hematocrit test
	Hearing loss	Hearing testing
	Visual loss	Comprehensive eye exam
Excessive menstrual flow	Anemia	Hemoglobin/hematocrit test
Inflammatory bowel disease, colorectal adenomatous polyps, breast, endometrial, ovarian cancer	Colorectal cancer	Digital rectal exam, fecal occult blood, sigmoidoscopy, colonoscopy, or barium enema
Blood transfusion between 1978 and 1985	HIV disease	HIV test
Diabetes mellitus	Vision loss	Comprehensive eye exam
	Urinary tract infection	Urinalysis test
	Influenza	Influenza immunization
	Pneumococcal disease	Pneumococcal immunization
Chronic pulmonary or respiratory disease	Influenza	Influenza immunization
	Pneumococcal disease	Pneumococcal immunization
Splenectomy, splenic dysfunction	Pneumococcal disease	Pneumococcal immunization
Renal dysfunction	Influenza	Influenza immunization
	Pneumococcal disease	Pneumococcal immunization
	Hepatitis B (if hemodialysis)	Hepatitis B immunization
Cirrhosis	Influenza	Influenza immunization
	Pneumococcal disease	Pneumococcal immunization

(continued)

326

HEALTH
PROMOTION
AND DISEASE
PREVENTION

Table 15.7
(continued)

Risk factor	Disease(s)	Preventive service(s)
Immunosuppression, including HIV, organ transplantation, medication induced	Influenza	Influenza immunization
	Pneumococcal disease	Pneumococcal disease
	Tuberculosis	Tuberculosis skin test
Lack of immunity to measles and born after 1956	Measles	MMR immunization
Lack of immunity to rubella, especially women of childbearing age	Rubella, congenital rubella sundrome in offspring	Rubella immunization
Cryptorchidism, orchiopexy, infertile or atrophic testes, ambiguous genitalia, gonadal dysgenesis, Klinefelter's syndrome (men)	Testicular cancer	Testicular exam
Sexual history		
Multiple sexual partners	HIV disease and other STDs	HIV testing and counseling STD testing and counseling
	Hepatitis B disease	Hepatitis B immunization
Homosexual or bisexual males	HIV disease and other STDs	HIV testing and counseling STD testing and counseling
	Hepatitis B disease	Hepatitis B immunization
Sexual partners who have been		
HIV positive	HIV disease	HIV test
Hepatitis B positive	Hepatitis B disease	Hepatitis B immunization
Heterosexually active, do not desire children	Unintended pregnancy	Contraception counseling
Prostitution, trading sex for money or drugs	HIV disease and other STDs	HIV testing and counseling, STD testing and counseling
	Hepatitis B disease	Hepatitis B immunization
Substance abuse history		
Alcohol abuse	Pneumococcal disease	Pneumococcal immunization
	Tuberculosis	Tuberculosis test
	Oral cancer	Oral exam
	Injuries	Injury prevention counseling
		Alcoholism counseling
Tobacco use	Oral and lung cancer	Oral exam
	Lung and other organ dysfunction	Smoking cessation counseling
Illicit drug use	HIV disease	HIV test
	Hepatitis B disease	Hepatitis B immunization
	Tuberculosis	Tuberculosis test
Social/living situation		
Inadequate fluoridation of water supply (<0.3 ppm if < age 3, <0.6 ppm if ≥ age 3)	Dental caries	Fluoride prophylaxis
Residence in or regular visits to a house built before 1960 with recent, ongoing, or planned renovations or remodeling or peeling or chipping paint (child)	Lead poisoning	Lead test

Table 15.7
(continued)

327

**ESTABLISHING A
PREVENTIVE CARE
PROTOCOL**

Risk factor	Disease(s)	Preventive service(s)
Residence near smelter, batter recycling plant or other industry likely to release lead (child)	Lead poisoning	Lead test
Household member being followed or treated for lead poisoning, adult member with hobby or job working with lead (child)	Lead poisoning	Lead test
Homelessness	Tuberculosis	Tuberculosis test
Institutionalization		
Criminals, developmentally disabled	Hepatitis B disease	Hepatitis B immunization
Elderly, chronic medical problems	Influenza	Influenza immunization
All	Tuberculosis	Tuberculosis test
Firearms in home	Injury and violence	Firearms and injury prevention counseling
Occupational/recreational history		
Migrant laborers	Tuberculosis	Tuberculosis test
Health care workers		
Contact with blood	Hepatitis B disease	Hepatitis B immunization
Might transmit influenza to persons at increased risk for complications	Influenza	Influenza immunization
All	Tuberculosis	Tuberculosis test
Staff of residential care facilities	Tuberculosis	Tuberculosis test
Exposure to increased		
Sunlight	Skin cancer	Skin exam and protection counseling
Noise	Hearing loss	Hearing test and protection counseling

[a]Adapted from *Clinician's Handbook of Preventive Services*, 1994. U.S. Government Printing Office.

    Computerized tracking systems have been found to be very effective at promoting the delivery of preventive services (McPhee *et al.*, 1991; Ornstein *et al.*, 1991). It is striking how little delivery of medical care is tracked by computers relative to the delivery of other seemingly less important commodities in our society, such as groceries in supermarkets or packages by delivery services. Several computerized systems for tracking preventive care have been developed and marketed. These systems have been reviewed by an expert panel (American Cancer Society Advisory Group on Preventive Health Care Reminder Systems, 1995). All "stand-alone" tracking systems for preventive care have the same serious drawback as paper flow sheets: they require double data entry. Either the clinician or staff has to take the time to enter data into the computer as well as manually writing it into patient charts.

    Clinicians entering practice should seriously consider using a totally electronic patient record that can track all aspects of patient care, including health maintenance services. Initial adoption of a totally electronic patient record will obviate the need to later convert written records into an electronic format. Data entry for electronic systems must now be done by keyboard, either by the physician or staff, but advances in voice recognition technology hold promise for simplifying this task.

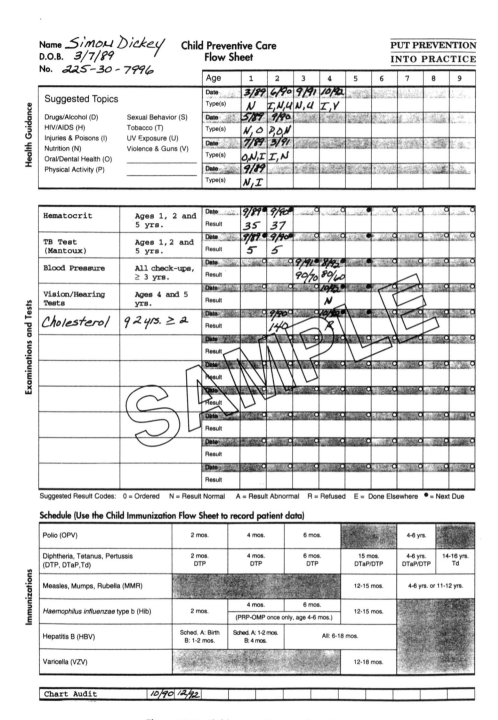

Figure 15.3. Child preventive care flow sheet.

The recent ascendance of managed healthcare will undoubtedly result in increased pressure on clinicians to provide ongoing accounting of preventive services provided to patients. The Joint Commission on the Accreditation of Healthcare Organizations has recently joined with the National Committee for Quality Assurance, which accredits health maintenance organizations, in requiring reporting on a number of practice parameters as part of the Health Plan Employer Data and Information Set (HEDIS). Four parameters address preventive services (mammography, Pap smears, cholesterol testing, and childhood immunizations). Pressure from managed care will probably help bring clinical accounting methods used by clinicians into the modern information age.

USING REMINDERS

Regardless of the tracking system used, it should be capable of generating reminders for the clinician and the patient about health maintenance. A number of studies have demonstrated that reminders both to clinicians and to patients are helpful in the timely deliver of preventive care (McPhee & Detmer, 1993). Reminders can take several forms. Letters generated by staff review of paper records or computer review of electronic records can be mailed to patients to remind them of needed preventive care. Letters or alert notices can also be prepared for clinician use at the time of patient visits. The more specific these reminders are as to each patient's health maintenance needs, the more effective they tend to be. Permanent, practicewide reminders can also be used, such as wall charts of preventive care protocols for examination and waiting rooms for easy patient and clinician reference.

Reminders are necessary because health maintenance, unlike illness care, does not call attention to itself if neglected. Illness symptoms tend to get worse, but the effects of neglected preventive care tend to be silent and insidious. By the time a woman who has not had a screening mammogram develops symptoms from a breast cancer, it may be too advanced to cure.

WORKING WITH NURSING AND OFFICE STAFF

The responsibility for preventive care must also be shared with nursing and office staff. Some authorities recommend designating a staff member to supervise and maintain the office system and the office milieu promoting the performance of preventive care (Carney *et al.,* 1992). Examples of functions of this person might include: maintaining the tracking system, sending out reminders to providers and patients, keeping educational materials about preventive care current and well stocked, and organizing in-service training sessions. Clinicians are often too busy responding to the acute care needs of the practice to ensure that such important activities occur.

CASE 15-7

Dr. J. is a family physician who set up practice of a retirement community in the desert Southwest. In the spring of his first year he did a small survey of 100 charts of patients over the age of 65 and was surprised to see that only 30% had received an influenza immunization during the winter, and those were mainly the ones who had been seen for an illness. He called a few patients who hadn't gotten flu shots and asked them why. Some typical answers were, "Those things don't work," "Flu shots give you the flu, so why should I want one?" and "I had a flu shot 2 years ago and thought I didn't need another one for 10 years."

It was clear to Dr. J. that his patients had a lot of misconceptions about influenza immunizations. In late summer he prepared a short letter to patients clearly explaining the potential benefits and side effects of influenza immunizations and asking patients to call and schedule an appointment for the immunizations. He also did a short public service message for a local television station in the area. Next spring when he repeated the chart survey he was pleased to find that 60% of his elderly patients had gotten immunizations. Other physicians in the community reported a slight increase as well and the administrator of the local hospital thought there were fewer hospitalizations for pneumonia than usual.

——— INVOLVING AND EDUCATING PATIENTS ———

Patients have a lot of interest in preventive care. They are, after all, the prime benefactors of good health. This interest can be utilized to help promote not only healthy behaviors but also performance of proper preventive services. All preventive care requires some active patient participation. At a minimum, patients have to come into the office or clinic, hopefully not only when acutely ill, and follow up with the performance of services, such as mammograms or fecal occult blood tests.

For some types of preventive care the lack of knowledge by patients is a major barrier. For example, the two main reasons given by women for never having had a mammogram in a series of National Cancer Institute studies were: they didn't know that they needed one and their physician had never told them to get one (NCI Breast Cancer Screening Consortium, 1990). Proper patient education is essential not only to help identify need, but also to help deal with fear and misunderstanding about services.

Patients can play a proactive role in their own preventive care by prompting their providers or self-referring for their own preventive services, such as mammograms or immunizations. With regard to the latter, influenza vaccinations for the elderly have been widely and successfully provided in community settings, as in Case 15-7. One approach, modeled on the childhood immunization card, is to give patients a protocol and tracking tool for their own preventive care. The Personal Health Guide and Child Health Guide are passport-sized documents recently published by the U.S. Public Health Service for this purpose (Dickey & Kamerow, 1994). Similar patient-held records have been tested and found to be well received by patients and helpful in promoting preventive care (Dickey, 1993).

For further information on patient education, see Chapter 10, Patient Education.

———————— CONCLUSION ————————

Health promotion and disease prevention are important aspects of modern medical care. As many as half of all deaths may be premature and the result of preventable risk factors. Even modest reductions in these risk factors through counseling and other behavior interventions in the clinical setting can result in a large number of years of life saved.

Clinical preventive services are of four major types: counseling, screening tests, immunizations, and chemoprophylaxis. It is important for the clinician to understand the basic principles underlying each of these types of care. It is also important for the clinician to understand how major authorities make recommendations regarding schedules for these types of care. In particular, the clinician should understand the process of scientific review of evidence.

Clinicians should decide on a protocol of preventive care that is based on science and fits the particular needs of their practice and patients. This protocol should be clearly displayed and explained to staff and patients. Office systems and practice routines should be instituted that aid in the timely delivery of appropriate preventive care. It is important to fully inform and involve patients in decision-making about and prompting of their own preventive care. Good health promotion and disease prevention practice requires team-work on the part of clinicians, staff, and patients.

CASES FOR DISCUSSION

CASE 1

Jane T. is a 45-year-old white female who has been coming to the clinic intermittently, every 2 to 3 years, for treatment of adult-onset diabetes mellitus, which has been relatively well controlled without insulin. Her medical history is otherwise unremarkable. A review of her family, social, sexual, substance use, and occupational/recreational histories reveals the following risk factors: she works as a nurse's aide in a nursing home and her mother died of breast cancer at age 55.

1. *What preventive services (don't forget counseling) will she need based on her age and sex? based on her diabetes mellitus? based on her other risk factors?*
2. *Given the intermittent nature of her visits, what types of office resources might you use to help ensure that she comes in at more appropriate intervals?*

CASE 2

John S. is a 5-year-old boy brought in by his mother for well-child care before starting kindergarten. He is healthy, lives in a modern middle-class neighborhood, received his last immunizations at age 2 years, and has no risk factors of relevance to his preventive care. His mother states that she would like him to have all of the testing and immunizations recommended by medical authorities and that she will pay for anything that her insurance does not cover.

1. *List all of the immunizations, screening tests, and counseling interventions that you could provide to him.*
2. *List only those that you are sure he needs.*
3. *How do you negotiate with parents about providing preventive services for their children that are recommended by some but not all authorities, particularly if evidence for those services is weak?*

CASE 3

You are the director of a student health service at a state college. The administrator of the college has read about the health consequences of genital chlamydia infections and requests that you study screening all 10,000 female students. You research the issue and find that the prevalence of genital chlamydia infections in similar populations is 5%. The sensitivity of the chlamydia test is 90% and the specificity is also 90%. Each test costs $20.

1. *Approximately how many cases of infection will the screening program be expected to detect? How many will the program miss?*
2. *How many false positives will occur during the testing?*
3. *What will be the cost per case of infection properly identified?*
4. *Assuming that it would only cost $5 to presumptively treat every female patient with tetracycline, would this be preferable to the screening program?*

CASE 4

Robert J. is a 35-year-old male who stopped smoking 1 month ago at your urging. He is struggling to avoid starting again.

1. *According to Prochaska, what "stage of change" is he in? What types of interventions are likely to be most helpful to him? What type least helpful?*
2. *How could you or your office staff be helpful to him between visits?*
3. *What screening examination(s) will he need as a result of his smoking?*

CASE 5

Mrs. J. is a 53-year-old white woman who is experiencing menopause. Although she does not have hot flashes or other symptoms, she tells you that she is interested in taking estrogen. You explain to her the potential health advantages and disadvantages of taking estrogen and counsel her that she should probably also take progestin if she elects to take estrogen.

1. *What diseases will hormone replacement therapy possibly help her avoid?*
2. *What diseases will hormone replacement therapy possibly put her at increased risk for?*
3. *Overall, do you think Mrs. J.'s life span will be increased by taking hormone replacement therapy?*
4. *Overall, do you think the quality of Mrs. J.'s life will be improved by hormone replacement therapy?*

RECOMMENDED READINGS

Prochaska JO, Norcross J, DiClemente C: *Changing for Good.* New York, William Morrow & Co, 1994.

Over the last decade the authors of this book have published a large number of excellent scientific articles detailing the stages people progress through in making behavioral and life-style changes. Because of their work, assessment of "readiness to change" has become a widely accepted component of counseling by health professionals of many types. This book, written as a self-help guide for the general public, is the first exposition of their model outside of the professional psychology literature. Although leaning a bit too far in the "pop psychology" direction, it is a useful and enjoyable introduction to their work for health professionals.

U.S. Department of Health and Human Services. *Clinician's Handbook of Preventive Services.* Washington, DC, US Department of Health and Human Services, 1994.

Part of the U.S. Public Health Service's Put Prevention Into Practice campaign, this book was designed as a "how-to" manual to complement the "what-to-do" information of the *Guide to Clinical Preventive Services.* Each type of preventive service recommended by any major U.S. authority is addressed in separate chapters. Five types of information are furnished: the burden of suffering of target conditions; the recommendations of all major U.S. authorities for the frequency of performance based on age, sex, and risk factors; the basics of how to perform the preventive service in simple steps corresponding to their temporal sequence in practice; current information on where to obtain patient and provider educational materials; and scientific references. The handbook was prepared by the U.S. Office of Disease Prevention and Health Promotion with input from every federal health agency and many professional and voluntary health organizations. This is a valuable reference for the busy practitioner and educational tool for health professionals in training. An updated edition was issued in the fall of 1996. It is available from the Superintendent of Documents, P.O. Box 371954, Pittsburgh, Pa 15650-7954 separately (Stock No. 017-001-00496-1) for $20 or as part of the Put Prevention Into Practice Education and Action Kit (see below). It is also published (Product No. 1980) by the American Academy of Family Physicians (1-800-944-0000) and International Medical Publishing, Inc (1-703-519-0807).

U.S. Department of Health and Human Services. *Put Prevention Into Practice Education and Action Kit.* Washington, DC, US Department of Health and Human Services, 1994.

In addition to one copy of the *Clinician's Handbook of Preventive Services,* this contains several copies of a variety of paper-based tools for implementing preventive care in the office or clinic. These include: the *Personal Health Guide* and *Child Health Guide,* passport-sized documents that provide patients and parents with basic information about preventive care and personal records for tracking preventive care; templates of flow sheets for patient charts; a variety of stickers for use on patient charts as reminders about different types of preventive care; a *Prevention Prescription* pad; and posters for examination rooms depicting preventive care for children and adults in timeline formats. The entire kit can be ordered for $57 from the Superintendent of Documents, P.O. Box 371954, Pittsburgh, Pa 15650-7954.

U.S. Preventive Services Task Force. *Guide to Clinical Preventive Services: Report of the US Preventive Services Task Force, Second Edition Baltimore,* Williams & Wilkins Co, 1996.

This new edition updates and expands upon the classic report produced by this expert panel in 1989. The scientific evidence regarding 70 different types of clinical preventive care has been exhaustively researched, evaluated, and clearly summarized for the practitioner, student, or policy maker. Recommendations for and against performance are presented based on patient age, sex, and other risk factors.

CHAPTER 16

Critical Appraisal of the Medical Literature

Warren P. Newton

At 10:00PM, the junior medical student on her medicine clerkship learns about her first admission of the night, a 34-year-old man with a history of alcohol abuse who now complains of epigastric pain and an inability to keep any liquids down. On physical examination, he is mildly uncomfortable, with orthostatic changes in pressure and pulse and significant epigastric tenderness. Lab results are normal except for an amylase of 324 mg/dl.

After examining the patient, the student is expected to prepare a formal written history and physical examination as well as a short oral presentation at morning rounds. For background information on pancreatitis, she looks in her textbook of medicine. Noting that the textbook was updated 4 years before, she goes to the **Index Medicus Bibliography of Medical Reviews** *and finds a more recent review.*

At morning rounds, she briefly summarizes the prognosis and treatment of pancreatitis, recommending IV fluids, pain control, and withholding an NG tube in view of his mild course. The patient recovers in 2 days and is discharged to outpatient alcohol rehabilitation.

—————————— **LEARNING OBJECTIVES** ——————————

At the conclusion of this chapter, the student will be able to:

1. Describe three sources of medical information and identify their strengths and weaknesses
2. Identify the principles of effective computer searching and apply them to actual clinical problems
3. Describe the criteria for critically appraising articles on diagnosis, prognosis, treatment, and causation of disease
4. Apply the principles of critical appraisal to specific clinical situations and specific articles

————————————— **INTRODUCTION** —————————————

Medical students, residents, and practicing physicians spend a great deal of time obtaining and evaluating medical information, but rarely get practical training in how to do this efficiently and effectively. Over the last 30 years, there has been an explosion of medical information available to physicians. Unfortunately, however, there has not been a similar expansion in the hours of the day available for physicians to review this information. As a result, practitioners have become increasingly like the rabbit in *Alice in Wonderland,* running ever faster to stay in the same place.

To make incorporating new information into practice more feasible, a group of physicians with training in epidemiology at McMaster University have developed techniques for "critical appraisal" of the medical literature (Sackett *et al.,* 1991). Based on the application of the principles of epidemiology to clinical research, critical appraisal allows physicians to prioritize the information available and systematically to review the quality of the information they receive. Using this approach, searching for appropriate literature is dramatically faster, and evaluation of what is found is substantially more rigorous.

CASE 16-2

As a part of a didactic seminar in the obstetrics and gynecology clerkship, a medical student is asked to present a 15-minute talk about epidural anesthesia: common techniques, mechanism of action, effectiveness, and adverse consequences. The talk is scheduled to be given in 1 week; the student reviews the relevant sections of his obstetrics text, as well as an anesthesiology text from the library. He also talks with the obstetric anesthesiologist to learn the techniques in use at this hospital and with the hospital business office to learn the current charges for epidurals. The talk goes well; the seminar leader, after praising the student's resourcefulness in learning the charges for epidurals, comments that his search was incomplete, in that his presentation did not address a major recent publication, a large randomized trial suggesting that epidurals doubled the rate of cesarean section (Ramen et al., 1995).

HOW MUCH TIME FOR WHAT KIND OF ANSWER?

Searching for medical information depends on both the time available for the search and the detail of the information needed. In Case 16-1, the student who has just admitted the patient with pancreatitis has overnight to learn the basics of pancreatitis—its differential diagnosis, prognosis, and treatment—prior to her oral presentation in the morning. Time is quite limited, but there is rarely the expectation that the junior medical student will need to know in detail the problems with Ranson's prognostic criteria or recent randomized trials on the management of pancreatitis. By contrast, the task given to the student in Case 16-2 allowed him ample time to search the literature and to review carefully primary research articles. The trade-off between the time available and depth of answer needed continues through residency and into practice. Practicing physicians often turn to *Facts and Comparisons* for a quick question about drug dosage, but may need to do more involved research when it is their turn to do Grand Rounds at their local community hospital or develop their group's practice guideline on a common medical problem.

Whatever the level of training, clinicians face a similar set of possible sources of clinical information. Most accessible and easiest to use are textbooks or recent review articles. Textbooks are portable, available wherever and whenever needed, and represent the best opinion of an "expert" in that field; disadvantages are that they are often out of date and they provide overviews that may be too superficial for specific clinical questions. In most cases, moreover, they have not been written from the perspective of "evidence-based medicine," that is, incorporating an assessment of the strength of the evidence behind specific recommendations (Rosenberg & Donald, 1995). Reviews published in journals possess advantages and disadvantages similar to textbook chapters, but are more likely to be up to date.

A second source of information are local experts, such as a colleague or consultant. Local experts are relatively easy to contact, know local conditions, and provide information more specific to the patient at hand. They may be more up to date than textbooks. However, there may be problems with the information provided by local experts. Most consultants have not been trained in evidence-based medicine, and their clinical experience since training has often been shaped by patients very different from those of the physicians who refer to them. Moreover, consultation may also include a direct monetary cost to the patient.

A third source of information is the primary medical literature, accessed by computer through Medline or manually through *Index Medicus*. A great advantage of this source is that it is as up to date as possible; this is particularly important when what is at issue is a recently recognized disease or problem, or when recent information is substantially better than what was known before. Another advantage of reviewing the medical literature personally is that the clinician can analyze the evidence directly, without looking through the lens of another reviewer. Original research reports, appropriately analyzed, remain the best information on which to base clinical practice. The major disadvantage of searching the primary medical literature is the time and effort necessary to retrieve, review, and synthesize the individual articles.

Practicing clinicians use all three sources of information regularly, switching from one to the other as the situation and their comfort with their sources vary. One of the goals of training in both medical school and residency is to become facile with the process of searching, including quickly deciding the best strategy for getting specific information and the tactics of searching a particular source.

COMPUTER SEARCHING OF THE LITERATURE

Computer searching of the medical literature has become increasingly important for clinicians, and it is important for students to develop good searching skills. The first step is a clear, focused clinical question. As much as possible, it is important to break down general questions into more specific questions. For example, rather than searching a very general topic like "knowing about Alzheimer's disease," it is important for the clinician to decide what aspects of its diagnosis, prognosis, or treatment she wants to know about. More specific questions make searching more efficient.

The clinician should also keep in mind what would be the ideal kind of evidence for answering her specific question. As will be discussed later, the ideal study will vary according to the kind of clinical question, but knowing what the ideal study would be greatly speeds the process of sorting "wheat from chaff." For example, for a question about the risks and benefits of treating isolated systolic hypertension, the best possible study will be a randomized clinical trial (RCT) or, possibly, a meta-analysis of randomized trials. Knowing this information means that the search process can focus on finding just RCTs, ignoring the many case series that have been published.

The next step is to consider how many years and what languages the search should include. Again, this decision will depend in part on the topic. For some clinical questions, e.g., the use of AZT in pregnant patients who are seropositive for HIV, it may make sense to limit your search to the last 5 years, but for other questions, e.g., the role of dietary restriction of purines in treatment of gout, searching back to the late 1960s and early 1970s may be more appropriate. For most clinical questions, it is not necessary to search other languages, but such a search may be necessary if the purpose is to prepare a research proposal or write a paper.

Once searching on line, the best strategy is to get as many citations as possible initially and then to narrow down. Start with only a disease term or a therapy and use the medical subject headings terms (MeSH) as much as possible. The MeSH headings are the terms used by the National Library of Medicine to code each article as it is entered into the computerized data base. MeSH headings are available in books in the library as well as in an on-line thesaurus in many searching programs. Using MeSH headings will improve retrieval of articles. For example, using our local system, PC OVID, to search 1992–1995 text and key words, *heart attack* yields 44 references, *MI* yields 6317, and the MeSH term *myocardial infarction* yields 11,203 references.

After getting a large pool of citations, the next step is to focus on the best articles for the clinical questions. Major MeSH headings, which select for articles with a major emphasis on the subject, are very useful, as are subheadings, like *drug therapy* or *prevention and control,* as well as the age of subjects or language of publication. Increasingly valuable is searching by publication type such as *meta-analysis* or by methodological terms, such as *randomized controlled trial.* Care must be taken not to weed too appropriate.

It is important to keep in mind that computer searching is sometimes insensitive, as medical students learn when they discover a critical article that should have been identified after they have made a presentation or handed in their paper! Even in the best of hands, with a clinician searching along with a librarian, using multiple data bases, a substantial number of references will be missed. The major cause for the insensitivity of searching is the human role in attributing subject headings to articles. With practice, and by using MeSH headings, searching several different ways, and, if necessary, following up the references in articles, the sensitivity of computer searching can be maximized.

CASE 16-3

Your family practice preceptors have developed a system for obtaining information from pharmaceutical representatives: In return for the purchase of medical textbooks, your preceptor and his partners have a bag lunch once a month over which they hear the sales pitches of the representatives. Today, the representative is from a company selling a calcium channel blocker. Her goal is to comment on a recent article (Furberg et al., 1995), which attributed a higher mortality rate to calcium channel blockers in routine use. She does not have a copy of the original article to give you, but she does have a public statement by a local cardiologist that the evidence is suspect and that clinical practice should not change at this point, "in view of the obvious effectiveness and safety that these agents have had over the years." The student does a search and retrieves the relevant articles but is still confused after reading studies that report conflicting results.

── CRITICAL APPRAISAL OF THE LITERATURE ──

GENERAL PRINCIPLES

Case 16-3 illustrates the need for critical appraisal of the medical literature. As popularized at McMaster University, critical appraisal is the application of clinical epidemiology to published human research. It has several key principles. First, there is an emphasis on the clinicians' perspective. Whereas traditional epidemiology focuses on the causation of disease, clinical epidemiology recognizes that there are a limited number of fundamental kinds of problems physicians face—diagnosis, prognosis, and treatment— and these problems typically require methodology that is specific to the clinical problem. Second, for each of these kinds of problems, there are some methodologies that are stronger than others, in the sense that they are more likely to get a valid answer for the patients in the study. Thus, for example, RCTs are in general stronger than cohort studies, which are stronger than case–control studies or case series. The third principle of critical appraisal is that there is little need to review studies that are methodologically weak if stronger studies are available. Time is crucial for busy clinicians, and critical appraisal allows them to focus their attention only on evidence that is worthwhile.

In practical terms, critical appraisal of the literature involves the application of a set of rules derived from epidemiology to specific articles. The particular set of rules will vary according to the kind of clinical question—e.g., diagnosis, prognosis, or treatment—being addressed. In general, the rules will address two different domains, internal validity and external validity or generalizability. Internal validity is the ability of the study to achieve a valid answer for the subjects in the study. Concerns of internal validity revolve around whether the design is randomized, whether the outcomes are appropriate, whether there are confounding effects, and so on. There is general consensus about what kinds of study designs are stronger, so that it is usually relatively easy to rank studies by quality, at least in a general way. Concerns of external validity revolve around the generalizability of the findings to the patient and clinical setting at hand. Are the subjects similar to those of the clinician asking the question? In contrast to the criteria related to internal validity, it is harder to rank studies based on their generalizability to the searcher's clinical context: there is no "scale" for "patients similar to mine"! Nevertheless, both internal and external validity are important, and the clinician should use both kinds of rules to assess the quality of the evidence relating to his or her clinical question.

CASE 16-4

An otherwise healthy 23-year-old woman presents with dysuria and urinary frequency for 12 hours, along with a subjective history of chills. Physical examination reveals no fever, costovertebral angle tenderness, vaginal discharge, or cervical motion tenderness; urinalysis shows 0–2 white cells/high-power field and trace leukocyte esterase. The preceptor asks the medical student how sensitive a test urinalysis is for urinary tract infection (UTI). The student finds the information in a text on laboratory medicine (Panzer et al., 1991), and reports that the sensitivity of urinalysis for UTI is between 60 and 80%—good, but not perfect. The woman is treated for a UTI and improves.

DIAGNOSIS

Questions about diagnosis occur frequently in both inpatient and outpatient settings. Typically, physicians are interested in articles evaluating a new diagnostic test or strategy [e.g., urinalysis to diagnose UTI in Case 16-4, prostate-specific antigen (PSA) for prostatic cancer, or the Michigan Alcohol Screening Test (MAST) questionnaire for alcoholism]; occasionally, the "diagnostic test" being evaluated is physician history taking (e.g., a history of angina for coronary artery disease) or physical examination (e.g., calf tenderness as a sign of deep venous thrombosis).

There are many texts available that describe various laboratory tests and list the diseases that can cause abnormalities, but most do not provide information on test performance. An exception is *Diagnostic Strategies for Common Problems,* which provides in-depth discussion of specific clinical questions with data about test performance (Panzer *et al.,* 1991). Computer searching the literature for diagnostic information can usually be done most efficiently by looking up the disease with a subheading of *diagnosis;* if this yields too many articles to scan, the methodological term *sensitivity and specificity* will select for methodologically stronger studies. Occasionally, meta-analyses of diagnostic tests are performed and can be found by searching by that term. For aspects of the history and physical examination, the recent *JAMA* series on the rational physical examination is an excellent source of information; computer searching should be supplemented by looking for references in textbooks of physical examination, since many of the references are older.

In order to understand how to evaluate articles on diagnosis, it is necessary to review some basic definitions. All diagnostic tests need to be evaluated against a *gold standard,* which is the best single test or combination of tests that is relevant to the particular diagnosis and should be applied to each subject who receives a diagnostic test. Thus, when thinking of exercise tolerance test as a diagnostic test for coronary artery disease, the gold standard would be angiography or autopsy. Gold standards may not be perfect—e.g., chlamydial culture, which is insensitive in clinical practice—and they may be impossible to obtain except under unusual situations such as autopsy. It is a clinical judgment about whether a particular gold standard is the appropriate one.

Articles on diagnostic tests should include the *sensitivity, specificity, positive predictive value,* and *negative predictive value* of the test, as defined in Chapter 4 on laboratory tests. Both sensitivity and specificity are characteristics of the test, and typically do not vary from setting to setting. By contrast, the *positive* and *negative predictive values* vary from setting to setting. It is the predictive value that physicians use when treating for a positive test and reassuring for a negative test. Statistics for a test are usually given in percentages, so that, for example, a 70% sensitivity for a new test for mycoplasma would mean that, on average, the test would read positive for 70% of women who have mycoplasma infections.

The predictive value of a test will depend on the prevalence of the disease in the population. According to the Bayes theorem, for diseases with high prevalence, the positive predictive value will be high; as the prevalence drops, however, the positive predictive value will decrease. The negative predictive value moves in the opposite fashion. In practical terms, given a particular test, if a clinician uses a diagnostic test in a high-prevalence setting, a positive test will be more likely to be truly positive than a positive test in a low-prevalence setting. For example, San Francisco gay males living in the Castro district have an HIV seroprevalence estimated to be at least 80%, while asymptomatic low-risk people from rural North Carolina have a prevalence of disease of <1%. A positive HIV screen in North Carolina is very likely to be a false positive; in a gay San Franciscan, the chances of a true positive are much greater.

Figure 16.1 summarizes the criteria for reading an article about a diagnostic test. The clinician should first decide if the test is one he might use in his clinical setting and whether the gold standard test was used for all subjects. If the answer to both of these questions is yes, the article is worth taking the time to read. Then the clinician should ask what the disease being tested for is. Usually, this is straightforward, but occasionally not, as, for example, when routine urinalysis is done as part of an annual physical examination to screen for infection, renal tumor, glomerular disease, and kidney stones. Next consider the gold standard test. Is it clinically appropriate? If not, the sensitivity and specificity reported by the study may be misleading. Then, review the sensitivity and specificity of the test; how does this test compare with other tests available? Most useful screening tests have sensitivities above 70%, e.g., mammography has a sensitivity of 75 to 85% and HIV testing has a sensitivity of 99%. Finally, compare the prevalence of the disease in the study

Is this article worth taking the time to read?

☐ Yes, because I use or might use the test regularly, a "gold standard" test was used on all subjects.

☐ No.

If yes, answer the following:

1. What disease is being looked for? What is the diagnostic test?

2. What is the "gold standard" test? Is it reasonable, and what are its limitations?

3. What is the sensitivity, specificity, and predictive value of the test?

4. In terms of prevalence of the disease, are the study subjects similar to your patients? Will the predictive value of the test be the same for your patients?

UNC Critical Appraisal Group; adapted from materials developed at McMaster University

Figure 16.1. Worksheet for articles about diagnostic tests.

with your own patients. Keeping the Bayes theorem in mind will allow an estimate of how the test will perform when you use it on your patients.

CASE 16-5

At a routine home visit 68 hours after delivery, the family physician notices that the baby he delivered is jaundiced in both the arms and the legs. The baby was a full-term product of an uncomplicated labor and delivery, with Apgars of 8 at 1 minute and 9 at 5 minutes. Neonatal course was uncomplicated, and the mother had requested discharge at 6 hours. The mother's first child had breast-fed to 15 months, and the mother has no concerns at this time. Except for the jaundice, results of the physical examination were reassuring; the infant was sucking well and was neurologically intact. Review of records shows that the mother is blood type A positive; the cord blood was Coombs negative. Laboratory examination of the newborn reveals a total bilirubin of 12, a normal hematocrit, and no evidence of hemolysis. The family physician asks the medical student accompanying him about the risk of kernicterus from hyperbilirubinemia as well as whether photo-therapy is indicated. A computer search with key terms jaundice, neonatal *and subheadings* therapy, complications *and publication type* practice guidelines, *yields recent practice guidelines (AAP, 1994) for the management of neonatal jaundice, as well as a recent reanalysis of a large study of prognosis (Newman & Klebanoff, 1993). Based on their findings from the computer search, the mother and baby are expectantly managed and do well.*

PROGNOSIS

Questions about prognosis are a common part of the practice of medicine in both inpatient and outpatient settings. Physicians use prognostic information to give patients advice about what symptoms to expect, when to expect them, and what the benefits of treatment are.

Unfortunately, there is much less information available in the medical literature on prognosis than on diagnosis and treatment. Textbooks and review articles will sometimes have citations of classic articles; for computer searches, combining the disease term with the subheading *prognosis* or the methodological terms *cohort study* or *prospective study* is the best approach. Also helpful are the control wings of randomized trials, although one haa to be careful that the patients enrolled are similar to one's own patients.

A good approach to describing what studies of prognosis ought to include is to describe a clinical question, imagine the best possible study to answer the question, and then extrapolate from this ideal. Regarding the issues raised by Case 16-5, as for most studies of prognosis, a randomized design is not possible, since one cannot usually randomize hazardous exposures like hyperbilirubinemia. As a consequence, the next strongest design would be a cohort study, in which people are identified and followed over years. Identifying the people at the beginning of a disease's course—an *inception co-hort*—allows better measurements of exposures and better tracking of the group and is stronger methodologically than identifying a group retrospectively. In the case of neonatal hyperbilirubinemia, it would be important to include patients who were similar to the patients the clinician is most concerned with—full-term babies without evidence of distress or sepsis, who are enrolled at birth rather than referred in, and to follow them for enough years to make sure that the clinically relevant outcomes (neurological abnormalities, school dysfunction, learning problems) have an opportunity to occur, at least 8 years. One would want to have enough numbers of patients to pick up rare outcomes like kernicterus, and keep track of all possible confounding variables, or the other factors that may influence outcomes. For neonatal jaundice, this may require tens of thousands of subjects. Finally, one would want to follow as many patients as possible to the end; if a

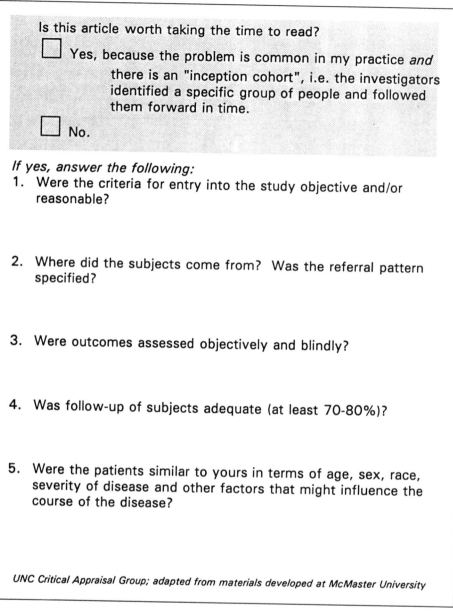

Is this article worth taking the time to read?

☐ Yes, because the problem is common in my practice *and* there is an "inception cohort", i.e. the investigators identified a specific group of people and followed them forward in time.

☐ No.

If yes, answer the following:

1. Were the criteria for entry into the study objective and/or reasonable?

2. Where did the subjects come from? Was the referral pattern specified?

3. Were outcomes assessed objectively and blindly?

4. Was follow-up of subjects adequate (at least 70-80%)?

5. Were the patients similar to yours in terms of age, sex, race, severity of disease and other factors that might influence the course of the disease?

UNC Critical Appraisal Group; adapted from materials developed at McMaster University

Figure 16.2. Worksheet for articles about prognosis.

study does not follow up at least 80% of the patients, the potential bias becomes very large, and the paper is not worth reading.

Obviously, this kind of "ideal study" could only rarely be done, but it does allow us to identify the key criteria for articles on prognosis. As Figure 16.2 depicts, the cardinal characteristics of studies of prognosis are use of an inception cohort and adequate follow-up. If neither of these features is present, the likelihood of getting valid information is so low that it is usually not worth the time to read the article. As it happens, most articles on prognosis in the medical literature do not meet this standard. Next, assess whether the subjects are similar to yours, both in terms of clinical characteristics required for entry into the trial as well as whether they represent a referral population. Prognosis may vary dramatically with clinical characteristics; patients who are referred to specialists and then followed may have a very different prognosis than other patients who are followed by their primary care physicians. Finally, did the estimates of prognosis take into account the confounding factors? These are factors that may influence outcomes significantly and should be accounted for in the analysis.

CASE 16-6

A 33-year-old male presents with a purulent nasal discharge, a temperature of 38.3° C, and right maxillary tenderness. The medical student diagnoses sinusitis and suggests treatment for 10 days with trimethoprim–sulfamethoxazole to the preceptor. The preceptor asks the student if there is any new information in the treatment of sinusitis. The student performs a literature search using the search terms sinusitis *(exploded) and publication type* randomized controlled trial, *and discovers a recent randomized trial showing that 3 days of antibiotic treatment has outcomes similar to 10 days (Williams et al., 1995). The patient is treated with decongestants and 3 days of antibiotics and recovers well.*

————— THERAPY —————

Therapy is any intervention made by a clinician to prevent, cure, or ameliorate disease. Thus, therapy includes not only medication, as in Case 16-6, but also other kinds of interventions as well, such as surgery, an exercise program to lower cholesterol, physician advice about screening mammograms, or over-the-counter medication for allergies.

Textbooks, reviews, and manuals are easily available and give therapeutic recommendations that are relatively applicable; in recent years, textbooks in obstetrics and pediatrics organized solely around the available randomized trials have been published. In situations in which you wish to look at the primary evidence for treating, a good first start for searching the literature is to enter the disease and a subheading, *drug therapy* or *therapy;* the specific drug or therapy can also be used. The publication-type term *randomized controlled trial* has the potential to increase the efficiency of the search dramatically, but not all randomized controlled trials have been given this subject heading, particularly in earlier years. For topics in which there have been many different randomized trials, such as hypertension or congestive heart failure, the publication term *meta-analysis* will be valuable.

To illustrate the principles underlying the critical review of articles on therapy, it is valuable to consider a hypothetical case. On a recent trip to Russia, the author visited the Russian National Institute of Physical Therapy, where a physician reported favorably on the therapeutic benefits of a particular type of mud found in the Crimea. She claimed that, when applied hot three to five times a week for up to an hour, this mud was useful for a variety of conditions, including psoriasis, hepatoma, and hypertension.

Consider a trial of the therapeutic benefit of mud for hypertension. Assuming adequate quantities of good-quality mud from the Crimea were available, the most important feature of this trial would be that it was *controlled*—or, in other words, that two groups are compared, one of which gets the new treatment and one of which does not. This sounds basic, but it is surprising how often new technologies or drugs are promoted on the basis of uncontrolled tests. Recent examples include single lung transplants in patients with COPD, diagnostic techniques such as chorionic villus sampling, and the use of buspar for smoking cessation.

Another important feature of a trial would be that the two groups be as similar as possible at the beginning of the trial, except for the therapy. To illustrate, suppose the group getting mud therapy started out with a diastolic blood pressure averaging 91 mm Hg, whereas the control group averaged 106 mm Hg. If blood pressure were measured at the end without making sure the two groups were similar at the beginning, the result might be attributed to the good effect of the mud rather than the fact they started out differently. An actual example of this is the old debate of medical or surgical management of esophageal varices. Early comparisons found that patients getting surgery did better. What was not addressed initially, however, was that, as a group, sicker patients did not go to surgery, so that better outcome was related to being less sick at the beginning of the study rather than the particular treatment.

Randomization is the best way to make the control and intervention groups similar. Why is randomization so powerful? Because it provides the best protection against unequal distribution of factors that may influence the outcomes. In the case of a randomized trial of mud therapy, with a large number of patients, age, race, dietary sodium intake, and other factors that are known to influence blood pressure will be relatively similar in the intervention and control groups. Randomization also protects against the influence of currently unknown factors that may influence outcomes. So, for example, it may be that a future study finds that a particular plasma renin greatly modifies the impact of hypertension therapy. In that case, the integrity of the mud therapy would probably be protected, because randomization would likely have made sure that the average renin level of those getting mud was the same as the average renin for those not getting mud, assuming adequate numbers of patients. An actual example of this is the Lipid Research Clinics Coronary Primary Prevention Trial. This trial was designed to test the hypothesis that lowering serum cholesterol would prevent myocardial infarctions. The two groups in this trial were randomized to receive either cholestyramine or placebo, resulting in a nearly identical distribution of known risk factors for myocardial infarction (e.g., cigarette smoking, hypertension). Now, almost two decades after the CPPT began, new data have suggested that persons who take aspirin are at lower risk for developing myocardial infarctions. Does this mean that the earlier observed results of the CPPT might be related to differences in aspirin consumption in the two groups rather than lowering cholesterol? Probably not, because the earlier study was randomized.

The next step in designing a clinical trial of mud therapy is to decide on which outcomes one wants to measure. The best way to choose outcomes is to apply clinical common sense. With respect to mud therapy for hypertension, blood pressure response is important insofar as it affects incidence of stroke and myocardial function, but other factors are also important, such as the cost in dollars and time and the quality of life of patients receiving the treatment. Frequent mud baths may be relaxing! Also important are side effects, which, in the case of mud therapy, might be burns from mud, time spent in treatment, and skin staining.

Who will measure the outcomes? It would be convenient, but probably not appropriate, to have a mud-room attendant measure blood pressure and other outcomes. Despite the best of intentions, there is a natural human tendency to bias recording to make what one is testing seem better than it is. This is the principle of *blinding* or masking: the people measuring or recording outcomes should not, if possible, know whether the subject was in the treatment or control group.

How long should the trial last? Ideally, of course, it would be nice to run a 20-year trial of the effects of mud therapy on the clinical outcomes of stroke and myocardial infarction, but limited resources dictate more limited durations. Use clinical common sense; in the case of mud therapy for hypertension, 2–4 weeks is probably too short and between 6 and 12 months would be much better. No matter what duration, all subjects should be accounted for at the end of the study. In analyzing the mud trial, it is not appropriate to compare the two groups if a large number of one of the groups dropped out. Subjects who drop out of studies tend to do worse than those who stay in; not paying attention to dropout may lead to the error of assuming that the treatment worked when in fact most of those who got it may have done so poorly that they went elsewhere.

Finally, in considering the results of the trial of mud therapy, it is important to distinguish between statistical and clinical significance. If the trail has 2000 subjects and finds that mud therapy lowers blood pressure by 1 mm Hg and that this finding is statistically significant, this would be nice to know, perhaps, but it would not be clinically useful. A 1 mm Hg change in blood pressure is clinically trivial. Only a trial that is both statistically and clinically significant should influence the clinician to adopt a new therapy. If the trial were negative—that is, if it was unable to show a significant effect of mud therapy on blood pressure—the first question to ask in interpretation of the results is: How large is the study? The *power* of a study is the likelihood that it has of showing a difference between the intervention and control groups; a small study may not have sufficient power to show a difference. In terms of the mud trial, suppose there were four cases treated with mud that showed a 14-mm decline in blood pressure and two placebo-treated subjects in which blood pressure dropped 6 mm. The difference, 8 mm, is clinically significant but, with the small numbers in the trial, may not reach statistical significance. One could imagine that a larger trial might confirm the 8-mm difference and if it did, we would herald a new age in the treatment of hypertension. A negative study might or might not be proof that the particular therapy does not work.

The last section discussed an *efficacy* trial of mud therapy for hypertension—that is, asking the question, "Under the best possible conditions, does mud therapy reduce blood pressure?" The best possible conditions include the best possible mud and physical therapists, physicians who are interested in the projects, subjects who are paid to get the treatments and stay in the trial, and carefully blinded assessment of multiple important clinical outcomes. Practicing clinicians, however, work in settings far removed from the hothouse atmosphere of well-funded clinical trials. Their patients are not homogenous, they don't necessarily show up, and high-quality mud may not be available. What they need to guide their actions are *effectiveness* trials, in other words, trials using more realistic conditions. Frequently, effectiveness trials have very different findings from efficacy trials; unfortunately, however, for most new technologies, drugs, and other medical interventions, effectiveness trials are not often done.

In addition to evaluating the methodological strength of studies, it is also necessary to assess the relevance or generalizability of the study to the clinicians' practice. Would the therapy be used or referred for frequently? If not, it is not often worth taking the time to read. Is the drug or therapy available locally? Even if the drug or operation is available locally, it may be used differently than the way it is reported. For example, initial advertising for ciprofloxacin cited a study of the effectiveness of ciprofloxacin in which the average dose was double what the sales representative was recommending. Are the patients similar to yours? Sometimes the patients are of substantially different age, gender, or ethnic background than yours. This is significant if these differences are related to differences in the biology of the disease, health-seeking behavior, or any other factor that will influence the effect of the therapy.

Figure 16.3 lists the criteria for evaluating articles on therapy. The cardinal criteria are: Is the therapy something you would use or refer for, and is the trial randomized? If the

---

Is this article worth taking the time to read?

☐ Yes, because I might use or recommend this treatment in my practice and treatment was randomly allocated to subjects.

☐ No.

If yes, answer the following:

1. Were the intervention and control groups similar?

2. Were all clinically relevant outcomes assessed?

3. Were all subjects accounted for at the end of the study? Were outcomes assessed blindly? Were other factors which might influence outcomes accounted for?

4. Are the results clinically as well as statistically significant? If a negative trial, was the power of the study adequate?

5. Are the patients similar to yours?

UNC Critical Appraisal Group; adapted from materials developed at McMaster University

---

Figure 16.3. Worksheet for articles about treatment.

answer to either question is no, it is usually not necessary to read the paper unless no other information is available. If the article is worth the time to read, systematically review the paper, looking first at subjects. Are they similar to yours? Did randomization work to divide the subjects into two similar groups? Was there good follow-up? Then look at the outcomes. Were all of the relevant outcomes chosen? Were outcomes assessed in a nonbiased way? Finally, look at the results. Are they clinically as well as statistically significant? Were confounding variables accounted for in the analysis?

CASE 16-7

A 53-year-old woman presents for her routine well-woman care. She has begun to develop mild hot flashes and wants to discuss the possibility of estrogen replacement. She tells the family physician that she has heard recent news reports and wonders whether estrogen causes breast cancer. She does not have a family history of breast cancer, but she is concerned. What does the physician tell her? A computer search with key words breast cancer, *with subheadings* prevention and control, etiology, *and* estrogen *yields the recent articles that have been in the press (Colditz et al., 1995) as well as a series of conflicting meta-analyses (Brinton & Schairer, 1993; Henrich, 1992; Steinberg et al., 1991). The family physician concludes that there is some good evidence that long-term replacement with estrogen increases the risk of breast cancer, and excellent evidence that estrogen reduces cardiac mortality and complications from osteoporosis. After discussion of risks and benefits, the patient decides to start estrogen replacement. The family physician documents the discussion of risks and benefits in the medical record.*

———— CAUSATION ————

As Case 16-7 illustrates, questions of causation come up frequently when physicians address prevention or give advice about life-style or other aspects of personal life, or when patients ask about medical studies reported in the popular press. While common, however, it is rarely as important for physicians to know the fine details of epidemiologic issues around causation, except insofar as they need to know them in order to form an opinion.

Information about causation is readily available but usually superficial in medical textbooks, and effective searching depends on review articles and computer searching. The best strategy is to search for the disease itself, with the subheadings *etiology* or *prevention and control*. Useful methodologic terms are *prospective study, cohort study, case–control* study; the publication term *meta-analysis* is also helpful for topics that have been the focus of a lot of research.

Critical appraisal of issues of causation is more complex than that of diagnosis, prognosis, or treatment, because the number of papers is greater, the study designs are often weaker, and final answers are less common than for many clinical questions. For most causal questions, true experiments are impossible for ethical reasons; for example, it would be impossible to randomly assign some people to smoke cigarettes to see whether lung cancer occurred. Determining causation is thus a judgment, based on a review of all of the evidence. To help with this judgment, epidemiologists have developed a list of criteria that may be used to judge when associations reflect causation. These criteria are listed in Table 16.1.

Table 16.1
Criteria for Causation

1. Temporality
2. Strength
3. Dose response
4. Consistency
5. Biologic plausibility
6. Specificity
7. Analogy

The most important criteria are temporality, strength of the association, dose response, and consistency. *Temporality* is the requirement that the exposure (smoking) precede the disease (lung cancer). This may seem self-evident, but some study designs like case–series and case–control studies often do not allow the assessment of temporality. The *strength of the association* is determined by the risk ratio or odds ratio; the higher the number, the more likely the association is causal. For smoking and lung cancer, many studies have put the risk ratio at between 4 and 16, whereas for alcohol and breast cancer, the risk ratio is probably less than 2. *Dose response* is the finding that more exposure leads to more of the disease, and *consistency* refers to whether the findings of one study are supported by findings in other populations.

Less helpful are biologic plausibility, specificity, and analogy. *Biologic plausibility* refers to what is known about the pathophysiology of disease; to suggest that a certain mechanism of disease is possible, however, falls well short of proving that it is the mechanism of disease. *Specificity* holds that one cause yields one effect, in the sense that an infectious agent like *M. tuberculosis* causes tuberculosis. This is less important for chronic diseases: Smoking causes COPD and myocardial infarctions as well as lung cancer, so the lack of specificity may be a weak argument against causality. Finally, *analogy* refers to the existence of a similar disease. The well-known consequences of thalidomide for developing fetuses suggest that other drugs can cause major developmental problems. Like specificity, however, analogy is a weak argument for causation.

Clinicians often have to review a single article that has been reported extensively, and usually incompletely, in the popular press. In this case, many of the principles discussed with other types of articles will hold true. More importantly, how strong was the study design? As noted before, randomized controlled trials are stronger than cohort trials, which are stronger than case–control studies. Beyond this question are the methodological details. Were the measures of exposure and disease appropriate and collected in a blinded fashion? Were other factors that might influence outcome accounted for in the design of the study, the baseline information, and the analysis? Are the risks strong and with evidence of a dose–response curve?

CONCLUSION

This chapter has provided a brief introduction to searching and critically appraising the medical literature. How should one continue to develop one's skills? To some extent, of course, medical students have no choice. At most medical schools, many clinical rotations require searching and interpretation of the literature in some fashion. Beyond medical school, residencies in most specialties have built journal clubs into their training programs. The formats vary greatly, but, typically, journal clubs meet every 1 to 4 weeks to review recent findings from the literature as well as to train skills in critical appraisal. As with any clinical procedure, practice is critical for proficiency, and these required exercises provide a good opportunity to improve skills. Beyond such required practice, however, should be the commitment to taking the time to improve skills. Improving the speed and effectiveness of searching and evaluating the medical literature becomes self-perpetuating, so that the clinician becomes more comfortable seeking out good-quality information.

The ultimate goal of critical appraisal is keeping up to date and in control of one's clinical practices. Practicing clinicians have a responsibility to keep current and to practice as effectively as possible, but changes in the volume of available information have made this increasingly difficult. Adding to the challenge is the format of traditional continuing medical education, in which practicing physicians receive didactic lectures, and which has very little impact on clinical practice.

To remedy the situation, dramatic changes have begun to appear in the way practicing physicians acquire new information. In the last several years, most journals have switched over to structured abstracts, which force the authors to name their methods at the beginning and allow clinicians to weed out quickly articles that are weak or not applicable to their practice. The National Library of Medicine has begun to pay more attention to clinical consumers of Medline, which has resulted in more attention to methodological terms as searching tools. Continuing medical education itself is changing, experimenting with formats to allow more involvement of data from physicians' own practice as well as an evidence-based format. Finally, the last 5 years have seen the popularization of practice guidelines published by the federal government, specialty societies, and insurers, some of which are evidence based.

Central to all of these efforts is critical appraisal of the literature. Critical appraisal empowers physicians by giving them the tools to cut through the reams of useless data that confront them every day; it facilitates the change of practice because it holds old practice up to the standard of evidence rather than tradition.

CASES FOR DISCUSSION

CASE 1

John Cotton is a 26-year-old man who comes to your office for evaluation of an ankle sprain. It happened in a pickup basketball game the night before. After going up for a rebound, he landed on someone else's foot and inverted his foot. Now there is no ecchymosis, but there is swelling and pain over the top of the foot. He asks you whether he needs an X ray. In recent years, the Ottawa rules have been promulgated as a guideline for this problem, but you don't remember the details.

1. *What are the Ottawa rules? Where can you find them?*
2. *How sensitive and specific are they?*
3. *Should you use them routinely? Should Mr. Cotton have an X ray?*

CASE 2

You are seeing Mrs. Walthrop, a 58-year-old woman with hypertension, who is well controlled on a long-acting preparation of diltiazem. An executive for a local software company, she pays close attention to the health information available in the local press and on the radio. At a routine visit, she mentions hearing that calcium channel blockers may lead to increased mortality in some patients. She asks you whether she should change medications. She has no other cardiac risk factors or symptoms and is otherwise healthy except for a sedentary life-style.

1. *How strong is the evidence against calcium channel blockers?*
2. *Should this evidence affect our prescribing for hypertension and angina?*
3. *What do you say to Mrs. Walthrop?*

CASE 3

You and your partners are discussing the health education information you will have routinely available to perimenopausal women considering estrogen replacement therapy (ERT). A key issue is the possible risk regarding ERT and breast cancer, and the consensus of the group is that you need to find or develop some material for patients that explains and assesses the possible risk. You volunteer to do that and you begin by reviewing the literature relating ERT to breast cancer.

1. *Is there a clinically significant risk of breast cancer with ERT?*
2. *What are the outcomes with the combined regimens now common?*
3. *How should this be expressed in a health education leaflet?*

CASE 4

Your staff model HMO is developing a practice guideline around the management of hypertension. Your assignment is to prepare a recommendation for the role of drugs in the management of mild hypertension. You decide to consult the recent JNC guidelines and search for studies of the treatment of mild hypertension.

1. *Should all patients with mild hypertension be treated?*
2. *What are the benefits, the risks, and the costs of treatment of mild hypertension?*
3. *What is the role of medication as opposed to other therapies in the management of mild hypertension?*

CASE 5

Thirty-year-old R. Perrin and his second wife come to your office for contraceptive counseling. Mr. Perrin has two children by his first marriage, which ended in divorce 10 years ago; his current wife has one child by a previous marriage. The couple has been married for 2 years and are emphatic about not wanting to have any more children. They are interested in the possibility of vasectomy and have come to you to discuss it. One of their questions is whether vasectomy causes prostate cancer.

1. *How strong is the evidence that vasectomy causes prostate cancer?*
2. *How should we incorporate that evidence into contraceptive counseling for our patients?*
3. *Specifically, what words would you use to describe the risk of prostate cancer to Mr. Perrin?*

Canadian Medical Association Journal. 1980, 123:499–504, 613–617; 1981, 124:555–558, 703–710, 869–872, 985–990, 1156–1162; 1984, 130:377–381, 1428–1433, 1542–1549.

The best introduction to critical appraisal is this series published in the early 1980s. It is relentlessly clinical, giving practical examples and providing "how to read" approaches for a variety of different questions; it is also very humorous.

Chalmers I, Enkin M, Keirse MJ: *Effective Care in Pregnancy and Childbirth.* London, Oxford University Press, 1989.

Using a file of all of the randomized trials in obstetrics, the textbook consists of a series of meta-analyses of topics in obstetrics. The result is the first evidence-based textbook; clinicians from all specialties should review it. It is now available on line and on CD.

JAMA. 1993, 270:2093–2095, 2598–2601; 1994, 271:59–63, 389–391, 703–707, 1615–1619, 272:234–237, 1367–1371; 1995, 273:1292–1295, 1610–1613, 274:570–574.

In recent years, the McMaster group has published another series. It is not quite as practical for practicing physicians, but it provides an excellent introduction to likelihood ratios, number needed to treat, decision analysis, practice guidelines, and other approaches that are used increasingly frequently.

Panzer RJ, Black ER, Griner PF: *Diagnostic Strategies for Common Medical Problems.* Philadelphia, American College of Physicians, 1991.

This is the best single text on diagnostic tests. It critically evaluates the usefulness of common diagnostic tests.

CHAPTER 17

Reducing Malpractice Risk

Richard G. Roberts

CASE 17-1

Dr. Newdoc, a resident physician on duty for the evening, answered a telephone call from M. I. Soot, a 38-year-old man who had never before been a patient in the residency practice. The man described severe indigestion and asked whether he should be seen that night or whether he could wait to see his usual physician the next morning. Dr. Newdoc reassured the caller that his symptoms most likely represented heartburn caused by acid reflux and advised him to use antacids. Eight hours later, Mr. Soot was admitted to the hospital with a myocardial infarction (heart attack). He eventually sued Dr. Newdoc, claiming that the incorrect telephone advice he was given delayed his presentation to the hospital and made him ineligible to receive medication that could have dissolved his artery clot and preserved more healthy heart tissue. At trial, Dr. Newdoc responded that Mr. Soot was not even a patient of the residency practice, that proper advice was given, and that he was going to have significant heart muscle damage regardless of any advice he might have offered.

EDUCATIONAL OBJECTIVES

After reading this chapter, the learner should be able to:

1. List the four elements the plaintiff must prove in a medical malpractice claim
2. Describe the traits of the suit-prone physician
3. Define risk management
4. Provide two examples for each of the four Cs of risk management
5. List the seven most common allegations against physicians

—— THE ESSENTIALS OF A MALPRACTICE CLAIM ——

While a medical malpractice suit can seem like an unwarranted affront to a physician, it can pose an insurmountable legal challenge for the patient. In order to understand how to reduce malpractice risk, it is first necessary to have an understanding of the essential elements of a successful malpractice suit. The patient-plaintiff must prove four essential elements to win a malpractice claim:

1. The physician owed the patient a duty.
2. The physician violated that duty through negligent care.
3. The negligent care caused the patient's damages.
4. Damages in fact were suffered.

Proving that the physician owed the patient a duty is usually easily accomplished by introducing evidence that the physician and the patient had a professional relationship. In Case 17-1, however, it is not clear whether the resident physician and the man had such a relationship; their only interaction consisted of a telephone call with no examination by the physician, no fees charged, and no expectation that their relationship would continue beyond the telephone conversation. In a case with facts very similar to those in Case 17-1, a California court ruled that the physician did owe the man a duty to provide competent professional advice because the man had been placed in a position to rely on the physician's advice and he suffered harm as a result. The case serves as a reminder of the importance of clearly and explicitly defining the relationship with a patient before providing advice (e.g., "I have been asked to help you with your bad back; you should ask your primary physician about your diabetes.").

The issue of negligence was also disputed in the case. The plaintiff's expert witnesses testified that the physician should have been aware of the possibility that a heart attack could present as indigestion and that the patient should have been urged to seek immediate medical attention and undergo an adequate examination. A telephone conversation is usually not a sufficient examination for a person at risk for a rapidly developing and potentially lethal condition. Negligence is proved by demonstrating that the physician's performance fell below the standard of care, which is the level of care provided by the average, not the best, practitioner in similar circumstances. Difficult questions regarding standard of care are present in Case 17-1. Should the resident physician have been expected to perform as well as the average resident physician, as well as the average practicing physician in that locale, or as well as the average cardiologist? The gradual evolution in U.S. courts has been toward a national standard of care, regardless of the physician's specialty. The policy underlying a national standard is that a patient should receive a similar level of care regardless of the physician's location or specialty because of the ease of consultation or referral when a physician does not feel competent to undertake the care of a particular problem. While it may seem straightforward, determining the standard of care is often the most contentious part of a case because physicians rarely agree on every aspect of the preferred approach for a given patient or condition.

The heart attack victim argued successfully that his delay in treatment, because of the physician's negligent advice resulting from an inadequate examination, caused him to suffer more heart muscle damage than he would have otherwise suffered which resulted in a worse prognosis for him. Causation, also known as proximate cause, is another controversial issue in many cases. Even when the physician is negligent, it may not be clear that the negligence caused the patient's injury. Powerful examples of this are "bad baby" suits. In the early 1980s, physicians frequently lost suits to children with cerebral palsy, mental retardation, or newborn seizures; these suits alleged that negligent "birth trauma" resulted in "perinatal asphyxia" and that the latter caused the neurologically handicapping condition. Improvements in scientific knowledge, however, revealed that the cause of such unfortunate outcomes for more than 90% of afflicted children was an unknown prenatal injury, rather than the delivery process (Freeman, 1985).

The final element that must be proved to prevail in a medical liability case is that damages in fact occurred. A frequent misconception among healthcare professionals is the notion that a large number of malpractice suits are frivolous. An analysis by the U.S. General Accounting Office (1987) demonstrated, however, that only about one in seven claims are for purely emotional reasons. Most malpractice claimants have substantial injuries.

CASE 17-2

Ms. Mamatobe was a 32-year-old woman who had been an infertility patient of Dr. N. Communicado for 3 years. She went from the heights of happiness to the depths of despair when she miscarried her first pregnancy at 14 weeks gestation. At the follow-up examination, Dr. Communicado spent most of the session explaining that the miscarriage was not his fault and that they should be able to try another in vitro *fertilization in about 2 months. Four months later, Ms. Mamatobe had not returned and had not responded to several requests to pay her bill, which had an outstanding balance of $4500. Dr. Communicado's staff then sent her account to a collection agency.*

THE UNHAPPY PATIENT AS UNPLEASANT PLAINTIFF

The most important requirement for any malpractice claim is an unhappy patient. People who are delighted with all aspects of their care do not sue. Their unhappiness may result from an undesired outcome (e.g., a miscarriage of a highly valued pregnancy) or from the process of care (e.g., a physician who seemed to care more about his own culpability than the patient's grieving or who placed the patient under significant financial pressure). While not a guarantor of results, the physician has a significant role in determining the overall satisfaction of the patient with the care process. Patients often enter the medical care system distracted by their symptoms, unrealistic in their expectations, and confused by the rituals and language of the healthcare system. Physicians, as well as other professionals on the healthcare team, can use reflective listening skills to validate a patient's "magical thinking" (Gutheil *et al.,* 1984) or to sort out the patient's real concerns (Shahady, 1990).

It can be understandable for a physician to withdraw from the patient when things are not going well or when conflict occurs. Certain patients, such as the hateful or difficult patient, can also tempt the physician to pull away (Groves, 1978). Patients who are rigid in their outlook with fixed beliefs or who have unrealistic expectations pose the greatest liability risk. Such difficult situations demand the most of the professional, but they also represent the greatest opportunities to best address the patient's needs. When a patient is critically ill or angry, that is the time when even more attention should be given to listening to the patient and family. A recommended consultation or referral can reassure a patient that the physician's primary concern is for the patient's welfare and satisfaction. Patients and families will more quickly forgive a lack of competence than a lack of caring.

Another common myth about patients who sue is that they do so because of an opportunity to take financial advantage of a bad situation. For many patients, nonpayment of the bill represents their final chance to express displeasure with the care they received. Thus, it may be important, before the patient is sent to collections, for the physician to personally inquire whether the patient has any financial problems, or dissatisfaction with care, that may be making it difficult to pay. The previously mentioned GAO study demonstrated that about two-thirds of plaintiffs had little or no income. A closer review of the data reveals, however, that most plaintiffs were children or women of childbearing age who were least likely to have reportable income, but who were the most frequent users of the healthcare system (i.e., being born and giving birth are the two most common reasons for hospitalizations). In fact, patients on medical assistance are less likely to sue than are patients who are not on Medicaid (Baldwin *et al.*, 1992). This finding reflects the likelihood that indigent patients may be unsophisticated in accessing the legal system, as well as in accessing the medical system.

CASE 17-3

Dr. Ty Wrant was known, and feared, by everyone on the hospital staff. A brilliant 42-year-old surgeon, he was given to outbursts of temper and was contemptuous of those staff with whom he worked, other physicians, and even patients. His surgical skills made for a very busy practice. His record keeping was sloppy and he was quick to anger when criticized. He was astounded when his malpractice carrier imposed a 100% surcharge on his insurance premium after he was named in his third suit.

THE UNPLEASANT PHYSICIAN AS UNHAPPY DEFENDANT

Dr. Wrant fits exactly the profile of the physician who is most likely to be sued. Physicians in their early 40s are at the height of their productivity—busy practices can result in oversights. Dr. Wrant's abusive personality made it less likely that patients, or fellow healthcare professionals, would be willing to forgive technical slips. Male physicians are more likely to be named in a suit than female physicians; this trend is felt to reflect the fact that more physicians are men than women and that the male–female differential is even greater when higher-risk (surgical) specialties are considered. The gender difference appears to be disappearing as the percentage of physicians who are women grows. Data suggest that inadequacies in interpersonal care (Hickson *et al.*, 1994) rather than quality of care (Entman *et al.*, 1994) describe physicians who are more likely to be sued. Having had prior claims, even if they are small or unpaid, does appear to predict and increase the probability that a physician will have future claims (Bovbjerg & Petronis, 1994) perhaps reflecting a high-risk or high-volume practice or a high-risk personality. There is evidence that the higher the volume, the greater the risk of suit, at least when it comes to delivering babies (Baldwin *et al.,* 1991).

Physicians go through a range of emotions when they are named in a suit: denial, anxiety, anger, and so on. The tort system exacts an enormous emotional toll on physicians: 96% of physicians experience emotional or physical symptoms as a result of a suit, 62% order extra tests, 57% believe their families suffer, 42% no longer care for certain kinds of patients, and 28% discontinue certain procedures (Charles *et al.,* 1984).

CASE 17-4

Ms. Fortune is a 44-year-old woman who had her left kidney removed in childhood because of a Wilms's tumor. She had a routine Pap smear performed by Dr. Bonnie Busy, a highly regarded obstetrician-gynecologist. The pathology report indicated that the smear was abnormal, showing moderate dysplasia. Dr. Busy never saw the report as it returned from the pathologist when she was on vacation and was filed in the patient's record. Nine months later, Ms. Fortune returned to see Dr. Busy with a complaint of vaginal discharge. Dr. Busy noted an abnormal cervix that proved to be an early carcinoma on biopsy. During her hysterectomy, Dr. Busy inadvertently ligated Ms. Fortune's right ureter, eventually causing the loss of her right kidney. Two years later, Ms. Fortune died of complications of renal dialysis while awaiting a kidney transplant. During the 2 years of dialysis, Dr. Busy turned her care over to a nephrologist and saw the patient only once. Dr. Busy's staff was most uncomfortable speaking with Ms. Fortune on the several occasions when she called the office. After her death, Mr. Fortune and his two children sued Dr. Busy for professional negligence and won a $6 million judgment.

RISK MANAGEMENT—IMPROVING CARE THROUGH A SYSTEMS APPROACH

Risk management is a style of practice that seeks to reduce patient injuries, malpractice claims, and malpractice claims losses. Ms. Fortune's tragic case illustrates a number of missed opportunities to reduce her chance for iatrogenic injuries, the likelihood that she or her family would sue, and the size of the claim if a suit did result. Her case would seem like a unique comedy of errors, except that a number of similar cases serve as reminders of how malpractice can occur when systems break down. A study of more than 30,000 New York State hospitalizations revealed that 3.7% of admissions resulted in an adverse event with 27.6% of the adverse events felt to be the result of substandard care (Brennan *et al.,* 1991). Yet the same study group showed that only 8 of the 280 patients who had an adverse event caused by medical negligence filed a lawsuit (Localio *et al.,* 1991). Studies such as this and others (California Medical Association, 1977) have led to the conclusion that there is more malpractice committed than is recognized, litigated, or compensated.

It is rare that healthcare professionals intend to do harm, and yet harm resulting from error occurs about 1 to 2% of the time. A major impediment to reducing the frequency of medical injuries is the failure to recognize that modern healthcare reflects a very complex system involving many individuals (Lucian, 1994). A systems perspective can be helpful in working through Ms. Fortune's case. The filing of the Pap smear report without Dr. Busy seeing it was the first system failure. The use of a simple system, such as requiring the physician to initial or sign every report before filing, could have reduced the chance that the report would have been filed without Dr. Busy becoming aware of it. A member of the office staff, such as the medical records technician, would usually be responsible for overseeing this step in the record keeping system.

A second system failure was Dr. Busy's failure to adequately identify the ureter at the time of surgery. The routine use of a preoperative imaging study (e.g., intravenous pyelogram), especially in a higher-risk patient such as Ms. Fortune, could have decreased the likelihood that the ureter would have been injured during surgery. Additional techniques (e.g., a ureteral stent during surgery) could have further protected the ureter. Careful postoperative monitoring of the kidney might have permitted earlier recognition of the ureteral damage with the possibility of reoperating and salvaging the kidney.

A third system failure was the response of Dr. Busy and her staff after the catastrophic sequence of events occurred. Rather than attempting to distance themselves from her, Dr. Busy and her staff should have put extra effort into attempts to communicate with Ms. Fortune and her family to express their concern for her well-being and their desire to help.

A convenient way to remember the general principles of risk management is the four Cs:

- Compassion
- Communication
- Competence
- Charting

COMPASSION

An old French aphorism states that the purpose of a physician is to "cure sometimes, alleviate suffering often, and comfort always." The phrase continues to offer good advice. Patients turn to physicians, as they have always done, not only for technical expertise but also to derive meaning from the experience of illness. They seek reassurance, comfort, and hope. If physicians are held only to objective outcome measures, such as death, then every physician is destined to eventually fail every patient, given the inevitability of death.

Compassion should also be shown to other members of the healthcare team. Taking care of patients is difficult and stressful work that demands the best possible performance of every member of the team. For example, it can be tempting to criticize the care provided by another when the only information available is the limited perspective of the patient or the patient's family. Finally, to function effectively as a member of the healthcare team, it is important to clarify responsibilities, to gain commitment to the team, and to be certain that team members share what they want so they get what they want.

COMMUNICATION

Effective communication is essential for good medical care and for malpractice avoidance. Patients who feel they have been heard, had their questions answered, and had their concerns addressed tend to be more satisfied with their care and less likely to sue

361

RISK
MANAGEMENT—
IMPROVING CARE
THROUGH A
SYSTEMS
APPROACH

(Levinson, 1994). There is also evidence to suggest that physicians who spend more time with patients are less likely to be sued (Adams & Zuckerman, 1984), although what seems to be more significant is the patient's perception of the time spent with the physician rather than the actual time spent (Di Matteo & Hays, 1980).

Communication between members of the healthcare team is as important as communication between the patient and individual team members. Keeping each other informed can minimize the risk of misinformation or misunderstanding, especially for higher-risk patients. As an example, a routine of signing out hospitalized or pregnant patients near term helps to avoid surprises for the patient and covering colleagues when a physician is unavailable. While such a routine may be self-evident and unlikely to need mention, the reality is that a disquieting number of patient injuries and malpractice claims arise at times when uninformed covering physicians are asked to respond to a patient who was likely to need the help of another physician during the absence of the attending physician. The key concept is that such communication needs to become routine, meaning every time.

COMPETENCE

The elaborate and prolonged training process needed to become a physician usually results in physicians taking on clinical problems for which they were well trained. A more vexing threat to competence is when the physician is distracted by fatigue, personal problems, or substance use. The ability to recognize one's limits at the moment they are encountered is the mark of a mature professional. There are other occasions when it may be reasonable to recommend a consultation or referral: when a patient is gravely ill or may die unexpectedly, when recovery is slower than expected, when the patient or family seem dissatisfied with the care given, or when the diagnosis remains obscure. On this final point, it can be helpful to set a limit to guide when to seek help for a diagnostic dilemma (e.g., three visits with no definitive diagnosis yet made).

CHARTING

Defense attorneys estimate that up to 40% of cases may be lost simply because the medical record was inadequate. The patient's chart is the one opportunity that a physician has to immortalize the attentive care that was provided to the patient. Physicians too often view the record as an unnecessary aggravation when it in fact represents the best chance to preempt a malpractice suit: Many an interested plaintiff's attorney has been dissuaded from filing what appeared to be a viable claim when confronted by a record that substantiates that good care was provided. The essentials of a good medical record include entries that were timely, legible, relevant, objective, and reflective of thoughtful decision-making. It can be as damaging to try to put too much in the record, and miss what is most important, as it is to put too little in the record, and offer no evidence of what was said, thought, or done. The record is so important because it is the only witness with sufficient memory to speak with credibility 4 to 7 years after the injury occurs when the case finally goes to trial. The record should always be honest: Any attempt to make dishonest entries, such as erasing prior entries, dooms the defendant. In those cases where a physician later remembers important information or discovers an error in the record, it is appropriate to add another entry so long as it clearly indicates that it is a late entry done to clarify or correct.

Ms. Liddy Gashun was a 30-year-old woman who was 10 weeks, pregnant with her fourth child in 5 years and had intractable vomiting. Dr. R. X. Mutch was her family physician and he prescribed an antinausea medicine that made her light-headed and caused her to fall onto her wrist. Dr. Mutch did an unshielded wrist X ray and determined that she had a sprained wrist. He advised her to do no heavy lifting for a few weeks. Throughout her pregnancy, Ms. Gashun worried about radiation damage to the fetus. Ms. Gashun continued to have severe wrist pain until after delivery at which time another X ray showed a nonunion (nonhealing) fracture of the scaphoid (navicular) bone of the wrist. She sued Dr. Mutch for failure to timely diagnose her fracture, negligent management of her pregnancy, negligent management of her fracture, failure to obtain timely consultation, negligent drug therapy, and failure to obtain informed consent.

COMMON ALLEGATIONS

Ms. Gashun's case touches on a number of the more common malpractice allegations made against physicians. It can be useful to review these common allegations because they help to focus attention on what areas physicians actually get sued. Physicians often justify decisions by invoking malpractice concerns (e.g., "If I don't do this test, then I'll be sued"), when in fact they usually have little data for such statements. In actuality, physicians are sued most often for common conditions, not for unusual ailments. Table 17.1 summarizes these common allegations.

FAILURE TO TIMELY DIAGNOSE

About one-third of cases allege a failure to timely diagnose a problem. Maintaining a high index of suspicion for common serious conditions will help guide the clinician. Nearly half of delayed diagnosis cases involve cancer, most commonly cancer of the breast, lung, colon, or testes. Every breast lump in a woman should be taken to diagnosis, either by observing its resolution after the next menses or with aspiration or by biopsing or excising it. A frequent mistake is to rely on a falsely negative mammogram and incorrectly reassure the woman that nothing is wrong. A mammogram is obtained not to

Table 17.1
Common Allegations

Failure to timely diagnose
Negligent obstetrical practices
Negligent management of fractures or trauma
Failure to obtain timely consultation
Negligent drug treatment
Negligent surgery/procedure
Failure to obtain informed consent

---

diagnose a palpated lump, but to screen the remaining breast or other breast for nonpalpable masses. Chest X-ray abnormalities should be followed to clearance in the case of pneumonia, or to tissue diagnosis if the abnormality does not resolve. An adult with bleeding per rectum who is over 40 years of age should be assumed to have colon cancer until ruling it out with endoscopy or contrast imaging studies. Men should be counseled to examine for testicular lumps and newly found lumps to be definitively diagnosed.

Other commonly misdiagnosed problems include myocardial infarct (do not be misled by a falsely reassuring ECG), pulmonary embolus (document adequate oxygenation with an arterial blood gas in a patient with significant shortness of breath), and appendicitis (assume abdominal pain to be a surgical condition until proven otherwise). In Ms. Gashun's case, her physician was mistakenly reassured by an apparently normal wrist X ray. Wrist fractures, particularly of the scaphoid/navicular bone at the base of thumb, may not appear on an X ray for the first several weeks after injury.

NEGLIGENT OBSTETRICAL PRACTICES

The probability of Ms. Gashun's fetus being harmed by the small dose of radiation involved in an unshielded wrist X ray is low, even though the exposure occurred at an especially radiosensitive period in the pregnancy. More common in pregnancy is to allege errors in decision-making based on inadequate dating of the pregnancy such as no pelvic examination before the second trimester or no ultrasound before the third trimester. Other frequent complaints include failure to adequately monitor the fetus during labor, to perform a timely cesarean delivery (within 30 minutes from the time of decision to incision), or to develop or follow a management plan for common complications, such as hypertension, diabetes, postdatism, or premature labor.

NEGLIGENT MANAGEMENT OF FRACTURES OR TRAUMA

Dr. Mutch should have known that navicular fractures are often not apparent on early X rays. He should have placed Ms. Gashun in a thumb spica cast to stabilize a possible fracture until follow-up later resolved the question of whether there was a fracture. Other fractures that are frequently missed are cervical spine and femoral head fractures. Immobilization should be maintained in suspicious clinical circumstances until additional radiographs or special studies (e.g., CT scan) can definitively rule out a fracture. Normal pulses and neurologic function should be documented distal to the site of significant trauma or fracture.

FAILURE TO OBTAIN TIMELY CONSULTATION

Ms. Gashun eventually came under the care of an orthopedic surgeon when her nonunion required surgical fixation of the bone. Dr. Mutch acted reasonably in attempting to care for her fracture only if he had sufficient training or experience with such injuries to adequately manage the problem. His failure to know that certain wrist fractures are not detectable on early X ray could be considered evidence that he should have referred Ms. Gashun to someone else earlier. Generalist physicians can manage conditions for which they have adequate training or experience, as is the case for limited practice specialists.

NEGLIGENT DRUG TREATMENT

In this case, liability on the negligent drug treatment allegation would turn on whether an average physician caring for a pregnant woman with unremitting vomiting would have used a similar medicine. The prevention of dehydration and electrolyte abnormalities in a pregnant woman with persistent vomiting may require medication. A frequent drug treatment error is the administration of a medicine to which the patient has a known allergy, often documented in the chart! Inquire about allergies each time a drug is to be prescribed. Other medications that can commonly cause problems include anticoagulants, psychoactive drugs, or certain cardiovascular medicines. The use of these drugs usually requires careful monitoring with bleeding studies, visits to check for medication side effects or electrolytes, respectively.

NEGLIGENT SURGERY/PROCEDURE

Proving that proper technique was used often depends on an accurate and sufficiently complete operative or procedure note. When a physician is undertaking a procedure for the first time, or because emergent circumstances require the procedure and no better qualified physician is available, then adequate documentation is even more important.

FAILURE TO OBTAIN INFORMED CONSENT

The omission by Dr. Mutch to warn Ms. Gashun of the frequent or serious side effects of the antinausea medication (i.e., dizziness) leaves him vulnerable to a claim of failure to obtain informed consent. The operative legal principle is that people have a right to control what happens to their body, and, in order to make good decisions about what they want to have happen to their bodies, they need sufficient information about the benefits, harms, and alternatives to recommended treatments. Some states impose an objective standard of informed consent ("What is it that the average physician tells to patients?"), while other states use a subjective standard ("What is it that the average patient would want to know?"). Sometimes consent is implied, such as when the patient is unconscious; other times it must be given by someone other than the patient, such as when the patient is deemed incompetent if a child or a person who is not mentally capable. The most important concept to remember regarding informed consent is that it reflects a relationship, not a piece of paper to be signed. The relationship is between two people, the attending physician and patient, and it should ensure that the patient's questions are answered and concerns are addressed.

CONCLUSION

Much like death and taxes, a medical malpractice lawsuit seems a painful inevitability for physicians. The odds are high that over the course of a 30- to 40-year career of high-risk decisions, particularly for surgical specialists, eventually a suit will occur. Focusing on the needs, especially the communication needs, of the patient and developing systems of care designed to reduce the chance of patient injury can yield fewer injuries and malpractice claims. A compelling example of a successful accident reduction program is anesthesiology. Standards for anesthesia monitoring have reduced anesthesia-related mortality rates from one in 10,000 to one in 200,000 over the past decade (Orkin, 1993).

Improved efforts by every member of the caregiving team to satisfy patients will lead to fewer liability suits. A shift in thinking must take place so that potential liability risks are approached from a systems perspective. Traditional approaches that focus on, or blame, only the physician will not succeed because the physician cannot and does not do everything when it comes to patient care. This will require a change in attitudes from one of errors as individual character flaws to one of errors as opportunities for system improvement.

A final word of advice regarding "lawsuit phobia." When bad outcomes do occur, caregivers, as well as patients, suffer. A lawsuit seems to add unnecessary insult to injury. It may represent, however, the patient's only chance to be made whole again, at least financially. Physicians who allow themselves to be paralyzed or tyrannized by fears of litigation will have very unsatisfying careers and most likely place themselves at added liability risk because they will try to practice medicine in a futile attempt to please an imagined lawyer rather than the real patient before them. While good medicine does not guarantee good legal outcomes, bad medicine rarely makes for good legal results.

——————— CASES FOR DISCUSSION ———————

CASE 1

Ms. O. Veight was an obese 37-year-old woman with a 3-month history of vague abdominal pain and bloating who was admitted to the hospital for a diagnostic laparoscopy. Outpatient evaluation over the past 2 months had included several visits to her physician and normal abdominal CT and ultrasound studies. At laparoscopy, she was found to have a large ovarian cancer with liver metastases. Over the following month, she developed fulminant liver failure and died in the hospital. Her husband, from whom she was separated, confronted her physician in the intensive care unit waiting room and shouted that he was going to sue.

1. *How should the physician respond?*
2. *Should the physician contact a lawyer? The malpractice insurance carrier? The hospital administrator?*
3. *Was this physician negligent?*

CASE 2

Timothy Cratchett was born at 32 weeks, gestation and developed seizures within the first 2 days of life. He was the product of a difficult 23-hour labor with 3½ hours of pushing. His Apgar scores were 3 at 1 minute and 4 at 5 minutes (normal is greater than 7). His parents asked for an explanation of his seizures and his prognosis.

1. *What should they be told?*
2. *Who should be with them when they are told?*
3. *Who should tell them?*
4. *Was the physician negligent?*

CASE 3

Billie Kramer was a 4-year-old who contracted Haemophilus influenzae *meningitis and was left with permanent hearing loss. Billie's first contact with the medical system for this illness was when he presented to a pediatrician's office about 30 hours after becoming ill. The physician immediately admitted him to the hospital, performed a spinal tap, and started appropriate antibiotics. Six months later, after being named in a suit filed by Billie's parents, the pediatrician discovered that a normal white blood cell count that was drawn in the office the morning of admission had not been included in the office visit's progress note.*

1. *What should the pediatrician do with the additional information?*
2. *Should the pediatrician change the progress note? If so, how?*
3. *Was this physician negligent?*

CASE 4

A 52-year-old newly remarried patient asked Dr. N. A. Binde whether he should have a prostate-specific antigen (PSA) blood test. The patient related that one brother had died at age 51 of prostate cancer, but that his 54-year-old brother had undergone prostatectomy and was left impotent, "a fate worse than death" according to the patient. Dr. Binde was aware that the American Cancer Society recommended annual PSA testing in men over 50 years of age, but that the United States Preventive Services Task Force recommended against PSA screening because of the lack of evidence that outcomes from prostate cancer were improved by early detection.

1. *What should Dr. Binde tell the patient?*
2. *Who should decide what to do?*
3. *Should a urologist be consulted? a radiation therapist? an oncologist?*
4. *What if the patient's insurance will not cover the cost of screening tests?*

CASE 5

Renee Runner was a 15-year-old runaway who was struck by a car and suffered massive internal bleeding. It was determined in the emergency department that her only hope for survival was massive blood transfusions followed by surgery. Her distraught parents arrived at the hospital, revealed that they were devout Jehovah's Witnesses, and insisted that Renee not receive any blood products.

1. *What should the emergency physician do?*
2. *What should the surgeon do?*
3. *Should anyone else be brought into the decision-making?*
4. *If the emergency physician transfused Renee and she survived, but sued later on, was the physician negligent?*

———————— RECOMMENDED READINGS ————————

American College of Obstetricians and Gynecologists. *Litigation Assistant: A Guide for the Defendant Physician.* Washington, DC, American College of Obstetricians and Gynecologists, 1986.

A nice primer that provides information on the litigation process and practical advice on how the defendant physician can mount the best defense.

Charles SC, Kennedy E: *Defendant: A Psychiatrist on Trial for Medical Malpractice.* New York, Free Press, 1985.

A gripping account of one psychiatrist's experience as a defendant in a medical malpractice case. Her experience caused her to become a leading researcher on the emotional impact of malpractice litigation on physicians and their families.

Ghitelman D: The natural history of malpractice. *MD* 4:59–81, 1987.

A fascinating reminder that malpractice, and physician discipline, are not new concepts. The author traces the history of malpractice from Babylonia to England to the colonial United States.

Robertson WO: *Medical Malpractice: A Preventive Approach.* Seattle, University of Washington Press, 1985.

Gathered from his extensive experience with a physician-owned liability insurance company, Dr. Robertson provides a number of examples of how risk management strategies can be applied to real-life cases. An excellent collection of examples of medical care gone awry.

CHAPTER 18

The Business of the Practice of Medicine

R. Martin Johnson

CASE 18-1

At a family gathering, three generations of physicians are discussing what organized medicine was like in their time. The grandfather, a general practitioner, describes being in solo practice, taking care of a community. The father, a surgeon, describes the independence that existed for him earlier in his practice, and his ability to make decisions and move forward. The daughter, an internist, is working for a health maintenance organization (HMO), and describes her role as a case manager.

——————— EDUCATIONAL OBJECTIVES ———————

At the conclusion of this chapter, the student will be able to:

1. Describe the six basic business structures seen in the practice of medicine, including their strengths and weaknesses
2. Describe four types of governance in the clinical setting, including their strengths and weaknesses
3. Describe the two basic types of physician compensation, and what their effect is on physician behavior
4. Describe three objectives of practice management

—————— INTRODUCTION ——————

Since 1950 there has been an ongoing revolution in healthcare technology. Daily there are new discoveries in the field of human physiology and pathology, as well as technological marvels that help treat disease. The rate of these changes is ever increasing. In contrast, the way healthcare delivery is organized and the way patients pay for it have, until very recently, been unaffected by these forces. Only recently has profound change begun to occur in the way healthcare is delivered in this country (Gabel *et al.*, 1987).

Medicine has traditionally been a cottage industry. It was composed of thousands of solo and small practices, accountable to no one, held together loosely by "guilds," called medical societies. This was "organized medicine." Before 1950, physicians' ability to cure was limited and care was relatively inexpensive. During the next 30 years scientific discoveries improved medical care. This explosion of knowledge and technology raised the possibilities and expectations for the prevention and treatment of disease. At the same time, changes in the payment mechanisms for healthcare, essentially indemnity insurance provided by employers, broke the direct financial link between the physician and the patient for the evaluation of cost versus benefits. By the 1990s, medicine was able to intervene more often than the nation was willing to afford, and perhaps more than a patient would even want. Evidence also surfaced that because of the lack of accountability for cost, there was a great deal of waste in all sectors of the delivery system (Eisenberg, 1989).

In 1994, the United States found that 14% of its gross national product was devoted to healthcare, whereas other industrialized countries were spending, on average, about 9%. With the highest costs in the world, it was a surprise that the United States lagged behind other countries in infant mortality, maternal death rate, immunizations of childhood, and other health statistics. In some U.S. communities, healthcare statistics were at the level of Third World countries. We found ourselves having both the best care in the world, and some of the poorest. This dichotomy is the setting for the changes in the healthcare delivery system that we are in the midst of now.

The organization of the healthcare delivery system is in the midst of a historic change from a cottage industry to big business, as described in Case 18-1. This change is occurring because of market forces. Employers and others who pay for health insurance are demanding accountability for cost and quality. Physicians need an understanding of the forces that are changing the delivery system. Most physicians will have little responsibility for the business of the practice of medicine, but will need to understand the principles. Administration will be done by business professionals and physician administrators. Clinical physicians will be free to treat patients, in an environment of accountability for the cost of care and the quality of their outcomes. This is an inevitable, irreversible change. Providers will be called to provide more care for less cost, at the same time giving better quality.

The physician family in Case 18-1 concluded their thoughts with three comments. All regarded their respective era to have been the most comfortable for them. Ultimately, however, they thought that the present changes will probably be beneficial for both providers as well as patients. They also believed that the transition will be painful for some physicians.

CASE 18-2

371

HOW WE
ORGANIZE
OURSELVES TO
PRACTICE
MEDICINE

Dr. New is in the last year of residency. She has received many offers of employment from diverse settings, ranging from a two-physician office in a very rural part of the country to a large multispecialty clinic. The physician wonders how she should choose a practice that is going to have the best chance of ensuring her professional success. She wonders what success is, who she will be responsible to, and how practice decisions are made.

HOW WE ORGANIZE OURSELVES TO PRACTICE MEDICINE

This section of the chapter will provide an overview of the business aspects of the practice of medicine in the hopes of offering a framework for selecting and evaluating practice opportunities for the new physician looking for employment.

SIX TYPES OF BUSINESS STRUCTURES

Solo practice has been the most common form of practice organization. It was the foundation of the cottage industry of medicine. In some rural parts of the United States, for awhile, it may still represent the only viable option. For most locations, however, solo practice provides independence, but leaves the practitioner relatively powerless, with problems of call coverage, lack of administrative support systems, inability to contract directly with HMOs, and difficulty raising capital for needed equipment and growth. The strength of solo practice is independence, and this too is its weakness. Solo means small—small capital, small systems, small negotiating power. Solo practice also cannot compete in attracting new physicians. For these reasons, in most specialties, and in most locations, the solo practice of medicine is no longer an acceptable alternative.

Small group practices are hard to precisely define. Certainly groups smaller than 35 providers are small. Groups with more than 100 are large. Between those numbers, whether groups are large or small would depend on their governance structures. Small groups have most of the characteristics of solo practice. Many of them are really collections of independent-minded physicians who have entered into an expense-sharing arrangement with others, but basically have retained a great deal of control over the bulk of their practice decisions. In these groups, decision-making can become a problem because it is not always possible to maintain consensus. Call is less of a burden than in solo practice. Such groups cannot compete with large groups in attracting new physicians because of their inherent weaknesses. For urban areas, small groups will probably have to merge into large groups to survive.

Independent practice associations (IPAs) are loose affiliations of small group practices and solo practitioners, which provide some enhancement to the physician's ability to contract with managed care payers. These entities are transitional and provide a bridge between solo and small group practices and large groups. The inherent problem with them, and the reason they are transitional, is that they are associations of independent physicians and not a true large group practice. Independent-minded and organized physicians cannot compete well in the managed care environment. They generally cannot discipline physicians, set work loads, evaluate quality, or raise and allocate capital.

Large single-specialty groups are becoming more numerous and larger. Such groups form to provide the geographic coverage, infrastructure, governance, capital, and contracting power to thrive in the managed care market. Particularly powerful groups in this category are the primary care groups, who are able to capture full capitation payments and then buy subspecialty services wholesale. Their primary weakness is a lack of coordination and inability to properly align incentives with the other providers of care. This weakness is partly overcome by strategic relations, contracting, subcapitation, and the development of "virtual" multispecialty groups. One advantage of the single-specialty clinic is a less complicated compensation plan, since all physicians' practices have a great deal of similarity. Basic incentives and goals within the group are aligned.

Large multispecialty groups of the past were, in many locations, top-heavy with subspecialists, lacking the primary care base to support them. Such groups depended on outside referrals to survive. As competition increased, their referral sources vanished. In order to thrive in the new medical marketplace, such groups will have to develop their own internal primary care base that will support all of its referral physicians. This type of group is the powerhouse of the future. They possess geographic coverage, strong governance, access to capital, and alignment of vision. Compensation systems are complex. Multispecialty clinics will not be able to maintain the great disparity of income that now exists between physicians of various specialties.

Unique types of groups. There are an increasing number of unique groups developing to meet the challenges of a managed care. These are special cases of large multispecialty clinics. Regional and nationwide *megagroups* exist, such as the Kaiser's Permanente group or the Med Partners–Mullikin Medical Centers, which began on the West Coast but is now nationwide. Such megagroups represent a new trend. They are very powerful as a result of their wide geographic coverage and ability to offer all of the primary care and specialty services necessary to managed capitated (full-risk) contracts. Such groups tend to become a dominant player in any market they enter, as their size makes negotiations with HMOs and insurance companies more balanced. Some megagroups, such as Med Partners–Mullikin, are publicly traded corporations.

The faculty of many *academic medical centers* have formed true medical groups to compete for managed care patients. Faculty members practice part time in these groups, and part time as faculty members. The success of this structure remains to be seen, as teaching is expensive and not funded by third-party payers. Faculty members also have many competing agendas, often causing them to be less effective caregivers than private physicians. Besides teaching, they are interested in research and internal politics. Using students as providers during teaching only serves to diminish their efficiency further.

Staff model HMOs represent a marriage between the insurance company and the providers, with total alignment of all segments, because they are all in one company. One company owns and manages the insurance business, owns and manages the hospitals, and hires the physicians. Physicians are simply employees. Physician productivity can become a problem in this environment, because they have no ownership, little control over clinic operations, and little rewards for hard work. These shortcomings, however, can be managed with proper incentives and attention to the work environment (Hale, 1988).

GOVERNANCE OF MEDICAL GROUPS

373

HOW WE
ORGANIZE
OURSELVES TO
PRACTICE
MEDICINE

How are practices governed? Governance is the process of decision-making. In general, groups are governed by their owners. Each type of organizational structure requires a different governance structure to be successful. There are four basic types of governance:

1. *Solo practice.* Solo practitioners are their own boss. They make all decisions about hiring and firing, capital expenditure, participation in managed care, marketing, and pricing, to the degree that these issues are under their control.

2. *Loose-knit associations.* There is an anarchy in expense-sharing small group practice arrangements and many IPAs. These groupings of independent physicians yield some governance to the larger body. Generally this governing group has little actual control over the basics of the practices. Without the ability to discipline a participating physician or raise and allocate capital, managing care, cost, and quality is difficult. Groups of independent physicians generally yield little actual power to the IPA governing body.

3. *Democracy.* Democracy is practiced by smaller groups. Meetings of the partners or shareholders decide key matters. If consensus can be maintained, this type of governance works well. If consensus is lost, there are winners and losers. Losers can sabotage action. It is difficult to maintain consensus in larger groups.

4. *Board of directors.* Boards manage larger groups. Directors are generally elected for long, staggered terms, and recall is difficult. Therefore, they are insulated from the fallout of the hard decisions they have to make. They have vast powers over compensation, discipline, establishing policies, allocation of resources, and contracting. Boards generally appoint a physician medical director to oversee day-to-day clinical activities, and an administrator to oversee the business. In a system such as this, it is important for the individual physician to have a clear idea of what areas the board rules, and in what areas individual or local sites have authority.

Ownership is not necessarily related to the type of organization. There are five types of ownership:

1. *Sole proprietorship* is the hallmark of solo practice, and it means that there is only one owner. Generally this is the solo practitioner. Situations exist where one physician will be the sole owner, but will hire other full- or part-time physicians. Loans represent the only source of additional capital. Most of the time there is no one to buy the practice when the practitioner retires, and the investment is thus mostly lost once the physician leaves the practice.

2. *Partnerships* are a common form of ownership of groups. They are less regulated than corporations. They do represent an increased risk to the estate of the partner if there is a loss. There are problems with access to and retention of capital. Survival in managed care situations, particularly in the capitation model, requires retention of capital to cover risk. Professionals newly joining the group are generally unwilling and unable to make an investment to buy out the departing partner. The group itself cannot afford to draw down its reserves to buy out the departing partner. Considering the need to preserve capital, groups moving into prepaid managed care tend to move out of this form of ownership.

3. Closely held *professional corporations* are very common. Generally the shareholders are the professionals. Individual estates are isolated from corporate losses that are not the result of malpractice claims. Entrance to and exit from the corporation is simpler. However, there is generally not a good market for the shares of a departing shareholder.

This is the same problem faced by the partnership. These organizations also are looking at alternative ownership arrangements in order to preserve capital, yet preserve a smooth transfer of physician assets on retirement, or when they leave the practice.

4. *Publicly traded corporations* are beginning to surface. These are physician groups whose shares are traded on the stock market. This provides an outside source of equity capital and a market for the shares of departing professionals. Generally these corporations try to retain control over the corporation by having the majority of shares held by its physicians. It remains to be seen if this will be possible as major shareholder physicians retire and sell their shares. These groups will be very sensitive to maintaining the value of their shares, which will add a new dimension to their corporate financial policy. Under this model, the new physician is not expected to make any contribution to capital. Over time there may be stock options given, and certainly the physician could buy public shares if he wants to make an equity investment in these corporations. Selling shares is as simple as calling a stock broker and ordering a sale. In most of these instances, there is an accompanying physician professional corporation, which has very minimal assets, that allows physicians a voice in medical matters. The buy-in to the professional corporation might be as little as $100, with no increase in value over time.

5. *Nonprofit organizations,* such as foundations, have become popular. These structures solve some major problems with previously described ownership arrangements. There is no buy-in, and no buyout. There is no ownership. As with the publicly traded corporations, there will likely be an asset-free professional corporation. Capital is raised by retaining earnings and also by donations.

COMPENSATION

How are physicians paid? There are all sorts of formulas and methods, but they all are a variation on one of two types:

1. *Productivity.* Productivity has been the traditional form. The more procedures that are done, the higher the charges. The more visits patients have per year and throughout the course of an illness, then the higher the gross billings and gross receipts, and hence more revenue available for compensation. The incentive is to do more. This payment mechanism creates pressures that are counter to current market demands. Groups of the future will generally not use this model because it encourages overutilization and excessive care.

2. *Salary and bonus.* Base salary and incentives are the method of choice for entities such as the staff model HMO and large group practices engaged in capitation. This type of compensation decreases the pressure to overutilize medical resources. Groups then establish the workload to ensure they get full value from each physician. Incentives are usually structured around issues of quality (patient satisfaction, use of preventive intervention, staff evaluation) and utilization (appropriate use of high-cost tests, following guidelines, appropriate referrals, availability).

Dr. New in Case 18-2 considered what she had learned about the organization of physicians who provide medical care. She also clarified her vision of success. For Dr. New, success would be a job that could last a lifetime, with a reasonable income, in a group that she would be proud to be a part of because it provided excellent clinical care and good quality of life for its staff. With those factors in mind, she drew up a check sheet for her ideal practice, and began the search. Some of the important items on her list were: large group, strong governance, access to capital, willing to take capitated risk, minimal investment required by her, and a vision that values quality care to its patients and quality

375

PRACTICE
MANAGEMENT:
THE IMPORTANCE
OF THE BUSINESS
ASPECT OF
MEDICINE

of life for its staff. She feels confident that, armed with her own personal mastery of her needs, and her check sheet, she can make a wise choice.

CASE 18-3

Dr. Martinez has decided to join a large primary care clinic after finishing his residency. The clinic has a large, well-functioning, administrative department that handles clinic operations, allowing physicians to devote their time to seeing patients. The majority of the patients seen at the clinic are in managed care plans, and capitation represents more than half of the clinic's income. Dr. Martinez wonders what economic forces drive the practice of medicine in this environment and whether those forces will facilitate or harm his ability to practice medicine.

PRACTICE MANAGEMENT: THE IMPORTANCE OF THE BUSINESS ASPECT OF MEDICINE

THREE OBJECTIVES OF PRACTICE MANAGEMENT

Business principles. Just like every other business, a medical practice must address typical aspects of starting and maintaining a business, including establishing a clear vision or purpose for the organization, hiring competent professionals who support the vision, and then ensuring that the business provides a return on the financial investment of the owners. Medical groups must always keep a focus on these issues. There are also some special objectives of the practice of medicine that require management attention. These have been standard issues in other types of business. Healthcare is just beginning to understand them.

Quality. The quality aspect of the practice of medicine also shares a great deal of similarity with every other business. Since medical care is the physician's life's work, medical organizations desire to create an environment that is a high-quality place to work, both for the professional and nonprofessional staff.

Physicians also expect that their organization will provide a high-quality place for patients to receive their care. Patients expect high-quality care, both in the delivery of service and with the clinical results of their care.

The chief way medical groups of the future will compete is on the basis of quality. Systems must be in place to ensure this quality effort.

Cost. To survive in a competitive environment, all businesses must control the costs of their products. Medicine is no different. Medical groups must be good stewards and be frugal in their use of medical resources. This frugality is achieved by finding ways to increase productivity, correctly choose the appropriate workup strategy, take cost into consideration when diagnosing and treating patients, and avoid unnecessary and futile care. Systems must be in place to manage utilization (cost).

Integration as a goal of practice management. Integration is a requirement of sound practice management. Healthcare is more than a series of encounters between a single care provider and a patient. There are many more players simultaneously involved. There are those who pay for healthcare insurance, such as the employers. There are those who pay the bills, such as the insurance companies. There are the hospitals, where some of the most expensive care is given. There is the public, who has other agendas and needs that compete with healthcare for the public's money. The cottage industry of medicine was only coordinated by degrees of collegiality. This was very expensive, wasteful, and produced poor patient care. The goal of integration is to address the needs of all of the players and to make them accountable to one another. Integration has several faces.

Multidisciplinary approach. We are becoming multidisciplinary in our approach to healthcare. In addition to multispecialty, we are seeing the addition into the mainstream of clinical life of doctors of osteopathy and midlevel providers, such as nurse practitioners and physician assistants. Traditional ancillary providers, such as optometrists, psychologists, podiatrists, and physical therapists, are also being integrated into large medical groups. Because of the market pressures of patient requests, nontraditional, alternative providers such as chiropractors are also making their way into medical groups. The net effect of this change is that as these providers are integrated into a care system, they are controlled as all providers are, to provide a demonstrated, quality product. With this integration comes accountability.

Delivery system major players. Integration of the major segments of the delivery system is occurring. Insurance companies, institutions such as hospitals, and provider groups find they have many common goals that they alone cannot accomplish. They also see that there are goals of the whole system to which they collectively need to respond. As such, the formation of various alliances between these players, to align incentives, develop shared vision, avoid duplication, and decide the allocation of resources, is occurring. Accountability of all of the major players to one another is key.

The medical record. The current medical record system is a major barrier to coordinated quality care. Traditional records are unsearchable, incomplete, illegible, and to a degree incomprehensible, leading to duplication, missed diagnosis, and wasted efforts. Some integration may have to wait until we have a single, permanent medical record utility that is universally accepted and implemented. Many large regional or national megagroups are actively addressing this issue.

Purchasers of healthcare. No mention of integration can be made without also considering the needs of those who pay for healthcare, i.e., the government and the employers. They are becoming very sophisticated buyers who are learning how to evaluate the quality of the services their clients receive. Quality, access, and cost are their focus. Delivery systems that are not responsive to the needs of the payers will find themselves out of business. More and more, payers are involved in the design of the delivery system and the evaluation of its day-to-day operation. One example of this is the development of the Health Employers Data Information Set (HEDIS) criteria to measure the quality of targeted medical care. HEDIS criteria were developed when employers, who buy health insurance, told the insurance companies that they want direct measurements of the quality of care given. Insurance companies collectively agreed on "report cards" of the degree of compliance to accepted HEDIS standards among providers of the insurance companies. The public will be given reports of the degree of compliance with these standards in the various health plans. Obviously medical groups and providers will be rated too as this system is fine-tuned. HEDIS standards have been set for items such as Pap smear and mammogram frequency.

Benefits of practice management. What will be the effect of all this on the physician? Will it be good or bad? Although the dramatic rapid change in the delivery system has caused major anxiety for many physicians, in the end it will be overwhelmingly good for Dr. Martinez and his colleagues in Case 18-3.

Practice guidelines will provide a rationalization of care, eliminating duplication and useless steps, and bring us to an end point of proper care sooner and at less cost. There will be a rationalization of physician income, with rewards for effort and education. The great discrepancy in income between various specialties will narrow a great deal. Administrators will manage the business, allowing physicians to devote the bulk of their time to seeing patients. Dr. Martinez knows that he has made an excellent choice of a work environment, in that his group is very attuned to proper management and economics. He has decided that these changes will allow him to focus his professional life on the joy that providing good care generates.

CASE 18-4

Dr. Black recently joined the prestigious City Clinic, a large multispecialty clinic in the state capitol. He has been appointed to the finance committee. City Clinic's payer mix includes nine HMOs, five of which have a fully capitated plan and four having discounted fee for service. They also participate in many different PPOs, all of which have discounted fee for service. The finance committee has been charged with determining which health plans to drop, to increase total reimbursement for the clinic. Dr. Black needs a basic understanding of reimbursement to be able to participate in this committee work.

REIMBURSEMENT ISSUES AND RELATED ETHICAL CONSIDERATIONS

A history of reimbursement for medical services is helpful in understanding the ethical issues involved.

Gratis. Gratis was the first model. Care was given as a gift. There were no ethical issues. Medicine was really not a science at this stage. The physician's role was that of an observer and comforter. Real intervention was almost nonexistent.

Patient pays all. The patient pays soon became the standard. The more the physician did, the more she earned. This conflict of interest was mitigated by the physician's professional responsibility to do good for the patients, and also the negotiation between the physician and the patient about the cost of care. For example, the patient and family might think twice when it looked as if they might use up their entire estate to pay for adding a few months to the end of life for a terminally ill family member.

Others pay. Someone else pays all or part of the bill is the insurance model. This is risk sharing. Here there is a break in the physician–patient relationship. The value judgment by the patient about what is received and at what price is not linked. Physicians tend to want to do more because it is being complete, and also because it pays more. Patients tend to want it all because it is free, they have earned it, and it is being complete. This is very inflationary. It has been our traditional model.

Who should pay for the insurance? The patient might pay by buying the insurance policy. Much is paid for by the employer, either directly or through insurance. The biggest single payer for healthcare is the federal government, through the military, Medicare, Medicaid, and veterans benefits.

There are several different payment mechanisms. In traditional fee for service, the physician determines the charge, the insurance company pays all or part of the bill, and the patient pays the balance. The insurance company has no relationship to the physician, only a relationship to the patient. There is no check on the physician's charges.

Most healthcare is now paid as discounted fee for service. Here the insurance company has a contractual relationship with the physician as well as the insured, and rates are negotiated. Sometimes, as with the government, the negotiations amount to: "This is what we pay; take it or do not treat the patient."

Capitation is the new and coming method. Groups are paid a fixed monthly rate for the total care of the patient. In this model the insurance risk is passed on to the medical group. Medical groups learn to live within a budget. These rates are negotiated and based on both market trends and actuarial data. Medical groups calculate the various health risks they expect to see in a year, negotiate the cost of care with subspecialists, and determine a budget for the year. If they meet or better their budget, there is a profit, and if their experience is worse than budget, they suffer a loss. This is the reason medical groups need capital reserves and stop loss insurance if they accept capitated contracts. In a way, the medical group has become an insurance company. Here providers are paid based on their effort, plus the profitability of the group.

EFFECT OF PAYMENT MECHANISM ON COST AND QUALITY OF CARE

Patient pays all. The patient pays model tends to limit the cost of care, because of the patient's limited willingness or ability to pay. Physicians and patients sit alone in the consultation room and decide. The quality of care can be adversely affected because of the same limitations. Physicians are drawn closer to their patients' total circumstances, and form closer bonds. There is a mutual accountability for the cost of care. Cost versus benefits are looked at closely. The focus is on episodes of care, not on long-term coordinated care. This focus can adversely affect quality.

Indemnity insurance. Indemnity insurance usually is accompanied by a copayment or deductible payment by the patient. This method preserves only a minor degree of patient accountability for the utilization of resources and cost of care. The physician is less accountable too for costs. Hence, costs tend to skyrocket. The focus here is also on episodes of care. Physicians give care to those patients who present themselves for care. Patients may not be seen for years, important preventive services neglected, and the physician would not know it because in this model there is no certain way to identify who, at any one time, are the physician's patients. This method also adversely affects quality.

Discounted fee-for-service insurance. Discounted fee for service is similar to indemnity insurance, except for the attempt at cost control the discount brings. However, even though fees are discounted, the incentive to do more procedures to maintain the revenue stream is still present, which is self-defeating. The Medicaid system is the classic case of the self-defeating nature of discounted fee for service. With reimbursement under Medicaid in many cases less than the cost of the overhead of a visit, some physicians did extra procedures of marginal values, such as a urinalysis or blood tests, if there was any justification for it at all, to cover their costs. To counter this trend, discounted fee-for-service payers developed utilization review methods. Battle lines developed between payers and physicians, with payers citing unnecessary procedures and physicians citing interference with their practice. Costs remain out of control, and there is minimal accountability for quality.

Capitation. The capitation model requires the physician to provide all and only (*all and only* is a key phrase in the emerging system) the care needed. Providing more care than needed will cause financial losses. Providing less care than necessary will also be associated with financial losses, for example, expensive hospitalization occurring when care is delayed, disenrollment (very expensive), peer review cases, or outside legal action. In this system, physicians will always know who their patients are because each month they will get a list of the names and a payment. Under capitation, physicians are accountable for the quality of their total care. Noncompliant patients can be identified, and corrective action taken.

Costs are better controlled in this model, because everything that is done is an expense to the person who best knows about the appropriateness of needed health services, the physician. Quality is monitored internally by the medical group. Payers monitor quality indicators to be sure they are receiving full value for their payment. Physicians and groups will be judged on how well they care for their patients, which will become public knowledge.

In Case 18-4, Dr. Black's committee considered the payment mechanisms for the various health plans and made a strategic decision. Their group would concentrate on capitation and normal fee for service. They would drop all discounted fee-for-service plans that were not transitional into full capitation. These plans would be dropped because they did not reward the medical group for excellent case management. Exceptions would be made on a case-by-case basis if the health plan had some form of strategic relationship to the group. Health plans would be given advanced warning, in hopes that they would be planning a transition to capitation. The finance committee recommended to the board of directors that they consider narrowing the number of health plans that the group participated in, to provide for some strategic relations with the health plans.

CASE 18-5

Dr. Black will need a basic understanding of the financial management of a practice if he is to do a good job on the finance committee of the City Clinic. The finance committee oversees the budget, monitors investment of capital and, monthly financial performance, and makes recommendations for action to the board of directors. They focus their attention on key performance indicators.

FINANCIAL MANAGEMENT

Purpose. The purpose of financial management is to stay in business. Practices have income and expenses. If income meets or exceeds expenses, the business is viable. If not, like any other business, the end comes. The objective of financial management is to increase revenue and to decrease expenses, while providing a high-quality environment and product.

Income sources. Sources of practice revenue include fee-for-service income, capitation income, return on investments (this includes interest income and the revenue generated by owned capital assets like a building, or in-house laboratory facilities, and so forth) and savings from insurance incentives programs, seen particularly in capitated programs.

Expenses. Practice expenses include facility costs such as rent and insurance, utilities, staff salaries and benefits, professional salaries and benefits, taxes, interest on loans, supplies, malpractice insurance, cost of goods sold such as braces and injectables, management services, systems such as computers, purchased services such as accounting, outside laboratory services, retirement plan costs, and depreciation of capital goods.

Methods. The methods and tools for financial management include an annual budget, regular financial reports, and cost accounting.

Annual budget. The annual budget is the foundational tool for financial management. This is a document prepared in advance, using knowledge generated from within and outside the organization, which predicts, in a very itemized way, both expenses and income. Capitation is all about living within a budget. In negotiations with health plans for the annual capitation rate, medical groups need to be able to predict the cost of care, including care for specialty care that is referred outside the group. They also need to be able to predict the cost of hospital care for the group. You can understand, then, how important historical and statistical data are to the group. The cost of referred care is based on the cost of a unit of service times the number of units of care. So, contracting rates with referral providers becomes important.

Financial reports generally are generated monthly. There are four standard reports that are regularly used by medical groups: balance sheets, income statements, cash flow analysis, and production analysis reports.

Balance sheets list the assets and liabilities of a company and establish the company's worth. Included in assets are cash in the bank, investments, funds owed the group, and fixed assets such as real estate and capital equipment such as an imaging machine. Liabilities include bills owed but not paid, balances on mortgages, and other loans. The difference between assets and liabilities is the company's net worth or value. Some of that worth may have been from contributed equity, and some of it may have come from retained profit. Year by year companies expect to increase their value. Balance sheets are helpful, but are of little value by themselves. They tell where a company is financially at a single point in time, but do not show what has happened to give that result.

The *income statement* itemizes the sources of income and the nature of expenses and arrives at a number that is the profit or loss for both the year to date and the month just passed. The budget document is a mirror of the income statement, so generally the income statement compares each item with budget, line by line, and reports whether the category is over of under budget for the time period. This is a very helpful tool for understanding the financial health of the group. Departments can be set up, such as laboratory services. In this way each department can be analyzed to determine its contribution to the profit of the group. If the contribution is less than desired, corrective action can be taken. Without this cost accounting, it is difficult to understand the profitability of the company.

The *cash flow analysis* keeps the financial department aware of the cash available to pay bills. It would be possible for a group to be earning a good profit, be on budget, but be out of cash to pay the monthly bills. Consider what would happen if a group that was making a good monthly profit bought some imaging equipment that was in the budget, and then paid for it with cash. The bottom line in the balance sheet would look the same. Cash would have been converted to another asset, the imaging machine. The income statement would look the same. This expenditure, since it was for a capital asset, would not show up as an expense. However, the cash available to pay bills might be gone. Cash flow reports generally make projections of the sources and uses of cash. The second example would be the clinic that has just enough cash in the bank, month by month, to pay their bills. However, 6 months in the future they have annual property taxes to pay, which is an extra $25,000. The cash flow analysis would pick up this coming shortfall of cash so that corrective action could be taken.

These financial reports are common to all businesses. *Production reports* are a special need for medical groups. These are reports that detail the financial results from the work of each physician. For sophisticated groups, these reports would include gross billings, by several categories, number of patients seen, ancillary services (lab, X ray) ordered, cost and frequency of referrals made, and number of active patients, capitation revenue, and fee-for-service revenue received. Since sophisticated groups generally fix the workload, and pay on the basis of salary and bonus, this information is partly used to determine the bonus.

Cost accounting is an attempt to allocate all costs in a business to its specific products and services, and then track the revenue from these products or services to find ways to increase profitability. This is a special case of the income statement. It is very complex and detailed. It might include costing out a telephone call to the physician about refilling a medication. This takes telephone equipment time, operator time, medical records time to get the record to the physician, physician time to give the response, and then a call to the pharmacy to authorize the refill, subsequently charting the action, and refiling the chart in medical records. There is cost but no revenue. How do you cover that cost? Cost accounting principles can be used to evaluate the performance of each capitated contract, to know if the capitation payment is adequate to cover the cost of services.

Dr. Black's finance committee, mentioned in Case 18-5, has evaluated the financial performance of the group for the past month, quarter, and year to date, as shown to them in the financial reports. Overall, the group's financial performance is better than budget. They have noted one capitated program that is losing money. It appears that in this program, the monthly capitation per enrollee, particularly the rate for women of childbearing age, is a bit low. They also note that one provider's production is below the third standard deviation from the mean. They report this information to the board of directors. Dr. Black feels good about the committee's work and his own role on the committee. He is pleased with the amount of very important information that is known in real time about the medical group.

CASE 18-6

After 2 years as an employee physician, Dr. Hing has become a shareholder and has been appointed to a 1-year slot on the governing body. This is a familiarization gesture for young physicians who have shown leadership potential. She is excited to serve, but knows little about medical practice governance.

COMPONENTS OF A SUCCESSFUL GROUP PRACTICE

The governing body. Medical groups cannot survive without strong governance. The role of governance is to provide the company with its direction. The governing body is generally the board of directors and the medical director. Governing bodies will be pressed to take unpopular action, such as imposing workload standards on physicians or salary modifications. These actions will be necessary to allow the group to compete and stay in business. Boards need to be insulated by powerful bylaws so that their members cannot be recalled when they take unpopular stands in different situations. A major task of the governing body is to make an accurate evaluation of current reality. Gaps between the vision and current reality create the driving force to move forward. Without a real-time, accurate view of current reality, businesses flounder.

Mission statement. The board of directors usually develops a mission statement, which is a very basic statement of why the organization exists. The basic mission of any business is to stay in business and provide jobs. When an organization loses its way or feels confused, it needs to revisit its mission statement. A mission statement can be as simple as:

> The mission of the Example Clinic is to provide a meaningful way for its employees to provide affordable, high-quality primary medical care to the people of our city.

Vision statement. The vision statement is the dream of what the company would like to create. To be valid, the vision statement needs to be clearly understood and shared by all employees. Governance needs to manage from this vision statement.

Value statement. The value statement is a capsule view of the culture of the organization. This is an itemization of the group ethics. It tells what values are important and by what means the company will move forward.

Business plan. A business plan developed by administration and approved by governance will propel the company toward its vision. Key indicators will be available to governance to evaluate progress. The business plan generally has a 3- to 5-year span. The business plan is not a financial document, although it will have financial components. It will include such items as growth, market penetration, strategic partnerships, quality goals, and introduction of new products or services.

Annual budget. An annual budget will be developed by administration and adopted by governance. This is a part of the business plan. To be successful, medical groups will need to learn to live within their budget.

Credentialing and peer review. Periodically the governing body will review the credentials of all of its providers to ensure they possess the skills necessary to do the work they are assigned. Peer review will be conducted by the governing body or its agent, when there seems to be cause for review. The purpose of the review is to ensure the competence of the professional staff and to take corrective action if necessary.

Quality improvement. The healthcare system is being called on to deliver more and better care for less cost. Estimates of the cost of waste in U.S. businesses run from 20 to 40% of the gross revenue. Achieving more for less (more for less is a key phrase in the emerging system) will require adoption of processes such as total quality management (TQM). TQM seeks to improve every facet of the life of the practice from janitorial service to clinical care of the patient.

Accreditation. Since medical groups will be paid by others to care for their patients, the payers and the public will demand that groups meet acceptable standards of performance. Medical groups will need to prove this by accreditation, just as hospitals have done for decades. National medical group accrediting bodies have already begun to function and develop standards.

Capital. A major challenge for a medical group is to attract, accumulate, and preserve capital. Groups need cash in the bank for several reasons. Groups expect to grow and growth takes cash. They are in a risk-taking mode. There will be times of adversity when they will need to dip into their reserves. Market fluctuations will produce years of good capitation payments and bad years. Since most groups will purchase medical services from other physician groups for some specialty care, they will need money on hand to pay bills that have been incurred but not reported (IBNR is an important term in accounting). There is an ongoing conflict in most groups between the pressures to raise professional salaries and to raise and retain capital.

The physician administrator. As medicine adopts the practices of big business and physicians are organized together in large medical groups, oversight of the clinical practice is essential. Only another physician can do this well. This is the role of the medical director or the chief medical officer. Medical directors are physicians who serve all or part of their time on the administrative side of clinic life. This is a new type of medical specialty, and training is not yet formalized. Some physician administrators have completed their master's degree in business or healthcare administration. They report to the board of directors, who reviews their performance. Duties of the medical director include the following:

1. *Utilization review and quality improvement.* Medical groups continually monitor the way they provide care. They want to be sure that they are providing all and only the care needed. There is a constant search for a new way to lower cost or to improve outcomes. A dramatic example of cost savings has been the reduction of the length of stay in the hospital for almost every type of admission during the past few years. An example of the improvement in quality has been the increasing frequency of vaginal births after cesarean sections rather than simply repeating the C-section. Utilization and quality problems are generally not individual but systems problems. Systems need to be in place to facilitate this work.

2. *Peer review and corrective action.* On occasion, individual physician performance warrants an investigation. Problems to investigate might relate to competence or behavior. An investigation is done according to the rules of due process, and is a responsibility of the medical director. If deemed necessary, appropriate corrective action can be taken. This action could be a warning, a requirement for continuing medical education, a fine, or even termination.

3. *Performance review.* Progressive medical groups provide periodic performance reviews of their providers. This review is done by the medical director. Since in many groups compensation is tied to performance, this is a very sensitive area.

Dr. Hing, in Case 18-6, will learn a lot about her medical group in her year on the board. Already she is impressed with the complexity of governance and the various issues requiring consideration. She is encouraged with the systems that are in place to manage the business and the physicians, and she is delighted with the vision of the company and its ideals.

CASE 18-7

James Chapman's father has been practicing general internal medicine for 30 years. He feels very uneasy with the changes in medicine and is disillusioned about the profession. His son James is in his third year of medical school. He knows his father's feelings and wonders why medicine is changing and what the effect of it will be on him.

CONCLUSION: THE FORCES AND DIRECTION OF CHANGE

We are in the midst of massive change in the manner in which healthcare is financed and delivered. The key driving force for change is cost control. A corollary to this force is the need to demonstrate quality. We are moving into the age of accountability. Physicians and healthcare delivery systems are being called to be accountable for these two issues, cost and quality. Their responsibility is also broadening beyond single episodes of care to encompass coordination of the health services in a patient population.

In response to these forces, the entire structure of the delivery system is undergoing massive change. Big integrated systems that use computer analysis, guidelines, and objective measurement of utilization and quality are developing to meet these demands. The financial risk of providing healthcare is being shifted from the receivers of care, and from the third-party payers, to the providers themselves. Large healthcare systems will compete intensely on the basis of cost and quality. These changes seem irreversible and unstoppable.

James, in Case 18-7, has had some rotations in clinical settings. One rotation was in a large prestigious multispecialty clinic nearby. What he saw there was a group on the cutting edge of the changes of the delivery system. He had close contact with physicians in the group. He found them pleased with their role as physicians and encouraged by the systems that surrounded them, enabling them to practice better medicine. James finds his new role as an agent of change, trying to help his father grow into the new reality.

CASES FOR DISCUSSION

CASE 1

You are a member of the compensation committee in your medical group. Sixty percent of your group's income now comes from capitation. This percentage has been increasing rapidly the past few years, and the group believes this increase will continue. The group's compensation for its physicians is based totally on their individual gross billings. The board of directors believes an overhaul of the compensation system might be in order. It has appointed a compensation committee to study the matter and make a recommendation to the board.

1. *If physicians are paid based on their total charges, what is the likely effect of this on work output and services provided?*
2. *If physicians are paid a straight salary, what is the likely effect of this on work output and services provided?*
3. *In a fee-for-service system, what is the effect of providing more or less than all and only the services that are medically necessary? What are the ethnical considerations?*
4. *In a capitated system, what is the effect of providing more or less than all and only the services that are medically necessary? What are the ethical considerations?*

5. If the group adopts a salary basis for compensation, how will the group ensure the physicians work hard, work smart, and provide good service to their patients? If you do this in the form of a bonus, what would be the basis of the bonus?
6. For both of the basic types of compensation listed, describe the physician work ethic and utilization patterns it would encourage and discourage, depending on the compensation plan.
7. What would your recommendation be to the board of directors?

CASE 2

You are a physician leader in a large medial group that is about to undergo rapid growth. The medical market in your community is very competitive and heavily dominated by managed care. To be able to survive in this market you know that your group will need to undergo many changes, including a revision of compensation. Salaries of the highly compensated specialists will have to come down, and for all, workload will have to go up. There are many quality issues that have to be faced because it is clear that competition in the future will be based on quality. To prepare for these changes, your group sees the need to revise its bylaws. You are the chairman of the bylaws committee.

1. What could happen to the leadership of your group if in 2 years the group had more than doubled in size and members of the board of directors were elected on an annual basis?
2. If the new board had a majority of members from the new groups, what might happen to the vision, the values, and the stability of the group? Would these changes be desirable?
3. Outline a governance plan, with methods of election and recall, for a 200-physician medical group, that would give the group the strong, effective, protected board of directors needed to thrive in a highly managed care, capitated environment.

CASE 3

Your medical group's main reimbursement has changed from fee for service to capitation over the past year. In times past, the annual influenza epidemic has been one of the most profitable seasons of the year. In the capitation model, your group realizes that next year the epidemic will be the most costly season of the year if it is business as usual. You are on a task force to study this and make a recommendation to the board of directors.

1. What is the "all and only" of the prevention and treatment of influenza? What are the roles of immunization, patient visits, antibiotics, imaging, laboratory studies in an influenza epidemic?
2. Develop a plan to immunize your patient population in the most cost-effective way. Include ways to monitor the percentage of the population immunized. What percentage of the "at risk" population could you immunize? How could you increase that percentage?
3. Using the tools learned in the chapter on practice guidelines, outline a plan to decrease the cost, and improve the quality, of the treatment of uncomplicated influenza in the normal yearly epidemic. Include consideration of treatment initiated by the patient as a result of patient education, telephone treatment by an advice nurse using clinic protocols, and visits to the clinic. If a patient is seen at the clinic, what level of provider could provide primary care?
4. Develop quality indicators to measure the effectiveness and patient satisfaction, as well as the cost, for the care of patients in this system, so that further improvements can be made the following year.

CASE 4

Your medical group receives the bulk of its income from capitated contracts. The group is mostly made up of primary care providers. Specialty care is referred out to specialists who are under a contract with your group. The group does not receive capitation for hospital care, but does share, on a 50% basis, the profit or loss of the hospital budget. The same arrangement applies to the cost of prescription drugs.

1. Outline the flow of cash to and from your group.
2. How will you determine how much to pay specialists? Will you pay them their billed charges in full, or discounted; will you develop your own fee schedule for them, or will you pay them a subcapitation payment, based on your enrollment? What would be the advantages and disadvantages of each method for both parties? Why would they be willing to accept anything less than full payment of their billed charges?
3. What financial tools would you use to monitor your group's financial health? Explain.
4. Explain the role of estimating IBNR (incurred but not reported) on the financial health of your group.
5. Why would your group need a large amount of available cash in its reserve account? What would be the risk of not having large enough cash reserves?
6. How would you deal with the temptation of the physicians to lessen the reserves and increase the compensation?

RECOMMENDED READINGS

Kongstvedt PR: *Essentials of Managed Health Care.* Gathersburg, Md, Aspen, 1995.

> This book outlines the effects of health reform, types of managed care organizations, and integrated healthcare delivery systems on the medical marketplace. Significant detail is provided regarding management of resources and contracting.

Medicare HMO/CMP Manual (HCFA Publication 75). Washington, DC, PB85-953899, 1985.

> This publication explains the requirements contained in the law and regulations for HMOs/CMPs/HCPPs.

Milakovich ME: Creating a total health care environment. *Health Care Manage Rev* 16(2):9–20, 1991.

> This article defines "total quality health care," describes poor-quality management practices, and suggests methods to measure costs and implement continuous quality improvement.

CHAPTER 19

Lifelong Medical Learning

Sonia J. S. Crandall

If physicians are to change . . . , their education will have to encourage reflection, personal development, and the growth of self-knowledge. The current environment of the medical school, with its information overload, frenzied activity and competitive ethos, in many ways discourages personal development of this kind. Medical scientists sometimes make reference to "the frontiers of knowledge." I think they have in mind a frontier that is "out there." The newest and most challenging frontier may be within us.

McWhinney (1989b, p. 40)

EDUCATIONAL OBJECTIVES

After reading this chapter, students will be able to:

1. Recognize the role of lifelong medical education in assuring, maintaining, and enhancing professional competence
2. Define continuing medical education
3. Define self-directed learning
4. Describe the three stages of physician development in obtaining new competencies
5. Define the attributes of a reflective practitioner
6. Design a plan for an individualized curriculum for lifelong professional education

INTRODUCTION

This chapter focuses on the vast differences between learning that occurs during medical school and learning that is necessary for the "real world" of medical practice. It will attempt to answer questions that many students may be asking themselves as they embark on a long and arduous course of study. How can students prepare themselves for the real world, regardless of how the real world may have changed after their training in medical school and residency? What can students do during medical training so that they will not be so overwhelmed when the primarily faculty-directed, medical school curriculum-driven learning becomes self-directed, physician-driven learning when they reach the real world? In other words, how does a physician remain competent during a career spanning 40 years after formal schooling is over, given the fact that medical knowledge doubles every 5 years, necessitating continual changes in clinical practice?

Except for the nursing profession, the education of physicians has been studied and written about more by educational researchers than any other profession. The size of this body of literature is immense, which indicates that many teachers and researchers believe this is an important topic worthy of their time and effort. A MedLine search of the literature from 1966 to 1995 of 3500 journals using the descriptors of "medical education" and "continuing medical education" yielded 18,689 and 2567 citations, respectively. The literature of medical education and continuing medical education has offered educators great insights into the processes of continuous lifelong learning in medicine and, more specifically, the strategies physicians use to remain up to date and acquire new skills.

It is the physician's utmost desire to remain competent and give the best possible care she can to her patients (Fox *et al.*, 1989). It is the very rare practitioner indeed who would disagree that the pursuit of lifelong medical education is an essential component to a productive and satisfying medical practice. "In medicine, the half-life of knowledge, the information explosion, new diseases, innovative diagnostic technology, advanced treatment methods, changing societal expectations and practice patterns, and the specific needs of individual practices" (Jennett *et al.*, 1994, p. 49) demand that practicing physicians devise an individualized, systematic approach for maintaining competence in an ever-changing healthcare environment.

CASE 19-1

"Recently, I moved my practice from a small house in the suburbs to a larger and more modern office downtown, closer to the hospital where I do most of my referral work. My patients were changing. Fifteen years ago, I started practice in the "growth area" of this community, the suburbs. Over the last ten years, however, I noticed that some of my "empty nest" patients were moving away, often into the core of the city. On top of that, many other new internists and subspecialists had come to the suburbs, competing for new patients. And it was getting harder to get to the downtown hospital where I practice, because of traffic. . . . We decided to move into a relatively new office building. . . . I feel very good about this change. I can get to the hospital in half the time, order laboratory tests and x-rays done in the same building . . . and my patients seem much happier as well. I have also noticed a shift in my patient load—more young unmarried

patients and geriatric cases, both of which have prompted some learning on my part." (Davis, 1989, pp. 99–100)

389

MANAGING
CHANGE IN
MEDICAL
PRACTICE

MANAGING CHANGE IN
MEDICAL PRACTICE

Probably the greatest challenge physicians face in their day-to-day practice is that of managing change (R. D. Fox *et al.*, 1994). The amount of medical literature to scan is unmanageable, and the rate of change of medical "facts" is overwhelming. Although there are concepts and principles that have remained static for the past 80 years, the techniques and practices that medical students learn will very likely be outdated by the time those same students complete their chosen residencies. This poses a great challenge for physicians in training to keep current and continuously acquire new skills.

In addition to the challenge of managing change in the clinical arena, societal trends regarding the delivery of healthcare in the United States are also necessitating change. Physicians are no longer in control of the healthcare enterprise. Physicians "will continue to be faced by more external regulation, increased competition from outside the field, intrusion of newer occupations [i.e., non-physician providers], louder public demands for more high-quality service at lower cost, and increasingly rapid and pervasive technological change that drastically alters practice" (McGuire, 1993, p. 15).

Many stimuli internal and external to the practice environment determine how physicians provide healthcare to their patients. Fox *et al.* (1989) identified ten forces that triggered change and facilitated new learning in the physicians who participated in their study. The forces identified by the physicians were intellectual curiosity, the desire for personal well-being, financial well-being, stage of career, the desire to remain competent, the clinical environment, relationships with medical institutions, relating to others in the profession, regulations, and family and community. The number of internal and external forces are balanced, but the internal forces may be more compelling to the practitioner who is contemplating a change in practice.

There are several approaches physicians use to cope with the amount of change they encounter in their practice life. And, there is no one perfect way to achieve and maintain stability. As described earlier, learning needs are brought about by multiple triggers, and several forces may come together to create a new need. Physicians use a smorgasbord of resources simply because no one resource meets all of their learning needs; making a change in practice is contextual and problem-specific (Gruppen *et al.*, 1987); and learning preferences and styles of physicians are diverse (Van Voorhees *et al.*, 1988).

Needs for information updates on "state-of-the-art" technologies and practices can be met by reading journals, talking with peers, and attending formal lecture/discussion-type continuing medical education (CME) programs. Needs for gaining new procedural skills can be met by participating in CME workshops and mini-fellowships, or by "apprenticing" with a colleague who is an expert in that area. It is very common for a physician to use three or more educational resources when adopting a change (Lockyer *et al.*, 1994).

The learning "of any physician is a dynamic interaction of multiple information-gathering strategies, both formal and informal, structured and unstructured" (Moore *et al.*, 1994). The ways physicians continue to learn include using printed materials from pharmaceutical representatives, interaction with colleagues, peers, and mentors, both locally and nationally, consultations with specialists, participating in formal CME programs, using nonprint media such as computer programs and expert systems, reading journals and books, participating in self-assessments, participating in practice audits, teaching students, residents, peers, participating as faculty for a CME event, and writing for medical audiences (Fox *et al.*, 1989; Manning & DeBakey, 1987; Means, 1984; Rothenberg *et al.*, 1982). Of equal importance is that physicians learn from their experiences with patients.

> To be effective, Continuing Medical Education, the third, and arguably the most important phase of medical education, can no longer be seen solely as a unidirectional educational delivery system. It must be aware of, and responsive to, the needs of the practitioner/learner, derived both from understanding of the principles of adult education, and from educational and cognitive psychology; must understand, work with, and even begin to direct the realities of practice and health care delivery, including patient forces, practice environment, exigencies; and continue to develop the delivery systems of continuing education in order that they be practice-based, appropriate, effective, and integrate with the practice and professional life of the physician. In order to accomplish this goal, it may be that a new phase is required in order to describe the vacuum which CME researchers and providers may fill—that between areas of the learner, practice environment, and educational delivery systems. This common domain may be called "medical practice education," or the discipline of CME but it is the expanding and intersectoral nature of the purview of continuing education which is most important to grasp. (Banff Summary Statement, 1989, p. 40)

——— CONTINUING MEDICAL EDUCATION ———

WHAT IS CME?

"[CME] involves physicians, practice environments, learning resources, and interventions designed to improve the ability of physicians to provide better medical care to patients" (R. D. Fox *et al.*, 1994, p. 17). The American Medical Association (AMA) definition of CME is as follows:

> Continuing medical education consists of educational activities which serve to maintain, develop, or increase the knowledge, skills, and professional performance and relationships that a physician uses to provide services for patients, the public, or the profession. The content of CME is that body of knowledge and skills generally recognized and accepted by the profession as within the basic medical sciences, the discipline of clinical medicine, and the provision of health care to the public. (American Medical Association, 1993, p. 1)

This definition makes it fairly clear that CME is related to professional practice and patient care, but it also indicates that any educational activity that helps a physician in his professional role is considered CME. For example, it is appropriate for medical school faculty to attend programs that help them become better teachers; those activities are considered CME. The AMA goes on to illustrate those continuing education activities that are not considered CME, such as personal financial planning and music or literature appreciation.

Mazmanian and Duff (1994) adapted from Liveright and Haygood (1968) "[a] gentler, more comprehensive and learner-oriented definition of CME" (p. 294) that considers the physician's need to be fulfilled personally and as a member of a community, as well as professionally. They say CME is:

> a process whereby (physicians) who no longer attend school on a regular full-time basis . . . undertake sequential and organized activities with the conscious intention of bringing about changes in information, knowledge, understanding, or skill, appreciation and attitudes; or for the purpose of identifying or solving personal, professional, or community problems. (p. 294)

FORMAL CME PROGRAMS

Attending formal CME programs is a norm among the majority of physicians. CME programs have been around in the United States since the early 1900s. Continuing education programs came into being to provide physicians with a vehicle for maintaining and gaining new competence, enhancing performance and improving patient outcomes, and giving patients a sense of well-being that their physicians were competent (Abrahamson, 1984).

The formal CME industry ("formal CME" denotes programs that offer AMA Category 1 credit) is a multi-billion-dollar enterprise. There are thousands of CME programs offered to physicians in every specialty every year. There are thousands of CME providers in the United States.

ACCREDITED SPONSORS OF CME

About 2500 CME providers are accredited in the United States; only 126 of those 2500 are medical schools (Wentz & Harrison, 1994). The accreditation process in the United States is voluntary, specific, for CME and is "directed at institutions and organizations, not specific, individual CME activities" (Wentz & Harrison, 1994, p. 5). A CME provider may be accredited if it meets the essentials set forth by the Accreditation Council for Continuing Medical Education (ACCME). Because CME providers are not limited to institutions whose principal mission is education, the range of accredited providers includes medical schools, state medical associations, specialty societies, subspecialty groups, hospitals, voluntary health agencies, pharmaceutical and medical device manufacturers, and a few for-profit organizations (Wentz & Harrison, 1994). This varied system of providers is not the norm in Canada. There are only 16 accredited providers in Canada, that is, the medical schools.

The accreditation process occurs basically on two levels, but the definitive accrediting body is the ACCME. The latter accredits some providers, about 517 (Wentz & Harrison, 1994), *directly,* for example, medical schools and state medical associations. Once accredited, state medical associations are give the authority by the ACCME to accredit hospital-based CME providers and other local sponsors. The American Osteopathic Association (AOA) and the American Academy of Family Physicians (AAFP) also provide systems for accrediting continuing education programs that are designed specifically to meet the needs of osteopaths and family physicians. In fact, family physicians must attend AAFP accredited programs to meet recertification requirements for their specialty board.

Physicians may receive CME credit for attending accredited CME programs, medical school or hospital grand rounds, specialty society programs, local/regional/national conferences and meetings, such as state academy meetings, teaching in CME programs, and in specific instances, precepting students and residents.

HOW DOES FORMAL CME WORK?

Accredited programs are allowed to give CME credit. "In 1968, the AMA announced its Physician's Recognition Award, by which was established a series of credit categories. Currently these are AMA PRA category 1 and category 2" (Wentz & Harrison, 1994, p. 6). The AMA PRA Certificate is awarded to any physician who accumulates 50 hours of CME credit in one year; two-year (100 hours) and three-year (150 hours) certificates may also be obtained. Sixty of those hours must be designated Category 1 and the remaining 90 hours may be either Category 1 or 2. Category 1 credit refers to CME provided by accredited sponsors. Category 1 activities include "lectures, seminars, use of self-study materials, self-assessment programs, mini-residencies, and use of audiovisual or computer based materials, so long as they are designated as AMA PRA Category 1" (American Medical Association, 1993, p. 8). Category 2 credit refers to all unsponsored educational activities, such as

> clinical consultations . . . , participation in patient care review activities, teaching of medical and other health care professionals, patient centered discussions with colleagues, journal club activities, use of self-assessment examinations and reviews . . . , use of databases and other computer based materials in connection with patient care activities, use of self instructional materials . . . , publication of medical or medically related articles and books, and preparation of exhibits. (American Medical Association, 1993, p. 8)

Since its inception, over 600,000 physicians have received the AMA PRA (Wentz & Harrison, 1994). Many specialty boards now mandate evidence of CME credit for continued certification of its physicians.

HOW CAN MEDICAL STUDENTS PREPARE FOR THE PROCESS OF CME?

Medical students should become aware of the CME process while still in medical school so that they will be properly prepared for the process after graduation. First, talk to physician faculty about the types of educational activities in which they participate. Second, talk to physicians in the community about how they learn and make changes in their practices. Third, get to know what the CME department at the medical school offers to physicians at the medical school and in the community. All CME departments offer programs locally, and many offer programs nationally and internationally via satellite. Tele-CME is becoming popular and will expand dramatically in the next 5 to 10 years.

While most medical students do not have time to participate in formal CME programs, knowing what is available will become increasingly important as residency and practice approach. Try to discover what other physicians do now to continue learning. Students need to think about how they learn best. Pay close attention to the types of learning experiences that have been most useful in gaining new knowledge, skills, and attitudes for you. Students should ask themselves, "Was this a significant learning experience for me?" "Why was it significant?" "What was different or unique about the experience that I remember it as significant?" Asking these questions will help you get to know how you prefer to learn and what works best for you.

Once physicians are in practice and need to participate in CME, there are ten criteria to consider when choosing whether a CME activity is an appropriate one. (These criteria were described in handout materials developed by David A. Davis, M.D., Associate Dean for Continuing Education, University of Toronto, for a workshop presented to medical students entitled "CME Skills: A Workshop For Lifelong Learners.") Rate each item on a scale of 1 to 10 to get an overall picture of the significance of the program for meeting specific learning needs.

- Does the program cover topics that I want to learn?
- Does the program cover topics that I need to learn?
- Is the program relevant to my practice environment and patients?
- Is the program convenient, and what does it cost?
- Are the program presenters known experts in the content areas?
- Does the program provide opportunities for me to interact with colleagues?
- Does the program provide opportunities for me to participate?
- Does the program provide opportunities for me to learn?
- What is the track record of the CME provider?
- What is the credibility of the program sponsor(s)?

CASE 19-2

"There's a medical-legal problem in taking an ECG [electrocardiogram] and not knowing that you don't know, when you're looking at it, that there's something wrong, and not getting a report back for a week. That's intimidating to have somebody leave the clinic, send the ECG off and not realize that there's some problem." (Crandall, 1990, p. 345)

INFORMAL CONTINUING MEDICAL EDUCATION

Dr. S. H., in Case 19-2, had been a physician for 33 years at the time of our interview. He worked in a freestanding ambulatory care clinic in a large southwestern city. Most of the patients who came to this clinic were between the ages of 18 and 50 and primarily had acute but common complaints. They rarely had serious or life-threatening problems. Once in a while Dr. S. H. needed to run an ECG to rule out a serious problem, but he was very uncomfortable interpreting the ECG. He did not read ECGs frequently enough to stay competent. Because Dr. S. H. was interested in enhancing his competence he purchased a cardiology textbook and started reading about interpreting ECGs. Each time he ran an ECG on a patient he would make an interpretation and then compare his diagnosis with the cardiologist's diagnosis when he received the report. Dr. S. H. continued to assess his skill level each time he received feedback from the cardiologist.

WHAT IS INFORMAL CME?

Informal CME is everything that is not formal CME. That statement is not meant to be pejorative, but to depict the variety of activities that can be called informal CME and to illustrate that the basic difference between formal and informal CME is the awarding of AMA PRA category 1 or 2 credit. Physicians participate in a great deal of learning for which no formal credit is offered. Case 19-2 illustrates a good example of how a physician may maintain or enhance her competence without attending formal CME. If physicians believe that they learn something new every day, then informal learning is the mechanism by which much of what they know is acquired.

It was mentioned earlier that lifelong learning is very individualized. It is a personal adventure. What constitutes informal learning activities includes conversing with colleagues and with consultants or specialists who have differing expertise, reading textbooks and journals, conversing with opinion leaders, discussing the latest therapies with pharmaceutical and equipment representatives, using computer programs and expert systems, i.e., medical decision support systems, to learn about diagnosis and management of disease, using computerized reminder systems and flowcharts, i.e., practice guidelines for specific conditions such as hypertension and diabetes, accessing and assessing the most recent medical literature pertaining to a specific patient problem to help make a clinical decision, fondly referred to today as "evidence-based" medicine, and using computerized systems to get feedback on individual practice outcomes compared with local or regional outcomes (Jennett *et al.*, 1994). However important all of these resources are, physicians claim that one of the greatest resources for informal learning, one that often leads to formal learning, is what the patient brings to the office. According to many physicians, learning from experience, from their practice environment and from their patients, is so memorable and significant that an entire section of this chapter is later devoted to that topic.

HOW DOES INFORMAL CME WORK?

There really is nothing magical about what has just been described. In fact, it may seem rather obvious how ubiquitous informal learning really is. Most medical students form study groups by the second week of medical school. Students hear their peers discuss ideas inside and outside of class and they absorb information like sponges from conversations with faculty and classmates and from readings outside of their medical textbooks. Many students join a student organization during school such as a family medicine interest group; some students are class officers. Many students volunteer some of their time to work in clinics that provide free healthcare to indigent populations. All of these activities contribute to medical student professional development although they are not part of *formal* schooling.

HOW CAN MEDICAL STUDENTS PREPARE FOR THE PROCESS OF INFORMAL CME?

Students cannot really prepare for informal learning; they are already experiencing it, just as they did before medical school. The purpose of this section is not so much to define informal learning, because it literally defies definition, but to create an awareness and openness to all of the opportunities that exist so students can take advantage of them.

CASE 19-3

Sandy Harris, a 29-year-old female, is brought to the emergency room after fainting twice at work.

Medical students who are participating in a problem-based learning tutorial group must solve the patient scenario described in Case 19-3. They form hypotheses relevant to the patient's situation and discuss both basic science and clinical issues pertinent to the case. Issues that are not answered by information students know are referred to as "learning issues" for the case and may include concepts and processes related to anatomy, physiology, biochemistry, pathology, pharmacology, behavioral science, and prevention. The students, not the faculty tutors, decide which issues to pursue depending on what students think they need to learn. Students decide which resources to use; they often refer to textbooks and journal articles but they may decide to consult with faculty experts and often invite experts to the tutorial group for discussions.

WHAT IS SELF-DIRECTED LEARNING?

Hammond and Collins (1991) state that self-directed learning (SDL) is

> a process in which learners take the initiative, with the support and collaboration of others, for increasing self- and social awareness; critically analyzing and reflecting on their situations; diagnosing their learning needs with specific reference to competencies they have helped identify; formulating socially and personally relevant learning goals; identifying human and material resources for learning; choosing and implementing appropriate learning strategies; and reflecting on and evaluating their learning. The immediate goal of critical SDL is to help learners take greater control of their learning. (pp. 13–14)

The reader might be wondering how SDL differs from the informal learning just described in the previous section. It is not different except that it is broader in scope; SDL can include formal learning activities as well as informal learning activities. In an SDL project, the learner, not the teacher, decides which educational activities (formal and informal) meet the learner's specific needs.

There is great debate about whether the medical school curriculum of traditional schools fosters SDL because of the great demand on students' time to learn the basic sciences and take exams (Vu & Galofre, 1983). There is little doubt that significant content overload exists in medical school and that this overload does not allow students to pursue personal learning goals or have much control over their learning (Vu & Galofre, 1983). The debate over curriculum content and educational process in medical schools continues. However, it is important to mention a popular alternative to the traditional curricula.

Several schools have implemented problem-based curricula where patient cases, similar to Case 19-3, are used to stimulate learning. Many medical educators believe that this type of curriculum fosters SDL and collaborative learning. Students in tutorial groups share the responsibility for learning and help the group grasp what is needed to resolve the patient scenario. Students also pursue personal learning goals and take initiative to identify resources they need to achieve their goals. Although this type of curriculum more closely resembles the process described by Hammond and Collins (1991), there are conflicting opinions as to whether problem-based learning is more effective than the traditional curriculum in fostering lifelong learning skills (Tolnai, 1991).

Colleagues   Reading   Programs

Assessing the need
for new competence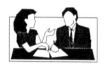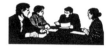

Gaining new
competence

Implementing
new competence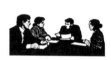

Figure 19.1. Self-directed curriculum for change. Adapted from Davis DA, Fox RD (eds): *The Physician As Learner: Linking Research to Practice.* Chicago, American Medical Association, 1994.

SELF-DIRECTED CURRICULUM FOR CHANGE

In the change study (Fox *et al.*, 1989) mentioned earlier, the researchers found that "physicians engage regularly in systematic processes to change their practices" (p. 19) because of personal (intellectual curiosity), social (family and community), or professional reasons (desire for competence). The process for adopting a change was fairly well articulated by physicians and described by R. D. Fox *et al.* (1994) as follows: (1) the reason for making a change triggered a mental image of the result; (2) once this "image" was perceived, a self-assessment process occurred to determine what skills were needed to facilitate the change and whether those skills were realistically achievable; (3) once the discrepancy between current competency and desired competency was known, learning resources were identified and strategies were employed to achieve new competence. These learning resources and strategies became a "self-directed curriculum for change."

Figure 19.1 depicts three stages through which physicians progress when adopting new practices and the types of learning resources they use to gain new competencies. At each stage a physician may use a combination of all of the resources mentioned in the sections on formal and informal learning. Figure 19.1 is an example of only one type of curriculum designed to meet one learning need. Each learning need may initiate a self-directed curriculum that looks very different from the curriculum in Figure 19.1. The resources a physician uses to assess the need for new competence (Stage 1) may be different from the resources he uses to gain (Stage 2) and implement the new competence (Stage 3).

397

SELF-DIRECTED
LEARNING
CURRICULUM

CASE 19-4

An interview between the author and a physician (J. R.).

JR: *[A] valuable CME experience that I can recall is going to learn how to do colposcopy which focused on an immediate practice need for me. I decided that I wanted to do that [colposcopy]. I had enough patients that needed it, and so I went. . . .*

SC: *So that was stimulated by what you thought was a need in your patient population?*

JR: *Right, and a desire on my part to offer them a broader range of services, and then going and learning that, and coming back . . . to put those skills to work.*

SC: *How did you go about learning how . . . to do colposcopy?*

JR: *. . . I did some reading. I went to a conference, a couple days conference, which I attended in full . . . because I was very motivated to learn. And then when I came back, there were people that I knew who were already doing that procedure, and I hung around them for awhile. They let me practice my skills under their supervision, and then I started doing my own.*

SC: *About how long do you think it took for you to feel comfortable doing them on your own?*

JR: *. . . Well, that's a relative question. How comfortable am I today? Comfortable enough to do it on my own, practicing in the way I knew it would be safe for a beginner. It probably took, seeing and helping with 10 or 15 procedures. And then when I started . . . part of what I had learned at the CME conference was kind of what the differences are between people who are new to the procedure [and] people who have been doing it for a long time. And that is the experience of being able to match what they see on the surface with what the biopsy results are. . . . So after about a month of helping other people do them, I felt qualified to do the procedure, keeping my own patients monitored. And then I had people I could talk to when I got biopsy results that I thought I needed some help, in terms of figuring out how to handle that. I could talk to a colleague who had been doing the procedure for a longer time for advice.*

SC: *Is it fair to say that the trigger . . . came from what you thought was a need in your patient population, and you knew there would be a way for you to meet that need?*

JR: *Yes. And I think having the CME experience and having . . . a network of physicians that I could be a part of made a big difference. And now I feel quite confident that I could go to Alaska or Siberia and do that [colposcopy] and I wouldn't need the collegial support in the same*

way. You know, I could call somebody, I wouldn't need to have them so
close. So having that network was also a very important part of adding
that procedure to my repertoire of practice. (Fieldnotes, March, 1995)

HOW DOES SELF-DIRECTED CURRICULUM
FOR CHANGE WORK?

J. R.'s curriculum for changing and learning in Case 19-4 included reading about the procedure, attending a formal CME event, discussing practice parameters with colleagues, apprenticing with experts, and building a network of peers who could support her while she was gaining confidence in her new skill. She assessed her need for new competence (Stage 1) by observing her practice and realizing that a need existed for her to offer a new service to her patients. She gained new competence (Stage 2) by reading, participating in CME, and working with colleagues whom she considered experts. She implemented the new competence (Stage 3) by relying on her network of peers (consultants) and getting feedback from them when she needed their advice.

HOW CAN MEDICAL STUDENTS BECOME
SELF-DIRECTED LEARNERS?

If one assumes that medical students are highly internally motivated, achievement oriented, curious, self-efficacious, and have the desire to develop as professionals (Mann & Ribble, 1994), then there should be a natural propensity for self-direction in learning. It just may not be obvious to individual students that they often engage in such a process. Medical students have a wealth of resources available to them; it just takes a little exploration. "Medical students do not survive on textbooks alone," to adapt a familiar phrase. Although students certainly will learn a great deal from their textbooks, aside from the faculty, the medical school library is one of the greatest resources students have handy. There are thousands of journals and books, literature-searching capabilities and resource people to help students search for topics of interest, and audio- and videotapes and interactive computer programs that help students learn, for example, anatomy or how clinical decisions are made. Students can get on the "information highway" (Internet) and link up with medical students and libraries in other schools. The resources available electronically are limitless. The student's world is restricted only by the time and motivation it takes to seek out these resources.

Technology will play a major role in the medical practices of the future. Students who are in medical school today are a generation of physicians who will have technology readily available in their practices in ways most physicians only dreamed of 10 years ago. Using an electronic medical record system will soon be the norm rather than the exception. Today, electronic systems exist in a few private physician offices, large hospitals, and managed care organizations. They are not pervasive in most academic medical center practices, but they are becoming more widespread as many academic practices are being integrated into managed care organizations. Using expert systems for diagnosis and management of many diseases and having practice guidelines available on line will be a routine for the next generation. Researching the medical literature and conferring with colleagues will occur on line and will take only minutes rather than days. These tools are available now, but many physicians, including those who have been in practice only 5 to 10 years, are not as familiar with the technology as the next generation will be.

The ability to observe and react appropriately to and learn from observation is an essential skill that burgeoning physicians must develop. As Mann and Ribble (1994) claim, "one learns from others and from interaction with the environment" (p. 76). Observe your role models; observe their actions and the outcomes of their actions. "The behavior modeled by others (in terms of information, values, attitudes, and skills) can also provide a standard against which to assess one's own performance" (p. 76). Seek out feedback from peers and faculty often, but especially when self-assessment reveals gaps in performance of a desired skill (Mann & Ribble, 1994). These are opportunities for medical students to learn and grow professionally and should not be viewed as negative experiences.

Search for a role model, someone to emulate. Faculty are generally very excited to have students involved in their research projects and patient care activities. Students should not be shy when they find physicians who would be good mentors. Faculty are *supposed* to mentor their students. However, not all faculty do this well. Observation is a key to choosing wisely.

CASE 19-5

I have a patient who is a very independent thinker, which she demonstrated by having her first child at the birthing center and her second child at home. . . . I saw her in the clinic, but she was hospitalized for hemolytic anemia. And she was being followed by hematology. They decided that she wasn't responding quickly enough to the prednisone therapy and that she should be; she should have a splenectomy. Well, she is kind of a low intervention type person. Her husband works in the physiology department, so he went and ran a literature search on splenectomy [in this situation]. So when they came to see me in this quandary, they had articles. . . . They were primed. And so essentially what we decided to do was to have her get a second opinion from a different hematology practice. And I read the articles they gave me which showed that there are very little findings to support doing a splenectomy in this situation. Needless to say she chose not to have the splenectomy, and she's fine. . . . And I didn't have, really, any background knowledge. I hadn't read a lot about splenectomy in that situation, so I learned about that from this woman. (Fieldnotes from interview with Dr. J. R., March 20, 1995)

————— LEARNING FROM EXPERIENCE —————

While the patient in the scenario above may be somewhat atypical, i.e., most patients will not bring a review of the literature on their specific illness to the office visit, physicians learn a great deal from their patient care experiences. Physicians change how they practice because of the experiences they have had and what those experiences have taught them (Fox, 1991).

Medical school teaches the basics, but physicians in training really start to learn when they begin interacting with patients, i.e., physicians learn by doing. As Sir William Osler (1945) pertinently said, "[i]n what may be called the natural method of teaching the student begins with the patient, continues with the patient, and ends his [or her] studies with the patient, using books and lectures as tools, as means to an end" (p. 315). Dr. Osler believed there really could be no teaching without a patient and the best teaching was that done by the patient.

While on their clinical rotations students will quite often hear that "patients rarely look like the examples in the textbooks." Textbooks unfortunately are limited in their ability to help learners, as they often describe only classic presentations of illness. Professional practice, however, is not routine, not textbook.

WHAT IS LEARNING FROM EXPERIENCE?

Fox and Craig (1994) distinguish learning from the teaching that occurs in the clinical setting from learning that occurs from the practice of medicine: "Learning from experience in the clinical setting is a way of both solving a clinical dilemma and generating a means for altering practices in similar situations. It is self-teaching with the clinical encounter as a learning resource and reflection on practices as a primary method" (p. 114). When medical students observe an expert clinician solve a complex patient problem, they are often amazed at the knowledge and skill the physician possesses and they wonder if they will ever reach a point when they, too, are expert clinicians. Much of the clinical know-how that expert physicians possess was gained because they built on each patient care experience.

SCHÖN'S MODEL OF REFLECTIVE PRACTICE

Donald Schön (1983, 1987) articulated the theory of what constitutes a reflective practitioner. His observations of professionals at work led to a description of a five-stage process professionals use to solve problems. Schön made the assumptions that professional practice was not routine and that there was always some conflict and ambiguity embedded in every episode of professional practice. Physicians, particularly primary care physicians, frequently admit that many patients leave their office with unresolved problems.

Schön's model translates well into the practice of medicine; Fox (1991) very succinctly interpreted it as follows:

> The first stage of learning from experience is what Schoen refers to as knowing in action. This is the physician's automatic and deeply [e]mbedded knowledge and skill that make up most of the practices of physicians. . . . Schoen makes the assumption that practitioners cannot practice effectively if they do not have this embedded, action-oriented knowledge. It is at this point that the uniqueness, conflict, or ambiguity come into play. These features present physicians caring for patients with surprises—the second stage of Schoen's model.
>
> Once surprised, physicians move to the third stage of the model, reflection in action. Reflection in action occurs when a physician is surprised during patient care and must reconstruct the knowledge, skills, and events that brought them to understand and hypothesize about the surprise. Reflection in action occurs during the patient–physician interaction. The physician reviews the practices, knowledge and information gleaned from the patient in an attempt to figure out exactly what it is that is different about this particular case and what should be done next. It may take the form of an odd answer to a usual question, followed by reconstruction of facts and information related to that patient in light of the knowledge and skill of the physician. The objective of reflection in action is to develop an appropriate response.

The fourth stage of Schoen's model is the experiment. Here, in the face of surprise and based upon their reflection in action, the physician decides to attempt something in an effort to gain more information or resolve some clinical dilemma. Experiments can be as simple as the rephrasing [of] a question or as complicated as the changing of medication dosages, surgical procedures, or therapeutic regimens. These experiments are ad hoc in nature. They reflect the ability of the physician to reconstruct the information, knowledge and skills needed to accommodate the unusual features of the case.

The fifth stage of Schoen's model occurs after the patient has left. The physician reflects back on what occurred in the patient-care episode. The purpose is to make sense of the surprise, the way he or she thought about that surprise (reflection in action) and the experiment at resolving it. Reflection on action has an impact on knowledge in action. In effect, reflection on action is the loop that brings what he or she has learned from recent experience to bear on general procedures and frame of reference for future cases. The loop presented by Schoen is provocative. It seems to encompass an area of learning that is free from the direct influence of formal or informal resources. In fact, the entire learning process may occur within the physician. (Reprinted by permission from the *Journal of Continuing Education in the Health Professions* 11(2):164–165, 1991)

CASE 19-6

An interview between the author and a physician (Dr. K. B.) who is reflecting on students' responses to the directive, "Tell me how you're going to keep up with advances in medical sciences over the next 30 years." (Reprinted by permission from the Journal of Continuing Education in the Health Professions *13(1):97, 1993)*

The majority of the time, [students] talk about reading their journals, and going to meetings, and a lot of them will say they want to be affiliated with the medical school, clinical assistant professor, whatever. Which is all well and good, but that . . . unfortunately tells me I haven't gotten my message through to them. It's probably not how your average practitioner is going to keep up. In reviewing your own cases and finding your frustrations, I think, is what stimulates you to learn and to do something different. . . . we try to have our students keep record of the patients that they interact with in the two months on the rotation. . . . I think practitioners need to do that as well. At the end of every year I, and a resident on the vascular service, go over all the vascular cases for the year. We look at the types of complications we've had and the numbers we've done. . . . It shows us a more global perspective [of] how we're doing. Recognizing frustrations, or problems, or patterns that we hadn't really seen in a day-in-day-out, week-to-week sort of review, stimulates us to look for better ways to do things and to keep up with what's going on. That's what I'd like to get the students to learn how to do.

HOW DOES LEARNING FROM EXPERIENCE WORK?

Dr. K. B. described a process of self-assessment for practitioners. This process could be called an informal practice audit. A particularly salient point he made was that this reflective process helps to identify patterns that a clinician may not recognize on a day-to-day basis. Dr. K. B. analyzed his patient outcomes along with a colleague and decided how to change practices based on his and his colleague's synthesis and evaluation of the patient information. In other words, he systematically learned from his experiences caring for patients.

HOW CAN MEDICAL STUDENTS LEARN TO LEARN FROM EXPERIENCE?

Manning and DeBakey (1992) offered physicians some suggestions to inspire them to learn from their clinical experiences:

> Some physicians keep a card file of lessons learned from instructive patients; others organize charts by diagnosis as well as patient name, as a guide to the conditions they are most likely to see. Some physicians exchange patient records with colleagues for an educational review and discussion of specific problems in diagnosis and therapy. (pp. 1135–1136)

It is easy to see how using a computerized medical record system would facilitate these types of learning strategies.

How does this information assist first-year medical students? Some of the earlier suggestions may be beneficial here, too. Medical students need to think about how they organize information. What works best? During the first year of school students have some opportunities to observe physician faculty and community preceptors in their clinical environment. Ask them how they keep track of their lessons learned. Do they study their patient outcomes in the way Dr. K. B. describes? How are their medical records organized? Ask them to recount a significant learning experience they had, what they learned, and what strategies they used to learn and change their practice. Their anecdotes are a wealth of knowledge that can help students to take advantage of their experiences. After 4 years of medical school students should have gathered several strategies they can adapt to their personal style of learning.

CASE 19-7

An interview between the author and a physician (Dr. M. D.) who is reflecting on the importance of keeping current and strategies for lifelong learning.

> *I think it [keeping current] sets one apart. It sets a good physician apart. I go to meetings and I read [about seven] journals [a month], and I continue to be fascinated by my patients. . . . Most specialties or fields are helped by their organizations. I know ophthalmology is quite helpful in continuing education. That's one of the main focuses of our academy. The people [who] are active in the academy can stay educated. Those that don't kind of drift away from it and stagnate.*
>
> *The state and local medical societies are also helpful. . . . I try to make one out-of-state meeting a year, but otherwise I do it [CME] locally within the state or within the city. There's a real smorgasbord out there between the hospital and the medical school, and then the county, and the state, and the national organizations. . . . I sometimes consult friends and other people in my specialty. Sometimes a patient spurs you to learn about a new treatment or how to better treat something.*
>
> *If you're having to convince somebody that lifelong education is necessary, I think it's a waste of time. I think you've failed at [the] admission level. What gets one*

through medical school? What makes one perform in medical school? Well, if you perform in medical school, you're going to continue to perform the rest of your career. And part of that performance is continuing education. Just like getting through medical school is education, getting through practice is continuing education. (Fieldnotes, December, 1994)

DESIGNING AN EFFECTIVE STRATEGY FOR LIFELONG MEDICAL LEARNING

Designing an effective strategy for lifelong medical education depends on an individual's ability to identify specific learning needs and acquire an understanding of his most effective strategies for learning. The first factor relies on the capability to self-assess one's learning needs.

What are the feelings? What are the signposts? What are the alarms that you have to recognize that say, "Hey, I'm there"? How do you recognize that you have holes in your knowledge [skill or attitude] that have to get filled? Students need to be able to reflect, and define their own needs. (Fieldnotes from interview with Dr. L. J., March 30, 1995)

How do medical students learn how to self-assess? Developing the ability to self-assess involves some risk taking because students have to be honest with themselves and accept feedback from others. Obviously the skill is learned and honed through experience. Self-assessment is part of the evaluation system for most of the problem-based curricula but students in traditional medical schools have the opportunity to develop this skill as well. One definite opportunity exists when students receive their exam scores. Students can get a sense of their strengths and weaknesses by reviewing exam questions.

Another opportunity for students to self-assess occurs when they are working with clinical faculty. Faculty usually provide their assessment of student progress. Students need to compare their self-assessments with preceptor assessments and openly discuss discrepancies in perceptions. It is easy to internalize the positive feedback received from preceptors; however, students need to be prepared to receive, accept, and act on negative feedback (that is the hard part); that is part of growing professionally.

The second factor is equally as tricky. Understanding which learning strategies work best involves gaining an awareness of learning preferences and styles. There is much controversy over the utility of knowing about the learning styles of students. Many adult educators believe that knowing something about their learning styles can be helpful to students *as long as they are willing to experiment with learning strategies that are unfamiliar to them*. Students may discover that these new strategies are quite effective, and students should avoid labeling themselves as particular types of learners.

CONCLUSION

What students have probably realized by reading this chapter is that all of the sections overlap; nice neat categories of learning do not really exist. The intent of the chapter sections was to explain concepts, not to put learning strategies into nice neat categories. Learning is a continuum and a cafeteria, which means students have many resources and opportunities for learning available, but students must take advantage of them.

There were four main themes to this chapter: Recognizing the role of lifelong medical education in ensuring, maintaining, and enhancing professional competence; identifying educational strategies that promote lifelong learning; distinguishing among the various types of formal and informal delivery systems for CME; and designing a plan for an individualized curriculum for lifelong professional education. In that context were described formal CME, informal CME, self-directed learning, learning from experience, and some strategies students can enlist now as they begin their professional development journey.

Unfortunately, there is quite a bit of evidence that medical school does not actually prepare students for the "real world" of practice (Cavanaugh, 1993). Academic medical centers are not viewed as the real world by most of the physicians who graduate from them, except for those who enter academic medicine. Students are typically exposed to complex clinical scenarios, or what the medical culture refers to as "zebras," on most rotations outside of family medicine, general pediatrics, and general medicine. However, students can learn a great deal if they adopt the strategies suggested herein and adjust them to fit their personal style; the transition from formal schooling to practice will be smoother and students will feel better equipped to pursue their lifelong challenge to care for patients and adapt to the ever-changing healthcare environment.

CASES FOR DISCUSSION

Cases were adapted from David A. Davis, M.D., course materials.

CASE 1

Dr. Daves, a 35-year-old emergency physician at an inner-city hospital, has been referred by the CEO of his hospital for "repair" of his interpersonal skills. He just cannot get along with patients, most of whom are indigent. He is short with them, intolerant of their questions, and unwilling to take time with them. "Content" competence issues have never been raised. It is presumed that racism is the problem. Chart audit results show a knowledge deficiency in emergency medicine problems. Interpersonal skills assessment shows a failure to include the patient in the encounter and a lack of interest in giving the patient information. Psychology assessment shows poor self-esteem.

1. *What potential educational needs are identified?*
2. *What educational intervention(s) would you recommend?*

CASE 2

Dr. Simon is a second-year internal medicine resident who just received the lab reports on one of her hemophilia patients. He is HIV positive. On his last visit the patient told Dr. Simon that he recently became engaged to be married.

1. *What potential educational needs are identified?*
2. *What educational intervention(s) would you recommend?*

CASE 3

*Dr. Foxfire is a family practitioner in a large HMO. For the third time this week he has encountered
a woman with a significant urinary tract infection (UTI), prompting him to think about different
treatment (e.g., single-dose therapy) and preventive strategies.*

1. *What would he need to do to change his practice?*
2. *What potential educational needs are identified?*
3. *What educational intervention(s) would you recommend?*

CASE 4

*The community you work in (18,000 population, 3-hour drive from a teaching hospital) has lost its
obstetrician to retirement. You enjoyed obstetrics in training, but have not done any in 2 years.*

1. *What would you need to do to change your practice?*
2. *What potential educational needs are identified?*
3. *What educational intervention(s) would you recommend?*

CASE 5

*While the rounds at your local hospital are good, and you do read journals, you and your partner
have agreed to get away for a CME course.*

1. *How do you choose the program?*

CASE 6

*Dr. Draper, a 41-year-old community medicine specialist with board certification in general sur-
gery, has worked at the public health department for 5 years. She has not practiced surgery for 10
years. She wants to reenter clinical practice but as a general practitioner working in emergency
medicine. She knows she has a problem with organization but otherwise is a very competent and
capable physician.*

1. *What potential educational needs are identified?*
2. *What educational intervention(s) would you recommend?*

—————— RECOMMENDED READINGS ——————

Close WT: *The Earth Is Not A Resting Place.* Salt Lake City, University of Utah School of Medicine, 1994.

> This book is the autobiographical adventure of Dr. William Close. Dr. Close's journey "reveals the
> gradual transformation of a gung-ho surgeon to a thoughtful and compassionate village doc" (p. xii). The
> book depicts three critical stages in Dr. Close's transformation: his 6 years as a surgery resident in New
> York City; his 16 years practicing in Zaire, Africa; and his 18, and still counting, years as a rural general
> practitioner in Wyoming. It is filled with colorful and emotional stories of the challenges met by a
> physician who is ever changing and ever learning about himself and about "being a doctor."

Davis DA, Fox RD (eds): *The Physician As Learner: Linking Research to Practice*. Chicago, American Medical Association, 1994.

This volume is a comprehensive, well-written review of the current state of the art in continuing medical education theory, practice, and research. Davis and Fox along with 21 colleagues who are some of the most well-known experts in the field provide their insights on future directions that CME must take to address new learning needs of physicians so that they can be proactive and responsive to ever-changing demands in healthcare delivery.

Fox RD, Mazmanian PE, Putnam RW (eds): *Changing and Learning in the Lives of Physicians*. New York, Praeger Publishers, 1989.

This book is a must for anyone who is interested in how physicians change and learn. The authors along with colleagues from 24 universities interviewed 340 physicians about how they perceived changes in their lives and what role learning played in implementing those changes. The chapters focus on ten types of forces that triggered physician changes. Anecdotes from many of the interviews are included to illustrate the motivation behind the changes. The book concludes with a model for changing and learning that is being tested in other professions outside of medicine.

PART IV

Advancing the Discipline
of Medicine

The practice of medicine is just that, a practice. Rarely do physicians find that their approach to a patient with a particular problem remains static, rather, it changes as medical knowledge advances, new skills are developed, and new ways of viewing the problem are formed. One of the most exciting skills a physician can develop is to participate in this renewal by training others to have more and better skills, researching new methods of clinical care, and developing clinical guidelines that enable physicians to more effectively integrate new medical research within their clinical practice. These chapters describe the skills needed by the clinician of the future to participate more actively in the grand experiment of medicine.

CHAPTER 20

The Art and Science of Teaching and Learning

Ric Arseneau and Daniel Pratt

CASE 20-1

Jack is a final-year medical student doing a clinical rotation in internal medicine. Dr. Brown is Jack's attending for the 6-week rotation. Jack is unclear about what is expected of him during this rotation. In addition, he finds Dr. Brown's hurried style not very conducive to learning. Jack's interest in the rotation wanes, and by the third week he resigns himself to the fact that this rotation will be a "waste of time." He learns the ward "routines" and satisfies himself with just getting by.

—————— EDUCATIONAL OBJECTIVES ——————

By the end of this chapter, learners should be able to:

1. Describe the relationship between beliefs, intentions, and strategies
2. Define what is meant by representation
3. Describe how concepts are constructed by learners
4. Define three types of knowledge (declarative, conceptual, and problem solving) and give examples of each
5. Explain the concept of bridging knowledge and provide examples from their own experiences
6. Explain the "driving the bus" metaphor and list some implications for themselves as learners
7. List the characteristics of "outstanding" learners
8. Define the concepts of stretching and feedforward

9. List the characteristics of effective feedback
10. Compare and contrast deep and surface approaches to learning
11. Demonstrate and apply the SQ3R strategy while reading
12. Compare and contrast a traditional apprenticeship from a cognitive (or intellectual) apprenticeship

---
INTRODUCTION

As the title implies, this chapter is about teaching and learning. The pairing of these two terms, teaching and learning, and the usual placement of the term *teaching* in front of *learning* is somewhat misleading. Can learning not occur without teaching? Is the best learning the result of teaching? And, does teaching necessarily result in learning? Consider the cartoon in which a boy tells his friend that he has taught his dog how to whistle. With his ear up to the dog's face, the friend says, "I don't hear him whistling." The boy replies, "I said I taught him. I didn't say he learned it" (Whitman, 1990). Teaching, we think, is only successful if it brings about learning. Learning, on the other hand, is only in part the result of teaching. Obvious, you say? We disagree. We have seen too many examples of teachers who think of teaching in terms of "performance," i.e., enacting a repertoire of teaching behaviors rather than focusing on student learning. We have also seen too many students who rely mostly (sometimes solely) on their teachers to bring about learning. Jack, in the introductory case, is a good example. When faced with a less than optimal learning environment, Jack gave up and simply relinquished the responsibility for his own learning.

The focus of this chapter is on learning and the student's role and responsibilities as a learner. We will also discuss how teaching can enhance learning. Therefore, this chapter is about learning and teaching (note inversion of terms). The discussion will focus on helping students identify and take advantage of outstanding teaching. More importantly, however, this chapter will help students take charge of their own learning in situations where the teaching is less than exemplary. This can be done through the use of specific learning strategies by students or by having students "elicit" good teaching behaviors from their teachers. However, learning and teaching are much more than a set of strategies or behaviors. They are both fundamentally influenced by intangible aspects, i.e., beliefs and intentions. Before we turn to anything as visible as strategies for either learners or teachers, it is important to look at the relationship to these intangibles. How do our beliefs and intentions affect our behavior?

THE RELATIONSHIP BETWEEN BELIEFS, INTENTIONS, AND STRATEGIES

Although all behaviors are guided by a set of beliefs and intentions, only a person's behaviors are visible to an observer. Consider the situation of a young woman standing alone on the sidelines at a school dance. Is she too shy to strike up a conversation with her schoolmates, or is she perhaps too arrogant and "stuck up"? We can make assumptions, but the only thing we can comment on with any degree of certainty is her behavior; she is standing alone. We can't comment on her beliefs; e.g., does she believe no one would be

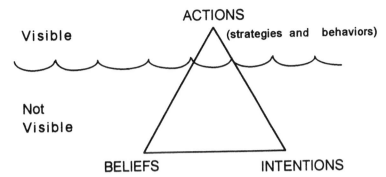

411

THE
RELATIONSHIP
BETWEEN BELIEFS,
INTENTIONS,
AND STRATEGIES

Figure 20.1. Beliefs and intentions are "invisible" to the extent that they cannot be observed directly. Like an iceberg observed floating, behaviors are supported by an impressive mass that cannot be seen.

interested in talking to her, that she is better than others, or is she simply preoccupied with other thoughts? Similarly, we don't know her intentions—is she trying to avoid the pain of rejection, or is she waiting for others to approach her? We don't know. Beliefs and intentions are "invisible" to the extent that they cannot be observed directly. Although we can inquire about them, there is no assurance that answers will be truthful. Like an iceberg observed floating, behaviors are supported by an impressive mass that cannot be seen (see Figure 20.1). Therefore, studying only learning or teaching strategies and behaviors is far too superficial to invite insight.

Consider three teachers. The first teacher believes his role is to inform. He wants to transmit as much of his expert information as he possibly can in the most efficient way possible. The second teacher believes that her role is to challenge students to think. She holds that current knowledge has a short "shelf life" and that students must be developed into independent thinkers. The third teacher believes that his role is to nurture students' self-esteem and motivation. He feels that students are "wounded" by prior bad educational experiences. He maintains that students need to feel good about learning first and foremost. Suppose each of these teachers decided to use questioning as a teaching strategy, i.e., an action. Although their visible behavior would be the same, asking questions, each of the three teachers would have a very different intention for the use of questioning based on what they believed. For instance, the first teacher might ask a question to see if the students received the information as transmitted. The second teacher might ask a different but related question to test students' ability to apply new information to solve problems. The third teacher would be concerned with establishing an atmosphere where students feel "safe" to risk answering questions; that teacher would likely handle wrong answers differently from another teacher who didn't share the same concern about students' self-esteem. The beliefs espoused by the three teachers above are not necessarily mutually exclusive. One teacher could easily hold all three beliefs and act accordingly. Nevertheless, it is apparent that beliefs and intentions govern actions in a crucial way.

The description above may give you the impression that we are aware of the beliefs that guide our actions; unfortunately, this is often *not* the case. More often beliefs are taken for granted; they are held as unconscious assumptions until these assumptions are challenged or we are presented with an alternative view. If you've ever traveled to any unfamiliar culture, you'll understand what we mean. Many people who have traveled away from their home culture often learn more about home than they do about the place they are visiting. The stark differences between the two places force them to reexamine previously held assumptions about how things work and what is culturally appropriate. They become acutely aware of previously held assumptions. In the same way, teachers may not be aware of assumptions they hold regarding their roles and responsibilities as teachers or assumptions they hold about students. And students, in turn, harbor equally unconscious assumptions about educational roles and responsibilities, both for themselves and for their teachers.

THE POWER OF BELIEF SYSTEMS

Beliefs are simply statements about what we consider to be true. They are *not* truth, only what we *consider* to be truth. Each one of us has had the experience of being truly committed to a belief, and subsequently having a "transforming" experience change that belief. We're sure that you can come up with several instances of beliefs you strongly held several years ago that you would be embarrassed to admit publicly today. Is it possible that beliefs to which you are strongly committed today could be changed by significant experiences in the future? Does "truth" change? Beliefs are simply a feeling of conviction, an idea or judgment held as true or valid. They are a state of mind in which we are free from doubt. But, they are not "truth," although we're sure you've been involved in arguments where beliefs have been presented as truth.

Beliefs do not exist in isolation; rather, they are usually organized into internally consistent systems called belief systems (BS). Given that beliefs are not truth, but our own special way of interpreting the world, the acronym "BS" seems amusingly appropriate. You can think of a BS as a set of lenses or filters through which we interpret the world. They allow us to "see" things a certain way; they allow us to interpret (i.e., impose meaning) on events. In addition, they can "screen out" or distort information. If you've ever tried on a friend's glasses, you may have found that the world looked unfamiliar or different. Our BS act in the same way; they are filters through which we "see" the world. Imagine that you are a crew member of the Starship Enterprise. You are relaxing in the Ten Forward lounge with your crew mates. Included in the group are a large number of Vulcans, whom you think incapable of lying and cheating, as well as some Ferengis, whom you consider deceitful and untrustworthy. Suddenly, you realize your scanner is missing and you're sure you had it with you only moments ago. Your BS helps you make sense of the situation. "A Ferengi must have stolen my scanner," you tell yourself. How might someone visiting from another galaxy with no knowledge of Vulcans and Ferengis react differently? Is it possible that a Vulcan-look-alike android has stolen your scanner? Is it possible that you've simply misplaced it? Beliefs about what you hold to be true may have "distorted" your vision. Perhaps a different set of lenses would have allowed you to interpret a different meaning of the same situation.

BS are very powerful. They allow us to interpret and make sense of situations. They are also the basis of our intentions. And, along with intentions, they are the foundation on which our actions are based. Therefore, attempts to understand learning and teaching "actions" (e.g., teaching "performance") are inadequate unless specific attention is paid to the beliefs and intentions that guide these behaviors.

As mentioned earlier, beliefs don't exist in isolation. Beliefs about learning and teaching can also be grouped into internally consistent BS. Suffice it to say that learning and teaching are based in particular sets of beliefs about:

413

BELIEFS ABOUT
THE NATURE OF
KNOWLEDGE
AND
UNDERSTANDING

- The nature of knowledge
- The roles and responsibility of the teacher
- The roles and responsibility of the student
- The learning process
- The teaching context

For you, as students, it is not essential to go into an exhaustive discussion of BS surrounding all of these, but it is important to investigate ideas about the nature of knowledge and how understanding is facilitated. For a detailed treatment of the other areas, see *Five Perspectives on Teaching in Adult and Higher Education* (Pratt, 1996). And, keeping in the back of your mind how beliefs affect how we interpret and act in the world, consider the implications in a learning/teaching situation when the teacher believes "knowledge" is created as described in the example below.

CASE 20-2

A senior medical student is asked for a brief summary of a recently discharged patient's case and what she learned from caring for this patient. The patient presented with an exacerbation of congestive heart failure (CHF). The student's summary misses only a few details. She reports having learned how to treat CHF. On questioning, the attending discovers that the student has learned a "recipe" approach, and despite having participated in this patient's care, she reveals a poor understanding of the rationale for the treatment choices. Further, she has a fragmented and incomplete conceptualization of CHF (Arseneau, 1995).

BELIEFS ABOUT THE NATURE OF KNOWLEDGE AND UNDERSTANDING

Close your eyes for a moment and imagine a dog; be specific. Which way is the dog facing? What breed is it? What color? When thinking about "dog," you have more than just the word *dog* in your head; you have a visual *representation* of a dog. It is only a representation, because you obviously don't have a dog in your head. But it's more than just a visual representation. If you were presented with a real dog of a different breed or a different color than the one you represented in your mind, you could still identify it as a dog. You must, therefore, have a *conceptual* representation of dog that allows you to interpret situations. You are able to make the distinction between "dog" and "not dog" based on your conceptual understanding of "dog."

How did you build, or *construct,* this concept? Perhaps, as a child, you were out with your parents one day. You came across a dog, and your parents pointed and said, "dog." What did you notice and understand at that moment? Was it the size? The color? Long ears versus short ears? What was it that you understood when your parents said "dog"? On another occasion, you may have come across a cat, and using your newly constructed concept to construe the situation, you proudly said, "Dog!" Your parents likely corrected you and said, "No . . . cat." At that point, you had to reconsider the accuracy of your internal representation for dog and readjust it accordingly: Not all small furry animals are dogs. With the help of your parents and others, you went through several iterative cycles of constructing and interpreting and each time refined your concept of dog. Your concept is now elegant enough for you to make the distinction that a German shepherd is more closely related to a Pekingese than it is to a wolf.

There are several important points to be taken from this example with implications for both learners and teachers:

1. The map is not the territory. Just as a map is simply a *representation* of the territory and not a reproduction *per se,* concepts are internal representations of an external "reality." (Remember, you don't have a dog in your head.)
2. Concepts, or internal representations, are not transferred. Your parents did not transfer the concept of dog into your head. They helped you *construct* it.
3. Concepts are refined and elaborated in the dual acts of constructing and construing (i.e., interpreting), often by interacting with others or with texts.
4. Concepts are by nature idiosyncratic, based on our "history" with a concept. We all have a specific and different understanding of dog based on the circumstances that allowed us to construct our internal representation. Perhaps one reader envisioned a friendly mongrel and another a snarling Doberman pinscher.
5. Concepts overlap sufficiently for us to understand each other. Given that we develop our idiosyncratic concepts with the help of others, they become similar enough for us to communicate with each other and come to a common understanding; i.e., knowledge is "socially constructed."

The concept of dog is unproblematic as we can all agree on what a dog is; we can all point to a dog. But, what about our concepts, or internal representation, of things that are more abstract and don't exist *per se,* things that are not concrete? What about beauty, justice, or health, for instance? Beauty is no different than "dog," in that it is an internal representation constructed by each individual used to construe the outside world. It is different, however, in that you can't point to beauty, justice, or health, only to examples of them. Based on our histories with these concepts we all carry subtle and not-so-subtle differences in our understanding and representation of these concepts. There is a larger leeway for difference and less overlap between different individuals' understanding of them. This is true for all more "abstract" notions within this belief system about knowledge.

Acting from this belief about knowledge has consequences for both students and teachers. It implies the important role of students in constructing their own knowledge base. Teachers' understanding of their roles shift, too. Since knowledge cannot be transferred, the teacher becomes a facilitator of learning rather than a repository of special knowledge to be "given" to students. Understanding that knowledge exists as concepts, i.e., representations, refutes an "all or none" itemized view of knowledge and facts. That is, "knowledge" does not exist pure and intact, at a distance from learners. Instead, it must be grasped incrementally and interactively in the form of representations. Concepts exist in degrees of sophistication, from misconception to relatively unsophisticated to elaborate and complex. For instance, "justice" is not a fact; it is a concept. The understanding of justice by children may be rather simple and even approximate an "all or none" representation. However, by the time they reach late adolescence, the concept has taken on shades of meaning and complexity.

Now that you have an understanding of how concepts are constructed and refined, we can consider one of the ways of looking at different types of knowledge. For our purposes, we will look at three types: (1) declarative, (2) conceptual, and (3) problem solving.

As the name implies, declarative knowledge is what you can declare or say. *Declarative* knowledge is those things for which you have words. Unfortunately, declarative knowledge does not imply understanding. For instance, just because a child can say the word *dog* does not mean that she understands the concept. Similarly, several laypersons know the term *congestive heart failure,* yet have little understanding of the concept. *Conceptual* knowledge, then, implies a deeper understanding of the meaning of a term. As mentioned earlier, conceptual knowledge is not "all or none"; it exists in degrees and reflects levels of understanding and sophistication. Believing that "dog" is equal to "small furry animal" is not completely wrong, but it is a relatively unsophisticated conception. Finally, and to the chagrin of many final-year medical students, conceptual understanding does not imply the ability to apply knowledge in practice. *Problem-solving* knowledge takes conceptual knowledge to a higher level. Problem-solving knowledge is usable knowledge in everyday practice. It includes the identification of causal connections and their application in analyzing and solving problems. It is conceptual knowledge that the person can adapt to changing circumstances.

Let's recap the levels of knowledge succinctly: Knowing *what* the symptoms of CHF are (declarative knowledge) does not imply knowing *why* these symptoms occur (conceptual knowledge). Similarly, having a deep and elaborated understanding of the symptoms of CHF (conceptual knowledge) does not imply knowing which distinctions are clinically useful and which are merely "interesting"; it also does not imply knowing how to use these concepts in practice (problem-solving knowledge).

Too often the focus of learning is on declarative knowledge. Students have the semblance of understanding because they know the lingo. But lingo is only borrowed language, a thin veneer that hides a lack of deeper understanding. Again too often, teachers accept the lingo, i.e., declarative knowledge, as evidence of learning and understanding. But, a few probing questions (especially "Why?" questions) can demonstrate the shallow level of learning and lack of understanding. Paradoxically, a student's ability to explain a concept without the use of technical jargon is evidence of a deeper understanding. A student who is able to describe a concept in her own words must have the necessary understanding to translate the jargon into something with personal meaning. The student in Case 20-2 is a good example of declarative knowledge masking the lack of a deeper understanding. When her attending asked probing questions, he unmasked her poor conceptual understanding of CHF. Further, her inability to provide a rationale for the treatment choices reveals poor problem-solving knowledge.

Remember our example of the three teachers, who all asked questions, but represented different beliefs and intentions about that strategy? Think about how the questions themselves would differ, depending on whether the teacher believed knowledge was "intact" or "constructed." And again, how they would differ, depending on whether a teacher sought evidence of declarative, conceptual, or problem-solving knowledge. From our experience, the most effective learning occurs in situations where teachers believe that knowledge is socially constructed and is learned by a process of transforming information into increasingly sophisticated concepts. Those teachers probe below the surface of declarative knowledge for evidence of understanding. Can the student explain, without jargon, a situation? Can the teacher ask questions that require a student to demonstrate both conceptual and problem-solving knowledge? In our definition, these kinds of knowledge represent understanding; to us, they are evidence of learning.

We believe that teaching must be approached from the learner's perspective. Good teaching has less to do with specific teaching performance than with student learning. Teaching is Machiavellian: "The ends justify the means." Frankly, we are perplexed by the many texts on teaching that fixate on the teacher's relationship to the content (i.e., material to be taught) or specific actions, rather than the relationship between teacher and student. In the former, teaching is reduced to a performance, not unlike the relationship between actor and script (teacher and content). Therefore, learning involves an active process on the part of the learner, and the only role for the teacher is in facilitating this process.

If you find this hard to grasp, reconsider for a moment, as an example, the story of how a child learns the concept of "dog." A parent can't "tell" a child what a dog is and hope that the child will immediately understand; the child must represent the concept internally and come to his own understanding. The parent, having an idea of how she would like the child to understand the concept, involves the child in a dynamic dialogue. The child has the opportunity to test and refine increasingly sophisticated conceptions and the parent has the opportunity to correct misconceptions and redirect the child's understanding. Eventually, the parent and child come to a common understanding of the concept of "dog." There is a specific quality to the child's interactions in refining its conceptions and discarding its misconceptions about "dog." Each refinement involves *linking:* i.e., adding new knowledge to what the child already knows, or making new connections between what is already known.

Learning and understanding develop as new knowledge "elements" are brought in and *linked* with the existing pattern of "connections" between elements of prior knowledge. Adding new elements will often stimulate the reorganization of the original pattern of connections as the learner reflects on the new knowledge and sees how it puts older knowledge in a different perspective. Obviously, students can't make meaningful links between two unknowns. Without some reference to what they already know, students may be forced to "invent" meaning and make links where none exist. This can lead to misconceptions. This often occurs when teachers make erroneous assumptions about students' prior knowledge. Teachers, therefore, need to start with the learner. They need an understanding of the range of learners' prior conceptions and misconceptions. Though the learners must be actively involved in constructing the links between new and prior information, it is the teacher's responsibility to adjust the content to the learners' prior understanding of it.

Thus, teaching that emerges from a belief about socially constructed knowledge is teaching that helps learners construct personal meaning. Approaches to learning aimed toward this end have been termed "deep" (i.e., an emphasis on meaning) in contrast to those methods of learning with a focus on reproduction (i.e., a surface approach) (Eizenberg, 1988; Marton & Saljo, 1984). According to this perspective, true learning and understanding can only occur when learners search for personal meaning by organizing information into an integrated and structured whole (i.e., use of a deep approach).

Mary has difficulty understanding the regulation of renal blood flow. Although she can recite her notes about afferent and efferent arterioles and angiotensin, she can't answer her attending's question about the mechanism by which angiotensin-converting enzyme (ACE) inhibitors cause renal failure in a patient with renal artery stenosis (RAS). Mary's attending sees the inability to answer this question as evidence of a poor conceptual understanding of the regulation of renal blood flow rather than a missing "piece" of knowledge. Instead of telling Mary the answer, she provides her with the following: "Suppose you had a garden hose with a series of small holes along its whole length—you know the kind that is used to water gardens. One end is hooked up to the tap and the other end is open and collapsible. How could I increase the height of the water coming out of the holes?"

Mary thinks for a moment and then replies, "You could turn up the tap to increase the amount of water coming in, or you could squeeze the other end and stop the water that is running through." "Very good," replies the attending. "Now, think of the glomerulus in the same way: the tap is the afferent arteriole and the other end is the efferent arteriole. The glomerular filtration rate (GFR) is the height of the water coming from the small holes. Imagine a situation where the afferent arteriole has a fixed and reduced "inflow"—as in RAS. How would you maintain the height of the water, that is, the GFR?"

"You would need to keep the other end—the efferent arteriole—constricted." Mary then has an "Ah ha" experience and continues, "I see. ACE inhibitors cause dilation of the efferent arteriole in this situation and the GFR falls!"

BRIDGING KNOWLEDGE

If you've seen the movie *Dances with Wolves*, you may recall the scene where Kevin Costner first encounters the natives. Initially, they try to communicate using their respective languages without success. In an attempt to bridge the communication gap, Costner searches for a point of common ground. He starts to imitate the buffalo while repeating the word *buffalo*. The natives watch him quizzically and question his sanity. Suddenly one member of the tribe understands and says, "Totonga." He too starts to imitate a buffalo. This becomes the first step in bridging their communication gap.

A similar gap often exists between students and teachers. Students, unfamiliar with a given topic, may not understand the "language" used by a teacher. If the teacher tries to explain concepts using the new technical language unfamiliar to students, she is likely to "lose" them. She too must attempt to find a point of common ground and bridge the gap.

Bridging knowledge is the knowledge teachers use to "transform" the content for the purposes of teaching. By transform, we mean any activity used by the teacher to move from her own comprehension of the subject matter to the variations of representation, narrative, examples, or association likely to initiate understanding in students. Bridging knowledge is often referred to as "pedagogical content knowledge" (Wilson *et al.*, 1987) or "content-specific pedagogy" (Reynolds, 1992) in the education literature.

Bridging knowledge is not, however, content as the experienced practitioner understands it. One belief, pervasive among medical educators, is that expertise is, in and of itself, sufficient for being a good teacher. Unfortunately, we have all been exposed to content experts unable to promote learning in their students. On the other hand, someone expert in the process of teaching, such as someone holding a Ph.D. in education, but unfamiliar with the content is also unlikely to promote learning. Therefore, good teaching requires more than expertise in the content area or in the process of teaching. It requires an expertise in helping students understand. Good teaching, then, assumes a knowledge of learners' starting points (existing conceptions—less sophisticated or misconceptions), a knowledge of where you want to take them [better or preferred conception(s)], and a knowledge of effective routes for the transition (i.e., bridging knowledge). The attending in Case 20-3 used a metaphor to explain the regulation of renal blood flow. She started with something Mary knew, a common everyday garden hose. Through this example she was able to create a bridge and lead Mary to a new understanding.

Bridging knowledge includes those things that make content more understandable. It includes such things as an appreciation for the "sticky points" and "conceptual stumbling blocks" that slow learners' understanding and require special attention and extra time. It includes a knowledge of the appropriate pace for introducing new and more complex concepts and an ability to notice cues from learners that the pace is too slow or too quick. Teachers with bridging knowledge speak the same language as their students; they don't make assumptions about what students know and don't know. They maintain a balance between the "big picture" and the "elements." Perhaps most importantly, they develop, collect, and use analogies, anecdotes, metaphors, and examples that are memorable, conceptually coherent, and provide insight.

Our favorite tool for achieving this is the metaphor:

> The metaphor is perhaps one of man's most fruitful potentialities. Its efficacy verges on magic, and it seems a tool for creation which God forgot inside one of His creatures when he made him. (José Ortega y Gasset)

If learning is the process of making new links between what is being learned and what is already known, metaphors are ideally suited because they provide a way of seeing how something we *don't* understand is like something we *do* understand.

As an example, consider our use of the metaphor "bridge" in talking about this kind of knowledge. Also, the attending in Case 20-3 helped Mary understand the regulation of renal blood flow with a garden hose metaphor.

Students stuck on one side of the bridge while their teachers are teaching from the other side can help the situation by helping their teachers find a common ground to start the journey over the bridge. The first and most important way is to ask for the clarification of unknown vocabulary. Teachers often forget what it is like "not knowing" and make assumptions about vocabulary that to them is common everyday parlance. We are often amazed how often students *don't* ask for clarification. They continue to listen to take part in discussions while "pretending to know." The most common feature of the "pretend to know game" is nodding in agreement, while not having a clue (Whitman, 1990). Unfortunately, learning often occurs in an ego-intensive environment where learners and teachers hate to admit what they don't know. In an effort to preserve self-esteem, learners may try to hide areas of deficiency in understanding. Be warned, though, this is not an effective means of developing mastery!

Other ways students can smooth the journey over the bridge to better understanding is to take some control over the pace of teaching and learning. They can bring "sticky points" and "conceptual stumbling blocks" to the teacher's attention. Students can ask for analogies, anecdotes, metaphors, and examples, or suggest some of their own, which will allow the teacher insight into their levels of understanding.

419
WHO'S DRIVING
THE BUS?

CASE 20-4

During the feedback session at the end of his medicine rotation, a clinical clerk expresses his disappointment in not having learned how to start IVs. The internal medicine program director is somewhat stunned. When he asks the student why he had not taken it on himself to seize an opportunity to learn this particular skill, the student remains silent and confused.

———— WHO'S DRIVING THE BUS? ————

Unfortunately, most adult learners take the passive approach to education. Like children they relinquish the responsibility for their education to the "system." They climb onto the "school bus" assuming that someone else has the big picture in mind and knows where they are going. But what if no one else is actually driving the bus? Those students who fail to realize that they're supposed to be driving the bus themselves either crash and burn or find themselves in a parked bus, unable to drive their own learning once their formal education is completed. Different skills are needed to be a good passenger versus a good driver. A student in the driver's seat is faced with two important questions: (1) Where am I going? (i.e., What are my goals/intentions?) and (2) How do I get there? (What strategies/behaviors will I need?).

In medical training, the need to become an active participant in learning cannot be overstated. The clinical clerk in Case 20-4 is a good example. He did not take charge of his own learning. Even more troubling, however, the idea itself that he could take charge of his own learning was novel and foreign.

However, it is important to note that students are not the only ones to blame for the passive roles they take in directing their own education. For many, like the student above, their role is a kind of "learned helplessness." Teachers have so often placed themselves in the driver's seat, and relegate students to passengers, that the arrangement becomes unconscious. A common example is the teacher who burdens himself with the impossible task of teaching everything about his area of expertise. Some would argue that anything teachers do, even if their intent is to help, that results in fostering dependence is counter-productive. We believe, instead, that teachers should see themselves as occupying a brief but important role in the student's development, not unlike a pair of training wheels on a child's first bicycle. Students, too, should be alert to their tendencies to become passive, as the shift in relationship can feel awkward to everyone. Indeed, teachers will (and should) feel increasingly unnecessary as their students take charge of their own learning. Unfortunately, teachers may mistake the feeling of being needed with that of being helpful.

From a practical perspective, teachers have three main ways of promoting learner autonomy (Candy, 1991): (1) helping learners develop a sense of personal control, (2) providing access to learning resources, and (3) helping learners develop the competence to take control of their learning. Imagine how you, as learners, would feel if teachers brought these competencies to all subject matter you are being "taught":

- Locating and retrieving information
- Setting goals
- Time management skills
- Question-asking behavior
- Critical thinking
- Self-monitoring and self-evaluation

And, perhaps the most important factor in promoting learner autonomy is helping learners "believe they can." Part of this is helping learners identify the sources of their successes and failures. Learner autonomy and confidence is enhanced when success is attributed to hard work rather than luck or favoritism, and failure is understood as resulting from lack of effort rather than lack of ability.

So far, this discussion has featured the beliefs, intentions, and some actions of learning and teaching. Now it's time to shift our focus directly to learners. What core beliefs and intentions do outstanding students hold? What strategies can they employ to get the most of the teaching they are exposed to?

CASE 20-5

John and Ann both did poorly on the last written internal medicine exam. John resigns himself to the fact that he just isn't good in internal medicine; he doesn't want to be an internist anyway. Ann, on the other hand, believes that her strategy for preparing for the last exam was misguided and plans to adopt a different approach next time. How do you think John and Ann did on the next exam? Why?

OUTSTANDING LEARNERS: BELIEFS AND INTENTIONS

Probably the most important belief of outstanding learners, discussed so far, is that *they are driving the bus!* Just as important are beliefs about ability. In other words, "they can because they think they can" (Virgil).

There is a saying that whether you think you can or you can't do something, you're right. *Beliefs* about ability are probably more important than ability itself (for a more complete discussion on "self-efficacy beliefs," see Bandura, 1977). This is related to the fact that success breeds success and vice versa, as shown in Figure 20.2.

Consider John and Ann in Case 20-5. If John believes, "I'm not a very good student" or "I can't," he will tap very little of his potential. He will take little action. And, he will get meager or no results. His lack of success will complete the vicious circle and reinforce his belief that he is a bad student and that he can't. Ann, on the other hand, sees herself as a "good student," and her beliefs about her ability empower her to deeply tap her potential and take action rather than quit when faced with challenges. Overcoming obstacles provides her with further evidence of her ability.

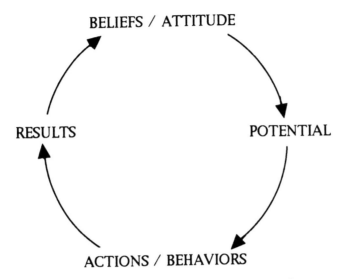

Figure 20.2. Beliefs about ability (and inability) can be self-fulfilling.

"Good" students also tend to be more flexible because they don't confuse ability with strategy. John believes *he* is not good at internal medicine. Ann believes her approach, or *strategy,* to learning internal medicine is not good. You can understand why John might give up, as the problem is with him, and therefore unchangeable. Ann can easily change her approach and try something else because she is not limited by a belief about ability. Further, "good" students are more likely to change their strategy if they aren't getting the results they want. Unlike their less successful colleagues, they understand that doing more of the same, just harder, doesn't always produce better results. Sometimes it's easier to switch approaches and climb over a wall instead of trying to push harder to get through. One successful inventor certainly thought so! In fact, he relished even mistakes as progress: "I am not discouraged, because every wrong attempt discarded is another step forward" (Thomas Edison).

How students deal with "failure" and challenges will shape their beliefs about themselves and their level of success almost more than anything else. In some ways "good" students are *less* demanding of themselves initially while they are learning something new. They understand that every new skill has a learning curve and don't expect themselves to be perfect right from the start. They learn from their mistakes and don't beat themselves up for not being good enough right away. They appreciate that success is often the result of having made many mistakes and that the only people who never fail are those who never try. They follow the dictum, "There are two types of experiences: successes and learning experiences." "Good" students appreciate that all learning starts with not knowing. They know that frustration often immediately precedes a breakthrough and that their efforts pay off.

Of course, teachers also play a role in students' belief systems about ability. This has been termed the "Pygmalion Effect" (the same effect that caused Eliza Dolittle to become a lady in *My Fair Lady*). Beliefs that teachers have about their students (positive or negative) can be very powerful and often end up as self-fulfilling prophecies (see *Pygmalion in the Classroom,* Rosenthal & Jacobson, 1968). In a classic experiment, teachers were told at the beginning of the year which students were the brightest and which were the weakest. The catch is that the students were picked at random rather than on ability. As you may have guessed, those students "labeled" bright at the beginning of the year did best while those labeled as weak did poorest. Another example of the Pygmalion Effect comes from the movie *Stand and Deliver*. This is the real life story of maverick teacher Jamie Escalente and his work with underprivileged inner-city kids. Escalente helped those adolescents develop a sense of pride in their ability to master things that others believed they never could. Not only did they learn calculus, but also the value of discipline, flexibility, and determination. Most of all, however, they learned to believe in themselves.

"Good" students, of course, also understand that success doesn't come without commitment. In the same way that they don't confuse ability with strategy, they don't confuse ability with commitment. The most successful individuals in any field are not necessarily the best or the most brilliant; they are often, however, the most committed. Intelligence is rarely the limiting factor. Likewise, "good" students expect more of themselves than anyone else does. They understand that "success" and "luck" are simply hard work in disguise. They create habits that serve their goals rather than enslave them. And they understand how habits grow and gradually define who they become:

> The beginning of habit is like an invisible thread, but every time we repeat the act we strengthen the strand, add to it another filament, until it becomes a great cable and binds us irrevocably, thought and act. (Orison Swett Marden)

Also, "good" students realize that they don't have to know or remember everything to use something. One anecdote about Einstein illustrates this approach. When asked what his phone number was, he went to a phone book to look it up. He said he never cluttered his mind with information he could find somewhere else. "Good" students, similarly, search for what is essential instead of getting bogged down in detail. They try to understand the main points and ideas; they look for distinctions or key features.

Finally, the metaphors students use to talk about learning are often telling of the underlying beliefs they hold. Some metaphors can be empowering, while others can be limiting. How would you complete the following sentences. "Learning is like . . . ." "School is like . . . ." Compare "learning is play" versus "learning is hell," or "school is like dance" versus "school is like torture." Metaphors hold emotional as well as conceptual power and can directly influence students' whole belief systems and actions regarding learning. For example, if a student likens medical school to a series of "piles of discrete elements in need of mastering," learning may feel like "moving stuff from the mountain of the unknown to the mountain of the known." This metaphor is limiting for at least two reasons. First, it leads to procrastination because the task seems so daunting, as it takes a lot of work to move a mountain. Second, it is incompatible with the concepts of learning presented earlier. Learning is not, as we argued, the accumulation of discrete bits of knowledge; therefore, it can't be assumed that once the elements are moved, or remembered, they are understood. This approach displaces the emphasis from the *links* between elements to the elements themselves. It also downplays the iterative cycles of learning that result in increasingly sophisticated conceptions. Such limiting metaphors are best replaced with more useful ones such as "learning is like training for a marathon." You can't train for a marathon the weekend before the big race! The training effect is in direct relationship to the development of good habits and the amount of effort exerted. As in a marathon, in learning, you can always strive to attain a new level, as you can always improve the degree of sophistication of your understanding.

But surely, no matter how constructive a student's belief system, underlying meta-phors, preparation, and habits of discipline, they still encounter a variety of teaching. How can outstanding students make the best of any teaching they are exposed to?

CASE 20-6

Dr. Smith is an accomplished cardiologist. She is leading a small group seminar for third-year medical students on reading electrocardiograms (ECGs). She projects ECGs on the overhead projector to provide students with an opportunity to develop their skills. Most of Dr. Smith's teaching experience is with residents and cardiology fellows. She becomes frustrated when the students are unable to interpret, what she believes, are common ECG findings. The students become frustrated because they had hoped to develop some basic skills in this unfamiliar area. Two-thirds of the students don't show up for Dr. Smith's next seminar.

——— OUTSTANDING LEARNERS: STRATEGIES ———

First and foremost, outstanding learners see themselves as responsible for their own education. Supporting that belief, we list some strategies here to enable learners to apply the strategies themselves, to identify those teachers who use them, and to elicit them in those teachers who don't. This section is by no means comprehensive. We hope that providing examples of how the above beliefs can be played out will stimulate readers to expand their own repertoire of learning and teaching skills.

"STRETCHING" STUDENTS

Suppose that you decided to start working out with free weights in the hopes of developing a Mr. Universe physique. In addition to selecting the appropriate combination of exercises, you would also need to choose the appropriate weight for each exercise in order to promote muscular growth. For instance, if you used a 2½-pound dumbbell to work out your biceps, you would unlikely see any growth and improvement, as the weight is too light. On the other hand, if you started out using a 120-pound dumbbell, you wouldn't even be able to lift it, as the weight is too heavy. Of course these two examples are extremes. But, in order to promote muscular growth, you would need to choose a weight that is just right, not too light, not too heavy. In fact, the best weight would be one at which your resources were not only being tapped, but being challenged. Therefore, the "right" weight is one that is just slightly heavier than your best last effort. If you did not exert yourself to this limit, you would likely maintain your current size but not grow. The same principle applies to learning (for more detail, see the discussion on zone of proximal development in Vygotsky, 1978). For instance, it would be inappropriate to assign similar reading assignments to undergraduate medical students and senior residents given that each is at a very different stage of professional development. Too often, students are referred to complex texts or journal articles before they have even grasped the basic ideas within a discipline. Similarly, students at the same level of training often differ in their ability to take over clinical responsibility for patient care. Disregard for a student's optimal "stretching zone" can overwhelm or lead to boredom and frustration.

Dr. Smith, in Case 20-6, had a set agenda for her seminar. Rather than become frustrated, she could have reconsidered the appropriateness of her agenda and assumptions about the third-year students, especially given her inexperience with this group of learners. Faced with similar situations, we have found it more fruitful to abandon a given agenda and fall back on the dictum, "start with the learner." Part of teaching a new topic, or a new group of students, involves finding the right starting point for that particular group of learners. Dr. Smith's students, on the other hand, could have brought up the issue with her, rather than give up altogether and not show up for the remaining seminars.

GIVING AND RECEIVING FEEDBACK

Feedforward?

The term *feedback* was coined in the 1940s where it was used by rocket engineers. Another common example of a feedback servo-mechanism is the thermostat in your home. An implicit and important component is often lost when feedback is translated to the educational setting, the idea of *goal seeking*. The rocket has a target and the thermostat has a set point. Unfortunately, students are often not told what is expected of them, especially during clinical rotations. It's very difficult to "hit the mark" when you don't have a clue what it is. Therefore, before you can interpret feedback, you need some "feedforward" (Osborn & Whitman, 1991).

Outstanding students recognize that before they receive feedback, they need a "road map" of the content and "big picture" of what they are being asked to accomplish. Just as important, outstanding students have specific ideas of what they would like to accomplish. Feedforward, what your clinicians and teachers expect of you, should be integrated to what you expect to get out of a rotation. In our experience, students rarely have specific goals for their rotations. If asked to give a list of their goals, students usually reply with silence and a dumbfounded look. In other instances, they simply provide a list of topics to be learned. Outstanding students move to the "driver's seat" by preparing a short written list of goals at the beginning of each rotation, being as specific as possible. You should do the same.

Too often, students are expected to "catch on" as quickly as possible when starting a new rotation. If you find yourself in a situation where no formal orientation is provided by your supervising clinician, suggest that the two of you sit down for a few minutes so that you can get an idea of what is expected of you, i.e., feedforward. At this time you can also let your clinician know what you hope to accomplish during the rotation, i.e., your own goals.

Ask and You Shall Receive

During clinical rotations, some students want (and need) more bedside teaching, others want more responsibility, and so forth. But few students make specific requests. Each student is different, with different backgrounds and needs. It is unrealistic to expect your clinician to "know" what you need. She may be a skilled clinician, but she isn't clairvoyant. We are not suggesting that you will always get more of the type of experience you want by asking for it, but it certainly is more likely than by not asking. Most things are negotiable.

One of the common areas of "mismatch" is clinical supervision. Clinicians and students without an appreciation of the concept of stretching, presented earlier, may encounter difficulties. This is one area where what is "just right" varies considerably between students. A student given too much responsibility may find himself scared and overwhelmed. Another student given too little responsibility may become bored and frustrated. Negotiation is the key. Ask your clinician for more help or responsibility, depending on the situation. Not all students progress at the same pace. This is not, however, an excuse to remain in your comfort zone. Remember, the idea is to stretch and to grow.

Feedback

Everybody likes to get positive feedback. It is important to remember, however, that positive feedback should be informative as well as make you feel good. Negative feedback, on the other hand, is often just as difficult to give as it is to receive. Too often, positive feedback is conceived as praise and negative feedback as criticism. When a person feels criticized, her energy may go into self-protection rather than self-improvement. Teachers may also avoid giving negative feedback for fear that it will harm the student's self-esteem or damage the student–teacher relationship. There can develop a tacit agreement between the teacher and learner not to give feedback and not to ask for it. Both the giver and the recipient of feedback need to appreciate the capacity for feedback to elicit an emotional response rather than avoid feedback. It is important for both to remember their common goal, namely, to improve understanding and practice.

It is not surprising that most students receive very little feedback during clinical rotations. The majority of students, therefore, are not only provided with little feedforward but also with little feedback. Like a rocket with no target and no feedback mechanism, this is a potential disaster. We suggest that you schedule not only a formal feedforward session, but at least two feedback sessions, one at the midpoint and the other at the end of a rotation. Remembering that feedback is not a statement about your personal worth, but only about your performance, may make it easier to deal with unflattering feedback. Some students want feedback only if it confirms their self-concept. In this sense they want "feeding" and not feedback. The most important thing about receiving feedback is listening. A feedback session is not meant to provide you with an opportunity to defend yourself. Listen instead.

Characteristics to help you identify constructive feedback (Ende, 1983) are as follows:
Constructive feedback

- Is descriptive rather than evaluative
- Is focused on behavior rather than on the person or personality
- Is specific rather than general (provides specific examples of behavior)
- Is directed toward behavior that the receiver can do something about
- Does not make assumptions regarding motives or intent
- Is well timed (i.e., soon after an "incident")
- Involves sharing of information
- Involves an amount of information the receiver can use (avoids overload)
- Is checked to ensure clear communication (e.g., the receiver is asked to rephrase the feedback)

Wondering why is probably one of the most important keys to learning. In our discussion on teaching and learning, we equated learning to understanding and the building of personal concepts. We emphasized that the *linking* of knowledge elements to prior knowledge was more important than the *accumulation* of elements, that understanding was more important than memorizing. We suggested the use of *deep* approaches to learning that stress meaning, organization, and integration, over the use of *surface* approaches to learning that emphasize reproduction. The "Why?" question is the most valuable tool to this end (White & Gunstone, 1992).

Unfortunately, the most common questions asked by teachers are "What?" questions. "What is the dose of captopril in CHF?" "What is the most common cause of acute renal failure?" Unfortunately, "What?" questions can often be answered with little or no conceptual understanding. The same is rarely true for "Why?" questions: "Why does captopril work in congestive heart failure?" or "Why does volume depletion cause acute renal failure?" "How?" and "What if . . . ?" can be just as powerful as "Why?" questions.

The preoccupation with "What?" questions may be borne out of a *Jeopardy* mentality. The game show *Jeopardy* presents the idea of knowledge and intelligence as the accumulation of facts and the ability to reproduce them on demand. The majority of answers begin with "What is . . ." (or the related "Who is . . ."). When was the last time you saw Alex Trebeck ask a question requiring the demonstration of a detailed understanding of a concept? Can you recall ever having seen an answer in response to a "Why?," "How?," or "What if . . . ?" question? Unfortunately, many teachers and students also carry a *Jeopardy* concept of knowledge.

"Why?," "How?," or "What if . . . ?" questions are important tools for learning. Not only are they effective for student learning, but they represent one of the best ways for teachers to assess student understanding, faulty reasoning, or misconceptions. It is amazing how often students get the "right answer for the wrong reason." Students should be challenged by being asked to support, justify, and defend their answers. Even their wrong answers facilitate learning in that they provide a window to misconceptions. It is more important to discover the faulty reasoning behind a student's wrong answer than to "replace" it with the correct one. By investigating wrong answers, teachers can map out learner deficiencies, inconsistencies, and misconceptions. Therefore, outstanding students should expect, look for, and elicit deep questions. Their active participation in grasping at concepts and reasoning may, of course, sometimes result in "wrong" answers. But the good student sees these as an integral step in developing conceptual mastery and deep understanding of complex information.

STUDENT READING AND STUDYING

Even if your teachers are not challenging you to answer "Why?" questions, remember to wonder why on your own time. Given that no one may be around to ask you such questions while you are reading and studying on your own, it becomes important to remember that your task is to understand rather than memorize. Often students don't get "the point" of what they are reading simply because they aren't looking for it. They are too busy trying to remember what they are reading instead. They are taking a *surface* approach to learning rather than a *deep* approach. *Look for the point!*

Following is a list of important characteristics of deep and surface approaches as they apply to a reading task (i.e., learning from reading) (adapted from Ramsden, 1988, p. 19).

Deep approach—the reader's intention is to understand, therefore he . . .

- Focuses on "what is signified" (i.e., "the point")
- Relates and distinguishes new ideas and previous knowledge
- Relates concepts to everyday practice
- Relates and distinguishes evidence and argument
- Organizes and structures content
- Has an internal emphasis: the reader is driven by personal and immediate reasons for learning this content

Surface approach—the reader's intention is to complete the task requirements, therefore she . . .

- Focuses on the "signs" (i.e., reproducing the text itself)
- Focuses on discrete elements
- Memorizes information and procedures for assessments
- Unreflectively associates concepts and facts
- Fails to distinguish principles from evidence, or new information from old
- Treats task as an external imposition
- Has an external emphasis: the reader is driven by the demands of assessments, and knowledge is cut off from everyday reality

SQ3R

One simple strategy to help students get the most out of independent reading assignments and facilitate a deep approach to learning is SQ3R (Survey, Question, Read/Recite/Review) (Adams, 1993).

Survey—obtain a basic orientation to the material

- Glance at headings, key words, diagrams, and the like
- Read summary, if one exists

Question—wonder why

- Turn the first heading into a question(s)
- Arouse curiosity (which increases retention)

Read

- To answer the question(s)
- Look for meaning (i.e., the point)
- Avoid "passive" reading

Recite

- The main point that you have learned—in your own words
- Provide examples (make them memorable)
- Jot notes in the margin, etc.

Repeat each of the three steps above with subsequent headings

Review (at the end of the reading assignment)

- Repeat the survey as a memory check
- Try to recall the main points from each heading
- Review any part you can't remember or don't really understand
- Grasp the "big picture"

A similar self-monitoring task during reading may be to continually ask yourself questions such as: What does this mean? What's the point? What does this mean for me (in my context)? What examples, from my own experience, can I think of? How does this relate to what I've read before in this subject and other subjects? How can I use this? The idea behind effective learning is personal understanding—making as many links as possible to what you already know and "restructuring" what you already know. *Effective* learning is not necessarily efficient in the sense that faster is better. In fact, the more time you take to "play around" with the information in your head, the better the outcome of your learning. If you find yourself coming to the end of a paragraph, or a page, and can't even remember what it was about, you may be reading the words using "cruise control." Unfortunately, it is possible to pay attention to the words rather than the message and gain little insight while reading. This can be likened to "passive" reading. Unless you are well versed in a subject, this type of reading is rarely instructive. Become an active reader intent on finding the message hidden among the words.

VISIBLE THINKING

Have you ever seen a master clinician at work? It looks like magic. She skillfully examines a patient, hears things you aren't hearing, sees things you aren't seeing, and somehow manages to come up with a diagnosis. In order to become a master clinician, you have to look for things you weren't seeing before, listen for things you weren't hearing before, feel for things you weren't feeling before, but most importantly *ask the questions* you weren't asking before. Expert clinicians are seeing, feeling, and hearing things because they are specifically looking for them; they are continually asking themselves questions while examining patients. The same applies to taking a history and problem solving. Expert clinicians are not simply collecting data. They are answering questions. The key to modeling master clinicians is to make their thinking "visible" (Collins *et al.,* 1991). Therefore, modeling expert clinicians involves modeling both manual skills and intellectual (i.e., cognitive) skills. We've seen how simply imitating performance, without appreciating the underlying beliefs and intentions of a practitioner, provides only limited and distorted "knowledge." So, if outstanding students want to learn by modeling after master clinicians, they must seek to make teacher thinking "visible."

Unlike traditional apprenticeships, the "work" of cognitive skills (e.g., problem solving) is not directly observable to students, and students must often make assumptions about the actual process. Students, therefore, do not have a "conceptual model" of the skill being learned. Take, for example, learning how to weave carpets in a traditional native apprenticeship. The apprentice (i.e., a student) can watch the procedure from beginning to end, so that he gets and idea of not only the process, but also the finished product. In contrast, taking a history and doing a physical examination in order to solve problems is an apprenticeship of a different sort. In this case, the apprentice (i.e., a medical student) cannot observe the process because it is actually going on in the master clinician's head. Listening to the questions as asked by the expert clinician and watching the physical examination only reveal part of the process, and not the more important part, at that. In addition, the "product" of the process, the solution to the problem, is a much less tangible end point than is a carpet. In a sense, you could describe a medical student's clinical work as a "cognitive apprenticeship." There are two essential requirements for this type of learning. First, the teacher's thinking needs to be made "visible" to the student. Perhaps the best example of this is "thinking out loud" and explaining. An outstanding student therefore asks the master practitioner, but also, in observations, focuses on wondering *why* she is asking a particular question, rather than simply trying to remember the question. What is she trying to get at? The second essential feature is to have medical students participate in real patient care, i.e., to have an opportunity to solve real-world problems.

In this way, cognitive apprenticeship is similar to a traditional apprenticeship. Both feature phases of modeling, scaffolding, fading, and coaching. Modeling allows learners to watch masters at work. "Support" for learners during actual practice is provided for in the form of scaffolding. As the name implies, this involves providing support for the learner and may include doing part of the work, giving advice, providing hints, and so on. Fading is just that; it implies providing increasingly less support, i.e., scaffolding. Coaching includes the first three aspects, i.e., modeling, scaffolding, and fading, as well as providing evaluation and feedback among other things. In short, coaching involves supervising students' learning. In addition, teachers must help students develop a "conceptual model"—a picture of the whole. As mentioned, unlike a finished carpet, cognitive skills have a much less tangible end point. Students need, however, a "big picture" of what they are trying to do in order to interpret the coaching provided by clinicians. For instance, we are always surprised that many senior medical students still think of the history and physical examination as a passive data-gathering activity instead of an intellectually active and dynamic process of problem solving.

You can see that being a master clinician and having an ability to make one's thinking visible are two quite distinct skills. Therefore, not all great clinicians are great clinical teachers. However, students with an understanding of cognitive apprenticeship can play a larger role in directing the process. First and foremost, such students are aware that the "performance" aspect of clinical skills, those they can see and hear by watching a master clinician in action, only tell half of the story. If your clinician is not forthcoming with the underlying thinking guiding his performance, you can ask questions to help him make his thinking visible. Rather than trying to memorize the important questions to ask a patient with chest pain, i.e., a surface approach, sort out *why* it is important to ask each question. What do you make of the answer? How does a particular answer change your thinking? What other information might you need to make sense of an answer? In addition to making thinking visible, you should seek out opportunities to practice your skills. Negotiate how much support you want and need rather than letting your clinician take over completely when you encounter difficulties. Being aware of the process gives you much more control and power over your own learning. Remember the old Chinese proverb: "I hear and I forget. I see and I remember. I do and I understand."

STUDENTS AS TEACHERS

We have often heard it said that we teach those things that we most need to learn. We can certainly vouch for this. The implication of this statement, though, is actually the converse: We learn best those things that we teach. As Joseph Joubert once said, "To teach is to learn twice." Students should not forget the powerful learning opportunity that comes from helping others, whether they are students having difficulties or patients in need of information and explanations. We suggested that an ability to explain things in your own words is evidence of learning and understanding. Perhaps, then, an ability to explain something in your patients' words is evidence of an even deeper understanding, as well as an example of bridging knowledge from a student physician's understanding to that of a patient's.

CONCLUSION

In this chapter, we have focused on learning and the student's role and responsibilities as a learner. We have tried to persuade you of the primacy of learning over teaching. Recall Jack in the introductory case. When faced with a less-than-optimal learning environment, Jack gave up and simply relinquished the responsibility for his own learning. Faced with a similar situation, we hope that you will make a different choice. To this end, we have provided you with a framework to think about learning and teaching in terms of not only behaviors, but also intentions and beliefs, the most important of which are beliefs about responsibility, "who's driving the bus," and beliefs about ability. We have also challenged you to reconsider what it means to learn and how learners construct their knowledge base. An appreciation for the different types of knowledge, declarative, conceptual, and problem solving, as well as the differences between surface and deep approaches to learning, can help you become a more effective learner. Remember to constantly wonder "why?" Concepts such as bridging knowledge, stretching, feedforward and feedback, SQ3R, and the intellectual apprenticeship were provided to help you develop learning strategies and elicit good teaching behaviors in situations where the teaching is less than exemplary.

If you've found the ideas presented in this chapter interesting but don't put them to use, then you've wasted both your time and ours. Don't treat this chapter as though it's from a novel. Instead, use it like a manual; come back to it several times, especially when you're feeling challenged. Adopt the beliefs and attitudes of an outstanding learner and practice the strategies. Appreciate exemplary teaching when you observe it, and elicit it when you don't. Play an active role in directing your own education. Remember, *you're driving the bus!* The renowned educator Marva Collins compares her role as a teacher to that of the wizard in *The Wizard of Oz*. She believes the most important thing she has to offer her students is the realization that what they want and need is already inside of them.

CASES FOR DISCUSSION

CASE 1

Recall Jack in the introductory case. Unclear about expectations and unhappy with his rotation with Dr. Brown, he satisfies himself with just getting by. About to embark on another clinical rotation, Jack is determined not to repeat this situation. He comes to you for advice.

1. *What should he consider even before starting the new rotation?*
2. *How should he prepare?*
3. *What are important considerations during his rotation?*

CASE 2

Sally is unhappy with her midrotation evaluation for internal medicine. Her attending recalled an incident from the first few days into the rotation that he was particularly unhappy about. He tells her that she is unmotivated and doesn't care. She needs to "work harder." He believes she has an "attitude problem." Sally is surprised, overwhelmed, and becomes defensive. She discounts her attending's feedback as "personality differences."

1. *How might this feedback session have been more fruitful?*
2. *Recall and reevaluate feedback sessions from your own experience.*

CASE 3

Tim, a third-year medical student, has just bought a copy of a major textbook of internal medicine. He plans to read it during his medicine rotation. The book is comprehensive with many details. He finds himself trying to memorize its many long lists. He becomes frustrated as he becomes increasingly aware that his book is not helpful for his understanding of medicine.

1. *What sorts of things would you be looking for in a "learning" text as opposed to a reference text?*

CASE 4

Heather is attending a seminar as part of her course work. The seminar leader is enthusiastic. He tries to engage her. He asks questions. Heather just doesn't seem to understand. The harder he tries, the more confused and frustrated she becomes. He obviously knows his stuff; he just can't get her to understand. Heather leaves feeling that she understands less than when she came in (Arseneau, 1996).

1. *How might you explain this situation?*
2. *What recommendations would you make, to both teacher and student, about improving the situation?*
3. *Define what is meant by bridging knowledge and provide examples from your own learning experiences.*

CASE 5

Cindy, a final-year medical student, is rounding with the residents and their attending, Dr. Jones. Dr. Jones makes sure to engage Cindy in all discussions about patients and tries to check that the level of the conversation isn't "over her head." Cindy, on the other hand, often "nods in agreement" even when she doesn't know or understand. She also has enough of the vocabulary to fool Dr. Jones into believing that she understands when she really doesn't.

1. *What is happening in the above situation? What are Dr. Brown and Cindy each trying to do?*

2. *Define the types of knowledge, declarative, conceptual, and problem solving, and give examples of each from your own experience.*

—————————— RECOMMENDED READINGS ——————————

Arseneau R, Rodenburg D: The development perspective: Cultivating ways of being, in Pratt DD (ed): *Five Perspectives on Teaching in Adult and Higher Education.* Huntington, NY, Krieger Publishing Co Inc, 1996.

This chapter looks at the developmental perspective of teaching, which is the flip side of a constructivist perspective of learning. This is a good place to start for new readers as it keeps educational jargon to a minimum and explains basic concepts.

Candy P: *Self-Direction for Lifelong Learning.* San Francisco, Jossey-Bass Inc Publishers, 1991.

Arguably the definitive text on self-directed learning. Despite its depth and breadth, it remains very readable.

Collins A, Brown JS, Holum A: Cognitive apprenticeship: Making thinking visible. *American Educator.* Winter:4–46, 1991.

This paper provides an in-depth discussion of some of the ideas underlying the "intellectual apprenticeship" discussed in the section, Visible Thinking, in this chapter.

Marton F, Hounsell D, Entwistle N (eds): *The Experience of Learning.* Edinburgh, Scottish Academic Press, 1984.

This book, which is unfortunately out of print, is one of the best books on research into learning we have come across.

Pratt DD (ed): *Five Perspectives on Teaching in Adult and Higher Education.* Huntington, NY, Krieger Publishing Co Inc, 1996.

This edited book looks at teaching from the perspective of five different belief systems as opposed to framing teaching as a set of behaviors. The five perspectives are (1) Transmission, (2) Apprenticeship, (3) Developmental, (4) Nurturing, and (5) Social Reform. It provides an in-depth discussion of some of the ideas presented at the beginning of this chapter regarding the relationship between beliefs, intentions, and strategies.

Ramsden P (ed): *Improving Learning: New Perspectives.* London, Kogan Page, 1988.

An excellent and practical book that looks at teaching from the learner's perspective. This book provides an in-depth discussion of surface and deep approaches to learning and teaching strategies that foster deep approaches to learning.

CHAPTER 21

Clinical Research

David A. Katerndahl

CASE 21-1

Because some children begin smoking prior to age 10, Fischer and colleagues wanted to learn whether preschool children recognize cigarette brand logos at a rate similar to logos of other children's and adult brands. Using a convenience sample of 229 preschool children aged 3–6, from preschools in Augusta and Atlanta, Georgia, children were asked to match logos with pictures of their products on a game board. The 22 logos used included ten children's brands, five noncigarette adult brands, and five cigarette brands. In addition, recognition of the Surgeon General's warning was also tested. The researchers found that the logo recognition for cigarette brands was intermediate to that of children's brands and noncigarette adult brands. Recognition rate increased with age such that by age 6 there was no significant difference in recognition rates between the Disney Channel and Camel's "Old Joe." Only 10% of children recognize the Surgeon General's warning. Thus, it appears that preschool children recognize cigarette brand logos to a high degree. Such advertisement by cigarette manufacturers may have an important impact on the children's later decision to smoke cigarettes (Fischer et al., 1991).

EDUCATIONAL OBJECTIVES

On completion of this chapter, the reader should be able to:

1. Describe the various roles that physicians may play in the research process
2. Define and contrast convenience, randomized, stratified, and probabilistic samples

3. Define "generalizability" and identify potential threats to generalizability
4. Define Type I and Type II errors
5. Outline the steps taken in planning and conducting a research study
6. Describe the ethical responsibilities of the physician-investigator

INTRODUCTION

Hippocrates said, "There are in fact two things, science and opinion; the former begets knowledge, the latter ignorance" (Strauss, 1968). It is only through the transformation of opinion into science that medicine advances. Yet the numbers of physician-investigators have been steadily decreasing (Cadman, 1994). In addition, as the emphasis on primary care increases, the need for new knowledge in this area increases. If that new knowledge is to be realized, it will fall on the practitioner to contribute to this search in a meaningful way.

The clinical literature is generally tertiary care based. Studies have shown that, although 75% of the population will suffer an illness in any given month and 25% will seek care from their primary care physician, less than 0.1% will receive care in a tertiary care hospital (White, 1980). Consequently, the generalizability of the literature is severely limited, particularly for the primary care setting.

Because of its generalist nature, primary care deals with all relevant aspects of a patient's health. This emphasis on breadth and the total patient enables primary care physicians to focus on the broad, high-impact questions that face our society. Case 21-1 emphasizes the role of primary care researchers in asking the big questions.

The pursuit of clinical research and new knowledge has benefits to the individual practitioner as well. It has been said that the "physician can reasonably expect to learn something, however slight, from every patient seen" (Geyman, 1978). This statement emphasizes the need for personal growth in the practitioner. In addition, the systematic approach to research enables the practitioner to sort out opinion and fact, thus providing for better patient care in the long run. In addition, the pursuit of scholarly activity provides a specialized interest that can help prevent physician burnout.

Because our scientific knowledge is less than perfect, medical care represents a blend of art and science. Indeed, all medicine *must be* a blend of art and science. One without the other produces poor patient care. Osler stated, "Medicine is a science of uncertainty and an art of probability." Unfortunately, experience without the systematic structured framework of investigation means that our clinical actions are based on a series of anecdotal events that serves to emphasize the most recent events or preconceived notions. Experience only becomes science when held up to the same strict standards of scientific method as any other research endeavor. While physicians must balance art and science, they must seek to turn the art of medicine into the science of medicine.

For those physicians working in an academic environment, research is a reality that must be faced and accepted if career advancement is to be achieved. The "coin of the realm" in academia is still the publication of research results in peer-reviewed journals. Failure to recognize this fact has often resulted in disillusioned, disgruntled academic physicians unable to achieve promotion or tenure.

Finally, as physicians, we each have an obligation to contribute to the knowledge base of our discipline. As physicians, we have the moral obligation to further our discipline as a way of promoting good patient care. We can only further that discipline through the advancement of new knowledge. Consequently, each physician has the duty and obligation to question, to investigate, and to increase our depth of understanding.

This chapter will review the process of patient-centered clinical research. The role of the physician-investigator will emphasize the varied obligations that the physician has depending on the level of participation. The research process will be reviewed, emphasizing the key concepts of sampling, generalizability, and probabilistic thinking. Finally, ethical issues involved in conducting research will be discussed, namely, ethics in research design, ethics in informed consent, and ethics in the role of the physician-investigator.

CASE 21-2

Believing that primary care physicians were managing patients with spontaneous abortions differently than were obstetricians, Green and colleagues sought to document the usual care provided in primary care for spontaneous abortions and its complication rate. Patients presenting to 49 primary care practices across the United States and Canada with spontaneous abortions were studied. This cross-sectional study of patients presenting during a 25-month period found that 40% of patients were managed completely as an outpatient and only 51% required dilation and curettage (D&C). D&C was more likely to be performed in patients with abortions later in pregnancy and for those with excessive blood loss. Although psychological consequences were the most frequent complication (24%), patients managed with or without D&C did not differ in the frequency of complications. The investigators concluded that selected patients with spontaneous abortion seen in primary care settings can be managed effectively as outpatients without the need for D&C (Green et al., 1988).

——————— ROLE OF THE INVESTIGATOR ———————

The role of the physician as an investigator may vary depending on the level of involvement in research. Although the physician may serve as the principal investigator, assuming all responsibility for a project, the option exists to serve as a coinvestigator or participant in a research network. Responsibilities vary depending on the role chosen.

As an independent or principal investigator, the physician is ultimately responsible for every aspect of the study. The question to be researched usually emanates from the principal investigator, who is responsible for designing the study and securing the necessary funding or support. During the conduct of the study, the principal investigator supervises data collection and analysis. This data management ensures that data are collected in the proper manner, recorded in a standardized fashion, and entered into the computer data base. The principal investigator must ensure that the quality of the data entered is good and, when inaccuracies are found, must supervise the "cleaning" of the data such that the ultimate data base is as accurate as possible. Finally, the principal investigator must ensure that the study results are analyzed appropriately and that the interpretations of the results are sound.

Once completed, the study results must be communicated to practitioners and other researchers. The principal investigator is ultimately responsible for the preparation of manuscripts and their accuracy. In addition, he or she must coordinate the presentation of results at conferences.

The principal investigator also must attend to relevant ethical issues. Therefore, the principal investigator must ensure that informed consent procedures are followed completely, that the data obtained are handled in a confidential manner, and that the analysis and presentation of results are made in the most accurate fashion.

Many physicians have neither the desire, the skills, nor the time to serve as a principal investigator. However, they are interested in serving as a coinvestigator or collaborator on a research project. In this capacity, the physician may be responsible for a particular aspect of a study, e.g., supervision of research assistants, or may simply lend his expertise in the design and analysis phases. Although not ultimately responsible for the entire project, the collaborator must feel free to share concerns about ethical issues, interpretation of results, and study conduct. Because all of those listed as authors on a manuscript bear responsibility for its contents, it is incumbent on every coauthor to fully read and support the results presented in any manuscript.

With the development of ambulatory research networks such as the Ambulatory Sentinel Practice Network (ASPN), primary care research developed a new tool for studying practice-based problems which should have greater generalizability than traditional tertiary care research as Case 21-2 showed. The number of research networks is ever increasing and these networks often vary in size, practice characteristics, and research focus. Practitioners may seek to become involved in research through participation in one of these networks. If considering joining network research, the practitioner should contact those networks of interest and seek more information. In addition, the practitioner should contact current network members to elicit their impression of the network and their level of satisfaction with involvement. Once the practitioners have committed to involvement in network research, they have responsibilities to patients and staff in addition to responsibilities to the project itself. The role of the research network participant in a particular study involves data collection. Not only do practitioners collect data on individual patients who are the subjects of the study, but they may also be required to keep age/sex registries on all of their patients. The accuracy of the data collected is essential to the success of the project.

In addition, as a member of the network, the practitioner must share ideas concerning current and future projects. Many successful network research projects have emanated from the network participants themselves. If the network is to remain viable, the participants must be involved in its direction and in the ideas for its studies.

Finally, research network participants must consider how any study will impact their practice. As subjects, the patients will undergo specific risks for participation. These risks may be potentially life-threatening, such as adverse reactions to medication or procedures, or they may simply involve potential loss of confidentiality as a result of the information collected. Practitioners must ensure that the safety of their patients is protected. In addition, many network-based studies seek to utilize office staff in the data collection process as much as possible. This minimizes the burden placed on the practitioner but may put considerable stress on the office staff. Practitioners must protect staff when committing to a network-based project. Hence, in the role of research network participant, primary care physicians must evaluate each study in terms of its practice feasibility and its impact on their patients and staff.

In order to develop a rational approach to the evaluation of a newly diagnosed hypertensive patient, Gifford sought to identify what proportion of hypertensive patients have secondary causes. Using 4939 hypertensive patients seen at the Cleveland Clinic in Cleveland, Ohio, a tertiary care facility, chart audits of patients with hypertension were performed. Approximately 10% of patients with the diagnosis of hypertension were found to have secondary causes. About 6% had potentially curable forms of hypertension. In order to identify 220 patients with renovascular lesions, 1256 selective renal angiograms were studied. However, only 67 patients had surgery with only 60% of those being cured. Similarly, to identify 9 patients with pheochromocytoma, 2775 tests were performed. Thus, this study found that approximately 10% of patients with hypertension have secondary causes. Consequently, newly diagnosed hypertensive patients should have a work-up for secondary causes (Gifford, 1969).

RESEARCH PROCESS

KEY CONCEPTS

Quantitative research relies heavily on statistical concepts. In fact, the validity of any quantitative research is heavily dependent on its statistical underpinnings. An understanding of key statistical concepts such as sampling, generalizability, and probabilistic thinking is essential to be able to interpret and develop clinical research.

Because researchers rarely can access and study all of the subjects of interest, they must generally rely on studying a sample of those subjects. Thus, the study "population" is the group to which the investigator wishes to generalize the study results, while the "sample" is the group of research subjects who actually participate in the study. The way in which the sample is selected determines the population to which the results can be generalized.

There are several methods used in selecting a sample. A "convenience sample" usually consists of subjects who are readily available, such as patients selected from a clinic population or research volunteers. Such samples are far from ideal because they are not selected from the population and often differ from the population in very significant ways. For example, volunteer subjects generally differ from nonvolunteer subjects in motivation and baseline characteristics (Marks, 1982).

A "randomized sample" is one in which the subjects are chosen from the population in a random manner such that each individual of the population has an equal chance of participating in the study. Randomized samples generally provide good representation of the population from which they are selected. In addition, randomization helps to control for unknown confounding variables that may affect the study results. However, the methods of randomization are important to ensure that it is a truly randomized process. Use of random number tables is appropriate. However, selection of subjects based on the day of the week that they present for care may not be a randomized process. The method of randomization used must be evaluated against potential confounding variables, variables that obscure the relationship between other variables.

When certain subject characteristics are important to the research question, it may be necessary for the sampling methods to oversample certain subgroups if these characteristics are rare in the population. In "stratified sampling," the population is divided into groups based on a key variable and a random sample is then selected from within each group. Similarly, "probabilistic sampling" oversamples segments of the population to adjust for any inequalities in the distribution. The use of these methods to deal with potential confounding variables relies on a prior knowledge of confounders. Frequently, however, confounders are not discovered until after the data are collected. In this situation, statistical analysis must be used to adjust for confounders during the analysis. The only way to deal with unknown confounders is through random sampling.

If the results of any particular research study are to be generalized to the desired study population, then the sample must be representative of that population based on important characteristics of the subjects. It is because of the issue of generalizability that the initial step in determining sample selection is to determine the intended study population. The method for selecting a representative sample is based on this intended study population. Therefore, if we wish to generalize the results of a study to the community at large, we cannot use a study sample selected from hospitalized patients and expect the results to be generalizable. In Case 21-3, the prevalence of secondary causes for hypertension was found to be 10% with 6% surgically curable. However, this study was conducted at the Cleveland Clinic, a tertiary care center. When a similar study was conducted in a general practice in Ontario, less than 6% of hypertensive patients were found to have secondary causes. Of these, only 0.6% were surgically correctable. Hence, generalizability becomes a key issue to the primary care physician.

Even if the sample is selected appropriately from the study population, there are other potential threats to generalizability. Subjects who drop out or are excluded may distort the sample and bias results. The reasons why subjects drop out or are excluded must be documented thoroughly in any study. The response rate of most cross-sectional surveys is less than 100%. However, nonrespondents may differ significantly from respondents in the prevalence of potential confounding variables. These considerations are especially important when the surveys are conducted on sensitive issues such as sexual behavior or illicit drug use. When the survey response is low, efforts must be made to compare respondents and nonrespondents on key variables to ensure that confounding differences have not affected their response.

The third key concept is that of probabilistic thinking. Statistical analysis cannot prove or disprove anything but provides a probabilistic frame of reference for judging results. It is up to the reader to make the final interpretation. Although researchers have access to the results of any particular study, they do not have access to reality. If the results of the study agree with reality, the correct conclusion will be made. If, however, the study concludes that there is a difference between treatment groups, but in reality there is no difference, then a Type I error is said to have occurred. As measured by the alpha level, the chance of a Type I error reflects the willingness to risk concluding that a difference exists when there is no such difference. This probability is reflected in the p value that is determined post hoc from statistical analysis. A p value of 0.05 means that if the study were repeated 100 times, a false conclusion would be obtained 5 times that a difference existed. A Type II error occurs when a false conclusion is made that no difference exists when indeed there is one. The probability of a Type II error is said to be the beta level. The statistical power, the ability to detect what researchers determine is a significant difference (the effect size), is determined by subtracting the beta level from 1.0. Generally, statistical powers of 80% are desirable. The sample size used in any particular study should be based on the desired alpha and beta levels as well as the magnitude of the difference between groups that the researchers are interested in being able to detect.

Effect size represents either the strength of association or the magnitude of the difference between two variables. Investigators must decide *a priori* what minimum effect size they wish to be able to detect. This minimum effect size is needed to determine the sample size required and is based on what difference the investigators feel is clinically important. The distinction between clinical significance, a difference important for the care of patients, and statistical significance, a p value less than the alpha level, must be kept in mind. For example, when comparing the efficacy of two antihypertensive agents, a large study may find a mean difference in diastolic blood pressures of 2 mm Hg with a $p \leq 0.05$. Although this small difference is statistically significant, few physicians would favor one agent over the other based on a 2 mm Hg difference, because it is not clinically significant. A minor difference can achieve statistical significance if the sample size is large enough.

PROCESS

The planning phase in conducting research is perhaps the single most important phase. Based on Sackett's classification of potential biases in research (Sackett, 1979), many biases occur during the planning and design phases (see Figure 21.1). The vast majority of all bias in research is not correctable once the study has been completed. This emphasizes the importance of the planning and design phases in any research project.

The first step in planning any research project is to identify a problem to study based on the researchers' personal interests and what they want to discover. At this stage, the investigator should be thinking about the population and variables to be studied.

The second step is the initial literature review, which should include both the conceptual literature and the research literature related to the problem in question. The conceptual literature should be used to focus on the theoretical background to the problem, while the research literature should emphasize secondary sources and review articles. This literature is used to identify whether your idea is a new one and thus worthy of further study.

The third step in planning research is to define a specific research problem and write a specific question to be answered. From the initial question, the revised study question should identify the patient population to be studied and the manipulated (independent) and outcome (dependent) variables to be measured. The final version of the research question should be in operationally defined terms with expected directions and results specified.

At this point, the investigator needs to estimate the potential for success of the project. First, the investigator needs to identify whether or not there is a need for this study. She must justify the study based on who would be interested in the results, why they would be important, and how the study will change standard practice. Second, the investigator needs to determine what resources are needed and what are available. Based on this assessment, the investigator should decide to either proceed, revise the question, or abandon the study altogether. Once the decision is made to proceed, the investigator returns to the literature for a detailed review of primary sources. This review focuses on study design, population, and variables used in previous studies and helps to identify what research approach, methods, and instruments are to be used.

Based on the study question, the investigator identifies the type of research project being proposed. The time frame, past, present, or future, is identified. In addition, the intent of the research, descriptive, comparative, evaluative, or predictive, is also identified.

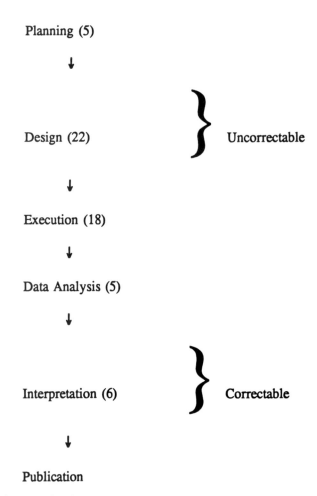

Planning (5)

↓

Design (22)   } Uncorrectable

↓

Execution (18)

↓

Data Analysis (5)

↓

Interpretation (6)   } Correctable

↓

Publication

Figure 21.1. Planning research: relative importance of research stages—based on the number of potential biases (shown in parentheses).

These are important concerns when identifying the research approach and the analysis to be used.

Specific operational hypotheses are now formulated. Although initially phrased in the null hypothesis format, assuming no difference between experimental and control groups, the alternative hypotheses are also composed. The benefits of stating hypotheses are that they (1) aid in the selection of methods and instruments, (2) predict results, (3) structure analysis, and (4) provide expectations.

At this stage, the study population and sample are identified. The sample must be representative of the population in all important aspects. At this stage, the selection method to be used to identify the sample is determined and criteria for subjects to be included or excluded from the study are also identified. Finally, the sample size needed is determined. This can be done through calculation using formulas, rule-of-thumb estimates, or, best of all, through power analysis based on the statistical power sought. The appropriateness of a sample size is dependent on several issues: representativeness of the sample, tradition, practicality, the type of study, the type of data, ethics, and cost.

The data-gathering method is next identified. Methods could include observation, measurement as in the use of instruments, and patient questioning. At this stage, the instruments that are needed and available should be identified.

The instruments to be used are selected or developed if not available. Because of the time-consuming nature of developing a new instrument and establishing its validity and reliability, the use of previously developed instruments is preferable if appropriate to the research question. When selecting or developing instruments, reliability must be considered. Reliability is the internal consistency of an instrument and its reproducibility between times and interviewers. In addition, the validity of an instrument—does it measure what it is supposed to measure?—is also considered. An instrument cannot have validity without reliability. However, it is possible to have a reliable instrument that is not valid. Acceptable instruments should have both reliability and validity.

The data-gathering plan needs to be designed. The data collection process is identified in terms of who collects the data and how they are collected. Practical considerations are important and the use of a flow diagram can be helpful. The research situation must also be identified, and, when research decisions are made, the reasons for these decisions need to be clearly recorded for future use. Finally, a timetable for conduct of the project should be completed.

Based on methodology and the research hypothesis, a data analysis plan should be designed. Specific statistical tests to be used should be noted and "mock" tables displaying results constructed. Choosing the appropriate statistical test is extremely important. Previous study of the published literature has suggested that 18% of articles fail to use statistical tests when needed and 7% use inappropriate statistical tests (Schor & Karten, 1980). There is a general trend toward a greater variety of tests. Choosing the wrong test can have important consequences: (1) loss of statistical power, (2) increasing the risk of concluding that a difference exists when it is simply the result of chance, (3) failing to address the stated hypothesis, and (4) invalidating your analysis. If possible, a parametric test should be used over a nonparametric test. Parametric tests are more powerful but make assumptions of normality and homogeneity of the data that nonparametric tests do not make. When choosing a specific statistical test, the choice is based on the type of sample, the purpose of the study, the level of observation in the data, and the power efficiency of the test (see Table 21.1).

At this point, the investigator determines whether the study is possible as designed. The investigator needs to. identify crucial elements to the success or failure of the study, sources of bias and invalidity to the study, and limitations on its generalizability. The decision at this point is whether to proceed as designed or redesign.

A pilot study may be necessary at this point. A pilot study is a ministudy of subjects not to be included in the final study. This is done to (1) test the methods and instruments for possible revision, (2) collect data to test the planned analysis, (3) estimate statistics needed for the final plan, (4) evaluate procedures, and (5) identify potential confounding variables. Pilot studies can be extremely useful to the design and revision of studies.

The study is next submitted to an Institutional Review Board (IRB) for review. Most IRBs focus on the question of risk versus benefits of the study. Studies using educational practices and tests, survey research, observational research, existing data, and those studies consisting of interviews and questionnaires may be exempted from IRB review. IRBs also examine ethical issues involved in study design to ensure that adequate informed consent is obtained (see the next section).

Once approval of the IRB is granted, funding for the study can be sought if needed.

Table 21.1
Choice of Statistical Test

Level of data	Parametric vs nonparametric	Purpose of study						
		Descriptive	Associative	Difference				
				One-sample case	Two-sample case		Many-sample case	
					Independent	Related	Independent	Related
Nominal	Nonparametric	Percentages Frequency distributions	Contingency coefficient	Chi-square Binominal test	Chi-square Fisher exact test	McNemar test	Chi-sqaure	Cochran Q test
Ordinal	Nonparametric	Median Range	Spearman rank correlation	Runs test Kolmogorov–Smirnov test	Mann–Whitney test	Wilcoxon test	Kruskal–Wallis ANOVA	Friedman ANOVA
Interval	Nonparametric	Mean Standard deviation	—	Kolmogorov–Smirnov test	Randomization test	Randomization test	—	—
	Parametric	Mean Standard deviation	Pearson correlation	Z test Student's t test	Student's t test	Paired t test	ANOVA	ANOVA with blocking ANCOVA

The study is then implemented and data are gathered and analyzed. Interpretation of the study is often difficult. The data are frequently interpreted as implying greater meaning than they actually contain. Interpretation should be based on acceptance or rejection of the null hypothesis.

In conclusion, planning high-quality research involves numerous steps. Attention to detail is extremely important to avoid loss of study validity and problems that are uncorrectable at a later stage.

CASE 21-4

Because of an ethical dilemma encountered during a research project, Slatkoff and colleagues documented ethical issues involved when practitioners allow their patients to become research subjects. Using 105 patients in a hospital neoplasia clinic and 268 control patients attending a university family practice center, a case–control study of the association between human papilloma virus (HPV) and cervical intraepithelial neoplasia (CIN) was performed. Early results suggested that patients with HPV were at high risk for developing CIN. Informing these patients of the risk and the need for follow-up produced a wide range of patient reactions from gratitude to bewilderment, panic, or anger. Final results of this study, however, found no association between HPV and CIN, raising several ethical questions, such as the need for an independent review committee to monitor study progress, a priori plans for sharing results with subjects, and plans for interventions based on findings. Because physicians engaging in research must be prepared to deal with discovered health risks, they must scrutinize the design and communication of results prior to inception of the study (Slatkoff et al., 1994).

———— ETHICS, COST, AND SAFETY ISSUES ————

Because research studies conducted by practitioners use patients who are vulnerable because of their relationship with the practitioner, ethical issues must be considered whenever embarking on a research study, especially when subjects will not necessarily benefit from participating in the study. The nature of the physician–patient relationship serves to coerce participation from patients and may compromise the basic tenet of patient care—first, do not harm.

Unethical practices in the design and analysis of experiments should not be encountered. However, one study of 295 articles in ten medical journals found that 39 articles had used the wrong study design for their hypothesis and 11 had improperly manipulated their data (Schor & Karten, 1980). Such studies are unethical because they unnecessarily place subjects at risk as these studies cannot answer the questions for which they were conducted.

From a treatment standpoint, the first ethical dilemma involves the use of placebo or conventional therapy in control groups. The traditional placebo-controlled group may not be ethical in all situations. If a conventional therapy has found some benefit for patients with the problem being studied, it is unethical to use a placebo in a control group. Conventional therapy should be the standard against which any new therapy is judged as long as the conventional therapy had some documented benefit. Second, the use of high-risk therapies, those known to entail severe side effects, should only be used in situations where the potential benefits warrant considering them. When there is already a good conventional therapy in use, the introduction of a high-risk therapy is probably unwarranted. Even in situations where no such acceptable current therapy exists in a condition with high morbidity or mortality, the use of high-risk intervention must be presented honestly to potential subjects. Subjects with severe disease are vulnerable to being exploited in such high-risk studies.

Because of the frequent misunderstanding of statistics by users of the medical literature, unethical practices in the statistical analysis and presentation of data are frequently seen in the medical literature. For example, the use of the standard error to describe the dispersion of a variable in a sample is inappropriate. The standard deviation is the correct measure of dispersion. However, researchers frequently use the standard error inappropriately in this situation, perhaps because the standard error by definition is a smaller value than the standard deviation. Second, researchers frequently ignore alpha and beta levels as well as effect size when planning and recording their study results. It is unethical to ignore these important statistical values. By ignoring the alpha level, we run the risk of making a Type I error, especially if multiple statistical tests are used. In this situation, we are almost assured that whether or not treatments differ, our analyses will find a difference in some category, suggesting a superior benefit from one treatment over the other. Similarly, statistical power and beta level are frequently ignored by researchers. Consequently, the lack of statistical significance may simply reflect the poor statistical power of our study. Furthermore, by not determining the minimal effect size of importance *a priori*, we run the risk of confusing statistical significance with clinical significance. Lastly, failure to recognize the importance of alpha and beta levels may result in sample sizes that are either too large or too small for the study's purpose. Thus, if the sample size is too small to produce an adequate statistical power, all of the subjects in the study have been placed at undue risk by participating. This is because the study had no realistic chance of finding a significant difference if one truly existed. Conversely, if the sample size is so large that even inconsequential differences between groups are statistically significant, we have also subjected a portion of the sample to unnecessary risk.

Also, the presentation of results can be skewed, thereby biasing the interpretation. This is especially true in the use of figures when the axes are not clearly defined or differ from the conventional axis, which starts at zero and proceeds in a nonlogarithmic fashion. Use of log scales may suggest a linear relationship to the reader if close attention is not paid to the graph and its axes.

Informed consent is the procedure by which potential research subjects are informed of the purposes of the study, the procedure, the risks to the subject, and the subject's rights. Except when the study presents minimal risk, subjects must give written signed consent that they understand and consent to participation in this study. The issue of informed consent becomes even more complicated when the age and condition of the patient are considered. For example, minor children cannot give informed consent; the parent or guardian must give the child's consent. Similarly, adults who are cognitively compromised, e.g., patients with Alzheimer's disease, cannot provide informed consent. Even under the best of circumstances, informed consent may not be all that informed and may not imply true consent. Investigators must make every effort to present a balanced description of the study, its risks, and the subject's rights before securing the subject's participation.

As demonstrated in Case 21-4, practitioners participating in research must fully understand the study design prior to committing their patients as potential subjects. This case demonstrates that preliminary review of the data collected can be dangerous, resulting in coming to false conclusions and interventions based on incomplete information that can produce significant anxiety in patients. As practitioners, we are committed to providing long-term patient care without doing harm. Unlike studies done in tertiary care centers, the subjects of the primary care researcher continue on in their physician–patient relationship with the researcher long after the study is completed. Consequently, any detrimental effects of participation in the study may have long-term effects on that relationship. The physician-investigator must consider these factors when planning or participating in a project.

CONCLUSION

In conclusion, there is a desperate need for expansion of the clinical, particularly primary care, research base. Such expansion must involve practitioners in the conduct of studies and must be practice based. Physicians willing to participate can assume a variety of roles from that of principal investigator to that of data collector. The exact physician role depends on experience, time, and commitment to the research question.

The planning and conduct of such studies must be carried out meticulously with the key concepts of sampling, generalizability, and probabilistic thinking kept foremost in our minds. The sampling strategy depends on resources, prevalence of the condition to be studied, and confounding variables. The particular strategy used will determine the extent to which results can be generalized to the population of interest. Because we do not know what the true answer is for any research question, probabilistic thinking is necessary to provide a frame of reference for interpreting results. When planning and conducting a research study, a stepwise approach based on these concepts is crucial to minimize bias. Founded on a well-defined research question, the sampling strategy is selected to enable generalization to the intended population. Identification of what data is to be collected and how to collect it is made to enable accurate determination of outcomes, interventions, and confounding variables. The method of analysis is based on the level of data, the purpose of the study, and sample characteristics.

The ethical burdens placed on the physician-investigator include ethics in design, analysis, and informed consent. In addition, the use of the practitioner's patients as research subjects must be kept in mind. The responsibilities as the patient's physician may conflict with the responsibilities as the researcher. Potential areas of conflict should be identified *a priori* to ensure appropriate patient care without compromising study results.

CASES FOR DISCUSSION

CASE 1

In order to determine whether routine prenatal ultrasound in low-risk pregnant women would reduce perinatal morbidity or mortality, 15,151 low-risk pregnant women receiving their prenatal care from 109 obstetrical and family practices were randomized to either a routine ultrasound screening group or a control group receiving ultrasound only for specific medical indications.

Although 45% of the control group had at least one sonogram for medical indications, only 2% had both ultrasounds that the experimental group had. There were no differences in any of the adverse outcomes when comparing the routine ultrasound group versus the control group (Ewigman et al., 1993).

1. How is this study an improvement over previous small, tertiary care-based studies that found similar results?
2. What are the potential limitations of the study?
3. What are the potential implications of this study for low-risk obstetrical patients, primary care providers, and society?

CASE 2

In order to examine the clinical characteristics of new headaches in primary care settings as well as the diagnostic and management strategies employed, 1331 patients presenting for new-onset headaches to practices in the Ambulatory Sentinel Practice Network were studied. Forty-eight percent of patients were diagnosed having a condition other than tension/vascular headaches with 15% remaining undiagnosed. Although 46% of patients met NIH criteria for receiving CT scanning, only 2% of patients received a CT scan. Although 72% of patients received medication and 59% received advice, only 1% were hospitalized (Becker et al., 1988).

1. What are the possible implications of the fact that 811 potential subjects were not included because follow-up data were incomplete?
2. What are the potential positive and negative implications of the discrepancy between the NIH indications for CT scanning (46%) and the actual use of CT scanning (2%)?
3. What are the implications of the fact that only 15% of patients included in the study made more than one visit to the primary care physician?

CASE 3

In the early 1900s, William Pickles, M.D., began observing and recording the prevalence of common diseases within his practice that included caring for patients in at least eight communities in England. By visually comparing the co-occurrences of varicella and herpes zoster, he established the close association of these two disorders. It was later determined that both disorders are caused by the same virus (Pickles, 1984).

1. Discuss the ability of epidemiologic studies to establish cause-and-effect relationships.
2. What are the potential difficulties in epidemiologic studies conducted in a single practice?
3. What specific tools can be used to record and evaluate the occurrence of common diseases in a particular practice?

CASE 4

In order to compare the efficacy of propranolol and alprazolam in the treatment of panic disorder, 55 volunteers were randomly assigned to placebo, propranolol, or alprazolam for 5 weeks. Subjects took up to 6 mg alprazolam and 240 mg propranolol per day. More patients receiving alprazolam had cessation of their panic attacks than those in either the placebo or propranolol groups. Of the 9 patients who dropped out during the study, subjects were more likely to drop out if they received the placebo or if they rated their panic attacks as severe (Munjack et al., 1989).

1. Discuss the generalizability of the results of this study.

2. *How might the differences in characteristics of patients who dropped out affect the overall results of the study?*

3. *Why is the fact that this is a double-blinded study important?*

CASE 5

In order to evaluate the influence of physician, patient, and resource characteristics on physician mental health treatment practices, a mailed survey of 107 primary care physicians was conducted. Physician self-rated confidence was related to referral, prescription, and counseling practices. These treatment practices were associated with admission rates, especially for substance abuse (Hendryx et al., 1994).

1. *Discuss the advantages and disadvantages of using a stratified sampling approach, as was done in this study.*

2. *Although the response rate was 52%, physician respondents and nonrespondents were similar demographically. Discuss the representativeness of the respondents.*

3. *What are the cause-and-effect implications of the results?*

———— RECOMMENDED READINGS ————

Gabel LL, Monk J: *Research Planning Guide.* Columbus, Ohio, Ohio State University, 1983.

   A short monograph outlining the steps taken in planning and conducting a research study. It can easily serve as a workbook for the beginning researcher. Because research basics haven't changed, it is still up to date on how to plan a study.

Hitchcock MA, Buck EL: Research roles for family physicians. *Fam Med* 22:191–195, 1990.

   A journal article discussing the varied research roles of practitioners from principal investigator to consumer of the literature. Each role is discussed in terms of its responsibilities and training requirements.

Hulley SB, Cummings SR (eds): *Designing Clinical Research.* Baltimore, Williams & Wilkins Co, 1988.

   This text provides a good overview of the research process and is particularly appropriate for the initial steps in the process. A good companion for the workbook by Gabel and Monk.

Norman GR, Streiner DL: *PDO Statistics.* Philadelphia, BC Decker Inc, 1986.

   A short text providing the basics in statistics. Written in a conversational and entertaining way, this book deals with everything from descriptive to multivariate statistics.

Reigelman RK: *Studying a Study and Testing a Test,* ed 2. Boston, Little Brown & Co, 1989.

   A basic text on research methods with practical medical examples from the literature. Clearly written with the novice in mind, this book covers all of the basics.

CHAPTER 22

Development of Clinical Guidelines

Julie Graves Moy

A 59-year-old white woman is working at her office when she experiences the sudden onset of chest pain, and then falls to the floor. Coworkers find that she is pulseless and apneic. Basic life support is instituted with positioning for proper airway, rescue breathing, chest compressions, and notification of the city's emergency medical system. An ambulance arrives, and the paramedics find that the pulse and respirations have been restored by the prompt and proper application of CPR. After intravenous access is established, she is transported to the hospital where electrocardiogram and cardiac enzymes show evidence of acute myocardial infarction. Intravenous streptokinase and nitroglycerine are administered. The cardiology fellow, the emergency room physician, and her family physician begin a discussion of management, with disagreement as to the appropriate subsequent medications, monitoring, imaging studies, length of stay in the coronary care unit, exercise testing, and rehabilitation planning. They differ over the use of calcium channel blockers and beta blockers in the acute phase, and over the use of nitrates for long-term therapy. The family physician believes that she needs to have only a monitor for cardiac rhythm and that her blood pressure should be taken manually, while the ER physician wants an intermittent automatic blood pressure device, and the cardiology fellow wants to place an arterial line for continuous blood pressure monitoring and a central line to monitor central venous pressure. The need for coronary angiography, nuclear imaging, and magnetic resonance imaging are discussed. Should she stay in the coronary care unit with intensive nursing for 12 hours? 24 hours? 48 hours? longer? The timing of the exercise tolerance test and whether a stress thallium study is superior to the modified

449

Bruce treadmill test are points of contention, and while one physician believes that cardiac rehabilitation begins in the hospital, another thinks that 2 weeks after the event is the appropriate time to begin.

EDUCATIONAL OBJECTIVES

At the conclusion of this chapter, students will be able to:

1. Know the definition, synonyms, sources, and methods for construction of clinical guidelines
2. Identify the method of construction for a guideline, its purpose, its degree of flexibility, its authors, and their potential and stated conflicts of interest
3. Approach a new guideline for prevention, diagnosis, or treatment with the questions "Is the guideline reliable?" and "Was the patient's interest placed first?"
4. Define the differences between implicit and explicit methods for developing guidelines
5. Define the differences between standards and guidelines

INTRODUCTION

Why do physicians disagree on the appropriate treatment for a given condition? Why is there a question as to the best medication, monitoring, testing, and rehabilitation for the patient in Case 22-1 who survived her heart attack? And why is there so little disagreement about the steps in CPR? Each of the components of the medical care given to the patient in Case 22-1 is the result of a clinical decision to perform or not to perform an intervention, and behind each decision about an intervention is a guideline.

The CPR given in her office and the initial care by the paramedics are outlined in the American Heart Association's Basic Life Support and Advanced Cardiac Life Support documents. First published in 1980, these documents are written by a panel of physicians and updated by a consensus conference process, held when new research findings lead to a need to change the guidelines (American Heart Association, 1987). A collaborative effort of the American College of Cardiology, American Red Cross, the National Heart, Lung, and Blood Institute, and American Heart Association, they are taught in hospitals, schools, churches, businesses, and community group settings (Montgomery *et al.*, 1986). The process of performing CPR has been studied, as have the outcomes of patients treated with it (Cummins *et al.*, 1991). Cities with strong educational programs that reach many citizens have lower death rates from cardiac arrest outside of the hospital (Cobb *et al.*, 1980; Cummins *et al.*, 1991). CPR guidelines are among the best we have in medicine, evidence-based, developed by a consensus method, taught to many people who may need to apply them, and then rigorously evaluated by studying the effect of using the guidelines on the health of the patients at risk.

But after CPR and initial cardiac care, the decisions about which interventions to select for the patient in Case 22-1 are not as clear. Is streptokinase or tissue thromboplastin the better thrombolytic agent? Is angioplasty or coronary artery bypass grafting surgery preferable? Should an exercise tolerance test, stress thallium, echocardiogram, or multigated pooled imaging (MUGA scan) be ordered? After how many days is it safe to go home? Post heart attack, should a woman take aspirin? A beta-blocker? What exercise program is safe? When is it safe to resume sexual intercourse? Why don't clear, reliable, tested guidelines exist for these issues?

How do physicians and their patients make decisions about clinical interventions? One option is for the physician to go to the literature, read everything published about the topic, present the information to the patient, and try to make a decision. This is usually impractical, since there may be hundreds of published articles about a given topic. Another is to recall what was taught in medical school or residency and choose that strategy. Or, the physician could select a textbook and follow its instructions. None of these strategies, although commonly used, seem optimal, considering the technology available to physicians today and the wealth of medical knowledge generated in the past 50 years. Ideally, the physicians should have an available guideline that has considered all published research, combining the results into a concise format that describes the state of knowledge and the clinical situations to which the guideline is applicable.

In the past, the physicians at our patient's bedside would not have disagreed so much. There were fewer tests, technologies, and treatments available, and their medical education and training were likely to have been similar, with one or just a few standard textbooks used for reference. New discoveries that changed practice occurred infrequently and were communicated at scientific meetings and via the few medical journals published. As medical science advanced and the nation grew, more and more frequent discoveries made changes in medical practice more common. More journals were published. Today, over 3500 medical journals publish more than 300,000 new articles each year (National Library of Medicine, 1995), making it impossible for an individual physician to keep up with all of the new information. With so many different recommendations coming from many sources, with the multiplication of training sites and therefore the professors' teachings and textbooks used, physicians began to diverge with respect to the decisions they made about clinical interventions. Adding to the confusion over appropriate care were new technologies, often widely adopted before effectiveness was established, such as electronic fetal monitoring (Hayward *et al.*, 1992a), and a patchwork, unregulated system of continuing medical education in which individual lecturers presented their own unevaluated opinions that many physicians accepted as truth without question.

Recently, studies examining the care provided by physicians have begun to note differences in medical care. Beginning in 1973, Wennberg and colleagues published a series of articles pointing out marked differences in rates for procedures such as tonsillectomy, hysterectomy, and carotid endarterectomy in different areas of Vermont, and marked variations in hospitalization rates and length of hospital stays for certain conditions in Boston, Massachusetts, versus New Haven, Connecticut, two demographically similar cities with most care delivered in university hospitals (Wennberg & Gittelsohn, 1973; Wennberg *et al.*, 1987, 1989). Hospital stays were 15% longer in Boston, but population-based mortality rates adjusted for age, race, and sex were virtually the same in the two cities. There was no evidence that an increased number of admissions to hospital or longer lengths of stay in these hospitals led to lower mortality, although the impact on quality of life remained unknown (Wennberg *et al.*, 1989). These "practice" variations attracted the attention of those who pay for healthcare, insurance companies and the federal and state governments, who wondered whether they were paying for unnecessary or inappropriate care. Numerous local initiatives have sprung up because of the discovery of this practice variation, some driven by a quest for improvements in healthcare quality,

Table 22.1
Synonyms for Clinical Guidelines

Old	New
Clinical pearls	Technology assessment
Indications	Clinical decision-making
Recommendations	Clinical epidemiology
Expert opinion	Critical appraisal
Medical necessity	Decision analysis
Utilization review	Medical effectiveness
Quality assurance	Clinical policies
	Practice parameters

such as the McMaster Evidence Based Medicine Group, and some driven by a quest for cost savings, such as some insurance industry efforts to decrease ordering of laboratory tests.

Clinical practice guidelines were one response shared by physician organizations, government, and the insurance industry alike, all of whom hoped that their use in medical practice would lead to reduced variation and thus lower cost and improved quality. New research methodologies such as meta-analysis and computerized calculation of Bayesian probabilities have made possible the combining of results from many previous research works into usable predictors of outcome that could be translated into new guidelines. By 1980, eight physician organizations had published 70 guidelines; by 1994, over 1600 guidelines had been published by 70 medical groups (Vibbert *et al.*, 1994). *Guidelines are statements issued for the purpose of influencing decisions about health interventions.* Health interventions consist of screening, diagnosis, or treatment and may include no action or watchful waiting (Eddy, 1992d). Unfortunately, many different terms are used to label guidelines, leading to some confusion over the appropriate terminology (see Table 22.1).

Federal and state governments, specialty societies, and insurance companies looked to practice guidelines as a strategy to increase control over medical practices and their costs (Bell & Roberts, 1989). Guidelines are intended to assist physicians with individual patient care decisions, to determine appropriateness prior to an intervention's occurrence, as insurance precertification, to review appropriateness after the intervention for payment decision or quality assessment, as utilization review and peer review, and to define community standards such as in credentialing, privileging, and in medical malpractice litigation.

CASE 22-2

A family physician is asked to chair a meeting to establish a hospital guideline for the care of well newborns. At the meeting a senior physician, influential in the community, immediately offers her set of routine orders, saying that she has used this approach successfully for years and believes the section could save a lot of time by just adopting them as the guideline. The family physician notices that the senior physician's standard orders include a routine blood glucose determination for every infant, routine feeding of formula to all infants whether the mother plans to breast-feed or not, and that they do not include any order regarding hepatitis B vaccine. The family physician mentions that her opinion differs on these issues, and the section members erupt into a heated discussion of whether these treatments are appropriate. The senior physician storms out of the meeting after telling the chair to go write her own guidelines, while she will continue to use her own orders.

THE DEVELOPMENT PROCESS

Development of a clinical guideline requires several steps. First is a precise definition of the problem. Next, the available evidence must be collected. This can be accomplished in several fashions, but perhaps the most convenient is an initial search of electronic medical data bases such as MedLine or Grateful Med, then a review of other resources such as Science Citation Index and the references cited in publications found in the electronic search. Textbooks, especially classic texts, can be helpful sources of references, and interested governmental agencies and healthcare organizations (such as the March of Dimes) can provide bibliographies on some topics.

In the past, guidelines were written at this stage. Traditionally, clinical guidelines resulted from the declarations of experts. The process used to create a policy was usually global subjective judgment, in which evidence from the identified references was combined intuitively by the author. Results were published as book chapters, review articles, or a standard protocol, and if a group was convened to develop the guideline, the results were published as a consensus statement. Group consensus was reached by voting, by persuasion by the more influential members, or by other methods that happen in the minds of the participants.

Guidelines are still being developed in this fashion. With this method, the experts subjectively assessed and weighed risks and benefits of a course of action and its alternatives. Global subjective judgment is an *implicit* method, which does not require experts to describe evidence, reveal bias, or justify decisions. Such a method is fast and relatively inexpensive, but there are risks that the developed guidelines will be wrong, and no way to determine where in the process the errors occurred. Individuals writing chapters or review articles might look at an incomplete collection of evidence or might ignore some evidence that doesn't fit their preconceived ideas. Conflicts of interest might arise, especially when consensus panel members are chosen because they have published in the field and are funded by pharmaceutical or device manufacturers. Bias by the authors of the guidelines cannot be determined when reading guidelines produced with this subjective, implicit method, and the risk that practice variations will magnify is high, especially when this strategy is used to produce local hospital or insurance company guidelines, since the process is likely to yield a different product depending on the experience and bias of the author or panel members. For some simple health problems, this may be appropriate, but for most health decisions, because of the complexity of diagnostic and treatment options and the vast amount of research information available, another method is needed to form a valid guideline.

More recently, authors have called for an orderly, prescribed *explicit* method for developing guidelines (Eddy, 1992d; Woolf, 1992). The advantages are that the product is reproducible and that all decisions made during the process are identified and described

Table 22.2
The Explicit Method for Guideline Development

1. Define the problem.
   Example: Do all infants need a blood glucose determination at birth? If not all, which infants do need it?
   a. Select interventions and alternative.
      Example: test all infants at birth, test no infants, test only large or small for gestational age infants, test those whose mothers have a positive diabetes test.
   b. Select the setting—patient, providers, and physical setting.
      Example: infants born to women cared for by obstetricians and family physicians, the local hospital.

2. List all relevant outcomes, especially those relevant to the patient.
   Example: infant endures a needle stick, hypoglycemia is identified so treatment can be initiated, possibly preventing seizures.

3. Develop evidence.
   a. Search the literature.
      Example: perform a search on the MedLine under headings "hypoglycemia," "neonatal care," "blood glucose determination," "large for gestational age infant," and "small for gestational age infant;" read the textbook *Effective Care of the Newborn Infant* (Sinclair & Bracken, 1992), which contains data from the Oxford perinatal trials; call the American Academy of Pediatrics and the American Academy of Family Physicians to ask if either group has published a guideline on the topic.
   b. Review and record the data.
      Example: make a chart that contains each intervention from 1a and each outcome from 2; enter information from the sources in 3a.
   c. Combine the data.
      Example: combine results from similar studies that use the same outcome variables, then redo the statistical tests; if necessary, consult a statistician at a local university, school of public health, or research organization.
   d. Assess expert opinion when necessary.
      Example: if information about some of the interventions or outcomes is not available, consult with experienced physicians and researchers.

4. List the outcomes by alternative on a balance sheet, include both probability and magnitude.
   Example: the balance sheet in Figure 22.1.

5. Assess preferences on the outcomes.
   Example: give the information from the balance sheet to several patients and ask whether they want their baby to get the glucose blood test; unfortunately, it is not possible to ask the baby's preference.

6. Write the policy.
   Example: in this case the policy might read: Term healthy-appearing newborn infants who weigh between 2500 and 4000 grams need not receive routine blood glucose determination.

for the reader to evaluate. The process of developing guidelines by the explicit method is outlined in Table 22.2 and Figure 22.1.

The explicit process starts with an evaluation of the available research to determine if the health intervention in question is effective and an estimation of the magnitude of the potential effort on outcomes important to the patient. This point usually requires emphasis to established physicians. In Case 22-2, many physicians justify the routine blood glucose test as defensive medicine used to help prevent malpractice suits or as information used to give the physician peace of mind by eliminating the possibility that a hypoglycemic infant will escape notice by physical examination. However, the parties whose outcomes are important are the parents and the infant. Physicians should not order health interventions for the purpose of making the physician feel better. During the process of comparing the benefits and harms of an intervention, the persons making the value judgments about the

BENEFITS	HARMS
Prevention of seizures by identifying all newborns with hypoglycemia	Pain and trauma of heel stick for infant - 100%
Incidence of hypoglycemia in newborns: 1.3 to 4.4/1000*	Parents' emotional distress - varies by parent
	Cost of the blood test
	Possible false positive test - varies with accuracy of laboratory

Figure 22.1. Balance sheet for routine blood glucose determination in healthy term newborns. *Data from Sinclair and Bracken (1992).

desirability of outcomes should be patients, if possible, or at least persons with some ability to imagine the likely wishes of the patient. Physicians are often not very good at estimating patients' values. Patients are more reluctant to take risks than physicians think they are (Eraker & Politser, 1982).

In the process of evaluating the available research, formal methods of combining the results of different studies may be needed. This process of combining research results is called meta-analysis, and it can employ the statistical techniques of pooling, effect size estimation, variance weighting, Mantel–Haenszel tests, and the confidence profile method of Bayesian meta-analysis (Eddy, 1992d). If uncertainty about the research results or the results of the combining of the various results exists, this should be stated clearly in the guidelines.

The fundamental difference between the explicit and implicit processes of development is the reproducibility of the method. Implicit methods such as global subjective judgment, consensus panels, review articles, and book chapters are simple, fast, and less expensive; however, bias is rampant, disputes are difficult to resolve, and gaps in knowledge and uncertainty are hidden. The explicit method is more expensive and time-consuming and requires sophisticated analytical skills and teamwork (Sussman *et al.,* 1993). The explicit method entails laying out the assumptions, the evidence, and the methods of decision-making that are involved. The intent is to produce policies based on the totality of knowledge that will be less arbitrary than traditionally developed policies and that should improve the quality of patient care.

CASE 22-3

The American Academy of Family Physicians convened a policy team to write a guideline for the management of labor when a woman's previous pregnancy had resulted in cesarean section. The policy team was chosen from members of the Academy's Task Force on Clinical Policies for Patient Care, and a methodologist who worked for the Academy served as the project's methodologist. The team met for several day-long sessions over a 2-year period. The teams defined the question precisely as, "Should an elective repeat cesarean section be scheduled when a woman has an uncomplicated term singleton gestation and has had one low vertical cesarean section previously?" The methodologist performed a computerized literature search; then team members reviewed article titles to determine which should be pulled for data collection. A data extraction form was developed, and the chosen articles were reviewed by two policy team members using the form to collect data. A team meeting was devoted to resolving differences between members about the data in individual articles. The data were combined by the methodologist into evidence tables. The team reviewed the available literature on patient preference, and after considering a new research project on preference, decided to use data from existing research in the policy instead. The team met to discuss the evidence and assigned sections of the policy for each team member to write. A final meeting was spent reviewing each section and developing a final document. This document was submitted to the Board of Directors of the American Academy of Family Physicians, who decided to adopt it as policy of the organization, and was submitted to a peer-reviewed medical journal for consideration for publication.

—————— SOURCES OF GUIDELINES ——————

GOVERNMENT

In 1989, the federal Physician Payment Review Commission recommended to the 101st Congress that expenditure targets be established to cap total federal health spending; during federal budget negotiations that year expenditure targets were not adopted, but the Agency for Health Care Policy and Research (AHCPR) was created to promote research on medical outcomes, and within it the Office of the Forum for Quality and Effectiveness in Health Care charged with developing clinical practice guidelines (Texas Medical Association, 1994; Wennberg, 1990) in hopes that these new guidelines would reduce health spending.

Clinical practice guidelines are developed and disseminated by several agencies of the federal government, including the Centers for Disease Control and Prevention (CDC-P), the Office of Disease Prevention and Health Promotion of the U.S. Department of Health and Human Services, the National Institutes of Health (NIH), and the AHCPR. The AHCPR uses panels of physician experts, methodologists, consumers, and health providers such as nurses, pharmacists, and psychologists who develop guidelines with the explicit approach (see Table 22.3). This agency also sponsors the Medical Treatment Effectiveness program, which includes funding for Patient Outcome Research Teams (PORTs) that perform clinical research needed to answer questions raised in the guidelines development process (Vibbert *et al.*, 1994). The NIH and CDC-P have traditionally convened consensus panels of designated experts and used an implicit methodology with no formal presentation of evidence, bias, or preferences, but recent panels have moved toward evidence-based approaches, though not yet explicit. The U.S. Preventive Services Task Force uses an evidence-based approach and rates the strength of evidence and the strength of the recommendation for each intervention (see Table 22.4). The Health Care

Table 22.3
Clinical Practice Guidelines Published by the Agency for Health
Care Policy and Research, 1992–1995

Acute pain management
Pressure ulcers—prediction and prevention
Urinary incontinence
Cataract in adults
Depression in primary care—detection, diagnosis, and treatment
Sickle-cell disease—screening, diagnosis, and management
Evaluation and management of early HIV infection
Benign prostatic hyperplasia—diagnosis and treatment
Management of cancer pain
Unstable angina[a]
Congestive heart failure
Otitis media with effusion
Mammography quality standards
Low back pain
Pressure ulcer treatment

[a]Cosponsored by the National Heart, Lung, and Blood Institute of the National
Institutes of Health.

Table 22.4
An Evidence-Based Approach to Guideline Development:
Rating the Strength and Quality of the Recommendations and Evidence[a]

Strength of recommendations
  A. There is good evidence to support the recommendation that the condition be specifically considered in
     a periodic health examination.
  B. There is fair evidence to support the recommendation that the condition be specifically considered in a
     periodic health examination.
  C. There is poor evidence regarding the inclusion of the condition in the periodic health examination, but
     recommendations may be made on other grounds.
  D. There is fair evidence to support the recommendation that the condition be excluded from
     consideration in a periodic health examination.
  E. There is good evidence to support the recommendation that the condition be excluded from
     consideration in a periodic health examination.
Quality of evidence
  I: Evidence obtained from at least one properly designed randomized controlled trial.
  II-1: Evidence obtained from well-designed controlled trials without randomization.
  II-2: Evidence obtained from well-designed cohort or case–control analytic studies, preferably from more
        than one center or research group.
  II-3: Evidence obtained from multiple time series with or without the intervention. Dramatic results in
        uncontrolled experiments (such as the results of the introduction of pencillin treatment in the 1940s)
        could also be regarded as this type of evidence.
  III: Opinions of respected authorities, based on clinical experience, descriptive studies, or reports of
        expert committees.

[a]Source: U.S. Preventive Services Task Force. *Guide to Clinical Preventive Services.* Baltimore, Williams & Wilkins Co, 1989,
pp 387–388.

Financing Administration (HCFA) developed its Health Care Quality Improvement Program, reshaping the Medicare Peer Review Organization structure that had previously used chart review to identify quality problems into a continuous quality improvement model that looked at patterns of care and outcomes instead. Recent efforts to import explicitly developed guidelines into the process used by HCFA have been applauded by clinicians who believed previous guidelines used by this agency were arbitrary.

PRIVATE MEDICAL ORGANIZATIONS

Many medical specialty societies have sponsored, organized, and constructed clinical guidelines. Among the first were the American College of Physicians (ACP) through the Clinical Efficacy Assessment Project started in 1981 (Vibbert *et al.*, 1994), the American Academy of Pediatrics with its many committee statements and the "Red Book" on infectious diseases, the American College of Obstetricians and Gynecologists through its Technical Bulletins, and the American Academy of Family Physicians (AAFP) with its recommendations for the periodic health examination and its Task Force on Clinical Policies for Patient Care. By the early 1990s, many groups including the ACP, AAFP, the American Urologic Association, and the American Psychiatric Association were using the explicit method to produce evidence-based guidelines.

Other groups involved in guideline production were collaborative medical organizations such as the American Heart Association, which sponsors the advanced cardiac life support guideline and consensus conferences on topics such as carotid endarterectomy (Moore *et al.*, 1995), the American Cancer Society, which produces guidelines for cancer screening by convening a group of experts in a multidisciplinary consensus conference, and the American Diabetes Association. Managed care companies and insurance companies were also early entries into the field of guidelines, although many were reluctant to release the details of the guidelines used for utilization review and were likely to use small groups or even individuals to construct their guidelines, using global subjective judgment. Hospitals, spurred by the Joint Commission on the Accreditation of Health Care Organization's 1987 Agenda for Change, began developing clinical pathways that set ideal length of stay for certain diagnoses and defined procedures in operating rooms, labor and delivery suites, newborn nursery, and emergency rooms (Vibbert *et al.*, 1994). Some independent research organizations, notably the RAND Corporation, were involved in collaborative projects with specialty societies, the government, insurance companies, and providers to develop and evaluate guidelines. From 1991, RAND employed an evidence-based method that relied on formal group judgment. A nine-point appropriateness rating scale was used by an expert panel in a strategy that still uses subjective judgment but that provides details about how each panel member thought about the problem (Vibbert *et al.*, 1994).

CASE 22-4

Decisions about care for a small child with fever, but no obvious source of infection, have been controversial for years. Physicians don't want to overtreat or overtest, but small children cannot communicate their symptoms adequately, masking life-threatening infectious illness. An expert panel convened to develop a guideline for this scenario was unable to agree on two aspects of care, so after

testing to be sure that most parents could understand the issues, they issued a
guideline with two options, namely, for low-risk infants, 28–90 days old, with a
temperature of 103°F or higher and no identifiable source of the fever:

> *Option 1: blood culture, lumbar puncture, and antibiotic injection in the*
> *thigh*
> *Option 2: careful observation at home and return in 24 hours for reevalua-*
> *tion*

More than 70% of parents studied chose option 2 (Oppenheim et al., 1994); under
Eddy's classification, option 2 would be issued as a guideline, since parents'
preference is known and over 60% agree. This panel chose to use the label of
option instead.

——— PRACTICAL ASPECTS OF GUIDELINES ———

FLEXIBILITY

Guidelines have met with some resistance by practicing physicians, some of whom
call them "cookbook medicine," and some who are reluctant to change established practices, because of fear of lawsuit, fear of losing income when lucrative procedures are no
longer indicated, or inadequate continuing education efforts. Those who label guidelines
as cookbook medicine have been noted to know little about cooking. Some recipes require
exact timing, oven temperature, and ingredients, like a soufflé, while others allow for
individual creativity, such as chili and marinara sauce (Baughan, 1993). Some practice
guidelines require strict adherence and are based on a well-defined body of research and
well-known patient preferences, such as Advanced Cardiac Life Support (ACLS). Others
are more flexible because the best course of treatment is not yet known or because
patients' preferences vary, such as neonatal circumcision, timing of cataract surgery, and
choice of antiarrhythmic agents.

Central to the cries of "cookbook medicine" is a failure to understand the degree of
flexibility intended in practice guidelines. Eddy (1992d) has described a system to classify
guidelines by degree of flexibility. ACLS protocols, for example, are standards and
should be followed without variation in all clinical situations in which ACLS is indicated.
A guideline is considered a *standard* if the health and economic outcomes of the alternative interventions are sufficiently well known to permit meaningful decisions and there is
virtual unanimity about which intervention is preferred. More flexible, but still requiring
justification for not following, is a *guideline*. For these guidelines, health and economic
outcomes of the interventions are sufficiently well known to permit meaningful decisions
and an appreciable but not unanimous majority agree which intervention is preferred, as in
Case 22-4. In clinical practice, variations will be relatively common, up to 40%, and in
some cases are justified by differences in individual preferences. Other terms used as
synonyms for this intermediate degree of flexibility are *recommendations, relative indica-*
tions and *contraindications, relative criteria, parameters,* and *procedures of choice*
(Eddy, 1992d).

In many cases, either (1) the health and economic outcomes of the interventions are
not sufficiently well known to permit meaningful decisions, (2) preferences among the

outcomes are not known, (3) patients' preferences are divided among the alternative interventions, or (4) patients are indifferent about the alternative interventions (American Academy of Family Physicians, 1994b). In these situations, the guideline should be labeled an *option,* and clinicians should work with patients to determine the best course of action. Widespread use of this or another uniform system of identifying guidelines by degree of flexibility should help to relieve the concerns of some who believe physicians will be punished if they do not follow a guideline to the letter (Woolf, 1993) and who worry that guidelines will eliminate the "art" of medicine and individual innovation and creativity. When guidelines are labeled as options, payers and regulatory agencies should not sanction physicians and patients who choose alternatives. When guidelines are labeled as standards, physicians should follow them except in very unusual circumstances, such as the refusal of lifesaving blood transfusion by an adult Jehovah's Witness. Also important is the designation of the permanence of a guideline. When new science emerges, old guidelines may need revision. The plan for evaluation and need for revision should be part of every guideline.

CONFLICT OF INTEREST

Since guidelines are involved in decisions on which hinge large sums of money in healthcare, the potential for conflict of interest exists in the development, evaluation, and implementation processes. Participants in guidelines panels should reveal direct financial interest in the results of the panel deliberation, as well as the use of a certain intervention in practice, any role in development of intervention, organizational commitment to certain interventions, or a commitment to research involving an intervention including research funding sources (Phillips, 1994). Guidelines have been distributed that recommended a medication manufactured by a company funding the dissemination of the guidelines (Berg & Moy, 1992) and that recommended laboratory tests that were developed by a panel member. Clinicians should be aware of potential conflicts of interest when deciding whether to adopt a particular guideline into practice.

LEGAL ISSUES

Concerns that the use of clinical guidelines in practice will lead to more malpractice litigation have been addressed by many authors and by several states. Maine enacted in 1990 legislation creating a 5-year demonstration project making compliance with a practice parameter an affirmative defense in anesthesia, emergency medical care, radiology, and obstetrics/gynecology. The plaintiff can sue for failure to comply with a guideline as well. The state government will track liability claims from 1992 to 1997 to determine the effect of guidelines on medical malpractice litigation (Vibbert *et al.,* 1994; Texas Medical Association, 1994). In 1992, Florida mandated development of practice parameters to provide for tort reform in a similar system where compliance with the parameter is a legal defense; Vermont and Minnesota established practice guidelines as standard for medical malpractice claims in 1992 (Texas Medical Association, 1994). The widespread use of terminology identifying the degree of flexibility physicians should have in applying various guidelines in the clinical settings should alleviate negative effects of guidelines on litigation. The ability to use adherence to a guideline, regardless of outcome, as a defense should assist physicians. Another potential legal problem arising from these guidelines is antitrust violation. Some groups have disseminated guidelines stating that only physicians of certain specialties should be privileged to perform certain procedures. Should this policy be adopted by a hospital or managed care organization, anticompetitive behavior could be alleged (Eddy, 1992d).

DOES THE USE OF GUIDELINES IN CLINICAL PRACTICE IMPROVE PATIENTS' OUTCOMES?

For many, this remains the critical question (Woolf, 1992, 1993). Initial studies of physician behavior after publication of guidelines for treating asthma, hypercholesterolemia, and chest pain have inferred that the appearance of a new guideline in the traditional medical journals is not sufficient to bring about change in practice (Rosser & Palmer, 1993; Gorton *et al.*, 1995; Lewis *et al.*, 1995). Widely cited works such as the Guideline to Clinical Preventive Services were known by only 60% of physicians in one study (Flocke *et al.*, 1994). Innovative methods of disseminating guidelines such as multimedia presentations, continual reminder approaches, and a "detailing" model of face-to-face or telephonic education about guidelines by another physician, similar to the sales methods used by pharmaceutical companies who wish to influence prescribing behavior, have shown better response, but are expensive (Gorton *et al.*, 1995). Traditional continuing education practices have consisted of day- or week-long lecture series, often sponsored by the specialty societies, state and local medical associations, hospitals, or the pharmaceutical industry. Information about guidelines is only beginning to appear in these formats for updating clinical skills. The availability of full-text guidelines on computer disk, CD-ROM, and on-line computer services may improve penetration of guidelines into the practices of those physicians who use computers in their continuing education. The American Medical Association has asked that guidelines meet minimum standards for acceptability by physicians before they are included on the National Library of Medicine's MedLine (Texas Medical Association, 1994; American Medical Association, 1995).

Large-scale studies that evaluate the effect of an implemented guideline on patient outcomes and cost are needed to determine whether guidelines will actually improve care (Goldberg *et al.*, 1994; Lomas, 1993). Projects are also under way to develop standards for assessing the quality of guidelines and to set a uniform style for presenting guidelines in abstract and in full format (Hayward *et al.*, 1992a,b; Vibbert *et al.*, 1994; Gorton *et al.*, 1995).

CASE 22-5

A multispecialty group practice that operates in a capitated managed care environment has spent more money than expected caring for patients with type II diabetes mellitus. The director of clinical guidelines for this group convenes a panel of physicians and other providers nominated by each section in the group to develop treatment policies for diabetic patients, including diet, medications, and exercise. The panel uses the explicit method to develop guidelines for use by primary care physicians, endocrinologists, dietitians, pharmacists, and physical therapists in the group.

The director of clinical guidelines then seeks input from each panel member as to how the guidelines should be introduced to the practice. It is decided to have each specialty section's representative bring the guidelines back to the sections during scheduled meetings, along with a set of options for evaluating the guideline. The evaluation strategies include counting hospital days for patients with diabetes mellitus, measuring total cost of care, counting days the patient misses work, and tracking complications of diabetes mellitus such as amputations, retinopathy, and myocardial infarctions. All group members are then asked to attend a meeting at which voting is used to determine which method is used to measure the guideline's effect on patient outcomes. The group decides to measure total cost of care and days the patient misses work. Significant disagreement is expressed over the time period needed to study the effect of the new guideline and the period to review for preguideline comparison.

At the group practice's annual meeting, a progress report notes that the guideline has been developed and implemented and that total cost of care is slightly lower while patient days at work has improved. A physician at the meeting asks whether patient satisfaction was measured. The group agrees to add this to the next phase of evaluation and to repeat the evaluation for a 1-month period each year.

CONCLUSION

Federal and state governments, specialty societies, and insurance companies now look to guidelines as a strategy to increase control over medical practice and cost. Physicians' views vary, often in relation to the degree of experience with guidelines. The field of clinical guidelines is out of its infancy, but is still in its adolescence, lacking a coherent approach to the process of development, inclusion of patient preference assessment methods, and methods to incorporate preference into guideline implementation. Many guidelines now in use have been developed using global subjective judgment, expert opinion, and administrative directive rather than newer, more reliable explicit, evidence-based methods. Guidelines with conflicting recommendations have been issued by different specialty groups, and no organized approach to resolving these disputes exists. Plans for updating are lacking from most guidelines. Many organizations including group practices are formulating their own guidelines, then using outcomes research methods to measure the effect of the guidelines on clinical practice, such as in Case 22-5. Outcomes are studied and the result used to redesign the guideline. This is an example of the total quality management (TQM) process.

Dissemination of high-quality guidelines is not yet a predictable part of continuing medical education, and those physicians not routinely accessing electronic media are often not aware of many published guidelines. Electronic medical records lag years behind electronic billing, even though technology could now support in-office implementation of guidelines with tracking of outcomes. Better use of research dollars to focus on studies needed to fill knowledge gaps in pertinent clinical areas and better use of the continuing education process to introduce physicians to guidelines and provide tools for implementation and tracking results will improve physicians' ability to provide high-quality care for patients. The number of clinical questions for which good-quality guidelines are available is relatively small. Over time, every medical textbook should be rewritten or perhaps phased out, with the traditional format of single authors for each chapter being abandoned. Ideally, the "textbook" of the future will consist of evidence-based guidelines developed with the explicit method by groups including primary care physicians, subspecialists, consumers, methodologists, and pertinent allied healthcare providers, available on-line with clear designation of flexibility, date of publication, and plans for updating.

---------------- CASES FOR DISCUSSION ----------------

CASE 1

A young professional couple are expecting their first baby, and during a prenatal visit with you express their plan for intermittent fetal monitoring and ambulation during labor. The hospital at which you deliver babies has a policy requiring continuous electronic fetal monitoring for all labors. The U.S. Preventive Services Task Force Report includes a chapter on screening for fetal distress. Their recommendation reads: "Fetal heart rate should be measured by auscultation on all women in labor to detect signs of fetal distress. Electronic fetal monitoring should not be performed routinely on all women in labor. It should be reserved for pregnancies at increased risk for fetal distress" (p. 233). The NIH consensus development conference recommended in 1979 that electronic fetal monitoring be used in high-risk pregnancies, and considered periodic auscultation acceptable for women at low risk for fetal distress. However, continuous electronic fetal monitoring is used in nearly half of all live births in the United States (Placek et al., 1984) and many physicians and nurses believe that using the electronic monitors lowers their risk of malpractice suit. Evidence that the decrease in ambulation and turning during labor for women with electronic monitoring leads to longer labor and an increase in the cesarean section rate has been ignored by many hospital staffs (Placek et al., 1984; McKay & Mahan, 1984; Leveno et al., 1986).

1. *How are most hospital policies made?*
2. *As this couple's physician, you believe that intermittent auscultation is appropriate and that the couple understands the risk and benefit involved in the decision. How will you approach the nursing director in the labor and delivery suite to assist the couple in having the birth experience they desire?*
3. *Is the risk of losing a malpractice lawsuit higher if electronic monitoring is not used?*

CASE 2

A 3-year-old son of divorced parents has had numerous ear infections and never clears the middle ear effusions that develop after acute infection. The custodial parent has been fired for missing work when taking the child to the physician. This parent demands that the physician refer the child for ear tube placement surgery. You have been taught in medical school that tympanostomy tubes should be reserved for children who are having hearing loss; this child is unable to cooperate with your office audiogram testing, and the state Medicaid program that insures this child will not pay for brain-stem audio-evoked response hearing testing. The AHCPR guideline entitled Managing Otitis Media with Effusion in Young Children *states that tube placement is appropriate if the effusion has not cleared in 6 months (Otitis Media with Effusion Guideline Panel, 1994). The American Academy of Pediatrics published a 1984 policy on middle ear disease and language development that recommends assessment of hearing and monitoring of development of language skills in children with frequently recurring acute otitis media and/or middle ear effusion persisting for longer than 3 months (American Academy of Pediatrics, 1984).*

1. *Despite your belief that a trial of suppression antibiotics may clear the effusion and your assessment that the child has normal language development, should you refer for surgery?*
2. *What are the benefits and dangers of ear tube surgery?*

3. *What are the costs of brain-stem audio-evoked response versus ear tube surgery? Should the state Medicaid program pay for the safer one if it is more expensive?*

CASE 3

You admitted a 58-year-old man to the hospital with the diagnosis of deep venous thrombosis. You have been taught that hospitalization for anticoagulant therapy is necessary until the prothrombin time is therapeutic. The hospital's utilization review nurse wants the patient to go home and have daily office visits for prothrombin time tests, since his insurance pays the hospital on a per-diagnosis basis. The patient wants to stay in the hospital since his wife's employer won't grant her time off work to care for him at home.

1. *Is it safe for patients to receive anticoagulants at home and travel to an office for lab tests?*
2. *What is the responsibility of the physician in disputes about length of stay and insurance reimbursement?*
3. *Is home healthcare nursing a safe alternative?*
4. *What policies have addressed the safety of home versus inpatient treatment of deep venous thrombosis?*

CASE 4

A patient with chronic pain after a crush injury to his leg has taken narcotics and nonsteroidal anti-inflammatory drugs for several years with only fair pain control. Some of the emergency room staff have voiced concern to you that the patient may be addicted to narcotics, since he has asked for refills from emergency room physicians. He has just had an emergency appendectomy, and as his surgeon you are concerned about postoperative pain control. One of the floor nurses tells you he knows the patient from the ER and that he does not want to administer any narcotics to the patient. You consult the AHCPR guideline on acute pain management and learn that restlessness and tachycardia can be caused by undertreated pain or opioid withdrawal, and that strategies for managing this patient's postoperative pain should include avoidance of opioid agonist-antagonist that might precipitate withdrawal, use of a "tamper-resistant" patient-controlled analgesia pump delivery system, adjunct therapies such as nonsteroidal anti-inflammatory drugs, transcutaneous nerve stimulators, and limits to the negotiation about drug choices (Acute Pain Management Guideline Panel, 1992). You ask that a physician from the hospital's pain management team consult regarding the patient's care.

1. *Why do some clinicians object to administering narcotic analgesics to patients in acute pain who have substance abuse problems?*
2. *What are the risks to a physician who prescribes narcotics to a patient who is addicted to them? To a physician who withholds narcotics to this patient in acute pain?*
3. *How can a clinical guideline assist in resolving the conflict between the nurse and patient in this situation?*
4. *How does a guideline assist in discussing treatment options with a patient?*
5. *How should this patient's substance abuse be treated during this hospitalization?*

CASE 5

A 35-year-old man in your practice has unipolar mood disorder and wants to take a medication with few side effects. He is afraid of fluoxitine because of media reports and wants to know if other medications would work as well with greater safety. The American Psychiatric Association's guide-

line on the treatment of depression recommends any serotonin-specific uptake inhibitor (SSRI) drug as first line, but the patient's insurance company will only pay for tricyclic antidepressants.

1. *What is the appropriate initial medication for this patient?*
2. *How does the physician choose among acceptable alternatives?*
3. *Considering the cost of the drug, cost of monitoring the drug, office visits, and the patient's well-being, are SSRIs more expensive than tricyclic antidepressants?*

RECOMMENDED READINGS

Eddy DM: *A Manual for Assessing Health Practices and Designing Practice Policies: The Explicit Approach.* Philadelphia, American College of Physicians, 1992.

> Dr. Eddy provides a comprehensive guide to policy development and discussion of statistical techniques, preference assessment, and other aspects of clinical guideline development.

Sackett DL, Haynes RB, Guyatt GH, Tugwell P: *Clinical Epidemiology: A Basic Science for Clinical Medicine,* 2nd ed. Boston, Little, Brown & Co, 1991.

> This text presents a valuable guide for literature searching strategies and provides the reader with tools for critical appraisal of the medical literature, skills vital to sound guideline formation.

U.S. Preventive Services Task Force. *Guide to Clinical Preventive Services,* 2nd ed. Report of the U.S. Preventive Services Task Force. Baltimore, Williams & Wilkins Co, 1996.

> The first comprehensive text to discuss the scientific evidence behind the many things physicians have done routinely for patients, this guide notes that many commonly used tests and treatments are not supported by research. The approach to prevention is presented in a patient-centered fashion, with age- and risk-specific strategies for effective preventive care provided.

References

Abernathy CM, Hamm RM: *Surgical Scripts: Master Surgeons Think Aloud about 43 Common Surgical Problems.* Philadelphia, Hanley & Belfus, 1995.

Abrahamson S: Research in continuing medical education: An historical review. *Mobius* 4:11–17, 1984.

Acute Pain Management Guideline Panel. *Acute Pain Management: Operative or Medical Procedures and Trauma. Clinical Practice Guideline.* Rockville, Md, US Department of Health and Human Services, Public Health Service, Agency for Health Care Policy and Research, 1992. AHCPR Publication No. 92-0032.

Adams EK, Zuckerman S: Variation in the growth and incidence of medical malpractice claims. *J Health Polit Policy Law* 9:475–488, 1984.

Adams WR: *Developing Reading Versatility,* ed 6. New York, Harcourt Brace Jovanovich College Publishers, 1983.

American Academy of Family Physicians, Commission on Public Health and Scientific Affairs. *Age Charts for Periodic Health Examination.* Kansas City, Mo, American Academy of Family Physicians, 1994a.

American Academy of Family Physicians. Positions on the clinical aspects of medical practice, 1994b.

American Academy of Pediatrics. Committee report on middle ear disease and language development, 1984.

American Academy of Pediatrics, Committee on Practice and Ambulatory Care. Recommendations for preventive pediatric health care. *Pediatrics* 96:373–374, 1995.

American Academy of Pediatrics. Practice parameter: Management of hyperbilirubinemia in the healthy term newborn. *Pediatrics* 94:558–565, 1994.

American Cancer Society. Report on the cancer-related health checkup. *CA* 30:194–240, 1980.

American Cancer Society. *Summary of American Cancer Society Recommendations for Early detection of cancer in asymptomatic people.* Atlanta, American Cancer Society, 1992.

American Cancer Society Advisory Group on Preventive Health Care Reminder Systems. Computerized health maintenance tracking systems: A clinician's guide to necessary and optional features. *J Am Board Fam Pract* 8:221–229, 1995.

American College of Obstetricians and Gynecologists. *The Obstetrician-Gynecologist and Primary Preventive Health Care.* Washington, DC, American College of Obstetricians and Gynecologists, 1993.

American College of Physicians. Periodic health examination: A guide for designing individualized preventive health care in the asymptomatic patient. *Ann Intern Med* 95:729–732, 1981.

American College of Physicians Task Force on Adult Immunization and Infectious Disease Society of America. *Guide for Adult Immunization,* ed 3. Philadelphia, American College of Physicians, 1994.

American Heart Association. *Textbook of Advanced Cardiac Life Support.* Dallas, American Heart Association, 1987.

American Medical Association Policy Compendium, 1995.

American Medical Association. *The Physician's Recognition Award: 1993 Information Booklet.* Chicago, American Medical Association, 1993.

Antonelli MA: Usefulness of a data-collection form in learning physical diagnosis. *Acad Med* 68:171, 1993.

Applegate WB, Blass JP, Williams TF: Instruments for the functional assessment of older patients. *N Engl J Med* 32:1207–1221, 1990.

Arseneau R: Exit rounds: A reflection exercise. *Acad Med* 70:8, 1995.

Arseneau R, Rodenburg D: The developmental perspective: Cultivating ways of thinking, in Pratt DD (ed): *Five Perspectives of Teaching in Adult and Higher Education.* Melbourne, Florida, Krieger, in press.

Asken MJ, Raham DC: Resident performance and sleep deprivation: A review. *J Med Educ* 58:382–388, 1983.

Baldwin LM, Larson EH, Hart LG, *et al:* Characteristics of physicians with obstetric malpractice claims experience. *Obstet Gynecol* 78:1050–1054, 1991.

Baldwin LM, Greer T, Wu R, *et al:* Differences in the obstetric malpractice claims filed by Medicaid and non-Medicaid patients. *J Am Board Fam Pract* 2:263–267, 1992.

Balint M: *The Doctor, His Patient and the Illness,* ed 2. New York, International Universities Press Inc, 1964.

Bandura A: Self-efficacy: Toward a unifying theory of behavioral change. *Psychol Rev* 84(2):191–215, 1977.

Banff Summary Statement. *Proceedings of the Banff Conference, Banff, Canada. Exploring New Frontiers in CME.* Hamilton, Canada, McMaster University Publishers, 1989, p 49.

Barsky AJ: The paradox of health. *N Engl J Med* 318:414–418, 1988.

Bass MJ, Buck CW, Turner L, Pickie G, Robinson HC: The physician's actions and outcomes of illness in family practice. *J Fam Pract* 23:43–47, 1986.

Bates B, Bickley LS, Hoekelman RA: *Physical Examination and History Taking,* ed 6. Philadelphia, JB Lippincott Co, 1995.

Bates GW: Faculty development: A continuing process. *J Med Educ* 63:490, 1988.

Baughan D: Assessing process. Agency for Health Care Policy and Research Primary Care Conference, Atlanta, 1993.

Becker E: *The Denial of Death.* New York, Free Press, 1973.

Becker L, Iverson DC, Reed FM, Calonge N, Miller RS, Freeman WL: The ambulatory sentinel practice network: Patients with new headache in primary care: A report from ASPN. *J Fam Pract* 27:41–47, 1988.

Beckman H, Frankel R: The effect of physician behavior on the collection of data. *Ann Intern Med* 101:692–696, 1984.

Beckman H, Markakis K, Suchman A, Frankel R: The doctor–patient relationship and malpractice: Lessons from plaintiff depositions. *Arch Intern Med* 154(12):1365–1370, 1994.

Beckmann CRB, Lipscomb GH, Williford L, *et al:* Gynecological teaching associates in the 1990s. *Med Educ* 26:105–109, 1992.

Belcher DW: Implementing preventive services; success and failure in an outpatient trial. *Arch Intern Med* 159:2533–2541, 1990.

Bell HA, Roberts R: American Academy of Family Physicians Clinical Policies Course, 1989.

Berg AO, Moy JG: Guidelines for the diagnosis and management of asthma: A policy review. *J Am Board Fam Pract* 5:629–684, 1992.

Berg I: *Family-Based Services: A Solution Focused Approach.* New York, WW Norton & Co Inc, 1994.

Bergus GR, Chapman GB, Gjerde C, Elstein AS: Clinical reasoning about new symptoms despite preexisting disease: Sources of error and order effects. *Fam Med* 27:314–320, 1995.

Berlin EA, Fowkes WC: A teaching framework for cross-cultural health care: Application in family practice. *West J Med* 139:934–938, 1983.

Bigos S, Boyer O, Braen G, *et al: Acute Low Back Problems Guideline Panel. Acute Low Back Problems in Adults. Clinical Practice Guideline, Quick Reference Guide No. 14.* Rockville, Md, US Department of Health and Human Services, Public Health Service, Agency for Health Care Policy and Research, AHCPR Publication No. 95-0643, December, 1994.

Billings J, Stoeckle J: *The Clinical Encounter.* Chicago, Year Book Medical Publishers Inc, 1993.

Birdwell BG, Herbers JE, Kroenke K: Evaluating chest pain. *JAMA* 153:1991–1995, 1993.

Blazer D: Depression in the elderly. *N Engl J Med* 320:164–166, 1989.

Blendon RJ, Edwards JN, Hyams AL: Making the critical choices. *JAMA* 267:2509–2520, 1992.

Boss P, Caron W, Horbal J: Alzheimer's disease and ambiguous loss, in Chilman C, Nunnally E, Cox F (eds): *Chronic Illness and Disability: Families in Trouble Series,* vol 2. Beverly Hills, Calif, Sage Publications Inc, 1988.

Boszormenyi-Nagy I, Spark G: *Invisible Loyalties: Reciprocity in Intergenerational Family Therapy.* New York, Harper & Row Publishers Inc, 1973.

Bovbjerg RR, Petronis KR: The relationship between physicians' malpractice claim history and later claims: Does the past predict the future? *JAMA* 272:1421–1426, 1994.

Bowen M: *Family Therapy in Clinical Practice.* New York, Jason Aronson Inc, 1978.

Brennan TA, Leape LL, Laird NM, *et al:* Incidence of adverse events and negligence in hospitalized patients: Results of the Harvard Medical Practice Study I. *N Engl J Med* 324:370–376, 1991.

Breslow L, Somers AR: The lifetime health-monitoring program: A practical approach to preventive medicine. *N Engl J Med* 292:601–608, 1977.

Brinton LA, Schairer C: Estrogen replacement and breast cancer risk. *Epidemiol Rev* 15:66–79, 1993.

Brock CD, Salinsky JV: Empathy: An essential skill for understanding the physician–patient relationship in clinical practice. *Fam Med* 25:245–248, 1993.

Brody H: *Ethical Decisions in Medicine,* ed 2. Boston, Little, Brown & Co, 1981.

Buckman R: *How to Give Bad News.* Baltimore, Johns Hopkins University Press, 1992.

Burns D: *Feeling Good: The New Mood Therapy.* New York, Avon Books Inc, 1980.

Byyny RL, Adams K: The logic of clinical problem solving: Differential diagnosis, in Beck P (ed): *Cases in Clinical Reasoning.* Chicago, Year Book Medical Publishers Inc, 1981, pp 14–15.

Cadman EC: The academic physician-investigator. *Ann Intern Med* 120:401–410, 1994.

California Medical Association. *Report of the Medical Insurance Feasibility Study.* San Francisco, California Medical Association, 1977.

Canadian Task Force on the Periodic Health Examination. The periodic health examination. *Can Med Assoc J* 121:1194–1254, 1979.

Canadian Task Force on the Periodic Health Examination. The periodic health examination: 2; 1987 update. *Can Med Assoc J* 138:619–628, 1988.

Canadian Task Force on the Periodic Health Examination, 1991 update 1. Screening for cognitive impairment in the elderly. *Can Med Assoc J* 144:425–431, 1991.

Candy PC: *Self-Direction for Lifelong Learning.* San Francisco, Jossey-Bass Inc Publishers, 1991.

Cantor JC, Baker KC, Hughes RG: Preparedness for practice: Young physicians' views of their professional education. *JAMA* 270:2035–2040, 1993.

Cantrell T: How do medical school staff learn to teach? *Lancet* 2:724–727, 1973.

Cappella JN: The management of conversational interaction in adults and infants, in Knapp JL, Miller GR (eds): *Handbook of Interpersonal Communication,* ed 2. Beverly Hills, Calif, Sage Publications, 1994, pp 380–418.

Carney PA, Dietrich AJ, Landgraff J, O'Connor GT: Tools, teamwork, and tenacity: An office system for cancer prevention. *J Fam Pract* 35:388–394, 1992.

Carney PA, Dietrich AJ, Freeman DH Jr, Mott LA: The period health examination provided to asymptomatic older women: An assessment using standardized patients. *Ann Intern Med* 119:129–135, 1993.

Carruthers A: A force to promote bonding and well-being: Therapeutic touch and massage. *Prof Nurse* 7:297–300, 1992.

Carter EA, McGoldrick M (eds): *The Changing Family Life Cycle: A Framework for Family Therapy,* ed 2. Boston, Allyn & Bacon, 1989.

Cassileth BR, Zupkis RV, Sutton-Smith K, March V: Information and participation preferences among cancer patients. *Ann Intern Med* 92:832–836, 1980.

Cavanaugh SH: Connecting education and practice, in Curry L, Wergin JF, *et al* (eds): *Educating Professionals: Responding to New Expectations for Competence and Accountability.* San Francisco, Jossey-Bass Inc Publishers, 1993, pp 107–125.

Centor RM, Meier FA, Dalton HP: Throat cultures and rapid tests for diagnosis of group A streptococcal pharyngitis. *Ann Intern Med* 105:892–899, 1986.

Charles SC, Wilber JR, Kennedy KC: Physicians' self-reports of reactions to malpractice litigation. *Am J Psychiatry* 141:563–566, 1984.

Chilman CS, Nunnally EW, Cox FM (eds): *Chronic Illness and Disability: Families in Trouble Series,* vol 2. Beverly Hills, Calif, Sage Publications Inc, 1988.

Christensen-Szalanski JJ: Discount functions and the measurement of patients' values: Women's decisions during childbirth. *Med Decis Mak* 4(1):47–58, 1984.

Clark LT: Improving compliance and increasing control of hypertension: Needs of special hypertensive populations. *Am Heart J* 121:664–669, 1991.

Cobb LA, Werner JA, Trobaugh GB: Sudden cardiac death: A decade's experience with out-of-hospital resuscitation. *Mod Concepts Cardiovasc Dis* 49:31–36, 1980.

Cohen-Cole SA: *The Medical Interview: The Three-Function Approach.* St. Louis, Mo, Mosby–Year Book Inc, 1991.

Colditz GA, Hankinson SE, Hunter DJ, Willett WC, Manson JE, Stampfer MJ, Hennekens C, Rosuer B, Speizer FE: The use of estrogens and progestins and the risk of breast cancer in post menopausal women. *N Engl J Med* 332:1589–1593, 1995.

Collins A, Brown JS, Holum A: Cognitive apprenticeship: Making thinking visible. *Am Educ* Winter:4–46, 1991.

Collins RD: *Differential Diagnosis in Primary Care*. Philadelphia, JB Lippincott Co, 1987, pp xii–xiii.

Combrinck-Graham L: A developmental model for family systems. *Fam Process* 24:139–150, 1985.

Council on Graduate Medical Education (COGME). *Recommendations to Improve Access to Health Care through Physician Workforce Reform: Fourth Report to Congress and the Department of Health and Human Services*. Washington, DC, US Department of Health and Human Services, January 1994.

Council on Scientific Affairs, American Medical Association. Users and uses of patient records: Report of the Council on Scientific Affairs. *Arch Fam Med* 2:678–681, 1993.

Crandall SJS: The role of continuing medical education in changing and learning. *J Cont Educ Health Prof* 10:339–348, 1990.

Cummins RO, Ornato JP, Thies WH, Pepe PE: Improving survival from sudden cardiac arrest: The chain of survival concept. *Circulation* 83:1832–1847, 1991.

Curtis P: Clinical reasoning in family practice, in Sloane PD, Slatt LM, Curtis P (eds): *Essentials of Family Medicine*. Baltimore, Williams & Wilkins Co, 1993.

Cutler P: *Problem Solving in Clinical Medicine: From Data to Diagnosis,* ed 2. Baltimore, Williams & Wilkins Co, 1985, p 199.

Davis DA: The clinical environment, in Fox RD and Maxmanian PE (eds): *Changing and Learning in the Lives of Physicians*. New York, Praeger Publishers, 1989, pp 99–109.

DeGowin RL: *Diagnostic Examination*. New York, McGraw–Hill Book Co, 1994.

DeGowin EL, DeGowin, RL: *Bedside Diagnostic Examination*. New York, The Macmillan Company, 1995.

DeNeef P: Selective testing for streptococcal pharyngitis in adults. *J Fam Pract* 25:347–353, 1987.

Department of Clinical Epidemiology and Biostatistics, McMaster University. Clinical disagreement: I. How often it occurs and why. *Can Med Assoc J* 123:499–504, 1980a.

Department of Clinical Epidemiology and Biostatistics, McMaster University. Clinical disagreement: II. How to avoid it and how to learn from one's mistakes. *Can Med Assoc J* 123(7):613–617, 1980b.

Depression Guideline Panel. *Depression in Primary Care*. 1993.

Dickey LL: Promoting preventive care with patient-held minirecords: A review. *Patient Educ Couns* 20:37–47, 1993.

Dickey LL, DiGuiseppi C, Atkins D: *Preventive Medicine I. Monograph, Edition No. 199, Home Study Self-Assessment program*. Kansas City, Mo.: American Academy of Family Physicians, December 1995. Updated from U.S. Dept. of Health and Human Services. Put Prevention into Practice education and action kit. Washington, D.C.: U.S. Government Printing Office, 1994.

Dickey LL, Kamerow DB: The put prevention into practice campaign: Office tools and beyond. *J Fam Pract* 39:321–323, 1994.

Dickey LL, Kamerow DB: Primary care providers use of office tools in the provision of preventive care. *Arch Fam Med* 1996, 5:399–404.

DiMatteo MR, Hays R: The significance of patients' perceptions of physician conduct: A study of patient satisfaction in a family practice center. *J Community Health* 6:18–34, 1980.

Doherty WJ, Baird M (eds): *Family-Centered Medical Care: A Clinical Casebook*. New York, Guilford Press, 1987.

Donnelly WJ: Righting the medical record: Transforming chronicle into story. *JAMA* 260:823–825, 1988.

Donnelly WJ, Brauner DJ: Why SOAP is bad for the medical record. *Arch Intern Med* 152:481–484, 1992.

Doyle DL, Stern PN: Negotiating self-care in rehabilitation nursing. *Rehab Nurs* 17:319–321, 326, 1992.

Eddy DM: Clinical decision making: From theory to practice. Cost-effectiveness analysis: Is it up to the task? *JAMA* 267:3342–3348, 1992a.

Eddy DM: Clinical decision making: From theory to practice. Cost-effectiveness analysis: Will it be accepted? *JAMA* 268:132–136, 1992b.

Eddy DM: Clinical decision making: From theory to practice. Cost-effectiveness analysis: The inside story. *JAMA* 268:2575–2582, 1992c.

Eddy DM: *A Manual for Assessing Health Practices and Designing Practice Policies: The Explicit Approach*. Philadelphia, American College of Physicians, 1992d.

Eddy DM: Clinical decision making: From theory to practice: Principles for making difficult decisions in difficult times. *JAMA* 271:1792–1798, 1994.

Egbert L, Battit G, Welch C, Bartlett M: Reduction of post-operative pain by encouragement and instruction of patients. *N Engl J Med* 270:825–827, 1964.

Eisenberg JM: Clinical economics: A guide to the economic analysis of clinical practices. *JAMA* 262:2879–2886, 1989.

Eizenberg N: Approaches to learning anatomy: Developing a programme for preclinical medical students, in Ramsden P (ed): *Improving Learning: New Perspectives.* London, Kogan Page, 1988, pp 178–198.

Ellis A: How to deal with your most difficult client: You. *J Ration Emot Ther* 1(1):3–8, 1983.

Ende J: Feedback in clinical medical education. *JAMA* 250:777–781, 1983.

Engel GL: The need for a new medical model: A challenge for biomedicine. *Science* 196:129–136, 1977.

Engel GL: The clinical application of the biopsychosocial model. *Am J Psychol* 137:535–544, 1980.

Entman SS, Glass CA, Hickson GB, *et al:* The relationship between malpractice claims history and subsequent obstetric care. *JAMA* 272:1588–1591, 1994.

Epstein O, Perkins GD, de Bono DP, Goodson A: *Clinical Examination.* London, Gower Medical Publishing, 1992.

Eraker SA, Politser P: How decisions are reached: Physician and patient. *Ann Intern Med* 97:262–268, 1982.

Ersek M: Examining the process and dilemmas of reality negotiation. *Image J Nurs Scholarship* 24:19–25, 1992.

Ewigman BG, Crane JP, Frigoletto FD, LeFevre ML, Bain RP, McNellis D: The radius study group: Effect of prenatal ultrasound screening on perinatal outcome. *N Engl J Med* 329:821–827, 1993.

Fischer PM, Schwartz MP, Richards JW, Goldstein AO, Riojas TH: Brand logo recognition by children aged 3 to 6 years. *JAMA* 266:3145–3148, 1991.

Fisher R, Ury W, Patton B: *Getting to Yes: Negotiating Agreement without Giving in,* ed 2. New York, Penguin Books, 1991.

Fishman E, Turkheimer E, DeGood DE: Touch relieves stress and pain. *J Behav Med* 18:69–79, 1995.

Fitzgerald FT: Physical diagnosis versus modern technology—A review. *West J Med* 152:377–382, 1990.

Flocke SA, Stange KC, Fedirko TL: Dissemination of information about the US Preventive Services Task Force guidelines. *Arch Fam Med* 3:1006–1008, 1994.

Folstein MF, Folstein SE, McHugh PR: Mini-mental state: A practical method for grading the cognitive state of patients for the clinician. *J Psychiatr Res* 12:189–198, 1975.

Fox RD: New research agendas for CME: Organizing principles for the study of self-directed curricula for change. *J Cont Educ Health Prof* 11:155–167, 1991.

Fox RD, Craig JL: Future directions in research on physicians as learners, in Davis DA, Fox RD (eds): *The Physician as Learner: Linking Research to Practice.* Chicago, American Medical Association, 1994, pp 111–118.

Fox RD, Mazmanian PE, Putnam RW: *Changing and Learning in the Lives of Physicians.* New York, Praeger Publishers, 1989.

Fox RD, Davis DA, Wentz DK: The case for research on continuing medical education, in Davis DA, Fox RD (eds): *The Physician as Learner: Linking Research to Practice.* Chicago, American Medical Association, 1994, pp 15–24.

Fox SA, Siv AL, Stein JA: The importance of physician communication on breast cancer screening of older women. *Arch Intern Med* 154:2058–2068, 1994.

Frame PS, Carlson SJ: A critical review of periodic health screening using specific screening criteria. *J Fam Pract* 2:29–36, 1975.

Framo JL: Family of origin as therapeutic resource for adults in marital and family therapy: You can and should go home again. *Fam Process* 15:193–210, 1976.

Freeman J (ed): *Prenatal and Perinatal Factors Associated with Brain Disorders.* Bethesda, USDHHS NIH Publication No. 85-1149, 1985.

Friedman LC, Nelson DV, Webb JA, *et al:* Dispositional optimism, self-efficacy, and health beliefs as predictors of breast self-examination. *Am J Prev Med* 10:130–135, 1994.

Furberg CD, Psaty BM, Meyer JV: Nifedipine: Dose related increase in mortality in patients with coronary heart disease. *Circulation* 92:1326–1331, 1995.

Gabel J, Jacich C, Williams K, *et al:* The commercial health insurance industry in transition. *Health Affairs* 6:47–48, 1987.

Gann PH, Hennekens CH, Stampfer MJ: A prospective evaluation of plasma prostate-specific antigen for detection of prostate cancer. *JAMA* 273:289–294, 1995.

Gartrell NK: Physicians report having sex, hearing about sex with patients. *Am Med News* 24:10, 1992.

Gendlin ET: *Focusing.* New York, Bantam Books Inc, 1981.

Gerteis M, Edgman-Levitan S, Daley J, Delbanco TL (eds): *Through the Patient's Eyes: Understanding and Promoting Patient-Centered Care.* San Francisco, Jossey-Bass Inc Publishers, 1993.

Geyman JP: Climate for research in family practice. *J Fam Pract* 7:69–74, 1978.

Gifford RW Jr: Evaluation of a hypertensive patient with emphasis on detecting curable causes. *Milbank Mem Fund Q* 47(2):170–186, 1969.

Glanville CL, Tiller CM: Implementing negotiating strategies into teen parenting programs. *J Natl Black Nurs Assoc* 4:45–54, 1990.

Glenn M: *Collaborative Health Care: A Family-Oriented Model.* New York, Praeger Publishers, 1987.

Goldberg HI, Cummings MA, Steinberg EP, Ricci EM, Shannon T, Soumerai SB, Mittman BS, Eisenberg J, Heck DA, Kaplan S, Kenzora JE, Vargus AM, Mulley AG, Rimer BK: Deliberations on the dissemination of PORT products: Translating research findings into improved patient outcomes. *Med Care* S32:JS90–95, 1994.

Goldman L, Goldman PA, Williams LW, Weinstein MC: Cost-effectiveness considerations in the treatment of heterozygous familial hypercholesterolemia with medications. *Am J Cardiol* 72(10):75D–79D, 1993.

Gorbien MJ, Bishop J, Beers MH, Norman D, Osterweil D, Rubenstein LZ: Iatrogenic illness in hospitalized elderly people. *JAGS* 40:1031–1042, 1992.

Gorton TA, Cranford CO, Golden WE, Walls RC, Pawelak JE: Primary care physicians' response to dissemination of practice guidelines. *Arch Fam Med* 4(2):135–142, 1995.

Gray DT, Fyler DC, Walker AM, Weinstein MC, Chalmers TC: Clinical outcomes and costs of transcatheter as compared with surgical closure of patent ductus arteriosus. *N Engl J Med* 329:1517–1523, 1993.

Green LA, Beck LA, Freeman WL, Elliott E, Iverson D, Reed FM: Spontaneous abortion in primary care: A report from ASPN. *J Am Board Fam Pract* 1:15–23, 1988.

Greenberger NJ, Hinthorn DR: *History Taking and Physical Examination: Essentials and Clinical Correlates.* St. Louis, Mosby–Year Book Publishers Inc, 1993.

Greenfield S, Kaplan S, Ware J: Expanding patient involvement in care. *Ann Intern Med* 102:520–528, 1985.

Greenfield S, Kayslan SH, Ware JE, Yamo EM, Frank HJI: Patient's participation in medical care: Effects on blood sugar control and quality of life in diabetes. *J Gen Intern Med* 3:448–457, 1988.

Griffith J, Griffith M: *The Body Speaks.* New York, Basic Books Inc, 1994.

Groves JG: Taking care of the hateful patient. *N Engl J Med* 298:583–587, 1978.

Grueninger UJ, Goldstein MG, Duff DF: A conceptual framework for interactive patient education in practice and clinic settings. *J Hum Hypertens* suppl 1:21–31, 1990.

Gruppen LD, Wolf FM, Van Voorhees C, Stross JK: Information seeking strategies and differences among primary care physicians. *Mobius* 7:18–26, 1987.

Gutheil TG, Burzstgia H, Brodsky A: Malpractice prevention through the sharing of uncertainty. *N Engl J Med* 311:49–51, 1984.

Guyatt GH, Pugsley SO, Sullivan MJ, Thompson PJ, Berman BL, Jones NL, Fallen EI, Taylor DW: Effects of encouragement on walking performance. *Thorax* 39:811–822, 1984.

Hahn DL, Roberts RG: PSA screening for asymptomatic prostate cancer: Truth in advertising. *J Fam Pract* 37:432–436, 1993.

Hale JA: *From HMO Movement to Managed Care Industry: The Future of HMOs in a Volatile Healthcare Market.* Minneapolis, InterStudy, 1988.

Hamm RM: Selection of verbal probabilities: A solution for some problems of verbal probability expression. *Org Behav Hum Decis Processes* 48:193–223, 1991.

Hammond M, Collins R: *Self-Directed Learning: Critical Practice.* New York, Nichols/GP Publishing, 1991, pp 13–14.

Hansson R, Remondet JH, Obrochta D, Bell L: The dissatisfied medical patient: Predictors of intent to change doctors. *Med Times,* 1988, pp 97–101.

Haynes RB, Taylor DW, Sacket DL (eds): *Compliance in Health Care.* Baltimore, Johns Hopkins University Press, 1979.

Hayward RSA, Steinberg EP, Ford DE, *et al:* Preventive guidelines. 114:758–783, 1991.

Hayward RSA, Tunis SR, Wilson MC, Bass EB, Rubin HR, Haynes RB: Guides for guidelines: Readers' guide to the critical appraisal of clinical practice guidelines. Working Paper for Johns Hopkins University School of Medicine and McMaster University Medical Center, February 26, 1992a.

Hayward RSA, Wilson MC, Tunis SR, Bass EB, Rubin HR, Levine DM, Steinberg EP: Clinicians' guide to guidelines: How to appraise and apply clinical practice guidelines. Practice guidelines workshop. Am Coll Physicians 73rd Annu Sess, March 28, 1992b.

Headache Study Group of the University of Western Ontario. Predictors of outcome in headache patients presenting to family physicians. *Headache* 26:285–294, 1986.

Helman CG: *Culture, Health and Illness: An Introduction for Health Professionals.* London, Butterworth–Heinemann Ltd, 1994.

Hendryx MS, Doebbeling BN, Kearns DL: Mental health treatment in primary care. *Fam Pract Res J* 14:127–137, 1994.

Henrich JB: The post-menopausal estrogen/breast cancer controversy. *JAMA* 268:1900–1902, 1992.

Herz F: The impact of death and serious illness on the family life cycle, in Carter EA, McGoldrick M (eds): *The Family Life Cycle: A Framework for Family Therapy*, ed 2. Boston, Allyn & Bacon Inc, 1989.

Hickson GB, Clayton EW, Entman SS, *et al:* Obstetricians' prior malpractice experience and patients' satisfaction with care. *JAMA* 272:1583–1587, 1994.

Hippocrates. *Hippocrates of the Epidemics.* Franklin, Pa, The Franklin Library, 1979.

Hitchcock MA, Ramsey CN Jr, Herring MA: Model for developing clinical teaching skills of family practice teachers. *J Fam Pract* 11(6):923–929, 1980.

Hoenig HM, Rubenstein LZ: Hospital-associated deconditioning and dysfunction. *JAGS* 39:220–222, 1991.

Holme I, Hjerman I, Helgeland A, Leren P: The Oslo study: Diet and antismoking advice: Additional results from a 5-year primary prevention trial in middle-aged men. *Prev Med* 14:279–292, 1985.

Hulka BS, Cassel JC, Kupper LL, Burdette JA: Communication, compliance, and concordance between physicians and patients with prescribed medications. *Am J Public Health* 66:847–853, 1976.

Illich I: The medicalization of life. *J Med Ethics* 1:73–77, 1975.

Imber-Black E: Rituals and the healing process, in Walsh F, McGoldrick M (eds): *Living beyond Loss. Death in the Family.* New York, WW Norton & Co Inc, 1991.

Inglehart JK: The struggle between managed care and fee-for-service practice. *N Engl J Med* 331:63–67, 1994.

Isselbacher KJ, Martin JB, Braunwald E, *et al* (eds): *Harrison's Principles of Internal Medicine,* ed 13. New York, McGraw–Hill Book Co, 1994, p 549.

Jackson LE: Understanding, eliciting and negotiating clients' multicultural health beliefs. *Nurse Practitioner* 18:30–43, 1993.

Jennett P, Jones DL, Mast TA, Egan K, Hotvedt MO: The characteristics of self-directed learning, in Davis DA, Fox RD (eds): *The Physician as Learner: Linking Research to Practice.* Chicago, American Medical Association, 1994, pp 47–65.

Johnson JD, Meischke H: Factors associated with adoption of mammography screening: Results of a cross-sectional and longitudinal study. *J Women's Health* 3:97–105, 1994.

Johnson K, Morrison EF: Control or negotiation: A health care challenge. *Nurs Admin Q* 17:27–33, 1993.

Judge RD, Zuidema GD, Fitzgerald FT: *Clinical Diagnosis: A Physiologic Approach.* Boston, Little, Brown & Co, 1989.

Kahneman D, Slovic P, Tversky A: *Judgment under Uncertainty: Heuristics and Biases.* London, Cambridge University Press, 1982.

Kalet A, Roberts JC, Fletcher R: How do physicians talk with their patients about risk? *J Gen Intern Med* 9:402–404, 1994.

Kaplan NM, Stamler J (eds): *Prevention of Coronary Heart Disease: Practical Management of the Risk Factors.* Philadelphia, Saunders, 1983.

Kasper JF, Mulley AG, Wennberg JE: Developing shared decision-making programs to improve the quality of health care. *Qual Rev Bull,* June 1992, pp 183–190.

Kassirer JP: Diagnostic reasoning. *Ann Intern Med* 110:894, 1989.

Kassirer JP, Gorry GA: Clinical problem solving: A behavioral analysis. *Ann Intern Med* 89:248–249, 1978.

Katon W, Von Korff M, Lin E, Bush T, Russo J, Lipscomb P, Wagner E: A randomized trial of psychiatric consultation with distressed high utilizers. *Gen Hosp Psychiatry* 14:86–98, 1992.

Katz S, Ford AB, Moskowitz RW, Jackson BA, Jaffe W: Studies of illness in the aged: The index of ADL: A standardized measure of biological and psychosocial function. *JAMA* 185:914–919, 1963.

Kazdin AE: *Single-Case Research Designs.* London, Oxford University Press, 1982.

Kern DC, Parrino TA, Korst DR: The lasting value of clinical skills. *JAMA* 254:70–76, 1985.

Kitchens J: Does this patient have an alcohol problem? *JAMA* 272:1782–1787, 1994.

Klachko DM, Reid JC: The effect of medical students of memorizing a physical examination routine. *J Med Educ* 50:628–630, 1975.

Kleinman AM: *The Illness Narratives: Suffering, Healing, and the Human Condition.* New York, Basic Books, Inc, 1988.

Kluckhohn FR: Variations in the basic values of family systems, in Bell NW and Vogel EF (eds): *A Modern Introduction to the Family.* Glencoe, Ill, The Free Press, 1960.

Koenig HG, Meador KG, Cohen HJ, Blazer DG: Self-rated depression scales and screening for major depression in the older hospitalized patient with medical illness. *J Am Geriatr Soc* 36:699–706, 1988.

Kong A, Barnett GO, Mosteller F, Youtz C: How medical professionals evaluate expressions of probability. *N Engl J Med* 315:740–745, 1986.

Koran LM: The reliability of clinical methods, data and judgments (two parts). *N Engl J Med* 293:642–646, 695–701, 1975.

Kottke TE, Battista RN, DeFriese GH, Brekke ML: Attributes of successful smoking cessation interventions in medical practice: A meta-analysis of 39 controlled trials. *JAMA* 259:2882–2889, 1988.

Kress DH: *The Cigarette as a Physician Sees It.* Mountain View, Calif, Pacific Press Publishing Assoc, 1931.

Krieger D: *The Therapeutic Touch.* New York, Simon & Schuster Inc, 1979.

Kroenke K, Mangelsdorff D: Common symptoms in ambulatory care: Incidence evaluation, therapy, and outcome. *Am J Med* 86:262–266, 1989.

Krumholz HM, Cohen BJ, Tsevat J, Pasternak RC, Weinstein MC: Cost-effectiveness of a smoking cessation program after myocardial infarction. *J Am Coll Cardiol* 22(6):1697–1702, 1993.

Kubler-Ross E: *On Death and Dying.* New York, Macmillan Publishing Co Inc, 1969.

Lachs MS, Feinstein AR, Cooney LM, Drickamer MA, Marottoli RA, Pannill FC, Tinetti ME: A simple procedure for general screening for functional disability in elderly patients. *Ann Intern Med* 112:699–706, 1990.

Lang F: Resident behaviors during observed pelvic examinations. *Fam Med* 22:153–155, 1990.

Larsen KM, Smith CK: Assessment of nonverbal communication in the patient physician interviews. *J Fam Pract* 12:481–488, 1981.

Lawton MP, Brody EM: Assessment of older people: Self-maintaining and instrumental activities of daily living. *Gerontologist* 9:179–186, 1969.

Leape LL: Error in medicine. *JAMA* 272(23):1851–1857, 1994.

Lee JM: Screening and informed consent. *N Engl J Med* 328:438–439, 1993.

Leedham B, Meyerowitz BE, Muirhead J, Frist WH: Positive expectations predict health after heart transplantation. *Health Psychol* 14(1):74–79, 1995.

Lefcourt HM: *Locus of Control,* ed 2. Hillsdale, NJ, Lawrence Erlbaum Associates, 1982.

Lester G, Smith S: Listening and talking to patients: A remedy for malpractice suits. *West J Med* 158:268–272, 1993.

Leveno KJ, Cunningham FG, Nelson S, Roark M, Williams ML, Guzick D, Dowling S, Rosenfeld CR, Buckley A: A prospective comparison of selective and universal electronic fetal monitoring in 34,995 pregnancies. *N Engl J Med* 315:615–619, 1986.

Leventhal H: Fear communications in the acceptance of preventive health practices. *Bull NY Acad Med* 41:1144–1168, 1965.

Levine DM, Green LW, Deeds SG, Chwalow J, Russell RP, Finlay J: Health education for hypertensive patients. *JAMA* 241:1700–1703, 1979.

Levinson DJ: *The Seasons of a Man's Life.* New York, Alfred A Knopf Inc, 1978.

Levinson DJ: A conception of adult development. *Am Psychol* 41:3–13, 1986.

Levinson W: Physician–patient communication: A key to malpractice prevention. *JAMA* 272:1619–1620, 1994.

Lewis CE: Disease prevention and health promotion practices of primary care physicians in the United States. *Am J Prev Med* 4(suppl):9–16, 1988.

Lewis LM, Lasater LC, Ruoff BE: Failure of a chest pain clinical policy to modify physician evaluation and management. *Ann Emerg Med* 25:9–14, 1995.

Ley P: *Communicating with Patients.* London, Croom Helm Ltd, 1988.

Like R, Steiner P: Medical anthropology and the family physician. *Fam Med* 19(2):87–92, 1986.

Lindeman C, Van Aernam B: The effects of structured and unstructured pre-operative teaching. *Nurs Res* 21:319, 1971.

Liveright AA, Haygood N (eds): *The Exeter Papers: Report of the First International Conference on the Comparative Study of Adult Education.* Boston, Center for the Study of Liberal Education for Adults of Boston University, 1968, p 8.

Localio AR, Lawthers AG, Brennan TA, *et al:* Relation between malpractice claims and adverse events due to negligence: Results of the Harvard Medical Practice Study III. *N Engl J Med* 325:245–251, 1991.

Lockyer J, Mazmanian PE, Moore DE, Harrison A, Knox AB: Adoption of innovation, in Davis DA, Fox RD (eds): *The Physician as Learner: Linking Research to Practice.* Chicago, American Medical Association, 1994, pp 33–45.

Logsdon DN, Rosen MA: The INSURE project on life cycle preventive health service: Feasibility and preliminary results. Presentation to the 112th Annual Meeting of the American Public Health Association, Washington, DC, 1984.

Lomas J: Retailing research: Increasing the role of evidence in clinical services for childbirth. *Milbank Mem Fund Q* 71:439–475, 1993.

Lorish CD, Parker J, Brown S: Effective patient education: A quasi-experiment comparing an individualized strategy with a routinized strategy. *Arthritis Rheum* 28(11): 1289–1297, 1985.

Lundberg GD: National health care reform: The aura of inevitability intensifies. *JAMA* 267:2521–2524, 1992.

Lynch J: *The Language of the Heart.* New York, Basic Books Inc, 1985.

Macklis RM, Mendelson ME, Mudge GH Jr: *Introduction to Clinical Medicine: A Student-to-Student Manual.* Boston, Little, Brown & Co, 1994.

Maclure M, Willett WC: Misinterpretation and misuse of the kappa statistic. *Am J Epidemiol* 126:161–169, 1987.

Mandelblatt J, Traxler M, Lakin P, Kanetsky P, Kao R: Mammography and Papanicolaou smear use by elderly poor black women: The Harlem study team. *J Am Geriatr Soc* 40(10):1001–1007, 1992.

Mann KV, Ribble JG: The role of motivation in self-directed learning, in Davis DA, Fox RD (eds): *The Physician as Learner: Linking Research to Practice.* Chicago, American Medical Association, 1994, pp 67–88.

Manning PR, DeBakey L: *Medicine: Preserving the Passion.* New York, Springer-Verlag, 1987.

Manning PR, DeBakey L: Lifelong learning tailored to individual clinical practice. *JAMA* 268:1135–1136, 1992.

Marks RG: *Designing a Research Project.* New York, Van Nostrand Reinhold Co, 1982.

Marton F, Saljo R: Approaches to learning, in Marton F, Hounsell D, Entwistle N (eds): *The Experience of Learning.* Edinburgh, Scottish Academic Press, 1984, pp 36–55.

Mathias S, Nayak US, Isaacs B: Balance in elderly patients: The get-up and go test. *Arch Phys Med Rehabil* 67:387–389, 1986.

Maynard D: Bearing bad news in clinical settings, in Dervin B (ed): *Progress in Communication Sciences.* Norwood, NJ, Ablex Publishing Corp, 1991.

Mazmanian PE, Duff WM: Beyond accreditation and the enterprise of CME: An alternative model linking independent learning centers and health services, in Davis DA, Fox RD (eds): *The Physician as Learner: Linking Research to Practice.* Chicago, American Medical Association, 1994, pp 283–312.

McConnell JD, Barry MJ, Bruskewitz RC, *et al*: *Benign Prostatic Hyperplasia: Diagnosis and Treatment. Quick Reference Guide for Clinicians.* Rockville, Md, US Department of Health and Human Services, Public Health Service, Agency for Health Care Policy and Research. AHCPR Publication No. 94-0583, February 1994.

McDaniel S: Collaboration between psychologists and family physicians: Implementing the biopsychosocial model. *Prof Psychol Res Pract* 26(2):117–122, 1995.

McDaniel S, Campbell T, Seaburn D: *Family-Oriented Primary Care: A Manual for Medical Providers.* New York, Springer-Verlag, 1990.

McGinnis JM, Foege WH: Actual causes of death in the United States. *JAMA* 270:2207–2212, 1993.

McGoldrick M, Gerson R: *Genograms in Family Assessment.* New York, WW Norton & Co Inc, 1985.

McGoldrick M, Pearce JK, Giordano J: *Ethnicity and Family Therapy.* New York, Guilford Press, 1982.

McGuire CH: Sociocultural changes affecting professions and professionals, in Curry L, Wergin JF, *et al* (eds): *Educating Professionals: Responding to New Expectations for Competence and Accountability.* San Francisco, Jossey-Bass Inc Publishers, 1993, p 15.

McKay S, Mahan CS: Laboring patients need more freedom to move. *Contemp Obstet Gynecol* 24:90–119, 1984.

McPhee SJ, Detmer WM: Office-based interventions to improve delivery of cancer prevention services by primary care physicians. *Cancer* 72(suppl):1100–1112, 1993.

McPhee SJ, Bird JA, Fordham D, *et al*: Promoting cancer prevention activities by primary care physicians. *JAMA* 266:538–544, 1991.

McWhinney IR: *A Textbook of Family Medicine.* London, Oxford University Press, 1989a.

McWhinney I: The need for a transformed clinical method, in Stewart M, Roter D (eds): *Communicating with Medical Patients.* Beverly Hills, Calif, Sage Publications Inc, 1989b, p 40.

Mead VP, Rhyne RL, Wiese WH, *et al*: Impact of environmental patient education on preventive medicine practices. *J Fam Pract* 40:363–369, 1995.

Means RP: How family physicians use information sources: Implications for new approaches, in Green JS, Grosswald SJ, Suter E, Walthall DB (eds): *Continuing Education for the Health Professions.* San Francisco, Jossey-Bass Inc Publishers, 1984, pp 72–86.

Mechanic D: *Medical Sociology*, ed 2. New York, Free Press, 1978.

Mechanic D: Health and illness behavior and patient practitioner relationship. *Soc Sci Med* 34(12):1345–1350, 1992.

Mengel MB: Physician ineffectiveness due to family of origins issues. *Fam Syst Med* 5:176–190, 1987.

Mengel MB, Holleman WL (eds): *Fundamentals of Clinical Practice: A Textbook on the Patient, Doctor, and Society*. New York, Plenum Press, 1997.

Mengel MB, Connis RT, Gordon MJ, Taylor TR: The relationship of family dynamics and social support to personal, emotional, and social functioning in diabetic patients on the insulin pump. *Fam Syst Med* 6:317–344, 1988.

Miller AB, Baines CJ, To T, Wall C: Canadian national breast screening study: 1. Breast cancer detection and death rates among women aged 40 to 49 years. *Can Med Assoc J* 147:1459–1476, 1992.

Miller RH, Luft HS: Managed care plan performance since 1980: A literature analysis. *JAMA* 271:1512–1519, 1994.

Miller W, Rollnick S: *Motivational Interviewing: Preparing People to Change Addictive Behavior*. New York, Guilford Press, 1991.

Minuchin S, Baker L, Rosman BL, Liebman R, Milman L, Todd T: A conceptual model of psychosomatic illness in children: Family organization and family therapy. *Arch Gen Psychiatry* 32:1031–1038, 1975.

Minuchin S, Rosman BL, Baker L: *Psychosomatic Families: Anorexia Nervosa in Context*. Cambridge, Mass, Harvard University Press, 1978.

Mold JW, Stein HF: The cascade effect in the clinical care of patients. *N Engl J Med* 314(8):512–514, 1986.

Mold JW, Holtgrave DR, Bisonni RS, *et al:* The evaluation and treatment of men with asymptomatic prostate nodules in primary care: A decision analysis. *J Fam Pract* 34:561–568, 1992.

Montgomery WH, Donegan J, McIntyre K: Proceedings of the 1985 National Conference on Standards and Guidelines for Cardiopulmonary Resuscitation and Emergency Cardiac Care. *Circulation* 74:SIV,1–3, 1986.

Moore DE, Bennett NL, Knox AB, Kristofco RE: Participation in formal CME: Factors affecting decision-making, in Davis DA, Fox RD (eds): *The Physician as Learner: Linking Research to Practice*. Chicago, American Medical Association, 1994, p 230.

Moore WS, Barnett HJM, Beebe HG, Bernstein EF, Brener BJ, Brott T, Caplan LR, Day A, Goldstone J, Hobson RW, Kempczinski RF, Matchar DB, Mayberg MR, Nicolaides AN, Norris JW, Ricotta JJ, Robertson JT, Rutherford RB, Thomas D, Toole JF, Trout HH, Wiebers DO: Guidelines for carotid endarterectomy. A multidisciplinary consensus statement from the ad hoc committee, American Heart Association. *Stroke* 26:188–201, 1995.

Moos R (ed): *Coping with Physical Illness: 2. New Perspectives*. New York, Plenum Press, 1984.

Morisky DE, Levine DM, Greene LW, Shapiro S, Russell RP, Smith CR: Five-year blood pressure control and mortality following health education for hypertensive patients. *Am J Public Health* 73:153–161, 1983.

Mullen PD, Green LW, Persinger GS: Clinical trials of patient education or chronic conditions: A comparative meta-analysis of intervention types. *Prev Med* 14:753–781, 1985.

Mumford E, Schlesinger H, Glass G, Patrick C, Cuerdon T: A new look at evidence about reduced cost of medical utilization following mental health treatment. *Am J Psychiatry* 141(10):1145–1158, 1984.

Munjack DJ, Crocker B, Cabe D, Brown R, Usigli R, Zulueta A, McManus M, McDowell D, Palmer R, Leonard M: Alprazolam, propranolol, and placebo in the treatment of panic disorder and agoraphobia with panic attacks. *J Clin Psychopharmacol* 9:22–27, 1989.

Mushlin AI, Fintor L: Is screening for breast cancer cost-effective? *Cancer* 69(suppl):1957–1962, 1992.

National Center for Health Statistics. *Advance Report of Final Mortality, 1990*. Hyattsville, Md, US Department of Health and Human Services, 1993. Monthly Vital Statistics Report, 41(7).

National Center for Health Statistics. *Health, United States, 1994*. Hyattsville, Md, US Public Health Service, 1995.

National Task Force on Training Family Physicians in Patient Education. *Patient Education: A Handbook for Teachers*. Kansas City, Mo, Society of Teachers of Family Medicine, 1979, pp 16, 33, 46.

NCI Breast Cancer Screening Consortium. Screening mammography: A missed clinical opportunity? *JAMA* 264:54–58, 1990.

Ness D, Ende J: Denial in the medical interview. *JAMA* 272:1777–1781, 1994.

Neugarten B: Adaptation and the life cycle. *The Counselling Psychologist* 6:16–20.

Newman TB, Klebanoff MA: Neonatal hyperbilirubinemia and longterm outcome: Another look at the collaborative perinatal project. *Pediatrics* 92:651–657, 1993.

Novey DW: *Rapid Access Guide to the Physical Examination*. Chicago, Year Book Medical Publishers Inc, 1988.

Oboler SK, LaForce FM: The periodic physical examination in asymptomatic adults. *Ann Intern Med* 110:214–226, 1989.

Oppenheim PI, Sotiropoulos G, Baraff LJ: Incorporating patients preferences into practice guidelines: Management of children with fever without source. *Ann Emerg Med* 24:836–841, 1994.

Orkin FK: Patient monitoring during anesthesia as an exercise in technology assessment, in Saidman LJ, Smith NT (eds): *Monitoring in Anesthesia,* ed 3. London, Butterworth Publishers Inc, 1993.

Ornish D: *Dr. Dean Ornish's Program for Reversing Heart Disease.* New York, Ballantine Books Inc, 1992.

Ornish D: Can lifestyle changes reverse coronary heart disease? *World Rev Nutr Diet* 72:38–48, 1993.

Ornstein SM, Garr DR, Jenkins RG, *et al:* Computer-generated physician and patient reminders: Tools to improve population adherence to selected preventive services. *J Fam Pract* 32:82–90, 1991.

Orr RD, Marshall PA, Osborn J: Cross-cultural considerations in clinical ethics consultations. *Arch Fam Med* 4:159–164, 1995.

Osborn LM, Whitman N: *Ward Attending: The Forty Day Month.* Salt Lake City, University of Utah School of Medicine, 1991.

Osheroff JA, Forsythe DE, Buchanan BG, Bankowitz RA, Blumenfeld BH, Miller RA: Physicians' information needs: Analysis of questions posed during clinical teaching. *Ann Intern Med* 114:576–581, 1991.

Osler W: The hospital as a college, in *Aequanimitas with Other Addresses to Medical Students: Nurses and Practitioners of Medicine,* ed 3. Philadelphia, Blakiston Co, 1945, p 315.

Otitis Media with Effusion Guideline Panel. *Otitis Media with Effusion in Young Children.* Rockville, Md, US Department of Health and Human Services, Public Health Service, Agency for Health Care Policy and Research, 1994. AHCPR Publication No. 94-0622.

Pacific Business Group on Health. Preventive services survey, 1993. Unpublished data.

Panzer RJ, Black ER, Griner PF: *Diagnostic Strategies for Common Medical Problems.* Philadelphia, American College of Physicians, 1991.

Parchman ML: A historical overview of patient care, in Mengel MB (ed): *Principles of Clinical Practice: An Introductory Textbook.* New York, Plenum Press, 1991, pp 3–19.

Paskett ED, White E, Carter WB, Chu J: Improving follow-up after an abnormal Pap smear: A randomized controlled trial. *Prev Med* 19(6):630–641, 1990.

Patterson CH: *Theories of Counseling and Psychotherapy.* New York, Harper & Row Publishers Inc, 1986.

Patton DD, Bodtke S, Horner RD: Patient perceptions of the need for chaperones during the pelvic exams. *Fam Med* 22:215–231, 1990.

Pederson LL: Compliance with physician advice to quit smoking: An analysis of the literature. *Prev Med* 11:71–84, 1982.

Penn MA, Bourguet CC: Patients' attitudes regarding chaperones during physical examinations. *J Fam Pract* 35:639–643, 1992.

Penn P: Coalitions and binding interactions in families with chronic illness. *Fam Syst Med* 1(2):16–25, 1983.

Perkoff GT: The boundaries of medicine. *J Chron Dis* 38:271–278, 1985.

Phillips WR: American Academy of Family Physicians Task Force on Clinical Policies for Patient Care. Clinical policies: Making conflicts of interest explicit. (letter) *JAMA* 272:1479, 1994.

Pickles W: *Epidemiology in Country Practice.* Exeter, England, The Royal College of General Practitioners, 1984.

Placek PJ, Keppel KG, Taffel SM, Liss TL: Electronic fetal monitoring in relation to caesarean section delivery, for live births and stillbirths in the U.S., 1980. *Public Health Rep* 99:173–183, 1984.

Pommerenke FA, Weed DL: Physician compliance: Improving skills in preventive medicine practices. *Am Fam Physician* 43:560–568, 1991.

Poses RM, Bekes C, Copare FJ, *et al:* What difference do two days make? The inertia of physicians' sequential prognostic judgments for critically ill patients. *Med Decis Mak* 10:6–14, 1990.

Pratt DD (ed): *Five Perspectives on Teaching in Adult and Higher Education.* Huntington, NY, Krieger Publishing Co Inc, 1996.

Prislin MD, Vandenbark MS, Clarkson QD: The impact of a health screening flowsheet on the performance and documentation of health screening procedures. *Fam Med* 18:290–292, 1986.

Prochaska JO, DiClemente CC: Transtheoretical therapy: Toward a more integrative model of change. *Psychother Theory Res Pract* 19:276–288, 1982.

Prochaska JO, Norcross JC, DiClemente CC: *Changing for Good.* New York, William Morrow & Co Inc, 1994.

Prochaska J, Velicer W, Rossi J, Goldstein M, Marcus B, Radowski W, Fiore C, Harlow L, Redding C, Rosenbloom D, Rossi S. Stages of change and decisional balance for 12 problem behaviors. *Health Psychology* 13(1):39–46, 1994.

Rabin D, Rabin PL, Rabin R: Compounding the ordeals of ALS: Isolation from my fellow physicians. *N Engl J Med* 307:506–509, 1982.

Ramen SM, Gambling DR, Lucas MJ, Sharma SK, Sidawi JE, Leveno KJ: Randomized trial of epidural versus intravenous analgesia during labor. *Obstet Gynecol* 86:783–789, 1995.

Ramsden P: Studying learning: Improving teaching, in Ramsden P (ed): *Improving Learning: New Perspectives.* London, Kogan Page, 1988, pp 13–31.

Ramsey CN: The science of family medicine, in Ramsey CN (ed): *Family Systems in Medicine.* New York, Guilford Press, 1989, 1989a.

Ramsey CN Jr (ed): *Family Systems in Medicine.* New York, Guilford Press, 1989b.

Redelmeier DA, Rozin P, Kahneman D: Understanding patients' decisions: Cognitive and emotional perspective. *JAMA* 270:72–76, 1993.

Reigelman RK: *Minimizing Medical Mistakes: The Art of Medical Decision Making.* Boston, Little, Brown & Co, 1991, p 73.

Reiser SJ: *Medicine and the Reign of Technology.* London, Cambridge University Press, 1978.

Reiss D: *The Family's Construction of Reality.* Cambridge, Mass, Harvard University Press, 1981.

Reiss D, Kaplan De-Nour A: The family and medical team in chronic illness: A transactional and developmental perspective, in Ramsey C Jr (ed): *Family Systems in Medicine.* New York, Guilford Press, 1989.

Relman AS: Medical practice under the Clinton reforms: Avoiding domination by business. *N Engl J Med* 329:1574–1576, 1993.

Reynolds A: What is competent beginning teaching? A review of the literature. *Rev Educ Res* 62(1):1–35, 1992.

Rivo ML, Saultz JW, Wartman SA, DeWitt TG: Defining the generalist physician's training. *JAMA* 271:1499–1504, 1994.

Robbins JA, Bertrakis KD, Helms LJ, *et al:* The influence of physician practice behaviors on patient satisfaction. *Fam Med* 25:17–20, 1993.

Roberts SJ, Krouse HJ: Negotiation as a strategy to empower self-care. *Holist Nurs Pract* 4:30–36, 1990.

Rogers A: *Luke Has Asthma, Too.* Burlington, Vt, Waterfront Books, 1987.

Rogers DE, Blendon RJ: The changing American health scene: Sometimes things get better. *JAMA* 237:1710–1714, 1977.

Roizen MF, Coalson D, Hayward RSA, *et al:* Can patients use an automated questionnaire to define their current health status? *Med Care* 30:MS74–MS84, 1992.

Rolland JS: Toward a psychosocial typology of chronic and life-threatening illness. *Fam Syst Med* 2:245–263, 1984.

Rolland JS: Chronic illness and the life cycle: A conceptual framework. *Fam Process* 26(2):203–221, 1987a.

Rolland JS: Family illness paradigms: Evolution and significance. *Fam Syst Med* 5(4):467–486, 1987b.

Rolland JS: Anticipatory loss: A family systems developmental framework. *Fam Process* 29(3):229–244, 1990.

Rolland JS: Working with illness: Clinicians' personal and interface issues. *Fam Syst Med* 12(4):149–171, 1994.

Roper WL, Winkenwerder W, Hackbarth GM, Krakaner H: Effectiveness in health care: An initiative to evaluate and improve medical practice. *N Engl J Med* 319:1197–1202, 1988.

Roper Reports. Report to Medicaid: What people do for minor health problems. New York, Roper Organization, 1986, pp 86–88.

Rose G, Hamilton PJ: A randomized controlled trial of the effect on middle-aged men of advice to stop smoking. *Journal of Epidemiology & Community Health* Dec 32(4):275–281, 1978.

Rosenberg W, Donald A: Evidence based medicine: An approach to clinical problem solving. *BMJ* 310:1122–1126, 1995.

Rosenthal R, Jacobson L: *Pygmalion in the Classroom.* New York, Holt Rinehart & Winston Inc, 1968.

Rosser WW, Palmer WH: Dissemination of guidelines on cholesterol. Effect on patterns of practice of general practitioners and family physicians in Ontario. Ontario Task Force on the Use and Provision of Medical Services. *Can Fam Physician* 39:280–284, 1993.

Rothenberg E, Wolk M, Scheidt S, Schwartz M, Aarons B, Pierson RN: Continuing medical education activities in New York County: Physician attitudes and practices. *J Med Educ* 57:541–549, 1982.

Rubenstein LV, Calkins DR, Greenfield S, Jette AM, Meenan RF, Nevins MA, Rubenstein LZ, Wasson JH, Williams ME: Health status assessment for elderly patients, report of the Society of General Internal Medicine Task Force on Health Assessment. *JAGS* 37:562–569, 1988.

Rubenstein LV, Fink A, Gelberg L, Berkowitz C, Robbins A, Inui TS: Evaluating generalist education programs: A conceptual framework. *J Gen Intern Med* 9(S):564–572, 1994.

Rubenstein LZ: Geriatric assessment: An overview of its impacts. *Clin Geriatr Med,* February 1987, 3(1).

Rubenstein LZ, Schairer C, Wieland GD, Kane R: Systematic biases in functional status assessment of elderly adults: Effects of different data sources. *J Gerontol* 39:686–691, 1984.

Ruffalo RL, Garabedian-Ruffalo SM, Pawlson LG: Patient compliance. *Am Fam Physician* 31:93–100, 1985.

Ruiz MS, Marks G, Richardson JL: Language acculturation and screening practices of elderly Hispanic women: The role of exposure to health-related information from the media. *J Aging Health* 4(2):268–281, 1992.

Sackett DL: Bias in analytic research. *J Chron Dis* 32:51–63, 1979.

Sackett DL, Haynes RB, Guyatt GH, Tugwell P: *Clinical Epidemiology: A Basic Science for Clinical Medicine,* ed 2. Boston, Little, Brown & Co, 1991.

Sacks O: *One Leg to Stand on.* London, Gerald Duckworth, 1984.

Sassetti M: Domestic violence, in Elliott B, Halverson K, Hendricks-Matthews M (eds): *Family Violence and Abusive Relationships. Primary Care* 20(2):289–306, 1993.

Schick FL, Schick R (eds): *Statistical Handbook on Aging Americans.* Phoenix, Ariz, Oryx Press, 1994, Table C2-4, p 119, and Table A1-9, p 8.

Schofield MJ, Sanson-Fisher R, Halpin S, Redman S: Notification and follow-up of Pap test results: Current practice and women's preferences. *Prev Med* 23(3):276–283, 1994.

Schön DA: *The Reflective Practitioner: How Professionals Think in Action.* New York, Basic Books Inc, 1983.

Schön DA: *Educating the Reflective Practitioner.* San Francisco, Jossey-Bass Inc Publishers, 1987.

Schor S, Karten I: Statistical evaluation of medical journal manuscripts, in Rimm AA, Hartz AJ, Kalbfleisch JH, Anderson AJ, Hoffmann RG (eds): *Basic Biostatistics in Medicine and Epidemiology.* New York, Appleton–Century–Crofts, 1980.

Schurman R, Kramer P, Mitchell J: The hidden mental health network: Treatment of mental illness by non-psychiatrist physicians. *Arch Gen Psychiatry* 42:89–94, 1985.

Seaburn D, Gunn W, Mauksch L, Gawinski A, Lorenz A (eds): *Models of Collaboration: A Guide for Mental Health Professionals Working with Health Care Providers.* New York, Basic Books Inc, 1996.

Seidel HM, Ball JW, Dains JE, Benedict GW: *Mosby's Guide to Physical Examination.* St. Louis, Mosby–Year Book Publishers Inc, 1996.

Seldin DW: The boundaries of medicine. *Trans Assoc Am Physicians* 94:75–84, 1981.

Seymour CA: *Introduction to Clinical Clerking.* London, Cambridge University Press, 1984.

Shahady EJ: Difficult patients: Uncovering the real problems of crocks and gomers. *Consultant* 10:49–56, 1990.

Shaughnessy AF: Considerations in antidepressant therapy. *Fam Pract Recertif* 17:31–37, 1995.

Shorter B: *Bedside Manners: The Troubled History of Doctors and Patients.* New York, Simon & Schuster Inc, 1985.

Siegel JE, Krolewski AS, Warram JH, Weinstein MC: Cost-effectiveness of screening and early treatment of nephropathy in patients with insulin-dependent diabetes mellitus. *J Am Soc Nephrol* 3(4 suppl):S111–S119, 1992.

Sigurdsson G: The medical record in general practice: Where art and science meet. *Scand J Prim Health Care* 2:113–116, 1984.

Simon GE, Von Korff M, Katon WJ: Balancing cost and effectiveness of antidepressant drugs in primary care: A randomized trial. Presented at the eighth annual NIMH international research conference on mental health problems in the general health care sector, September 7–9, 1994, McLean, Va, pp 72–73.

Simpson M, Buckman R, Stewart M, Maguire P, Lipkin M, Novack D, Till J: Doctor–patient communication: The Toronto consensus statement. *BMJ* 303:1385–1387, 1991.

Sinclair JC, Bracken MB: *Effective Care of the Newborn Infant.* London, Oxford University Press, 1992.

Slatkoff SF, Curtis P, Coker A: Patients as subjects for research: Ethical dilemmas for the primary care clinician-investigator. *J Am Board Fam Pract* 7:196–201, 1994.

Smith AC, Kleinman S: Managing emotions in medical school: Student's contacts with the living and the dead. *Soc Psychol Q* 52:56–69, 1989.

Sox HC Jr: Preventive health services in adults. *N Engl J Med* 330:1589–1595, 1994.

Sox HC, Blatt MA, Higgins MC, Marton KI: *Medical Decision Making.* Boston, Butterworths, 1988.

Spiegel D: *Living Beyond Limits.* New York, Times Books, 1993.

Spiegel D, Bloom JR, Kraemer HC, Gottheil E: Effect of psychosocial treatment on survival of patients with metastatic breast cancer. *Lancet* 2:888–891, 1989.

Stamler J, Farinaro E, Mojonnier LM, Hall Y, Moss D, Stamler R: Prevention and control of hypertension by nutritional-hygienic means: Long-term experience of the Chicago Coronary Prevention Evaluation Program. *JAMA* 243:1819–1822, 1980.

Stein HF: An argument for more inclusive context in clinical intervention: The case of family medicine, in Stein HF, Apprey M (eds): *Context and Dynamics in Clinical Knowledge.* Charlottesville, University Press of Virginia, 1985, pp 48–91, 1985a.

Stein H: *The Psychodynamics of Medical Practice.* Berkeley, University of California Press, 1985c.

Stein HS: Whatever happened to countertransference? in Stein HF, Apprey M (eds): *Context and Dynamics in Clinical Knowledge.* Charlottesville, University Press of Virginia, 1985b.

Stein HF: *American Medicine as Culture.* Boulder, Colo, Westview Press, 1990.

Steinberg KK, Thacher SB, Smith SJ, Stroup DF, Zach MM, Flanders WD, Berkelman RL: A meta-analysis of the effect of estrogen replacement therapy on the risk of breast cancer. *JAMA* 266:1358–1360, 1991.

Stephens G: A family doctor's rules for clinical conversations. *J Am Board Fam Pract* 7:179–181, 1994.

Stetten D Jr: Coping with blindness. *N Engl J Med* 305:458–460, 1981.

Stewart M, Brown JB, Weston WW, McWhinney IR, McWilliam CL, Freeman TR: *Patient-Centered Medicine: Transforming the Clinical Method.* London, Sage, 1995.

Stiell IG, McKnight RD, Greenberg GH, *et al:* Implementation of the Ottawa ankle rules. *JAMA* 271:827–832, 1994.

Stillman PL, Swanson DB: Ensuring the clinical competence of medical school graduates through standardized patients. *Archives of Internal Medicine* 147(6):1049–1052, 1987.

Stratton BF, Nicholson ME, Olsen LK, *et al:* Breast self-examination proficiency: Attitudinal, demographic, and behavioral characteristics. *J Women's Health* 3:185–195, 1994.

Strauss AL: *Chronic Illness and the Quality of Life.* St. Louis, CV Mosby Co, 1975.

Strauss MB (ed): *Familiar Medical Quotations.* Boston, Little, Brown & Co, 1968.

Strull WM, Lo B, Charles G: Do patients want to participate in medical decision making? *JAMA* 252:2990–2994, 1984.

Stuart M, Lieberman J: *The Fifteen Minute Hour: Applied Psychotherapy for the Primary Care Physician,* ed 2. New York, Praeger Publishers, 1993.

Stuck AE, Siu AL, Wieland GD, Adams J, Rubenstein LZ: Comprehensive geriatric assessment: A meta-analysis of controlled trials. *Lancet* 342:1032–1036, 1993.

Suchman A, Roter D, Green M, Hepkin M, and The Collaborative Study Group of the AAPP. Patient satisfaction with primary care office visits. *Med Care* 31(10):83–92, 1993.

Sudarsky L: Geriatrics: Gait disorders in the elderly. *N Engl J Med* 322:1441–1445, 1990.

Susman JL, Crabtree BF, Essink G: Depression in rural family practice: Easy to recognize, difficult to diagnose. *Arch Fam Med* 4:427–431, 1995.

Sussman J, Berg AO, Moy JG: Critiquing clinical policies. Society of Teachers of Family Medicine Annual Conference, San Diego, May 1993.

Swartz L: The politics of black patients' identity: Ward rounds on the 'black side' of a South African psychiatric hospital. *Culture Med Psychiatry* 15:217–244, 1991.

Swartz MH: *Textbook of Physical Diagnosis: History and Examination.* Philadelphia, WB Saunders Co, 1989.

Tabar L, Fagerberg CJG, Gad A, *et al:* Reduction in mortality from breast cancer after mass screening with mammography: Randomized trial from the Breast Cancer Screening Working Group of the Swedish National Board of Health and Welfare. *Lancet* 1:829–832, 1985.

Talmadge KS: *Focus on Steroids, A Drug-Alert Book.* Frederick, Md, Twenty-First Century Books, 1991.

Tang PC, Fafchamps D, Shortliffe EH: Traditional medical records as a source of clinical data in the outpatient setting. *Proc Annu Symp Comput Appl Med Care,* 1994, pp 575–579.

Taylor TR, Gordon MJ, Ashworth CD: A systems perspective on clinical management. *Behav Sci* 29:233–247, 1984.

Texas Medical Association Hospital Medical Staff Section Subcommittee on Practice Parameters. *Practice Parameters: A Primer,* 1994.

Tinetti ME: Performance-oriented assessment of mobility problems in elderly patients. *JAGS* 34:119–126, 1986.

Tinetti ME, Ginter SF: Identifying mobility dysfunctions in elderly patients. Standard neuromuscular examination or direct assessment? *JAMA* 259:1190–1193, 1988.

Tinetti ME, Speechley M: Prevention of falls among the elderly. *N Engl J Med* 320:1055–1059, 1989.

Tolnai S: Lifelong learning habits of physicians trained at an innovative medical school and a more traditional school. *Acad Med* 66:425–426, 1991.

Tombaugh T, McIntyre NJ: The mini-mental state examination: A comprehensive review. *JAGS* 40:922–935, 1992.

Tsevat J, Weeks JC, Guadagnoli E, *et al:* Using health-related quality-of-life information: Clinical encounters, clinical trials, and health policy. *J Gen Intern Med* 9(10):576–582, 1994.

US Department of Health and Human Services. *Clinician's Handbook of Preventive Services.* Washington, DC, US Department of Health and Human Services, 1994.

US General Accounting Office. *Medical Malpractice: Characteristics of Claims Closed in 1984.* Publication No. GAO/HRD-87-55, 1987.

US Preventive Services Task Force. *Guide to Clinical Preventive Services: An Assessment of the Effectiveness of 169 Interventions.* Baltimore, Williams & Wilkins Co, 1989.

US Preventive Services Task Force. *Guide to Clinical Preventive Services, Second Edition.* Baltimore, Williams & Wilkins Co, 1996.

US Public Health Service. *Healthy People 2000: National Health Promotion and Disease Prevention Objectives.* US Department of Health and Human Services Publication No. PHS 91-50212, 1991.

US Public Health Service Recommendations for Human Immunodeficiency Virus: Counseling and Voluntary Testing for Pregnant Women. *Morbidity and Mortality Weekly Report* 44(FF-7):1–14, 1995.

US Public Health Service recommendations for human immunodeficiency virus: Counseling and voluntary testing for pregnant women. *MMWR* 44(RR-7):1–14, 1995.

Vander Zanden JW: *American Minority Relations,* ed 4. New York, Alfred A Knopf, 1983.

Van Voorhees C, Wolf FM, Gruppen LD, Stross JK: Learning styles and continuing medical education. *J Cont Educ Health Prof* 8:257–265, 1988.

Veith I: *The Yellow Emperor's Classic of Internal Medicine.* Berkeley, University of California Press, 1972.

Verbeek ALM, Hendricks JHCL, Hollan TR, *et al:* Reduction of breast cancer mortality through mass screening with modern mammography: First results of the Nijmegen Project, 1975–1981. *Lancet* 1:1222–1224, 1984.

Vibbert S, Migdail KJ, Strickland D: *1995 Medical Outcomes and Guidelines Sourcebook. A Progress Report and Resource Guide for Outcomes Research and Practice Guidelines: Developments, Data and Documentation.* New York, Faulkner & Gray, 1994.

Vogt HB, McHale MS: Testicular cancer. Role of primary care physicians in screening and education. *Postgrad Med* 92:93–101, 1992.

Voigt LF, Weiss NS, Chu J, Daling JR, McKnight B, VanBelle G: Progestagen supplementation of exogenous oestrogens and risk of endometrial cancer. *Lancet* 338:274–277, 1991.

Vorhies D, Riley B: *Deconditioning, Geriatric Rehabilitation, Clinics in Geriatric Medicine,* vol 9, No 4. Philadelphia, WB Saunders Co, 1993.

Vu NV, Galofre A: How medical students learn. *J Med Educ* 58:601–610, 1983.

Vygotsky LS: *Mind in Society: The Development of Higher Psychological Processes.* Cambridge, Mass, Harvard University Press, 1978.

Walker G: The pact: The caretaker-parent/ill-child coalition in families with chronic illness. *Fam Syst Med* 1(4):6–29, 1983.

Wallis LA, Tardiff K, Deane K: Evaluation of teaching programs for male and female genital examinations. *J Med Educ* 58:664–666, 1983.

Walsh F: Conceptualization of normal family processes, in *Normal Family Processes,* ed 2. New York, Guilford Press, 1993.

Walsh F, McGoldrick M (eds): *Living beyond Loss: Death in the Family.* New York, WW Norton & Co Inc, 1991.

Wasson JH, Cushman CC, Bruskewitz RC, Littenberg B, Mulley A, Wennberg JE, and the Prostate Disease Outcome Research Team. A structured literature review of treatment for localized prostate cancer. *Arch Fam Med* 2:487–493, 1993.

Weed LL: Medical records that guide and teach. *N Engl J Med* 278:593–657, 1968.

Weiss L, Meadow R: Women's attitudes toward the gynecologic practices. *Obstet Gynecol* 54:110–114, 1979.

Wennberg JE: Outcomes research, cost containment, and the fear of health care rationing. *New England Journal of Medicine* 323:1202–1204, 1990.

Wennberg JE, Freeman JL, Culp WJ: Are hospital services rationed in New Haven or over utilized in Boston? *The Lancet* 1185–1189, May 23, 1987.

Wennberg JE, Freeman JL, Shelton RM, Bubolz TA: Hospital use and mortality among Medicare beneficiaries in Boston and New Haven. *New England Journal of Medicine* 321:1168–1173, 1989.

Wennberg J, Gittelsohn A: Small area variations in health care delivery. *Science* 182:1102–1108, 1973.

Wentz DK, Harrison A: Forces for change in the CME environment, in Davis DA, Fox RD (eds): *The Physician as Learner: Linking Research to Practice.* Chicago, American Medical Association, 1994, pp 1–13.

White JE, Begg L, Fishman NW, Guthrie B, Fagan JK: Increasing cervical cancer screening among minority elderly: Education and on-site services increase screening. *J Gerontol Nurs* 19(5):28–34, 1993.

White KL: Information for health care. *Inquiry* 17:296–312, 1980.

White KL: *The Tasks of Medicine: Dialogue at Wickenburg.* Menlo Park, Calif, The Henry J Kaiser Family Foundation, 1988.

White R, Gunstone R: *Probing Understanding.* London, The Falmer Press, 1992.

Whitman N: *Creative Medical Teaching.* Salt Lake City, University of Utah School of Medicine, 1990.

Wiener S, Nathanson M: Physical examination. Frequently observed errors. *JAMA* 236:852–855, 1976.

Wilkerson L, Armstrong E, Lesky L: Faculty development for ambulatory teaching. *J Gen Intern Med* 5:44–53, 1990.

Williams JW, Holleman DR, Samsa GP, Simel DL: Randomized controlled trial of 3 vs 10 days of trimethoprim/sulfamethoxazole for acute maxillary sinusitis. *JAMA* 273:1015–1021, 1995.

Willms JL, Schneiderman H, Algranati PS: *Physical Diagnosis: Bedside Evaluation of Diagnosis and Function.* Baltimore, Williams & Wilkins Co, 1994.

Wilson DM: Assessment of an intervention in primary care: Counseling patients on smoking cessation, in Tudiver F, Bass MJ, Dunn EV, Norton PG, Stewart M (eds): *Assessing Interventions: Traditional and Innovative Methods.* Beverly Hills, Calif, Sage Publications Inc, 1992, p 139.

Wilson J, Braunwald E, Isselbacher K, Petersdorf R, Martin J, Fauci A, Root R (eds): *Harrison's Principles of Internal Medicine.* New York, McGraw–Hill Book Co, 1991.

Wilson SM, Shulman LS, Richert AE: '150 different ways' of knowing: Representation of knowledge in teaching, in Calderhead J (ed): *Exploring Teachers' Thinking.* London, Cassell Education, 1987, pp 104–124.

Wolin SJ, Bennett LA: Family rituals. *Fam Process* 23(3):401–420, 1984.

Woolf SH: Practice guidelines, a new reality in medicine. II. Methods of developing guidelines. *Arch Intern Med* 152:946–952, 1992.

Woolf SH: Practice guidelines, a new reality in medicine. III. Impact on patient care. *Arch Intern Med* 153:2646–2655, 1993.

World Health Organization. The constitution of the World Health Organization. *WHO Chronicle* 1:29, 1947.

World Health Organization. *International Classification of Impairments, Disabilities, and Handicaps: A Manual of Classification Relating to the Consequences of Disease.* Geneva, World Health Organization, 1980.

Wortman C, Silver R: The myths of coping with loss. *J Consult Clin Psychol* 57:349–357, 1989.

Yesavage JA, Brink TL, Rose RL, Lum O, Huang V, Adey M, Leirer VO: Development and validation of a geriatric depression screening scale: A preliminary report. *J Psychiatr Res* 17:37–49, 1983.

Index